Toward Equity
in Health

Barbara C. Wallace, PhD, is a tenured Professor of Health Education and Founding Director of the Research Group on Disparities in Health within the Department of Health and Behavior Studies at Teachers College, Columbia University. As a licensed psychologist, Dr. Wallace has been honored by the American Psychological Association with the status of Fellow within both Division 50 (Addictive Behaviors) and Division 45 (Society for the Psychological Study of Ethnic Minority Issues). She also directs the Annual Health Disparities Conference at Teachers College, Columbia University and is Editor-in-Chief of the electronic *Journal of Equity in Health* (www.JEHonline.org/).

Her books include: *Crack Cocaine: A Practical Treatment Approach for the Chemically Dependent* (1991), *The Chemically Dependent: Phases of Treatment and Recovery* (Editor, 1992), *Adult Children of Dysfunctional Families: Prevention, Intervention and Treatment for Community Mental Health Promotion* (1996), *Understanding and Dealing with Violence: A Multicultural Approach* (with Co-Editor Robert T. Carter, PhD, 2003), *HIV/AIDS Peer Education Training Manual: Combining African Healing Wisdom and Evidence-Based Behavior Change Strategies* (2005), and *Making Mandated Addiction Treatment Work* (2005).

Dr. Wallace was enstooled as a Queen Mother (African Traditional Ruler) in 2000 at Larteh, Ghana. She is now also known as Nana Ohemaa Oparebea Agyiriwa, II—the Abradehemaa, and is actively involved in philanthropic activities to support health education and HIV/AIDS prevention in Africa.

Toward Equity in Health

A New Global Approach to Health Disparities

Barbara C. Wallace, PhD
Editor

SPRINGER PUBLISHING COMPANY
New York

Springer Publishing Company, LLC
11 West 42nd Street
New York, NY 10036
www.springerpub.com

Acquisitions Editor: Sheri W. Sussman
Production Editor: Shana Meyer
Cover design: Joanne E. Honigman
Composition: Aptara Inc.

07   08   09   10/5   4   3   2   1

Library of Congress Cataloging-in-Publication Data

Health Disparities Conference (1st : 2006 : Columbia University)
   Toward equity in health : a new global approach to health disparities / edited by Barbara C. Wallace.
      p. ; cm.
   Papers from the first annual Health Disparities Conference, held March 2006 at Columbia University and organized by the Research Group on Disparities in Health of Teachers College, Columbia University.
      Includes bibliographical references and index.
      ISBN 978-0-8261-0313-0 (hardback)
   1. Health services accessibility–Congresses. 2. Equality–Health aspects–Congresses. 3. Community health services–Congresses. 4. Health education–Congresses. 5. World health–Congresses. I. Wallace, Barbara C. II. Columbia University. Teachers College. Research Group on Disparities in Health. III. Title.
      [DNLM: 1. Health Services Accessibility–Congresses. 2. Cross-Cultural Comparison–Congresses. 3. Health Policy–Congresses. 4. Health Promotion–Congresses. 5. World Health–Congresses. WA 300 H43383t 2008]

RA418.H3894   2006
362.1–dc22

                                                                                    2007029926

Printed in the United States of America by Bang Printing.

Dedication

This book is dedicated to the memory of Janene Martha Murray (January 13, 1959 to May 14, 2007), Princeton University, Class of 1982.

May Janene know the deep gratitude I hold for all she did to support and contribute to my developmental trajectory as a researcher, scholar, writer, and professor.

Of note, Janene died at age 48 from a health condition where there are major disparities for African Americans, Native Americans, and Latinos. May her physical end signal a beginning: one wherein a new paradigm prevails; all enjoy respect, acceptance, empathy, and equal access to opportunity; and there is a new social justice and civil rights movement for the achievement of equity in health for all.

> *No man is an island, entire of itself; every man is a piece of the continent, a part of the main. . . . Any man's death diminishes me, because I am involved in mankind; and therefore never send to know for whom the bell tolls; it tolls for thee.*
> —John Donne, 1624

May we hear the bell toll and awaken! Once awake, may we become involved in mankind, view ALL as part of the main, and take action to bring about equity in health for all! BiakoYe! Unity!

Contents

Part 3: The Legacy and Role of Racism—Implications and Recommendations for Research and Practice

Part 4: Collaborations, Partnerships, and Community–Based Participatory Research

Part 5: New Internet Technology—Achieving Wide Dissemination and Global Reach

Part 6: Training Community Health Workers and Peer Educators

Part 7: Closing Gaps in Health for Special Populations

Part 8: Closing the Education and Health Gaps—Addressing Dual Inter-Related Disparities Through Effective Engagement

Contributors

Diane L. Adams, MD, MPH, CHS-III
Founder & Chair
Health Informatics Information Technology
  (HIIT)
Special Primary Interest Group (SPIG) of the
  American Public Health Association (APHA)
Senior Health Policy Fellow and Consultant
Georgia Centers for Advanced
  Telecommunications Technology (GCATT)
Silver Spring, MD

Collins O. Airhihenbuwa, PhD, MPH
Professor, Department of Biobehavioral
  Health
College of Health and Human
  Development
The Pennsylvania State University
University Park, PA

John P. Allegrante, PhD
Professor of Health Education
Department of Health and Behavior Studies
Teachers College, Columbia University
New York, NY

Shaffdeen A. Amuwo, PhD, MPH
Associate Dean for Urban Health and
  Diversity Programs
Clinical Associate Professor of Public Health
  Sciences
University of Illinois
CEO/President
Public Health Associates, LLC
Chicago, IL

Nana Akomfohene Korantema Ayeboafo
Chief Creative Officer
StarSpirit International, Inc.
Philadelphia, PA, and Larteh, Ghana

Amrita Bahl, MA
Project Director
Social Education & Health Advocacy Training
  (SEHAT) Project
India Vision Foundation
New Delhi, India

Beatrice L. Bridglall, EdD
Research Scientist & Editor
Institute for Urban & Minority Education
Teachers College, Columbia University
Adjunct Assistant Professor
Department of Health and Behavior
  Studies
Teachers College, Columbia University
New York, NY

David R. Buchanan, DrPH
Professor of Community Health
  Education
School of Public Health and Health
  Sciences
University of Massachusetts
Amherst, MA

Angela Campbell, EdD
Executive Director
Academic Pathways
New Rochelle, NY

Adrienne Chew, EdD
Principal
Academy at Palumbo
Philadelphia, PA

Waiwah Chung, RN, MA
Consultant
Staten Island, NY

James W. Collins, Jr., MD, MPH
Division of Neonatology
Children's Memorial Hospital
Chicago, IL

Madonna G. Constantine, PhD
Professor of Psychology and Education
Department of Counseling and Clinical
    Psychology
Teachers College, Columbia University
New York, NY

Richard J. David, MD
Associate Professor of Pediatrics
College of Medicine
University of Illinois at Chicago
Chicago, IL

Nabila El-Bassel, DSW
Professor
Director
Social Intervention Group
Columbia University School of Social Work
New York, NY

Shameka Faulkner, BS
Study Coordinator
David Geffen School of Medicine
Department of Medicine
Division of Endocrinology
UCLA
Los Angeles, CA

Angela D. Ferguson, PhD
Assistant Professor
Director
Counseling Psychology Program
Human Development and Psychoeducational
    Studies
School of Education

Howard University
Washington, DC

Senaida Fernandez, PhD
Postdoctoral Scientist
Center for Behavioral Cardiovascular Health
Division of General Medicine
Department of Medicine
Columbia University College of Physicians &
    Surgeons
New York, NY

Yves-Michel Fontaine, MA, EdM
Doctoral Candidate
Health and Behavior Studies
Department of Health and Behavior Studies
Teachers College, Columbia University
Project Director
Connect With Pride
Social Intervention Group
Columbia University School of Social Work
New York, NY

Anderson J. Franklin, PhD
Honorable David S. Nelson Professional Chair
    and Professor
Department of Counseling, Developmental,
    and Educational Psychology
Boston College
Lynch School of Education
Chestnut Hill, MA

Mindy Thompson Fullilove, MD
Research Psychiatrist
New York State Psychiatric Institute
Professor of Clinical Psychiatry and Public
    Health
Columbia University
Director
Community Research Group
New York, NY

Louisa Gilbert, MSSW
Codirector
Social Intervention Group
Columbia University School of Social
    Work
New York, NY

Edmund W. Gordon, PhD
Richard March Hoe Professor Emeritus of
　Psychology and Education
Founding Director
Institute of Urban and Minority Education
　(IUME)
Teachers College, Columbia University
New York, NY
John M. Musser Professor of Psychology,
　Emeritus
Yale University
New Haven, CT

Sheila V. Graham, BA
Doctoral Student
Department of Counseling and Clinical
　Psychology
Teachers College, Columbia University
New York, NY

Beverly Greene, PhD, ABPP
Professor of Psychology
Department of Psychology
St. John's University
Jamaica, NY
Certified Clinical Psychologist
Diplomate in Clinical Psychology
American Board of Professional
　Psychology

Monique Guishard, MA
Doctoral Candidate
Social-Personality Psychology
The Graduate and University Center of the
　City University of New York
New York, NY

Brenda D. Hayes, DSW, MPH, MSW
Research Assistant Professor
CHPM
Director
Grant and Proposal Development
OSRA
Director
Community Partnership Development
COEHD
Morehouse School of Medicine
Atlanta, GA

Henrietta Ho-Asjoe, MPS
Center for the Study of Asian American
　Health
New York University
Institute of Community Health and Research
New York, NY

Joyce Hunter, PhD
HIV Center for Clinical and Behavioral
　Studies
New York State Psychiatric Institute
New York, NY

L. Philip Johnson, EdD
Assistant Director
Research Group on Disparities in Health
Department of Health and Behavior
　Studies
Teachers College, Columbia University
New York, NY

Richard M. Keller, PhD
Director
Office of Access and Services for Individuals
　with Disabilities
Teachers College, Columbia University
Assistant Professor of Psychology and
　Education
Department of Clinical and Counseling
　Psychology
Teachers College, Columbia University
New York, NY

Mai M. Kindaichi, EdM
Doctoral Student
Department of Counseling and Clinical
　Psychology
Teachers College, Columbia University
New York, NY

Joe P. King, MA Candidate
Teachers College, Columbia University
Intern
Office on Disability
Department of Health and Human
　Services
Washington, DC

Ansumana Richard Konuwa, EdD
Postdoctoral Fellow
Research Group on Disparities in Health
Department of Health and Behavior Studies
Teachers College, Columbia University
New York, NY

Kenny Kwong, PhD
Director of Research and Evaluation
Charles B. Wang Community Health Center
New York, NY
Adjunct Assistant Professor
Hunter College of the City University of
    New York
School of Social Work
New York, NY

Kajal Lahiri, PhD
Distinguished Professor of Economics, and
    Health Policy, Management and
    Behavior
Department of Economics
University at Albany-SUNY
Albany, NY

Natalie Langston-Davis, MD, MPH
Assistant Clinical Professor
Department of Pediatrics
Montefiore Medical Center
New York Children Health Project
New York, NY

Brenda A. Leath, MHSA, PMP
President
National Consortium for African American
    Children, Inc. (NCAAC)
Chair
Health Informatics Information Technology's
    (HIIT's), Community Outreach
    Committee of the American Public Health
    Association (APHA)
Washington, DC

Cindi Melanson, MPH, CHES
Health Scientist
Office of Public Health Research
Office of the Chief Science Officer

Centers for Disease Control and Prevention
    (CDC)
Atlanta, GA

Marie L. Miville, PhD
Associate Professor of Psychology and
    Education
Department of Clinical and Counseling
    Psychology
Teachers College, Columbia University
New York, NY

Frank Moretti, PhD
Executive Director
Columbia Center for New Media Teaching and
    Learning
Columbia University
Professor of Communications
Teachers College, Columbia University
New York, NY

José Nanín, EdD, CHES
Assistant Professor
Department of Health, Physical Education,
    and Recreation
Kingsborough Community College
Brooklyn, NY
Director of Education and Training
Center for HIV Educational Studies and
    Training (CHEST)
Hunter College, City University of
    New York
New York, NY

Gbenga Ogedegbe, MD, MPH, MS
Assistant Professor of Medicine
Center for Behavioral Cardiovascular Health
Division of General Medicine
Department of Medicine
Columbia University College of Physicians
    & Surgeons
New York, NY

Titilayo A. Okoror, PhD
Assistant Professor of Public Health
Department of Health and Kinesiology and
    African American Studies Research
    Center

Purdue University
West Lafayette, IN
Chair
HIV/AIDS International Workgroup
American Public Health Association
Washington, DC

Sweene Oscar, MA
Doctoral Candidate
Clinical Psychology
The Graduate and University Center of the
    City University of New York
New York, NY

Betty Perez-Rivera, EdD, CHES
Director,
East Harlem Centers of Excellence,
Bureau of District Public Health Office
New York City Department of Health and
    Mental Hygiene
New York, NY

James O. Prochaska, PhD
Director
Cancer Prevention Research Center
Professor of Clinical and Health
    Psychology
University of Rhode Island
Kingston, RI

Zulkarnain Pulungan
Doctoral Student
Department of Economics
University at Albany–SUNY
Albany, NY

Jamila R. Rashid, PhD, MPH
Team Leader
CDC Research Agenda and Promotion
Senior Advisor for Special Populations
Department of Health and Human Services
Office of Public Health Research
Office of the Chief Science Officer
Centers for Disease Control and Prevention
Atlanta, GA

Margaret Rosario, PhD
Department of Psychology

The City University of New York
The City College and Graduate Center
New York, NY

Denise E. Ross, PhD
Associate Professor of Psychology and
    Education
Program for Applied Behavior Analysis
Teachers College, Columbia University
New York, NY

Antoinette Schoenthaler, MA
Postdoctoral Scientist
Center for Behavioral Cardiovascular Health
Division of General Medicine
Department of Medicine
Columbia University College of Physicians
    & Surgeons
New York, NY

Eric W. Schrimshaw, PhD
Doctoral Program in Psychology
The City University of New York
Graduate Center
New York, NY

Elizabeth L. Skillen, PhD, MS
Health Scientist
Office of Public Health Research
Office of the Chief Science Officer
Centers for Disease Control and Prevention
    (CDC)
Atlanta, GA

Yemonja Smalls, PhD
Chicago Professional School of Psychology
W. A. Howe Center
Chicago, IL

Robin M. Wagner, PhD, MS
Associate Director for Research Planning
    and Evaluation
Office of Public Health Research
Office of the Chief Science Officer
Office of the Director
Centers for Disease Control and Prevention
    (CDC)
Atlanta, GA

Bailus Walker, Jr., PhD, MPH, FACE
Professor of Environmental and
  Occupational Health
Howard University College of Medicine
Washington, DC

Nicole L. Watkins, MA
Department of Counseling and Clinical
  Psychology
Teachers College, Columbia University
New York, NY

Susan S. Witte, PhD, LCSW
Associate Professor
Columbia University School of Social Work
Associate Director
Social Intervention Group
Columbia University School of Social Work
New York, NY

Sally Sukman Wong, MS, RD, CD
Department of Nutrition, Food Studies, and
  Public Health
New York University
New York, NY

Kyungmi Woo, RN, MA
Predoctoral Fellow
Research Group on Disparities in Health
Department of Health and Behavior
  Studies
Teachers College, Columbia University
New York, NY

Ann Zauber, PhD
Associate Attending Biostatistician
Memorial Sloan-Kettering Cancer
  Center
New York, NY

Preface

This volume seeks to launch a new field of equity in health, as a new global approach to inequities in health. The goal is to shift the discourse toward a focus on moving from *InEquity in Health* to *Equity In Health* and spur a global movement in response to the major civil rights issue of the twenty-first century involving injustice in health. This contribution also seeks to serve as a tool for training global leaders for this movement—whether professionally trained members of transdiciplinary teams, community health workers, or peer educators.

The origin of the vision for bringing about equity in health for all, fostering a major paradigm shift, and training global health leaders who are capable of working with cultural competence on collaborative transdiciplinary teams arose in January 2003. At that time, I provided leadership in founding the Research Group on Disparities in Health (RGDH) at Teachers College, Columbia University within the Department of Health and Behavior Studies. The RGDH was envisioned as a setting in which to provide support, nurturance, and systematic mentoring for those junior colleagues, and pre- and post-doctoral fellows committed to reducing and eliminating health disparities, toward the goal of forging equity in health for all. The goal was for them to emerge as culturally competent researchers not only equipped with the knowledge, attitudes/beliefs, and skills/behaviors to be model researchers and health educators addressing disparities in health, but also to emerge as global health leaders.

Given this vision, a weekly Research Seminar in Disparities in Health was launched, attracting the participation of pre- and post-doctoral fellows from diverse places across the nation and around the globe. Fellows of every race, ethnicity, religion, sexual orientation, and socioeconomic status have sat around the table at the research seminar and worked out their personal vision for the trajectory of their careers—typically articulating a commitment to addressing disparities in health with a goal to realize equity in health for all through teaching, training, research, practice/interventions, and service.

Within the setting of the RGDH, in the spring of 2005, an annual research conference was envisioned for bringing together a national and international audience similarly committed to health disparities and bringing about equity in health for all. A model for what was envisioned existed: the long-standing Annual Winter Roundtable on Cross Cultural Psychology and Education at Teachers College, Columbia University—founded by Dr. Sam Johnson in 1982, and subsequently directed by Dr. Robert Carter, and now Dr. Madonna Constantine. The Annual Winter Roundtable on Cross Cultural Psychology and Education has evolved into the nation's premier cross-cultural conference. In 1982, as a poor graduate student, I yearned to attend the First Annual Winter Roundtable, yet was unable to do so, lacking funds. However, I eventually presented as a Teachers College faculty member in 1994, and each year since then—even organizing the volume that arose from the 1998 conference as coeditor of the proceedings with Dr. Carter. In this manner, I discovered the potential of a conference to be a significant setting in which participants can present new and cutting edge research, theory, and practice, while receiving expert feedback that contributes to the systematic evolution of one's work being renewed, revitalized, and inspired in the process.

My vision was to create the same kind of annual forum for addressing health disparities. A collective was essential to the formation of the vision and charting of the mission so a conference planning committee was formed, constituting a transdiciplinary team (i.e., Edmund Gordon, Robert Fullilove, Gbenga Ogedegbe, Lisa Lewis, and numerous predoctoral fellows with the RGDH).

With Teachers College, Columbia University as the ideal platform, and its Center for Educational Outreach and Innovation (CEO&I) as the ideal partner—the Spring 2006 First Annual Health Disparities Conference was launched. The theme for the First Annual Health Disparities Conference, held the second weekend in March 2006, was "Declaring a Decade of Health Disparity Reduction: Toward Evidence-Based Approaches." The March 2006 conference was hailed by the staff of CEO&I as the most successful first-time conference in the history of Teachers College. It was also during the first day of the two-day event that the conference body collectively declared "A Decade of Health Disparity Reduction," putting forth a powerful call during a plenary session.

Among those things that concretely and immediately reflected the power of the conference call and declaration was an oral publishing agreement for this edited volume by 4:00 p.m. the first day of the 2006 conference. The result is the present edited volume—representing, in large measure, the proceedings of the conference, insofar as it includes mostly invited papers from among the many presented at the conference.

Intended Audience

The intended audience for the book includes all those interested in closing gaps in health, addressing disparities in health, and moving from the current widespread inequity in health to the achievement of equity in health for all, within a twenty-first century civil rights movement for health. This includes all those working in health education, health promotion, disease prevention, public health, the health care delivery system, and both patient- and population-level health.

Thus, the broad audience for whom this volume is intended includes policy makers, funders, providers, researchers, interventionists, educators, and community members—whether government officials, epidemiologists, health care administrators, leaders in health care insurance systems, physicians, psychologists, health educators, social workers, nurses, anthropologists, lawyers, demographers, economists, sociologists, computer/information technology specialists, teachers, community health workers, or peer educators. All will find a vision translated into roles and functions for each within the field of equity in health. Moreover, the training this volume provides will prepare them for service as global leaders on the transdiciplinary teams that must engage in collaborative work alongside community members, forging equity in health for all within a twenty-first century global civil rights movement.

Overview of the Book

The introduction to the volume identifies the forces driving and embodied within a new field of equity in health (chapter 1, Wallace), while also identifying these as the thirteen guiding principles for the new field. Part I of the volume introduces new theory, paradigms, and perspectives, starting with the work of Walker (chapter 2) who provides a comprehensive overview of the challenges involved in eliminating health disparities. In chapter 3, Airhihenbuwa and Okoror offer a compelling example of the kind of new perspectives needed to guide the field of equity in health, specifically offering an Africanist perspective that highlights the important role of evidence-based and culturally appropriate models for reducing global health disparities. Prochaska puts forth in chapter 4 new paradigms for inclusive health care, articulating the need for both individual patient and population health approaches, while highlighting the role of home-based interactive computer technology in having a wide impact.

Part II introduces new procedures and policies deemed vital for a new field of equity in health, specifying some of the implications for funders, researchers, and policy makers. Buchanan and Allegrante (chapter 5) discuss the tensions between scientific and ethical considerations when it comes to evaluating public health proposals, specifically discussing the types of proposals that agencies should be funding and the types of evidence that should matter—offering recommendations in this regard. Lahiri and Pulungan illustrate in chapter 6 the new kind of sophisticated data analysis that examines income related health disparities and their determinants, focusing on New York state, while making racial/ethnic and geographical comparisons; these point toward a need to redistribute income via equal access to educational or employment opportunities. In addition to these kinds of detailed and highly sophisticated data analytic strategies being valued in the field of equity in health, along with such pointed conclusions, so is the need for a new generation of research that searches for those underlying mechanisms which may be contributing to disparities, including factors such as provider bias—as covered by Ogedegbe, Schoenthaler, and Fernandez in chapter 7. Beyond the need for new procedures in research, there is also a need for new policies to counter those that have been destructive to communities, led to the incessant displacement of communities, and effectively created the social context for the emergence of health disparities; Fullilove provides a thorough discussion of such policies in chapter 8.

In Part III, contributors review the legacy and role of racism in contributing to disparities, while also discussing the implications and recommendations for research and practice. Constantine, Kindaichi, Graham, and Watkins offer in chapter 9 strategies for reducing disparities in African Americans' receipt and use of mental health services. David and Collins (chapter 10) explore whether the field should be pursuing the contemporary trend to focus on genetics (too often reflecting our racist legacy) or social forces, concluding how public health planners need to look to social and environmental rather than genetic differences in any campaign to eliminate health disparities; and, what is essential in the United States for understanding health outcomes is a model that incorporates both race as a social construct and social class, while solutions may involve the development of a broad political unity, or class unity, that challenges the status quo. The legacy of racism may also be seen in the distrust of African American patients, subtly influencing the level of attention they pay to health messages prompting them to pursue screenings for conditions such as colon cancer, while Franklin, Oscar, Guishard, Faulkner, and Zauber (chapter 11) frame the behavior of such patients within a psychosocial model of resilience, underscoring the role of adaptive coping strategies. Through the chapters in Part III, both the legacy and role of racism in contributing to the manifestation of health disparities emerges, as well as implications and recommendations for the types of new theories, models, and approaches needed to guide research and practice.

Part IV of the volume covers the key role of collaborations, partnerships, and community-based participatory research in the field of equity in health. In this regard, Rashid, Anuwo, Skillen, Melanson, and Wagner (chapter 12) call for collaboration on national research priorities to eliminate health disparities. Drawing upon the pioneering work across decades at Moorehouse College in developing the model of community-based participatory research and collaborative relationships with partners in the African American community, Hayes (chapter 13) outlines the process of successful grant-writing to obtain funds to support community-based health disparities research and services. With regard to collaborations developed in New York City to benefit Chinese immigrants, Kwong, Ho-Asjoe, Chung, and Wong (chapter 14) describe how cardiovascular health disparities were addressed via the Chinese-American Healthy Heart Coalition, while distilling principles for effective collaborations that others may follow; they emphasize the use of a community-wide multipronged integrated approach to providing culturally competent and linguistically appropriate health education and health care services for medically underserved Chinese immigrants, as well as the use of an asset-based community development intervention approach focused on increasing social capital. Illustrating the very best within the tradition of federally funded community-based participatory research, including community members in every project phase, El-Bassel, Witte, and Gilbert (chapter 15) provide an example of the best case scenario outcome: a new emergent evidence-based model for reducing HIV/AIDS risk with serodiscordant couples worthy of dissemination, and adaptation to new culturally distinct populations.

The next part of the book, V, presents new Internet technology for use in achieving wide dissemination of health information, interventions, and training that attains a global reach. In this regard, Moretti and Witte (chapter 16) describe the use of new media designed by education technologists to improve learning; they illustrate the potential of such media to disseminate an evidence-based model for HIV/AIDS risk reduction, enrich the training experience, and expand the possibilities for disseminating content arising from various fields. Adams and Leath (chapter 17) describe a role for health informatics and information technology in shaping a global research agenda to eliminate health disparities, covering international developments. Woo (chapter 18) describes how evidence-based approaches can be integrated to frame the creation of an online multimedia peer education smoking cessation program for Korean youth, while seeking to engage them in her program via a film script writing contest soliciting stories on quitting smoking.

Part VI of the book covers the training of community health workers and peer educators, suggesting how they play a vital role in the field of equity in health. In chapter

19, the authors (Wallace, Konuwa, & Ayeboafo) describe a model of training community health workers and peer educators for HIV/AIDS prevention in Africa, one that integrates African Healing Wisdom and evidence-based behavior change strategies. Bahl (chapter 20) responds to the crisis, common to many parts of the world, involving the incarcerated population and their need for interventions to address their health, especially HIV/AIDS prevention, describing her work in India implementing a peer education training program—one developed while a graduate student at Teachers College, Columbia University. Indeed, several chapters (19—Wallace, Konuwa & Ayeboafo; 20—Bahl; and 18—Woo) all reflect the challenge put forth by the editor of this volume for future global health leaders training at the university to go beyond the acquisition of mere knowledge about evidence-based approaches, and to design, implement, and evaluate interventions for the vulnerable and at-risk populations "back home" in their countries of origin. What is essential to the new field of equity in health is the training of such future global leaders who "go back home" to forge equity in health—not constituting a "brain drain"—while the Research Group on Disparities in Health (RGDH) at Teachers College constitutes a magnet attracting those seeking training to guide the design of evidence-based approaches to research and intervention. In chapter 21, the authors' (Johnson & Wallace) work, which is rooted in the same RGDH training model, results in the development of an approach to training peer educators within urban America where Black men who have sex with men (MSM) are a particularly vulnerable group; yet, through training, Black MSM can emerge as leaders and valued partners in conducting ethnographic community-based participatory research. Thus, the training of peer educators and community health workers—who may emerge as ideal partners in community based participatory research—emerges as central within the new field of equity in health.

In Part VII, attention is turned to other special populations also considered the most vulnerable and what it will take to close gaps in health. With regard to men who have sex with men (MSM), Nanín, Fontaine, and Wallace (chapter 22) recognize how they are currently living at the intersection of two epidemics—one involving HIV/AIDS and another involving Methamphetamine drug use, while going on to offer recommendations for researchers and clinicians working with this special population. The vulnerability of lesbian and bisexual women of color is contextualized as involving exposure to the multiple threats of racism, heterosexism, and homophobia—all of which contribute to health care disparities, while Greene, Miville, and Ferguson (chapter 23) offer a recommended intervention and research agenda in light of all of these factors. Moving from special subpopulations of men and then women within the larger Gay, Lesbian, and Bisexual community to the youth, Rosario, Schrimshaw, and Hunter (chapter 24) open a window into their lives, exploring ethnic/racial disparities in gay-related stress and health. Next, Keller and King (chapter 25) explore health disparities impacting people with disabilities, underscoring the need for future global health leaders to embrace the value of pursuing equity in health for all within a movement that also represents the needs of the special population of people with disabilities.

Finally, Part VIII of the volume covers the task of closing the education and health gaps by addressing these dual inter-related disparities through effective engagement. First, Ross and Smalls (chapter 26) discuss the kind of classroom-based interventions that hold the promise of closing the gap, or reducing academic disparities between low- and high-income students; at the core of interventions is the learn unit—which can be measured as the key component of effective engagement for learning, while suggesting a meaningful interaction between a teacher and a learner wherein successful transmission and acquisition of knowledge occurs. Next, Bridglall and Gordon (chapter 27) describe the role of supplementary education—typically, a form of additional structured education that takes place outside of the school classroom—and how it can prepare learners for high academic achievement and effective engagement in the process of learning that is key to academic success. Toward the goal of closing the academic achievement and health gaps, an example of a supplementary education program rooted in an academic, community and faith-based coalition is described; key program features include ensuring effective engagement in the learning process via the use of marbles given to reward/shape behavior, and youth involvement in community service via the National Association for the Advancement of Colored People (Campbell & Wallace, chapter 28). Next, a peer mentoring/tutoring program for at-risk urban youth attending a college preparatory high school is described, emerging as an effective intervention, especially having success in reducing academic failure in the major subject areas of math and science for Black males (Chew & Wallace, chapter 29). In the next chapter, 30, Perez-Rivera and Langston-Davis illustrate the manner in which schools may also be settings for the infusion of health education across the curriculum in response to an epidemic such as asthma, highlighting the importance of face-to-face engagement to foster learning; at the same time, linguistically and culturally appropriate materials that physicians can use in educating patients and their families also find a central role in comprehensive community-wide health education.

To conclude the volume, the future of the field of equity in health is discussed, in light of all that has been organized and presented (Wallace, chapter 31). The volume effectively establishes the foundation for a new field of equity in health, while training global leaders for work within a twenty-first century global civil rights movement for equity in health for all.

Barbara C. Wallace, PhD

Acknowledgments

First, I must express my gratitude for all those who made this book possible, starting with Sheri W. Sussman who rapidly grasped the nature and promise of the vision, and secured the contract for this book with Springer Publishing Company, LLC. Next, I must acknowledge the many contributors to this edited volume, and all with whom they work. In addition to the Divine Creator, I must acknowledge and express gratitude to my personal spiritual pillars—Nana Asi, Nana Anima, Nana Asuo Gyebi, Nana Okomfohene Akua Oparebea, Nana Boafo Tigare, the Mmotia, and Nana Akomfohene Korantema Ayeboafo. I must acknowledge my family pillars, starting with my parents, Cynthia Comer Wallace and Uriel Hamilton Wallace, Jr., as well as my siblings and large ever-growing extended family. I must also thank my family at Teachers College, Columbia University, including my many colleagues, students, training fellows within the Research Group on Disparities in Health, and vital support staff for the inspiration, and foundation they provided.

—Barbara C. Wallace, PhD, Editor

Introduction: The Forces Driving and Embodied Within a New Field of Equity in Health

Barbara C. Wallace

Introduction

Health is a state of well-being with physical, emotional, mental, and spiritual dimensions that serves as an essential foundation for human life with implications for how all other aspects of life are pursued and evolve. It is also an essential resource to be valued by individuals, families, communities, and our larger global community. Health may vary in how it is defined, qualified, and pursued within diverse communities and for individuals. Not all enjoy a good state of health, and there are vast differences with regard to the markers and indicators of this state, with health varying across races/ethnicities, diverse groups, special populations, socioeconomic classes, geographic regions, and countries within our global community. It is often through contact with others and via processes of simple social comparison or complex statistical analyses that we arrive at an awareness of how states of health can profoundly vary across groups and locals.

There are implications for what it means to be a global community with the capacity to: (1) travel, observe, and use technology to broadcast images suggesting states of health for groups scattered over vast regions around the globe; (2) rapidly mobilize to take action and quickly respond to a health issue or crisis in literally any region around the globe, dispersing resources where needed; and (3) differentially interpret what is being observed, what we elect to broadcast, and how we choose to respond, given historical legacies and contemporary forces of oppression, domination, and discrimination. Vital differences and distinctions also emerge with regard to: (1) our potential to act as a global community with a keen sense of our interdependence, the essential right to health, and what social justice dictates that we do as vital social action (i.e., the Asian Tsunami of December 2004) on the one hand; and (2) our potential to allow forces of oppression, domination, and discrimination to serve as a barrier to our responding appropriately to all health crises (i.e., the case of Hurricane Katrina in August 2005) on the other hand.

Because of vast differences with regard to access to the resources associated with the pursuit and maintenance of health, there is a need for a global health transformation—one wherein we value and pursue equity in health for all as a global interdependent community with vast resources at our disposal for sharing and deployment to any group in need located on any part of the globe. To value and pursue equity in health means that we engage in fair play, act with impartiality, and allow a sense of social justice to guide us as we ensure that all human beings are free to enjoy the right to health and pursuit of physical, emotional, mental, and spiritual well-being—consistent with how any diverse groups may define it and elect to pursue it. This brings to mind the indigenous people who apparently wanted to be left alone in the aftermath of the Asian Tsunami, shooting arrows at hovering helicopters to underscore this point. Thus, acceptance of and respect for diversity and the right of cultural groups to determine their own health, health standards/outcomes, and way of life suggest constant principles of the highest order. Such overarching ever-present guiding principles are essential in this new era of expanded awareness of and contact with the multiple groups in our global community.

Meanwhile, historical legacies and contemporary forces of oppression, domination, and discrimination compromise the pursuit of equity in health. It requires paying special attention to the needs of those groups that have suffered injustice, and taking action to improve their health, in particular—to ensure they enjoy the right to health and social justice. This may even include new policies for the distribution of resources and access to opportunities.

Some use the terms "health disparities" or "health equity" interchangeably, while noting how there is little consensus about the meaning of the terms "health disparities," "health inequalities," or "health equity" (Braveman, 2006, p. 167). Also noted is how "health equity" is a term rarely encountered in the United States, although one more familiar to public health professionals outside of America. Braveman (p. 181) defines health disparities as "systematic, potentially avoidable differences in health—or in the major socially determined influences on health—between groups of people who have different relative positions in social hierarchies according to wealth, power, or prestige." Moreover, since "these differences adversely affect the health or health risks" of "groups already at a disadvantage by virtue of their underlying social positions, they are particularly unfair" (p. 181). Consistent with the focus in this edited volume, Braveman (p. 181) provides additional clarification "by noting that pursuing health equity—that is, striving to eliminate health disparities strongly associated with social disadvantage—can be thought of as striving for equal opportunities for all social groups to be as healthy as possible." However, totally justifiable is a "selective focus on improving conditions for those groups who have had fewer opportunities" (p. 181). This may involve "removing obstacles for groups of people—such as the poor, disadvantaged racial/ethnic groups, women, or persons who are not heterosexual—who historically have faced more obstacles to realizing their rights to health and other human rights" (p. 181).

Consistent with this perspective, this volume seeks to forge equity in health for all. The volume seeks to be a milestone in the study of health disparities, marking a major paradigm shift, while launching a new field of equity in health—as a new global approach to health disparities. One goal of the volume is to foster movement toward framing the discourse in the United States as one focused on the achievement of equity in health. Another goal is to encourage and train researchers and interventionists in the United States to view the national and international health domains as intricately inter-related and include both in their purview, taking a global approach. Our further discussion, as evidenced in this text, demarcates the nature of the shift in the guiding paradigm, the nature of the desired movement toward equity in health, the parameters of the new field of equity in health, while illustrating how researchers and interventionists may practically approach the reality of our interdependence as one global community.

In seeking to be a milestone in the year 2007—the publication date of this volume— it is important to recognize other key milestones. Prior key milestones in the field of health disparities are noted (Satcher & Pamies, 2006) as including (1) the 1985 U.S. Department of Health and Human Services' *Report of the Secretary's Task Force on Black and Minority Health*, citing a continuing disparity in the burden of death and illness by race (blacks and minorities compared to American population as a whole) (p. xix); (2) the January 2000 *Healthy People 2010 Report* which "targeted the elimination of health disparities in health as two of its primary goals" (p. xix); (3) the publication of the 2003 Institute of Medicine (IOM) report, *Unequal Treatment*—which allowed health disparities to emerge "as a topic of national importance and worthy of much attention and discussion" (p. xix); (4) the resulting charge issued by Congress to the Agency for Healthcare Research and Quality to compile "an annual report on the status of disparities," as well as resulting increases in "research funding from the government and foundation community" for the study of health disparities (p. xix); and (5) more sophisticated analyses of health disparities being published in leading health journals (p. xix).

We are living in a distinct historical period in time, one which Ayeboafo (2005) describes as the time of milestones and the weeding out of the destructive forces. Oddly, some of the prior milestones contain that which may need to be weeded out as a destructive force.

For example, consider how Levine et al. (2001) take as the point of departure for their analysis the two overarching goals of Healthy People 2010—to increase the quality and years of healthy life and to eliminate health disparities (i.e., disparities between African Americans and other population groups)—as goals assumed to be attainable based on absolute improvements in health during the twentieth century; and, more specifically, improvements since 1979 when the first objectives were published. Levine et al. (2001) investigated the validity of the hypothesis that future success could be built on the foundation of past success, concluding there has been "no sustained decrease in black-white disparities in either age-adjusted mortality or overall life expectancy at birth at the national level since the end of World War II" (p. 480). Moreover, this is "despite decades of funding for social, health-related, and other programs designed to reduce racial disparities" and even regular "assurances in support of Healthy People objectives" which appear in just about "all requests for research applications from federal health agencies over the past two decades" (p. 480). Optimistic forecasts for the future are deemed "poor regardless of whether inequality is measured by relative overall age-adjusted mortality, relative life expectancy, or lags in either measure, and regardless of whether the 1940 or year 2000 standard population is used for age-adjustment" (p. 480).

With regard to the value of other evidence of improvements, Levine et al. (2001) assert that "it would be illusory to consider national public health programs a success based on other indicators as long as inequalities in mortality and life expectancy fail to improve" (p. 480). Moreover, they argue that "the millions of premature deaths among African Americans over the course of the twentieth century challenge the hegemony of current models designed to improve health" (p. 480). They conclude that major change is needed, encompassing "the ways that medical and public health practitioners are trained, compensated, and evaluated" (p. 481). Also needed is "further research on the translation of prevention studies into practice," and "meaningful evaluation of federally funded research in terms of its impact on the inequality trends" they observe in their research (p. 481). More pointedly, they envision how "the aim of public health should not be simply elimination of disparities, but rather attainment of the best health for all people regardless of race, ethnicity, or social class" (p. 482).

Hence, as another milestone, the work of Levine et al. (2001), assists in broadening and shifting the discourse beyond eliminating health disparities—consistent with this volume's goal: to shift the national discourse in the United States beyond a focus on simply the elimination of disparities, and call for movement toward equity in health for all. This book seeks to be a milestone by also facilitating the weeding out of anything that constitutes a destructive force—whether a paradigm, model, theory, approach, or practice, resulting in a clearing for new growth.

This book's context is now anchored in over two decades of pertinent research with regard to health disparities, as well as other critical bodies of research and knowledge. There is also a great momentum for change from the twentieth century civil rights, social justice and human rights movements. Indeed, a global movement *From InEquity in Health to Equity In Health* is called for, given what Washington (2007, p. 3) cites in two powerful quotes: the declaration of Donna Christian-Christensen, MD, a Delegate to Congress and Chair of the Congressional Black Caucus Health Braintrust, that "Health disparities are the civil rights issue of the 21st century." Moreover, the leader of the civil rights movement in the United States, Martin Luther King, Jr. placed this civil rights issue we now face in the twenty-first century within context, stating, " Of all the forms of inequality, injustice in health is the most shocking and the most inhumane" (Washington, 2007, p. 2).

Given the impetus for a twenty-first century global health civil rights movement, there is justification in launching a new field of equity—one driven by thirteen guiding principles reflective of contemporary forces driving the change this volume embodies, as listed below: (1) The Drive for a Major Paradigm Shift; (2) The Drive for New Models of Health Care and Training; (3) The Drive for New Theories, Perspectives, and Identities; (4) The Drive for Evidence-Based Approaches; (5) The Drive for Transdisciplinary Teams and Community-Based Participatory Research; (6) The Drive for Globalization and Global Collaboration; (7) The Drive for Cultural Competence and Cultural Appropriateness; (8) The Drive for Health Literacy and Linguistic Appropriateness; (9) The Drive to Ensure the Right to Health; (10) The Drive for Social Justice and Acknowledgment of Forces in the Social Context; (11) The Drive to Protect and Support the Most Vulnerable; (12) The Drive to Repair Damage, Restore Trust, and Take Responsibility; and (13) The Drive to Redistribute Wealth and Access to Opportunity. This chapter will introduce the scope of this volume by reviewing these thirteen guiding principles for a new field of equity in health.

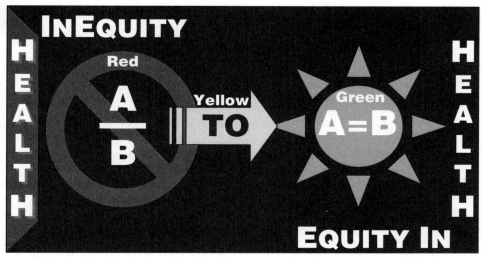

The symbol of the Research Group on Disparities in Health; Reflecting a recommended paradigm shift *From Health InEquity to Equity in Health.*

(1) The Drive for a Major Paradigm Shift

There is a symbol representing the drive for a major paradigm shift. This symbol represents the following: the Research Group on Disparities in Health (RGDH—founded and directed by the author); and, the annual conference the RGDH sponsors and out of which this volume grew (i.e., the Annual Health Disparities Conference at Teachers College, Columbia University) (see Figure 1.1). Therefore, this symbol is also on the back cover of this edited volume, being accompanied by the motto guiding the suggested twenty-first century global health civil rights movement *From InEquity in Health to Equity In Health.*

Red for Stop the Old Paradigm

With regard to this symbol, located at left there is a red circle with a diagonal slash combined with *A/B*. The red reminds us to stop that which does not work any more: the paradigmatic thinking, behavior, and ways of being in the world associated with hierarchical domination, symbolized by *A/B*; more specifically, given any actor *A* and any actor *B*, we may conceptualize the problematic interpersonal dynamic of unacknowledged domination and hierarchical authority in all forms that foster oppression (Wallace, 2003). The symbolic formula includes a dividing line with A in the top position and B in the bottom position, suggesting how a line is drawn (/), thereby depicting all forms of hierarchical domination as *A/B*. This captures the generic problem of a line drawn to subjugate and oppress *any* human based on any characteristic, trait, belief, or behavior (e.g., slavery, colonialism, genocide, ethnic cleansing, racism, classism, homophobia, heterosexism, disregard of people with disabilities). The formula conveys how A subjugates and denies the basic humanity of B; it captures how many people repeatedly and compulsively assert the privilege of acting in the role of the dominant superior, A, by placing B in a subordinate position as the inferior—to be controlled and dominated (Wallace, 2003).

Yellow for Take Caution in Moving "To" or Forward

Moving from left to right, at the center of the symbol is a yellow arrow with the word "TO," providing direction; it directs us to move "TO" or forward with caution. This embodies the process of moving across stages of change or identity statuses (Wallace, Carter, Nanín, Keller, & Alleyne, 2003)—as individuals, organizations, professions, and societies—toward a new paradigm. This draws upon an integration of the stages of change—*precontemplation, contemplation, preparation, action, maintenance*—of Prochaska and DiClemente (1983, 1992) and the use of motivational interviewing to enhance intrinsic motivation to move across the stages of change toward taking action (Miller & Rollnick, 1991, 2002); the yellow arrow suggests this integration and a reality. First, there is the reality of how individuals, organizations, professions, and societies may be in different stages of change or readiness to move forward and shift to a new paradigm: some may be in *precontemplation*, and not even thinking about a paradigm shift; others may be in *contemplation* and only thinking about it; others in *preparation*, having made a determination that it is important to shift to a new paradigm; others are in an *action* stage, having taken actions consistent with the new paradigmatic ways of thinking, behaving, and being in the world—for less than 6 months; and, others are in a *maintenance* stage, having engaged for more than 6 months and perhaps many years in the new paradigmatic ways of thinking, behaving, and being in the world (Wallace, 2003, 2005a; Wallace et al., 2003). Second, we can use motivational interviewing principles and techniques to foster movement toward taking action and shifting to the new paradigm—whether on the level of individuals, organizations, professionals, societies, or a global community (Wallace, 2003, 2005a; Wallace et al., 2003). An individual, organization, academic field, research discipline, or overall society might be characterized by stage of change with regard to the task of moving "TO" or forward toward a new paradigm; and/or stopping all the problematic paradigmatic ways of thinking, behaving, and being in the world associated with the old paradigm (A/B). This implies work on identity and our guiding theories and models and approaches to research, so they all move toward being in accord with a new paradigm.

The yellow associated with caution also suggests the new heightened state of awareness and alertness associated with a conscious attempt to recondition ourselves by doing the following: (1) stopping old paradigmatic ways of thinking, behaving, and being in the world; (2) potentially consciously catching or observing one's self or organization engaging in the habitual execution of old paradigmatic ways of thinking, behaving, and being—even if this is a temporary lapse or relapse; (3) after stopping the old paradigmatic ways of thinking, behaving, and being, going on to create a space or clearing for the emergence of something new, and then consciously directing one's self to execute new ways of thinking, behaving, and being in the world that are consistent with the new paradigm; and, (4) systematically rehearsing and refining over time new paradigmatic ways of thinking, behaving, and being in the world so that they become automatic natural responses from which a sense of natural reinforcement and gratification arises. All of us living in the aftermath of centuries of domination and oppression are in need of such a reconditioning process which may transpire over time. Not surprisingly, this process in many ways parallels that of reconditioning a survivor of abuse and trauma; this process is rooted in an integration of theory (see Wallace, 1996 for details).

Also symbolized by the yellow arrow, among the things that we are moving toward is the cultivation of social capital (see Kwong, Ho-Asjoe, Chung, & Wong, chapter 14) and global leadership capable of overcoming the legacy of practices of domination and oppression that have transpired in places such as the United States and around the globe. Moreover, the new paradigm needs to be firmly established, or to take root in the very foundations of our individual beings, families, professions, disciplines, institutions, and local and global communities.

Green for Go: The New Paradigm

All of these foundations (e.g., individual, disciplines, communities, etc.) may each be symbolized as a green circular whole (at the far right of the symbol). At the core of a green foundation is the symbol of the new paradigm: $A = B$, suggesting a relationship of equality, freedom, justice, and the conditions for all reaching their full human potential prevailing (Wallace, 2003). The goal of interpersonal relationships reflecting a *non-hierarchical state of equality*—a term put forth by Taylor (1994)—is recommended by the $A = B$ formula. This non-hierarchical state of equality constitutes the desired status to be reached and reflected in all levels of human interaction—ranging from the personal to the global.

Of note, the whole green circle as the foundation for the new paradigm, $A = B$, also has rays spanning out, reminiscent of a sun, or arrows suggests the multi-pronged actions that may follow from the new paradigm—spreading out in all directions and reaching all parts of the global community. The green symbolizing "go" also suggests that all is clear for movement and action, within an approach that is holistic, inclusive, and supports resources being distributed, reaching out to all. This is also consistent with a global collaborative approach and sense of our interdependence, reminding us of our vast potential to collaborate, share, and disperse resources to literally any place on the globe; this also suggests a new definition and reconceptualization of globalization.

Researchers and interventionists may need to first undergo their own personal paradigm shift, and then provide leadership in ensuring their academic disciplines, models, and theories also pursue a paradigm shift, searching for new models and ways of conducting the business of their profession. Even as entire fields and/or academic disciplines, such as public health or psychology, must seek a restructuring, there may be paradigms that are of great value and must be retained; a need to integrate and combine some paradigmatic approaches; and need to forge entirely new ways of thinking and doing the work of a one's profession, including the design of new interventions and research strategies (see Buchanan & Allegrante, chapter 5; Prochaska, chapter 4). There are also implications for how we must shift to a search for underlying mechanisms influencing health outcomes (see Ogedegbe, Schoenthaler, & Fernandez, chapter 7), as we seek to identify and uproot all past influences of the old paradigm.

The results of a major paradigm shift also include new policies and procedures. This includes eliminating those policies and procedures that are destructive to our communities (see Fullilove, chapter 8), and pioneering new ways of analyzing data so our conclusions speak to the need to restructure how we distribute resources in society—and even how to tailor our resulting approaches by race/ethnicity given how the data speaks to us (see Lahiri & Pulungan, chapter 6). Thus, a shifting in our personal paradigms, and the subsequent shifts in our professions, may interact with larger societal shifts that all reflect the new paradigm based on a non-hierarchical equality prevailing on all levels and in all interactions.

(2) The Drive for New Models of Health Care and Training

The shift to a new paradigm necessarily includes a drive to create new models of health care and training, while also having implications for evaluation and research. As Levine et al. (2001) have asserted, new models of health care and training are needed. They pointed out how all models of health care that devalue prevention are inadequate. Equally inadequate are simple assurances of equal access to care or equality in "curative and/or palliative care services once access is achieved" (p. 481). Comprehensive prevention needs to achieve "parity as an integral part of regular care" (p 481).

Levine et al. (2001) bolster their argument for valuing prevention, given how more than 80% of the U.S. population visits a health care provider in any given year. They categorize this as unsurpassed opportunity for the initiation of solutions that may involve primary, secondary, and/or tertiary prevention. However, our health care system must be redesigned to accomplish such a mission, while providers must be trained in new ways to work within such a new system. Moreover, Levine et al. (2001) point out how the vast majority (9 out of 10) of the leading health indicators established for Healthy People 2010 (i.e., physical activity, overweight and obesity, tobacco use, substance abuse, responsible sexual behavior, mental health, injury and violence, environmental quality, and immunization) are amenable to prevention. They underscore the need to go beyond a current primary focus on curative and/or palliative treatment which dominates today, also being reactive, and serving to increase "the overall prevalence of disease" (p. 481). Such an increase occurs because "it prolongs the duration of illness while having little impact on incidence." Within such a model, "black people can be expected to continue to have higher mortality rates than white people, because the higher occurrence of preventable risk among blacks will continue to produce higher risks of becoming ill or injured in the first place" (p. 481).

The extent of their challenge to the hegemony of current models designed to improve health in the United States suggests how Levine et al. (2001) are assisting in fostering a major paradigmatic shift. Not only are changes needed in the entire medical system infrastructure and medical practice, but also in research.

Change is also needed in how public health programs are constructed. "A public health program can be defined as a structured intervention with the intent of improving the health of the total population or a subpopulation at particularly high risk" (Brownson, Baker, Leet, & Gillespie, 2003, p. 4). Thus, the overall health care system, medical field, and public health systems should change in response to the drive for new models of health care and training (e.g., see Johnson & Wallace, chapter 21; Moretti & Witte, chapter 16; Wallace, Konuwa, & Ayeboafo, chapter 19; Woo, chapter 18).

(3) The Drive for New Theories, Perspectives, and Identities

The new paradigm also requires new theories and new perspectives (see Airhihenbuwa & Okoror, chapter 3; Walker, chapter 2), as well as a menu of integrated theories and approaches from which we may choose, selecting that which is most appropriate, given diversity, for example, and different needs for diverse groups at various times (Wallace, 2005b; and, see Nanín, Fontaine & Wallace, chapter 22).

An important goal is to avoid engaging in "blame-the-victim" or "deficit-oriented" research. It is also vital to avoid locating key variables—seen as deficits or evidence of an inherent inferiority—within the individual. And, it is absolutely important to appreciate the role of factors located in the social context; this includes the role of factors associated with the old paradigm of A/B, or hierarchical domination, and the forces of oppression that followed from it.

It is important to avoid theories that over-emphasize genetics (see Walker, chapter 2). Such theories betray their racist roots (see David & Collins, chapter 10).

Airhihenbuwa (2006, p. 34) cautions against a "focus only on individuals and their attitude or actions," given how such "individual-based theories undermine the cultural and political contexts that shape behaviors." Indeed, it is a flaw of Western theories that they focus on the individual and their agency as individuals (Airhihenbuwa, 2006). Nairn, Pega, McCreanor, Rankine and Barnes (2006) have also highlighted critiques of theories with individualist, pathologizing roots.

Kwong et al. (chapter 14) demonstrate the value of using the asset-based community development approach, as these frameworks give rise to interventions that can significantly enhance social capital and increase community assets and resources for a particular neighborhood. Such approaches can ultimately alter the social milieu and economic position at a community or neighborhood level, demonstrating the importance of going beyond a focus on the individual.

Diderichsen, Evans, and Whitehead (2001, p. 14) also critique how the "pervasive clinical orientation of epidemiology has resulted most often in the identification of "individual" attributes that differentiate health risk (e.g., age, dietary habits, etc.). However, Diderichsen et al. suggest, instead, how any "practical framework must capture the idea that the physiological end-pathways leading to an individual's ill health are inextricably linked to the social setting" (p. 14).

Also, epidemiology lacks theory development, while other theories are far too reductionistic, individualistic, or partly biomedically driven, as Elder (2001) underscores and explains. Even some psychosocial theories used in health psychology and health education may not be appropriate globally when approaching country- or population-level health issues; they may also not gel well with indigenous or traditional cultures, let alone the value placed on community identity versus the individual level. An emphasis on health communication, learning theory, media advocacy, or community self-control strategies involving careful monitoring of selected behavior in light of selected goals may be more appropriate in the global context (Elder, 2001; and see fuller discussion in Wallace et al., chapter 19).

Diderichsen et al. (2001, p. 13) discuss how some tend to "blame the trend in health care and medical research toward an excessive focus on individuals—their biological and behavioral risks of illness—to the relative neglect of population groups and the societal forces that create health divides." Meanwhile, one result is a focus on proximal causes of illness. On the other hand, there are those who think gains in health will best be achieved by seeking a better understanding of more distal or upstream determinants. Instead, Diderichsen et al. assume the position that adequate understanding of and interventions against social inequities in health requires both looking upstream into "the mechanisms of society," as well as "downstream into the mechanisms of human biology and the clinical issues of how people cope with disease and disabilities" (p. 13).

A viable recommended approach is to structure research in such a way as to investigate multiple relationships, drawing upon multiple theories as needed. This may guide the examination of the relationship between certain selected factors in the larger social context, or the experience of specific sources of stress in the social context, or the prevalence of certain adaptive strengths in the population under study, as well as demographic and other subject variables. This is what this volume strongly advocates. In this manner, researchers are encouraged to follow important trends valuing theory to guide such research—whether Multiculturalism, Positive Psychology, a Strengths-Based Approach, Optimistic Thinking/Learned Optimism (Wallace, 2005b), or the Psychosocial Theory of Resilience (see Franklin, Oscar, Guishard, Faulkner, & Zauber, chapter 11), or PEN-3 Model (see Airhihenbuwa & Okoror, chapter 3).

The goal is to be able to conceptualize and document subjects' strengths and evidence of resiliency, as well as to view many problem behaviors as merely attempts to cope and adapt in a stressful social context. Also recommended is a focus upon which attempts to cope with stress in the social context reflect maladaptive affective, behavioral, and cognitive coping responses versus those that seem to reflect adaptive affective, behavioral, and cognitive coping responses (Wallace, 2005a). In this manner, a population can be approached as being able to reveal much more than the prevalence of a disease entity or problem behavior. The population can be approached as holding important information about both the prevalence of maladaptive and adaptive coping responses, given a theoretical framework that encompasses adaptive strengths in response to stress and other factors in the larger social context. Information on adaptive coping responses can serve as evidence of strengths and resilience, as well as form the basis for recommendations with regard to the content of future health education and health promotion targeted for delivery to individuals with the same or similar characteristics as those who were studied; findings might generalize in this manner. The resulting content for health education and health promotion may also be utilized in consultation work, community-based media campaigns, or social marketing efforts striving to disseminate "what works" or constitutes adaptive coping for those facing certain kinds of stress in the larger social context.

Theories guide how we understand and approach disparities in health. In this regard, Airhihenbuwa (2006, p. 37) notes how the United States has spent "tens of millions of dollars" on "projects for researchers to eliminate racial and ethnic health disparities." However, the entire endeavor has failed to follow the wisdom of W.E.B. Du Bois (1899/1996) and his study of *The Philadelphia Negro*, dating back to 1899; therein, Du Bois concluded that any data or health statistics need to consider the absolute condition of Negroes, instead of focusing on their relative status—merely comparing Blacks to Whites. Airhihenbuwa emphasizes how only a focus on the absolute condition, or the larger context would allow an adequate analysis of social–cultural infrastructure.

In the process, one might identify that which "nurtures a state of resilience among many African Americans such that they are able to cope and thrive in social and political contexts where the assault on their identity remains chronic and systemic" (p. 37). Theories are needed that consider the social–cultural infrastructure, as well as coping and adaptation.

This is not to deny that some attempts to cope may be deemed more or less adaptive or maladaptive. Thus, another guiding rationale involves seeking to identify the underlying mechanisms that may be creating or sustaining disparities in health—such as potential maladaptive coping responses by providers to patient diversity, racism, or health practitioner behavior/bias/stereotypes—as information which might inform how these factors can be addressed in order to reduce health disparities (see Ogedegbe et al., chapter 7). Theories or the guiding rationales they provide for research need to encompass such underlying mechanisms operating in the social context.

Kunitz (2007, p. 6) reviews a large body of contradictory findings, illustrating how "anomalous findings need to be acknowledged and not ignored, as so often happens." These findings are typically ignored because of the manner in which scientists tend to be "wedded to their theories," holding "deeply held preexisting values" that effectively shape their "interpretation of data and the abstractions inferred from them" (p. 6). This serves to blind scientists from even acknowledging anything that contradicts their view. It is only when an overwhelming body of contradictory evidence accumulates that a shift to a new paradigm occurs, and the inherited ideas embodied in theories which have been long influencing interpretations of data should give way to something new.

This something new should be a full appreciation of the larger social context and the forces operating within it. For example, Airhihenbuwa (2006) identifies four concentric circles spanning out from around the person: (1) spouse, family, community, culture; (2) information, education, language, communication; (3) schools, curriculum, institutions, policy; and (4) housing, employment, environment, and government. This description of four concentric circles suggests the larger sociocultural context. However, we need to stop primarily targeting the person at the center of these concentric circles, and debunk "individual-based preventive models and embrace a focus on the confluence of factors in the concentric outer circles that collectively circumscribe the health decisions of the individual" (Airhihenbuwa, 2007, p. 150). Such a focus on the outer circles "addresses the root causes of individual problems" (p. 151).

Indeed, a more appropriate approach is to start with government policy which "exacts the most impacting influence on social change that can transform the outer layers for the benefit of individual health outcomes even when individuals have no intention of changing" (Airhihenbuwa, 2007, p. 159). Secondly, one needs to focus on socioeconomic status (SES), and "SES is influenced to a great degree by government policy," while the poor are the most vulnerable—even as SES, independently, does not explain inequality (p. 160). Third, absolutely crucial is a focus on the role of culture so as to understand the contexts of preventive health behavior (p. 161). Fourth, gender relations are vital (especially for an epidemic such as HIV/AIDS, and issues such as condom negotiation or a male's multiple partners). Fifth, spirituality, which tends not to be actively or sufficiently engaged in prevention (pp. 162–163). We need new theories and guiding models that adequately acknowledge these five contextual domains, as does the UNAIDS/Penn State framework, providing a basic structure for HIV/AIDS prevention in places such as Africa (Airhihenbuwa, 2007).

Or, we need theories and models such as the PEN-3 model (Airhihenbuwa, 2007), which encompasses the domains of (1) Cultural Identity, (2) Relationships and Expectations, and (3) Cultural Empowerment (see Airhihenbuwa & Okoror, chapter 3). Such a model also allows us to understand and respect the cultural identity of the people in a community where research is being conducted. The PEN-3 model is a cultural model vital in enlisting community voices to inform the development, implementation, and evaluation of programs; and, in guiding attention to the positive and existential behaviors within communities, effectively building on strengths located in the communities and people who live there when working on changing a behavior of interest. Thus, in all instances we should appreciate how there is also a cultural context where issues of identity for both the people and the researcher are pertinent. For "global health issues are identity and social issues;" moreover, they "should be analyzed using frameworks that can be derived from the social and behavioral sciences" (Airhihenbuwa, 2006, p. 32).

The transformation of the identity of the researcher to be consistent with the new paradigm advanced in this volume is also vital. Indeed, all who seek to work with communities around the globe should first and foremost assume personal responsibility for deconstructing an identity rooted in Western theories, and for reconstituting and rearranging their own identity, following the analysis and promptings of Airhihenbuwa (2006, 2007, chapter 3). The goal is to create an identity so they can perceive that which is of value in a social cultural context that is new to them, and actively seek to approach or enter that social cultural context via what Airhihenbuwa (2006) eloquently refers to as the "gate" or point of reference of those people in that social cultural context.

The era of generating research and delivering interventions in a multiplicity of settings, communities, and countries, following a misguided "one size fits all" approach is over, as is the legitimacy of acting as if our Western theory extends to all globally (Airhihenbuwa, 2006). Instead, this outdated approach should be declared as yielding to a much-needed paradigm shift and reconstituting and rearranging process, as we sort through our theories—weeding out that which is destructive (Ayeboafo, 2005). We should weed out what is destructive in our theories and, therefore, in our own perspectives and identities which are closely tied to our theories.

Airhihenbuwa (2006) speaks to the nature of the challenge facing many Western educated researchers and practitioners who now seek to be a part of the new era, given how attached to and deeply engrained they may be within an approach that is part and parcel of their very identity. For so many, theory may be akin to an opiate, with theoreticians "behaving as a drug addict," given how "problems are defined and solutions sought in the social and behavioral sciences" (p. 40). There is a compulsive tendency to "define problems and solutions as sharing common gateways to all cultures leading to the conclusion that what works in the United States or Europe should work in Africa or, for that matter, anywhere" (p. 40). Hence, a vital error is made in ignoring the "critical roles of social cultural contexts that nurture such behaviors" (p. 40).

Also, there is a "need to debunk Westernized theorizing about African health issues" (Airhihenbuwa, 2006, p. 36). And, a corresponding need to recognize how such Westernized theorizing does not apply with a multitude of groups within our global community. In addition to considering issues of identity, we must consider the intersection of multiple identities and related issues of stigma in the social context (see Greene, Miville, & Ferguson, chapter 23; Johnson & Wallace, chapter 21; Nanín et al., chapter 22; Rosario, Schrimshaw, & Hunter, chapter 24). However, even where disease causation is multi-factorial, many of the factors are rooted in social injustice (Levy & Sidel, 2006b, p. 11). Hence, our theories should also encompass a viable approach to social injustice.

The drive for new theories, perspectives, and identities emerges as an essential guiding value for the field of equity in health. We should evolve to the point where we have a menu of approaches and theories from which to choose when designing research and interventions (Wallace, 2005b).

(4) The Drive for Evidence-Based Approaches

It is also crucial to move toward a menu of evidence-based approaches (Wallace, 2005b) for each health challenge we face. This is now the standard in many fields that have systematically evolved over decades (Hester & Miller, 2003; Wallace, 2005b). This volume's approach is rooted in the value that the field of equity in health generates a growing menu of evidence-based approaches to reducing disparities—decade by decade. All of this is consistent with assertions that we are living in an age of evidence-based practice (Sammons, 2001).

This book's approach seeks to value and promote the very best of patient and population level research (see Prochaska, chapter 4), and the very best research within the traditions of the National Institutes of Health and the Centers for Disease Control that has led to the identification of evidence-based models (see El-Bassel, Witte, & Gilbert, chapter 15; and Rashid, Amuwo, Skillen, Melanson, & Wagner, chapter 12). However, despite the prevalence of "new evidence-based guidelines for clinical preventive services, many patients are not receiving scientifically proven interventions" (Brownson et al., 2003, p. ix).

Evidence is important for many reasons. There are certain primary uses of evidence (Fielding, 2003), such as the following: first, public health practitioners, particularly those with executive and managerial responsibilities, may want to know "what is the evidence for alternative strategies, be they policies, programs, or other activities" (p. v). Sometimes practitioners are so busy they fail to inquire with regard to "the most important things I can do to improve the public's health" (p. v). Population-based data may provide direction as to what a practitioner can do, especially if it addresses factors such as "health status, health risks, and health problems for the overall population" (p. v) or specific subpopulations. There may be other important data on a "population's attitudes and beliefs about various major health problems" (p. v). Of great importance are data on potential interventions, including the menu of available options and what is known about each one, in terms of evidence—as well as "their individual and conjoint effectiveness in improving health in the populations" being served (p. v). In sum, the result may be a "rational prioritizing of opportunities, constrained only by resources and feasibility" (p. v).

The implication is that there is a role for the integration of theories, or their selection for use, depending on factors such as client characteristics or attitudes or preferences. A menu of options permits tailoring interventions in light of multiple client characteristics (Wallace, 2005b).

Toward the goal of making the practice of public health more evidence based, Brownson et al. (2003, p. 4) suggest how evidence-based "public health involves the development and implementation of effective programs and policies" wherein a public health program can be defined as a structured intervention. Here the intent may be to improve the health of "the total population or a subpopulation at particularly high risk" (p. 4).

Taking from the evolution of evidence-based medicine, Brownson et al. (2003) note how key skills "include the ability to track down, critically appraise, and rapidly incorporate scientific evidence into a clinician's practice" (p. 5). Differences between evidence-based approaches in medicine and public health include the quality and volume of evidence. For example, Brownson et al. explain how

> medical studies of pharmaceuticals and procedures often rely on randomized controlled trials of individuals: the most scientifically rigorous of epidemiological studies. In contrast, public health interventions are likely to rely on cross-sectional studies, quasi-experimental designs, and time-series analyses. These studies sometimes lack a comparison group, which may limit the quality of evidence for some interventions.... (pp. 6–7)

Brownson et al. recommend a six-stage sequential framework to promote greater use of evidence in day-to-day decision making: (1) develop an initial statement of the issue, perhaps identifying gaps between some current status of a program or organization and desired goals, and, ideally stating "the health condition or risk factor being considered, the population(s) affected, the size and scope of the problem, prevention opportunities, and potential stakeholders" (p. 13); (2) quantify the issue by identifying sources of existing data, such as vital statistical data, perhaps from a survey—ideally with a representative cross section of the population of interest—permitting quantification of prevalence of "behaviors, characteristics, exposures, and disease at some point (or period) of time in a defined population" (p. 15); (3) accumulate knowledge about previous and ongoing strategies to address the issue, such as via a formal literature review; (4) develop a list of options, given the prior three steps, listing intervention options, also prioritizing them; (5) develop an action plan and implement intervention, via strategic planning, including the identification of goals (long-term desired change) and objectives—"a short-term, measurable, specific activity that leads toward achievement of a goal"—as well as the course of action, or plans for how to achieve what is desired (pp. 16–17); and (6) evaluate the program or policy to determine the degree to which "program or policy goals and objectives are met"—even as they note how "the strongest evaluation designs acknowledge the roles of both quantitative and qualitative evaluation" (p. 16).

Brownson et al. (2003) present an array of strategies for how to select, implement, and evaluate evidence-based programs, interventions and policies, requiring multi-disciplinary teams that design the overall action plan. Options include those that reflect the highly valued standard of community-based participatory research (see El-Bassel et al., chapter 15; Hayes, chapter 13), and enlisting community voices and participation to ensure cultural appropriateness (see Airhihenbuwa & Okoror, chapter 3).

When discussing how to translate evidence into recommendations and public health action, Brownson et al. (2003) recommend the use of expert panels and consensus conferences (to review scientific evidence)—a mechanism "used by the National Institutes of Health (NIH) since 1977 to solve important and controversial issues in medicine and public health" (p. 69); practice guidelines, or recommendations, typically offering advice on how to improve effectiveness and impact of interventions—effectively translating research findings and results of demonstration projects into "accessible and usable information for public health practice," (p. 71) whether for clinical or community settings; "best practices" in public health—reviews describing discoveries of what worked best in a practitioner's experiences, or via some grass-roots approach, or results of an evidence-based or expert opinion regarding what works (pp. 75–76).

Thus, there are many uses for and types of evidence. Sources of evidence may also be multiple.

Consider the use of quantitative and qualitative data, or "triangulation" in the data collection and analysis process. This involves multiple methods of data collection and/or analysis to determine points of commonality or disagreement; on the one hand, quantitative data may show how variables are related for large numbers of people, but not why these relationships exist; on the other hand, qualitative data may help to explain or give meaning to quantitative findings (Brownson et al., 2003, p. 207).

There are also approaches to acquiring evidence that are controversial. For example, in the United States, there is a dominant tradition that focuses on racial/ethnic differences in health or health care by largely comparing racial/ethnic groups (Braveman, 2006). This is despite the warning of W. E. B. Du Bois (1899/1996) over a century ago, as shared earlier through the work of Airhihenbuwa (2006), that seeking to understand the relative status of groups, instead of the totality of the conditions that creates vulnerability to high rates of morbidity and mortality, is not an adequate data collection approach.

However, within the tradition of seeking to understand the relative status of groups, Braveman (2006) offers a recommended evidence-based approach. Braveman explains how definitions impact data collection and policy. First, there are "different approaches to defining health disparities/equity" and corresponding measurement implications (p. 188). Such a discussion is important, because there can be important implications for health policy and the taking of action. Experience has shown that "a definition can have a significant impact on policies, particularly when resources are scarce and the definition is vague" (p. 188). For example, in the United States, the term "health disparities" is "generally assumed to refer to racial/ethnic disparities," while there is also the prevalent erroneous belief that "such disparities are rooted in biological and/or "cultural" differences rather than underlying social disadvantage." In such cases, explicit guidance is needed with regard to what constitutes an adequate measurement approach—"not only for research on specific research questions but also for ongoing surveillance to assess the magnitude of the health gaps and how they change over time in relation to policies and conditions in all sectors that influence health" (p. 188). Braveman goes on to acknowledge how public health surveillance "is certainly not sufficient to reduce health disparities, but without monitoring how the size of disparities between more and less advantaged social groups changes over time in relation to policies, there is a lack of accountability for the differential effects of policies on vulnerable groups" (p. 188). Hence, a kind of moral imperative to take seriously "what we should measure and monitor and why" emerges (p. 188).

Of note, consider the following (Braveman, 2006):

> While epidemiology—the study of the distribution of diseases and risk factors across different populations—is concerned with health differences in general, which are important, the terms "health disparities" or "health inequalities" refer to a very specific subset of differences deemed worthy of special attention because of social values, including ethical concepts of distributive justice and core human rights principles (p. 188).

Braveman (2006) offers a recommended evidence-based approach within the context of what has traditionally been done in the United States. It may be summarized as follows: First, select the health or health-related indicators of concern and categorize people into social strata (by social position); and, secondly, calculate rates of the health indicator in each social stratum and display this graphically. More specifically, calculate rate ratios (e.g., relative risks) and rate differences to compare each stratum with the a priori most advantaged stratum that corresponds to it (e.g., all other income groups compared to the highest income group). Next, proceed to examine any changes over time in the rate ratios and rate differences. Moreover, if feasible, use a summary measure to assess multiple parameters at the same time. Finally, conduct multivariate analyses in the overall sample and within strata shown to be at elevated risk compared to the most advantaged stratum, to identify particular issues warranting further attention through research or action (p. 187).

The work of Kunitz (2007, p. 3) also analyzes influences on the kind of evidence we value and collect: for example, consider the "way inherited ideas about industrial growth, economic expansion, social change, and causes of disease have shaped explanations of the health of populations"; and, how "inherited ideas have become assimilated to political ideologies that influence how epidemiologic and demographic data are understood, causal inferences made, anomalies ignored, and abstractions drawn." In other words, it is the "inherited ideas about the consequences of social and economic change and of causes of disease" and how these ideas have been "assimilated into different political ideologies that influence the choices we all make of the evidence we accept and ignore" (Kunitz, p. 175) that create a contemporary challenge and danger.

Thus, the drive for evidence-based approaches lies at the core of the field of equity in health. The goal is to arrive at a menu of evidence-based options for specific health challenges (Wallace, 2005b), as we move forward decade by decade.

(5) The Drive for Transdisciplinary Teams and Community–Based Participatory Research

There is also a drive for research to be conducted from the multiple perspectives that are brought to the table when there are transdisciplinary teams, as well as critical stakeholders, at the table. New forms of collaboration among all such parties are vital for future research envisioned (see El-Bassel et al., chapter 15; Hayes, chapter 13; Rashid et al., chapter 12; Walker, chapter 2).

Brownson et al. (2003) explain how a "stakeholder is anyone who is involved in program operations, is served by the program, or will use the evaluation results," while stakeholders should be representatives of all these groups; and, they should be actively involved in "the design of the program or policy as well as in the design, implementation, and interpretation of evaluation results" (p. 196). This is consistent with the latest standards for community-based participatory research (see Hayes, chapter 13; and, El-Bassel et al., chapter 15).

Key stakeholders must bring the perspective of the cultural community in which research and interventions will be conducted. Community members should be seen as "working alongside" professionals, researchers, and interventionists (Comas-Diaz, Lykes, & Alarcon, 1998), consistent with the new paradigm and value of a nonhierarchical equality prevailing. Ideally, professionals and community members enjoy a mutual respect and recognition, as well as a free-flowing dialogue among equals—as other vital aspects of the new paradigm (Wallace, 2003).

There is a strong rationale for the use of transdisciplinary teams (see Walker, chapter 2). Consistent with this, Brownson et al. (2003) discuss how public health relies on a number of disciplines, and people in public health have no one single academic credential, also working on multidisciplinary teams, while engaged in problem solving that depends on the expertise of group members bringing "diverse experiences and educational" backgrounds (p. 11). Professions represented might include "management and administration, epidemiology, biostatistics, behavioral science, environmental health, and health economics (p. 11). All of this is consistent with their overall vision of what constitutes and characterizes evidence-based decision making. The best possible science is drawn upon, while problem solving is multidisciplinary, drawing upon the expertise of a diverse team. A variety of planning frameworks and behavioral science theories are applied, such as ecological or systems models that consider how changes in the social environment will produce changes in individuals; and environmental changes may be brought about by supporting individuals. Meanwhile, problems need to be addressed at multiple levels with attention paid to interaction and integration of factors within and across all levels—"individual, interpersonal, community, organizational, and governmental" (p. 12). Also, the goal is embraced of moving toward healthy community environments where health-promoting information and social support is provided so people achieve a healthier way of living and being (p. 12). All of this suggests a role for community members as key stakeholders, helping to determine how to best accomplish such goals.

Transdisciplinary teams with community stakeholders at the table also follow sound evaluation principles. This includes systematic evaluation—both formative and outcome evaluation, permitting that which emerges as lacking effectiveness to be discontinued; that lacking effectiveness will not be continued merely because of "historical or political considerations" (Brownson et al., 2003, p. 12). Such historical or political considerations tend to prevail when one perspective, group, or discipline dominates. In addition, results are disseminated to others who need to know, allowing them to "enhance their own use of evidence in decision making"—sharing the news via publications, media, or meetings and hearings with policy makers (p. 12). Once again, community members as key stakeholders have an essential role to play in determining the format, shape, and content of what is disseminated, along with diverse transdisciplinary or multidisciplinary team members.

Moreover, such practices, consistent with community-based participatory research, effectively serve to "ensure that all voices are considered in the evaluation and that all will benefit" from it (Brownson, et al., 2003, p. 196). Results may include staff developing "skills and abilities in evaluation design and interpretation" (p. 196). Moreover, Brownson et al. note the following:

> There are also other evaluation designs (participatory, collaborative, or empowerment evaluation) where stakeholders are seen as equal partners in all evaluation decisions from questions asked to types of data collected and participate in analysis and

interpretation of results. Some of these designs emphasize stakeholder participation as a means of ensuring that the evaluation is responsive to stakeholder needs while other designs involve stakeholders to increase the control and ownership.... (p. 197)

The work of Airhihenbuwa (2006) further reinforces why transdisciplinary teams and key stakeholders who are community members from the cultural context play such a vital role. The approach that is needed should draw upon "the experiences of scholars from multiple fields of specialization in ways that render a single disciplinary focus inadequate" (Airhihenbuwa, p. 32). By bringing stakeholders, community members, and members of transdisciplinary teams to the table in conceptualizing the approach to research, there is hope for averting critical errors of misrepresenting the reality of a group of people (Airhihenbuwa; also, see Airhihenbuwa & Okoror, chapter 3).

A drive for transdisciplinary teams and community-based participatory research must be at the core of the field of equity in health. This is essential in order to function effectively in our global community where diverse cultures abound.

(6) The Drive for Globalization and Global Collaboration

There is also a drive for globalization and global collaboration. The Internet and new technologies serve to bind us together as a global community (see Adams & Leath, chapter 17; Moretti & Witte, chapter 16).

The Internet is not the only force that binds us as a global community (Carr-Chellman, 2006), nor is the reality of our interdependence (Ayeboafo, 2005). As a global community, we are bound by the forces of globalization, including the multidimensional integration of the world economy, politics, culture, and human affairs—all of which are fundamentally changing world health dynamics (Chen & Berlinger, 2001, p. 35). Kawachi and Wamala (2007a) cover the challenges and opportunities that come with globalization, the resulting health threats, and various approaches that can be taken in contemporary times, given the global organizations in existence and reality of globalization; most importantly, they note how globalization is "breaking down economic, political, cultural, social, demographic, and symbolic barriers across the world at a pace hitherto unseen in the history of civilization" (p. 3).

This globalization is an inescapable reality, corresponding to our current phase of historical development, while having the power to fulfill many human wants (Chen and Berlinger, 2001). Kawachi and Wamala (2007b) summarize the key aspects of contemporary globalization that make it unique historically. This includes how more than $2 billion is exchanged in the world's currency markets, the presence of new actors (e.g., the World Trade Organization [WTO] with authority over national governments, multinational corporations with more economic power than many states, as well as the global networks of nongovernmental organizations), and new rules of governance (e.g., multilateral agreements on trade and intellectual property). Moreover, there are also "new forms of communication (e.g., the Internet, satellite television), and the global movements of populations (whether as economic migrants, refugees, or trafficked individuals)" (pp. 3–4).

Consistent with the multiple influences of globalization, others have offered global approaches. For example, Merson, Black, and Mills (2006) compile the voices of many to articulate the full scope and dimensions of international and global health, shedding light on what nations around the globe are doing, including the challenges being faced, and how health systems are emerging in response to these issues, including their connection with the economic development of countries—providing many case studies for purposes of illustration.

The physical space that separates us is bridged by the rapidity with which technology can disperse information across time, linking those who share this planet in ways that suggest it is now a rather intimately shared space. Images and news of what is happening in one corner of the world can rapidly reach us, while we can just as quickly travel to another continent around the globe—potentially taking our infections and rapidly spreading them to others.

Kawachi and Wamala (2007b, p. 4) point out how "both travel and migration have helped to spread contagious diseases such as HIV/AIDS and SARS, while the Internet has provided a convenient vehicle for the global illicit traffic in laundered money, drugs, women, and weapons." Given the impact of globalization, Kawachi and Wamala (2007a) put forth strategies (i.e., tools) for monitoring and evaluating these impacts, including health impact assessment techniques, the kind of global solutions needed, the role of global organizations (i.e., World Bank, IMF, WTO, WHO, the G8, other national governments), while stressing the opportunities that globalization also presents (e.g., globally coordinated efforts to combat the SARS outbreak, applications of technology) via health dividends (pp. 13–14).

Given the inescapable reality of globalization and the forces that will ensure it continues, we can maximize the potential for good through global collaboration on problems. If weapons and armed forced can be rapidly deployed, so can resources to ensure equity in health for all. Meanwhile, global warming is yet another phenomenon that speaks to how what one country does or sanctions affects other countries, if not all members in the global community. The emergent reality is that "what affects one, affects all" in our global community, suggesting our interdependence (Ayeboafo, 2005).

A New Definition of Globalization

This suggests a new definition of *globalization* as an awareness of how "what affects one affects all," or a consciousness of our fundamental interdependence as a global community, as well as the resulting process of learning to work collaboratively and share and disperse resources within our global community to ensure social justice, equity, the protection of human rights, and the sustainability of the planet.

Such a consciousness and process can also guide the weeding out of the destructive forces to which Ayeboafo (2005) also refers. We should collaborate to fully actualize that which is constructive.

The drive for globalization, as newly defined, and global collaboration is at the center of the field of equity in health. The reality of our interdependence necessitates constructive collaboration.

(7) The Drive for Cultural Competence and Cultural Appropriateness

There is also a drive for cultural competence and cultural appropriateness. Scholarship and recognition are growing with regard to what constitutes cultural competence and its impact, underscoring the importance of obtaining training in cultural competence (Núñez & Robertson, 2006). Núñez and Robertson (p. 371) explain cultural competence as the "ability of health-care providers to interact with patients who are different from themselves," encompassing "knowledge, attitudes, and skills (educational perspective) about health-related beliefs and cultural values (socioeconomic perspective), disease incidence and prevalence (epidemiologic perspective), and treatment efficacy (outcomes perspective)." In addition, cultural competence has been defined as "a set of behaviors, knowledge, attitudes and polices that come together in a system, organization, or among health professionals that enables effective work in cross-cultural situations" (p. 371).

However, cultural competence may also be discussed in the context of training not only practitioners or interventionists, but also researchers, teachers, trainers, policy-makers, administrators, and organizational leaders. Both individuals and organizations can be assessed for their level of organizational cultural or multicultural competence (Wallace, 2000).

Also, consider how some within the field of psychology have provided tremendous leadership, allowing us to amass a critical body of knowledge on how to foster, train, and educate for multicultural competence, cultural competence, and the overcoming of racial prejudice, discrimination, and hate; this body of knowledge also covers how to identify, respond to and redress unintentional and covert forms of racism and oppression, as well as pursue social justice—having implications for the training of counselors, psychologists, teachers, those working in various other disciplines/fields, as well as ordinary community members (Carter, 2005; Constantine & Sue, 2005, 2006; Pedersen, 2006; Pedersen, Draguns, Conner, & Trimble, 2002; Sue, 2003; Sue & Sue, 2003; Sue & Torino, 2005; Vera, Buhin, & Shin, 2006; Wallace, 2003, 2005a, 2005b).

While the field of psychology has provided critical leadership with regard to the fostering of cultural competence, more recently the field of medicine and training of medical professionals has also made great strides. There has been recognition of the role of cultural sensitivity, cultural appropriateness, and cultural competence as factors related to good quality health care (IOM, 2001). Indeed, there is now widespread recognition of the importance of cultural competence (Betancourt, Green, Carrillo, & Park, 2005). Cultural competence emerges as a core strategy for eliminating health disparities.

Betancourt et al. (2005, p. 499) explain cultural competence as "a strategy to improve quality and eliminate racial/ethnic disparities in health care;" in addition, it can lead to the creation of a health care system and adequately trained workforce—one capable of delivering "the highest quality care to every patient regardless of race, ethnicity, culture, or language proficiency" (p. 499). Reporting on the results of interviews with experts on cultural competence from a variety of fields, Betancourt et al. found evidence of a widely perceived link between cultural competence and health disparities; however, also found was a consensus that cultural competence alone would not reduce disparities—as they are rooted in multiple factors/causes; and, cultural competence alone was viewed as insufficient to address the problem of disparities.

Betancourt et al. (2005) also recognize the role of the Liaison Committee on Medical Education (LCME) in fostering progressive change, given their cultural competence accreditation standard; specifically, the LCME has established the requirement for all medical schools to integrate cultural competence into their curricula. Also fostering change is the Association of American Medical College's (AAMC) newly developed tool, specifically designed for the assessment of cultural competence training (Tool for Assessing Cultural Competence Training, TACCT) within medical schools; the goal is to assist medical schools in meeting the new standards. Furthermore, residency programs have responded to the Accreditation Council of Graduate Medical Education's (ACGME's) cultural competence standards; and cultural competence training has substantially increased in recent years due, in part, to both the increasing diversity of the patient population, and pressure from the ACGME. Meanwhile, the Institute of Medicine has also recommended that cross-cultural curricula be part of the training of clinicians from the undergraduate level through continuing medical education (CME). Collectively, these developments provide hope that the new drive for cultural competence is "evolving from a marginal to a mainstream health care policy issue and as a potential strategy to improve quality and address disparities" (Betancourt et al., p. 503).

There is also contemporary discussion about what is culturally appropriate with regard to research, prevention, interventions, training, and treatment (Wallace, 2000). Engaging in that which is deemed culturally appropriate when interacting with diverse patients is also of vital importance (LaVeist, 2005). Underlying mechanisms may be at play (see Ogedegbe et al., chapter 7). For example, LaVeist provides a summary of key findings in this regard: Black and Hispanic patients are less likely to be treated by providers from the same culture, while Whites enjoy the highest rates of race concordance with their physicians; and patients who were race concordant with their physicians rated their visits with physicians as more participatory compared to those who were race discordant; and, that African American patients who were race concordant with their physicians rated them as excellent and reported receiving needed medical care and preventive care; and, those patients reporting the highest level of satisfaction were race concordant with their health care provider (pp. 121–124).

Hence, discussions of cultural competence and what is culturally appropriate inevitably need to include calls for more training for researchers, practitioners, and interventionists (see Franklin et al., chapter 11; Walker, chapter 2). Meanwhile, the field of equity in health incorporates as its core the drive for cultural competence and cultural appropriateness.

(8) The Drive for Health Literacy and Linguistic Appropriateness

There is also a drive for health literacy and linguistic appropriateness at the core of the field of equity in health. For example, the Association of American Medical Colleges (AAMC) seeks to ensure training that produces both cultural and linguistic competence (Betancourt et al., 2005).

Health literacy and linguistic appropriateness are vital considerations, particularly with regard to delivering health information—as a task distinct to medical practitioners and health education/disease prevention specialists (see Perez-Rivera & Langston-Davis, chapter 30). Interventions must be tailored in light of language and culture—as the two critical dimensions of cultural tailoring (LaVeist, 2005).

Zarcadoolas, Pleasant, and Greer (2006) bridge health education, health promotion, and health literacy through the model they advance from a public health perspective, including standards for how to develop and evaluate health communications materials. They offer definitions of three terms often used interchangeably: *health promotion* is a process of enabling people to increase control over their health, thereby also improving it; *health education* involves a multiplicity of activities where the communication of vital health information to people is at the core of all activities, while seeking to bridge the gap between what people know and what they do; and *health communication* involves the use of "human and mass or multimedia and other communication skills and technologies to educate or inform an individual or public about a health issue and to keep that issue on the public agenda" (in an era when consumers want more and better health information) (p. 5). Also of note, *social marketing* involves the "merging of traditional marketing and advertising strategies to persuade people to act in specific ways on social issues such as health and the environment" (p. 5); *consumer decision making* involves the "cognitive and emotional roles individuals play in attending to, evaluating, and acting on health information" (p. 5); and *health literacy* "is the wide range of skills and competencies that people develop to seek out, comprehend, evaluate, and use health information and concepts to make informed choices, reduce health risks, and increase quality of life (pp. 5–6).

Furthermore, Zarcadoolas et al. (2006) explain how health and literacy are linked, as low levels of literacy are strongly linked with poor health and early death both nationally and globally; and the greater the health literacy the greater the level of health (p. 21). At our current historical juncture in time, "there is an urgency to identify relevant characteristics of individual and groups in order to design effective health messages and campaigns" (Zarcadoolas et al., p. 42). Culture, language, and level of health literacy are key characteristics being given due consideration.

Zarcadoolas et al. (2006) explain how health literacy involves "people's abilities to understand and use health information, most often in print (p. 46). Also, a person can have "high fundamental literacy but have low or insufficient health literacy and vice versa" (p. 46). Zarcadoolas et al. (p. 260) also note how language "is clearly not the sum total of culture, but at times the two are inseparable." Zarcadoolas et al. advocate for "efforts at communication" at "the appropriate level of linguistic difficulty" with all materials "crafted with the appropriate cultural characteristics" of individuals and group being kept in mind (p. 260). "Culture, and by extension cultural literacy as a component of health literacy, is clearly part of a successful equation to improve health care, promote healthy decisions, and prevent unhealthy behaviors" (p. 260). Most importantly, it is vital that medicine and health care "consistently include culture as a component in the design of health care, health promotion, and health communication efforts" (p. 261). In order to do this effectively, knowledge and understanding of the language and literacy needs of an audience should be acquired through a "combination of quantitative and qualitative research" (p. 290). Many sources of health information currently available, including that available on the Internet is "poorly designed in terms of the ability to help people with low literacy and health literacy skills" (p. 309).

Hence, the drive for health literacy and linguistic appropriateness emerge as vital to ensure equity in health—lying at the core of the field of equity in health.

(9) The Drive to Ensure the Right to Health

The drive to ensure the right to health is also at the core of the field of equity in health. Closely aligned with the right to health is the right to determine what constitutes health, health standards/outcomes, and way of life, while we accept and respect members of diverse cultures and their right to self-determination—as an overarching ever-present principle.

As evidence of a drive to ensure the right to health, Braveman (2006, p. 183) explains how the foundations for addressing health disparities and pursuing health equity "come not only from ethics but also from the field of international human rights." Elaborating further, human rights are described as "that set of rights or entitlements that all people in the world have, regardless of who they are or where they live" (p. 183). Even if we tend to think of certain civil and political rights (e.g., freedoms of assembly and speech and freedom from torture and cruel or arbitrary punishment), the reality is that these "human rights also encompass economic, social, and cultural rights"; this encompasses things such as the right to a decent standard of living, adequate food, water, shelter, and clothing—indeed, all requisite for health, "as well as the right to health itself" (p. 183).

Bambas and Casas (2003) cite the Universal Declaration of Human Rights, asserting that it established "a benchmark of standards against which to assess equity in health" (p. 321). Bambas and Casas (p. 321) focus on the assertion in article 25 that "Everyone has the right to a standard of living adequate for the health and well-being of himself and his family, including food, clothing, housing and medical care and necessary social services, and the right to security in the event of unemployment, sickness, disability, widowhood, old age or other lack of livelihood in circumstances beyond his control." Equally important for Bambas and Casas (p. 321) is what is set forth in article 2: "Everyone is entitled to all rights and freedoms set forth in this Declaration, without distinction of any kind, such as race, colour, sex, language, religion, political or other opinion, national or social origin, property, birth or other status."

Bambas and Casas (p. 333) acknowledge how "the pursuit of equity is necessarily linked to issues of governance, which includes accountability, transparency, decision-making procedures, and the ability of the political sphere to allow for broad representation and the effective exercise of choice by all" in that society. Bambas and Casas conclude as follows: "Once a society embraces a political foundation of egalitarianism, whereby all citizens of a country are due equal regard under the law and have equal political voices, societies themselves become the ultimate arbitrators of equity in health or any other sphere" (p. 333).

Levy and Sidel (2006b) also acknowledge the value of an approach rooted in "the Universal Declaration of Human Rights and the International Declaration of Health Rights, as these provide a foundation for "reducing, and ultimately eliminating, social injustice" (p. 13). In this regard, Satcher (2006) notes the following: "From the founding of the United States to the present day, the right to good health and well-being has been a basic tenet the nation holds dear" (p. 547). Despite this, it is also true that currently, "the United States stands alone among industrialized countries in not providing universal access to health care"—as just one dimension of a rather poor ranking, overall (Satcher, p. 554).

Thus, we need more than guiding ideals. We need concrete actions that reflect the drive to ensure the right to health.

(10) The Drive for Social Justice and Acknowledgment of Forces in the Social Context

The drive for social justice and acknowledgment of forces in the social context is also key within the field of equity in health. Any discourse on equity goes hand in hand with that on not only the "right to health," but also "social justice," while drawing necessary attention to the social context. Social justice also goes hand in hand with training that inculcates the development of a professional and personal identity that encompasses the taking of social action for social justice (Wallace et al., 2003).

Levy and Sidel (2006b) define social injustice as "the denial or violation of economic, sociocultural, political, civil, or human rights of specific populations or groups in the society based on the perception of their inferiority by those with more power or influence" (p. 6). In all cases and with all types of social injustice, the hallmarks involve "a lack of fairness or equity, often resulting from the way that society is structured or from discrimination by groups or individuals within the society" (Drucker, 2006, p. 6).

Peter and Evans (2001) discuss the ethical dimensions of health equity, placing emphasis on the link between the pursuit of health and the pursuit of social justice; they view health equity as embedded in the more general pursuit of social justice, while efforts to ensure social and economic justice are key. Also, Hofrichter (2006, p. xviii) compiles a chorus of voices in his book on health and social justice in order to support a core argument that forging "health equity requires a coherent strategy that addresses social and economic inequality, as well as the ideologies that support and sustain it." Also worthy of acknowledgment are the many "imbalances in political power and the institutions that maintain those power relations," as these should be seen as "primarily responsible for producing inequities, apart from other uncertainties and immeasurable factors" (p. xviii). In essence, the resulting task of eliminating health inequities becomes "a matter of social justice" (p. xviii). Attention to matters of social justice remains essential, as merely implementing "enhanced social services or other interventions aimed primarily at effects cannot eliminate the sources of health inequities" (p. xviii). As a consequence, it emerges as vitally important to rethink "how we might create health equity or at least overcome barriers to achieving it" (p. xviii). Toward this goal, it emerges as equally important "to identify the social determinants of health—social and economic conditions that improve community health; to examine the political implications of differing paradigms and perspectives used to explain health inequities; and to explore alternative strategies for eliminating health inequities" (p. xxi). Thus, an emphasis on social justice forces us to pay attention to the social context and the social determinants of health, leading to potential points of entry for their remedy, reduction, and elimination.

Kunitz (2007, p. 183) points out how understanding and predicting health is "much more likely to result from stitching together all that one can know about the context—institutional, cultural, political, epidemiological—in which particular populations live and work"; even if such a view is "disquieting for those who equate doing science with having a theory that makes possible accurate predictions" (p. 183); (also, see Walker, chapter 2). What is needed is an acceptance of how all "generalizations about the social determinants of health and disease begin in the lived reality of particular people and places" (Kunitz, 2007, p. 185). This may include the impact and legacy of injustice embodied in the social context. For example, Williams and Jackson (2005) emphasize the social sources of disparities in health, noting how factors in the social environment initiate and sustain racial disparities in health.

The link between inequity in health and social injustice has also been discussed in terms of the fundamental social basis of disparities in health. Diderichsen et al. (2001) elaborate on the relationship between the social context and how individuals are sorted into certain social positions, asserting this is central to the issue of social differentials in health. It emerges as crucial to articulate effective actions to redress health inequities; this is contingent on elucidating the pathways through which social context and position are linked to health outcomes, as well as being linked to the social consequences of disease. Diderichsen et al. (2001) identify four mechanisms they view as playing a role in generating inequities: factors affecting social stratification; differential exposure to health damaging factors; differential vulnerabilities/susceptibility that lead to unequal health outcomes; and differential consequences of illness.

In a similar vein, LaVeist (2005) discusses the role and function of social risk factors. LaVeist identifies variables such as "racism, sexism, socioeconomic status, social support, population density, housing quality, racial segregation, stress, or residence in a neighborhood with a high crime rate" as having all been "demonstrated to be associated with health" (p. 27). Within the model of LaVeist, also recognized as impacting health, illness behaviors, and overall health status is "the culture of an ethnic group" (p. 27). Also included in the model are societal factors impacting health, illness behavior, and health status, given how these "place constraints on an individual's ability to engage in health or illness behaviors that are protective of health" (p. 27). For example, societal factors may include how "race may lead to lower socioeconomic status, which may lead to underutilization of health services," even as "one might inaccurately ascribe such a finding to a person's race when it is really an effect of social class" (p. 27). The real danger that LaVeist's (2005) model seeks to correct is erroneous thinking that might "lead to the assumption that there is something about a person's skin color that makes the person engage in risky behavior" (p. 27). What is really at issue is the effects of a social category.

Edelman (2006) similarly notes how the current gaps in health "thrive in a climate of economic and social inequities," which includes an adverse impact on "the health of individuals and communities by denying individuals and groups the equal opportunity to meet their basic human needs" (p. vii). Levy and Sidel (2006b) also note how social injustice has a negative impact on both individuals and communities, while also constituting a violation of fundamental human rights. In order to substantiate this claim, Levy and Sidel (2006a, p. ix) compile the voices of many in their edited volume; they do so in order to offer a "comprehensive approach to understanding social injustice and its impact on public health," given how "social injustice underlies many public health problems throughout the world." Moreover, Levy and Sidel (2006b) note how the origin of social injustice is often rooted in how "those who control access to opportunities and resources block the poor, the powerless, and those otherwise deprived from gaining fair and equitable access" to vital opportunities and resources; meanwhile, "those in the upper class receive a disproportionate share" (p. 11). Allen and Easley (2006) assert that the equitable provision of health care is the "most important immediate action in response to social injustice against racial and ethnic minorities that leads to disparate health outcomes" (p. 63).

The new field of equity in health must incorporate the drive for social justice and acknowledgment of forces in the social context.

(11) The Drive to Protect and Support the Most Vulnerable

The drive to protect and support the most vulnerable is also at the core of the field of equity in health. The characteristics (e.g., the poor, powerless) of those who tend to experience social injustice emerge as meaningful and key.

According to Levy and Sidel (2006b, p. 6), the most vulnerable tend to be populations of groups "defined by racial or ethnic status, socioeconomic position, age, gender, sexual orientation, or other perceived population or group characteristics." Moreover, these groups tend to be negatively stereotyped and stigmatized, as well as "targets of hate and violence" (p. 6). Thus, groups with certain key characteristics emerge as among the most vulnerable to forces of domination, oppression and discrimination.

Those oppressed because of their race emerge as among the most vulnerable (see Constantine, Kindaichi, Graham, & Watkins, chapter 9; Franklin et al., chapter 11). Allen and Easley (2006, p. 62) emphasize the importance of addressing institutionalized racism such that institutionalized structures "no longer support racism."

House and Williams (2003) also analyze how racism affects disparities in health: the impact of racism in the larger society is such that it can lead to "systematic differences in exposure to personal experiences of discrimination" which "may be an important part of subjectively experiences stress that can adversely affect" physical and mental health for a broad range of racial/ethnic minority populations, as also reflected in self-reported measures of health (p. 107); racism and related systematic discrimination "can also affect the quantity and quality" of medical care and health services received (p. 107); "the prevalence of negative stereotypes and cultural images of stigmatized groups can adversely affect health status" (p. 107); "racism restricts and truncates socioeconomic attainment" (p. 106); the impact of economic discrimination produced by large-scale societal structures are reflected in racial differences in SES and poorer health; racial segregation and residential segregation create and reinforce racial inequality, and operate to determine access to educational and employment opportunities—which leads to "truncated socioeconomic mobility for blacks and American Indians" (p. 106); next, living in segregated neighborhoods "can lead to exposure to environmental toxins, poor-quality housing, and other pathogenic living conditions, including inadequate access to a broad range of services provided by municipal authorities" (p. 106); moreover, these living conditions "importantly account for the large racial difference in homicide," together with the "combination of concentrated poverty, male joblessness, and residential instability" that account for variation in violent crime levels (p. 106); research is also impacted, insofar as racism has an influence on SES indicators such that they are "not commensurate across racial groups, which makes it difficult to truly adjust racial differences in health for SES"; as a result, it is vital to recognize "racial differences in the quality of education, income returns for a given level of education or occupational status, wealth or assets associated with a given level of income, the purchasing power of income, the stability of employment, and the health risks associated with occupational status" (p. 107).

People with disabilities are another vulnerable group (see Keller & King, chapter 25). Thus, the most vulnerable are also sometimes referred to as special populations, possessing special needs, necessitating extra protection and support.

All working in public health should work to ensure that "disability issues are included in all phases of public health education and practice" (Groce, 2006, p. 158). Making an analogy to women, Groce recalls how 30 years ago there was little being done in public health with regard to women—beyond maternal and child health, while, today, the considerations of women are routine. Groce anticipates the day that such considerations people with disabilities will be just as routine. What must be transformed is the "denial of human rights to people with disabilities, their lack of equitable access to public health and social service resources, and their disproportionate rates of poverty"—which are all socially determined "threats to social justice" which can be "socially redefined" (p. 158).

Mutaner and Geiger-Brown (2006) also discuss how the LGBT population is another vulnerable group, being at risk for unjust treatment, given how they suffer from homophobia and heterosexualism (see Greene et al., chapter 23; Nanín et al., chapter 22; Rosario et al., chapter 24). Lombardi and Bettcher (2006) similarly discuss the impact of social injustice on the health of the LGBT population, given the stigmatization and marginalization that they face; they indicate a need for legislative and other policies explicitly prohibiting discrimination and violence against the LGBT population; and, the transgender/transsexual also need legislation and policies that legitimize their lives and identities, while covering practical matters such as changing legal documents, and access to affordable medical care for procedures related to their identity.

Another vulnerable population suffering great social injustice includes those who are incarcerated around the globe (see Bahl, chapter 20), and especially in the United States. Drucker (2006, p. 161) acknowledges how among those factors damaging community cohesion is mass incarceration, while also detailing the damage done to opportunities for "work, education, housing, and a stable family life, undermining many of the foundations of personal health and well-being." Contemporary U.S. incarceration policies and practices are appropriately likened to being "the modern heir to our long legacy of state mechanisms that perpetuate social and racial injustice" (p. 161). These include slavery, segregation, discriminatory immigration, trade union, and social welfare policies. Moreover, incarceration is likened to a plague because of the "striking economic, ethnic, and racial disparity in its application," disproportionately impacting African American males, in particular. And, the incarcerated population suffers from health disparities common to low-income populations (e.g., sexually transmitted diseases, viral hepatitis, HIV/AIDS), as well as from trauma and abuse while incarcerated.

The incarcerated emerge as more than worthy of protection and support (e.g., Mauer & Chesney-Lind, 2002; Restum, 2005). The over-representation of Black males in prisons suggests their vulnerability, in particular, within the socio-cultural-political context of the United States. This serves to justify early interventions that begin as early as possible, such as in elementary school, and focus upon the most at-risk, such those experiencing the largest gaps in academic achievement, lagging behind. In this regard, attempts to close the gaps in academic achievement are now increasingly focusing on Black males; these efforts include culturally tailored components and mentoring designed to meet the needs of Black males and reduce their risk for a range of negative outcomes—from special education placements, to school dropout, and incarceration (Hu, 2007). Interventions that effectively engage such at risk students show promise for closing the education gap between Whites and Blacks (see Ross & Smalls, chapter 26). Supplementary education (see Bridglall & Gordon, chapter 27) may target Black males, in particular, or utilize strategies that effectively this group in the learning process (see Campbell & Wallace, chapter 28). Other interventions that provide peer mentoring and tutoring may also benefit Black males more than any other group, consistent with how the needs of urban adolescent males at risk of school drop-out are also the most pronounced (see Chew & Wallace, chapter 29).

Global policies also create new vulnerable groups. Pertinent polices include those that lead to "war, violence, global warming, government corruption, lack of access to essential public health or medical services, erosion of civil liberties and freedoms, restriction of education/research/public discourse" as well as other "actions that adversely affect the societal conditions in which people can be healthy" (Drucker, 2006, p. 6). The resultant vulnerable groups who suffer the most include "the poor, the homeless, the ill or injured, the very young, and the very old" (p. 6).

Not to be forgotten are those displaced from their homes or homelands, those injured and maimed who end up disabled, refugees forced into camps, child soldiers who are traumatized, and victims of sexual violence/exploitation and rapes within the context of war. All emerge as especially vulnerable within the global social context.

A drive to support and protect the most vulnerable is essential to the field of equity in health.

(12) The Drive to Repair Damage, Restore Trust, and Take Responsibility

The drive to repair damage, restore trust, and take responsibility for what needs to be done in the aftermath of the damage done is also at the core of the field of equity in health. The damage done includes a host of negative consequences experienced by those subject to domination, oppression, and discrimination. Typically, it involves damage experienced most acutely by the most vulnerable populations.

For example, Levy and Sidel (2006b) point toward "adverse health consequences, as reflected in disparities in health status and access to health services within or between populations" (p. 7); there are also "increased rates of disease, injury, disability, and premature death because of increased risk factors and decreased medical care and preventive services," as well as "poverty, inadequate education, and inadequate health insurance" (p. 10); and, poorer nutrition, greater exposure to unsafe water, increased contact with infectious disease agents, more exposure to occupational and environmental hazards, higher rates of complications of chronic diseases, more use of alcohol/tobacco/drugs, decreased social support, and increased physiological and immunological vulnerability to disease. Furthermore, there is less access to comprehensive diagnostic, therapeutic, and rehabilitative services and lower quality of health. And, there is less access to clinical preventive services (i.e., screening and counseling) and to community-based preventive measures (p. 10).

Regarding repairing the damage done, House and Williams (2003) identify numerous avenues: "socioeconomic policy and practice and racial/ethnic policy and practice are the most significant levers for reducing socioeconomic and racial/ethnic disparities and hence improving overall population health in our society, more importantly even than health care policy" (p. 111). They also note how "intervening in or changing one or a few major risk factors for health (including inadequate medical care) can have only a limited effect on socioeconomic and racial/ethnic disparities in health" (p. 122). However, they also indicate that this "effect is clearly enhanced if interventions or changes are attentive to the broader social forces that produce these disparities" (p. 122). Most important among the avenues for repair of the damage done there is the "potential for reducing socioeconomic and racial/ethnic disparities in health and improving overall population health" by improving socioeconomic status and "reducing invidious racial/ethnic distinctions themselves, especially among the more disadvantaged portions of the population" (p. 122). Thus, both "economic growth and development and progress toward greater racial/ethnic equality have had and can have dramatic effects on individual and population health" (p. 122). This is the case, "especially if these changes impact the more disadvantaged socioeconomic and racial/ethnic groups in our society" (p. 122).

Other avenues for repairing the damage done emerge through the work of LaVeist (2005, p. 285) who presents a model similar to that of Benzeval, Judge and Whitehead (1995), who presented a four-level framework for addressing health disparities: (1) improving the physical environment; (2) addressing social and economic conditions; (3) improving access to appropriate and effective health and social services; and, (4) reducing barriers to adopting healthy lifestyles. Hence, these are all avenues for repairing damage done.

There is also a need to restore trust, given the damage done (see Constantine et al., chapter 9; Franklin et al., chapter 11). In this regard, the research of LaVeist (2005) locates lower rates of health care use in issues of level of trust of health care institutions. For example, citing the research of van Ryn and Burke (2002), African Americans endorsed at twice the rate of Whites items indicating that hospitals often seek more personal information than needed, and that "hospitals have sometimes done harmful experiments on patients without their knowledge" (LaVeist, 2005, p. 117). Also, nearly three times as many African Americans perceived, when compared to Whites, that racial discrimination in a doctor's office is common (p. 117). Meanwhile, other evidence reveals good reasons for distrust, given how physicians "consistently reported more negative attitudes toward African American patients than toward White patients" (p. 120). More specifically, this included perceptions that African Americans were more likely to abuse alcohol or drugs, be noncompliant with medications, while Whites were perceived as more likely to strongly desire a physically active lifestyle, had adequate social support; and, White patients were more likely to be the "kind of person" the physician could see being friends with (p. 120). Other negative perceptions of African Americans held by physicians included being less likely to see them as very intelligent, or at least somewhat educated; meanwhile, Whites were more likely to be viewed as very pleasant and very rational.

Others take a historical view in locating the roots of distrust. Randall (2006) locates the destruction of trust in the medical and health care system, as well as in medical personnel and researchers within the long history of medical experimentation in the United States on Blacks, prisoners, and members of the armed forces in America. As a consequence, Randall (2006, p. 124) asserts that such episodes of abuse are stored within the collective Black consciousness. The result is a deep-seated distrust that currently influences Blacks' attitudes toward the health care system, contributing to disparities in health.

In the same vein, Washington (2007) details the practice of "medical apartheid" in the United States, meaning the history of medical experimentation on Blacks, dating back to colonial times and the abuse of enslaved African Americans; it continues up to the present via forced experimentation on prison inmates and soldiers in the armed forces, and the erosion of informed consent so experimental procedures are used in emergency rooms on non-consenting victims—many of whom end up dead. The result is not only a lack of trust, but even a deep seated fear "of medical professionals and institutions"— something Washington (p. 21) calls iatrophobia, being "coined from the Greek words *iatros* ("healer") and *phobia* ("fear"). Black iatrophobia is the fear of medicine" (p. 21).

Damage has been done, and trust destroyed through a more modern legacy of research with mostly African Americans, and some Hispanics that Washington (2007, p. 5) details: suspended research "at such revered universities as Alabama, Pennsylvania, Duke, Yale, and even Johns Hopkins"; and, "experimentation-related deaths at premier universities, from Columbia to California," and revelations of researchers lying through "falsified data or fictitious research agendas" involving scientists from "the University of South Carolina to MIT."

One theme running throughout Washington's (2007) analysis is that, while African Americans have either been specifically selected and targeted or suffered disproportionately because of their presence in prisons, the armed services, or urban emergency rooms, all of America has suffered and paid a high price, especially White middle class Americans paying for the health cost burden, creating an American tragedy. However, Washington's analysis goes beyond the borders of the United States to how Western researchers turn to the Third World or developing countries, and Africa in particular, and engage in unacceptable ethical practices that would not be allowed by Institutional Review Boards (IRBs) if the subjects were here in the United States. "American IRBs treat Africans as second-class subjects and employ different standards for evaluating study designs in Africa than those used in the United States (Washington, p. 394). Thus, there is a resultant global damage, including a profound distrust.

Avenues for rebuilding trust and repairing the damage done is also described by Washington (2007, p. 396). Despite the legacy of abuse, African Americans are strongly advised to "embrace new medical research—after judicious inquiries of their own into any study they are considering;" this is recommended, even as "there are still issues that must be addressed," requiring that they "embrace medical research warily" until these issues are "rectified" (p. 396). In particular, there is a vital need for "more and better research into black health care" (p. 399). There is also a need to do the following: ban the erosion of consent, specifically a ban on exceptions to informed consent, such that physicians face an imperative to treat patients as if the physician had no research protocol "to worry about"; this will leave physicians in a position where they must use the best-known treatment, not the one offered via a research protocol (p. 403); institute a coordinated system of mandatory subject education, covering the "ethical and practice conduct of biomedical research," just as the National Institutes of Health and Office of Research Integrity require of every practicing medical researcher (p. 403); embrace a single standard of research ethics, ending the practice of championing "human rights in medical research" in the United States, but ignoring them abroad, while following "informed-consent strictures abroad that are as restrictive as those governing their research on American shores;" also, the "federal government should take advantage of its legal right either to force manufacturers to lower their prices [of lifesaving drugs] or to suspend patent enforcement" in poor countries (p. 403).

Offering yet other avenues for repair of the damage done, Washington (2007, p. 403) offers a vision of medical-research education. Within her vision, accessible lay education on medical research and assistance navigating clinical trials via "brochures, Web sites, and access to experts" is made readily available. There is also a role in this work for "church health fairs, social organizations, and community activism" (p. 403). This includes community members working to "bring medical-research education to the fore of the American health agenda," as well as joining Institutional Review Boards and asking "the hard questions of physicians who are recruiting in your community, and to join appropriate clinical trials once you have satisfied yourself that they are worthwhile and relatively safe" (p. 403).

These recommendations begin to suggest how the taking of responsibility is also being advanced by Washington (2007)—even among those who were historically the most vulnerable and suffered the most damage. Further suggestive of what is involved in rebuilding trust and taking greater responsibility, African Americans are challenged to "effect a transformation of our attitudes toward medical research," demanding "our place at the table to enjoy the rich bounty of the American medical system in the form of longer, healthier lives" (p. 403).

Others acknowledge the loss of trust, regardless of race, across America, and view the rebuilding of trust as a vital task, while also offering viable solutions. Shore (2007a), as Founding Director of the Trust Initiative at the Harvard School of Public Health, asserts that there is a lack of trust in health care (Shore, 2007b). The edited volumes goes on to discuss in detail both causes and consequence of declining trust in health care. In his opening chapter, Shore (2007b, p. 3) explains how trust "in the professionals and institutions that provide healthcare in America has been eroding over time," being at "an all-time low." Consequences include endangering "patients' lives and well-being," while stripping the health care system of what is vital to a "well-functioning system" (p. 3).

Whether the patient who takes a medication (that would be toxic if taken in large quantities), or the patient stripped naked and knocked unconscious for surgery, trust is essential (Shore, 2007b). Specifically, "trust entails two distinct but equally important elements. If I am to trust you, I must believe that you are competent to do what needs to be done," having requisite skills and resources "to do what you say you will do, and that your actions are likely to help me rather than to hurt me" (p. 4). Second, "I also must believe that you have my best interests at heart and that your judgment and actions are not compromised by a financial (or any other) motive that would put me at risk" (p. 4). Most importantly, the lack of trust may mean that patients "don't do what they are supposed to do and they don't tell their caregivers the truth about what they actually do" (p. 4).

Shore (2007b) explores what steps might be taken by providers and the health care organizations in the process of rebuilding trust. First they would have to address service quality, having to establish and monitor high levels of quality, and provide consistent high quality—just like a "power brand" (pp. 14–15); this includes everything from a friendly receptionist to a clean environment, to the physician's manner, to how billing is handled.

Secondly, "trust-seeking organizations must be learning organizations. They must learn from experience what builds trust and what destroys it"—such as rigid gatekeeping, or responses to crisis (e.g., the cover-up) (p. 15). In health care, a third factor is cultivating brand identity with the hospital corporation needing a brand "that means something to people," since "perception is reality," justifying "using all the tools and techniques of branding to build a power brand" (p. 16).

Blendon (2007) discusses how the dynamics of declining trust in health care "correspond very closely to the dynamics of declining trust in government"—citing three kinds of scandal: (1) the medical error where a "doctor or a hospital makes a mistake, and a patient dies"; (2) the impaired physician, whether by drugs, alcohol, or mental illness—doing "terrible things to patients"; and, (3) the "doctor or hospital found to be billing insurance companies or Medicare, fattening his or her own purse at the expense of premium payers or taxpayers" (p. 24).

Blendon (2007) explains that getting trust "back is not magic. It involves leadership that does not ignore problems, that reacts firmly and ethically to scandals the minute they break and does not try to cover them up, and that understands how the consequences of seemingly small decisions can loom large" (p. 30). Leaders need to take the "long view" and "take the steps necessary to build trust" (p. 31).

In concluding his analysis, Shore (2007b) asserts that health care is at a "tipping point" that is hoped to be a "turning point." Shore (p. 16) asserts how everybody "has an interest in building trust: patients, clinicians, organizations, government," while all will also benefit from increasing levels of trust. Most importantly, the problem "is being named and analyzed, and solutions are being offered. Providers and healthcare organizations can pick these up and run with them" (p. 16).

Levy and Sidel's (2006b) view of what needs to be done further suggests how we have reached a tipping point or turning point. Also, striking a hopeful note, they observe how humanity has entered an era, perhaps "for the first time," wherein we actually possess the requisite "technical capacity and the human and economic resources to address poverty, ill health, human rights violations, and the social injustice that helps spawn and promote these problems" (p. 13). Thus, if we take responsibility, we can restore trust and work to repair the damage done.

Although humanity now possesses "the way" to solve these problems, the "will" to do so is not a universal trait. Instead, those enjoying privilege may resist sharing their greater proportion of resources. In such cases, Levy and Sidel (2006b) see a role for "social or legal action for their prevention or correction" (p. 13). Even this requires the taking of personal responsibility by individuals and communities.

Elder (2001) also describes a new public health era—one in which societies and individuals have to take responsibility for health, rather than waiting for changes to be made for them. Also, suggesting the taking of responsibility, Washington (2007, p. 403) concludes by asserting that above and beyond all of her recommendations, most important "is the need for African Americans to set their own research agendas—as an ultimate avenue for taking responsibility." This taking of responsibility is consistent with a final charge to "change," given how survival goes to "the one most responsive to change"—with Washington (pp. 403–404) quoting Charles Darwin to underscore this point.

In this manner, there is a drive to repair damage, restore trust, and take responsibility—as a core and essential guiding principle for the field of equity in health.

(13) The Drive to Redistribute Wealth and Access to Opportunity

Finally, there is a drive to redistribute wealth and access to opportunity, as a guiding principle for the field of equity in health. In this regard, Kubzansky et al. (2001) underscore how the United States has the dubious distinction of ranking first among industrialized nations in inequalities in both income and wealth. There is a growing trend of growing socioeconomic inequalities in the United States that have widened considerably over the past two decades. There is a robust effect of income on health; it is evident in all age, racial/ethnic, gender, and income groups; moreover, it persists across two different markers of health status—premature mortality and disability. Those with less income— when compared to their counterparts with more income—consistently live more disabled and less healthy lives, while also dying at younger ages (Kubzansky et al., 2001, p. 116). Kubzansky et al. thereby underscore "both the relative unfairness and the burden of poor health in the United States" (p. 119). They view this type of documentation of "contingent inequalities in health" as being of the utmost importance, as it may lead to action to "reduce these inequalities and improve health equity" (p. 120)

In a similar vein, Kawachi, Daniels, and Robinson (2005) identify historical, political, and ideological obstacles that have prevailed in blocking adequate analyses of race and class as codeterminants of disparities in health. What they perceive as needed is a whole new second front and new approach to the elimination of health disparities by addressing class, in addition to race (Kawachi et al., p. 350). First, they reject an approach based in pseudo-science—one that views racial disparities in health as linked to innate biological inherited differences in susceptibility to disease—such as notions that Blacks were inferior and only suited to be slaves, justifying slavery; in rejecting this approach they advise others to consider how much skepticism is warranted with regarding to "pinning our hopes on the biological account of disparities in health" (p. 343). Secondly, they view the practice of viewing race as a proxy for class as unwarranted; it is race that influences class, and not vice versa. They support a third approach, a model that accounts for the "independent and interactive effects of both class and race" in producing disparities in health (p. 346). And, racial disparities in health should not be analyzed without simultaneously considering the contribution of class disparities. Meanwhile, the information infrastructure necessary to measure and monitor both race and class is currently lacking in the United States. Hence, they recommend health equity impact statements, following the British model, which could influence policy initiatives. This same call for a focus on race as a social construct and social class is also put forth in this volume (see David & Collins, chapter 10).

There is also a need to link efforts to address the "injuries of race and class simultaneously" (Kawachi et al., 2005, p. 351). We may also have to face certain consequences. For, political "struggle is unavoidable, and the contest involves questions of equity and reallocation, if not redistribution, of vital resources. So there are formidable obstacles to making class inequalities in health a focus of policy reform" (pp. 349–350). Nonetheless, Kawachi et al. (p. 350) hold fast to their assertion that "major progress against either form of health inequalities (by race or class) requires linking efforts to address them, not separating such efforts." They even explain the possible motivations in keeping the focus on race, while eliminating class. For example, a function of racism in the United States is to "divide people with common class interests so that they are less able to struggle politically in their common interest" (p. 347). There is also an attempt "to make race a highly visible feature of public policy while hiding or disguising anything that resembles class" (p. 347). Indeed, there is "a long-standing ideological effort to suppress any consciousness of class" (Kawaichi et al., p. 347).

A corresponding pattern of elevating whiteness and negatively stereotyping blackness in the United States has weakened support for "more redistributive policies," historically undermining class solidarity (Kawaichi et al., p. 348). In sum, poor Whites and Blacks end up divided so they "fail to see their common interests" (p. 349), such as the benefits of a policy of wealth redistribution in the United States. A focus on racial inequalities allows them to be discussed as a "violation of basic human rights" as well as being seen within a "moral and legal framework of equal opportunity that many associate with U.S. culture;" this makes it "easy to point to racial disparities as unjust because the only explanation for them is unjust social policy" (p. 349). Different challenges emerge when it comes to class. For, "class inequalities either are not seen or understood, or are obscured by rationales that provide some apparent justification for them" (p. 349).

Braveman (2006) acknowledges disputes about the extent to which a given condition could be influenced by policies. "For example, some people might argue that it is impossible to enact policies in the United States that redistribute resources in favor of less advantaged groups, given this country's deep-rooted ethos regarding individual responsibility and entrepreneurship" (p. 182). There is also recognition of a "relative lack of tradition of social solidarity in the United States" (p. 182).

Regardless, more and more contemporary data analyses lead to the conclusion that a response to health disparities needs to include policies that redistribute income, such as via equal access to educational or employment opportunities (see Lahiri & Pulungan, chapter 6). Such data analyses include explicit suggestions that even more studies need to link health outcomes to explicit social, economic and political processes; moreover, there is hope that social class unity—across racial lines—could develop over time, making possible deep political change (see David & Collins, chapter 10).

In this regard, there are even guiding ethical principles for policies of wealth redistribution or equalization of access to opportunity. For example, the following: a concept of "distributive justice," meaning "the equitable allocation of resources in a society;" a guiding value wherein "the most disadvantaged in a society" have their needs attended to; and, the "egalitarian distribution of resources for the essentials of life (such as health) could be justified" (Braveman, 2006, p. 183).

In this manner, there is a drive to redistribute wealth and access to opportunity that is also at the core of the field of equity in health.

Conclusion

The thirteen guiding principles embodied as driving forces within the field of equity in health, as discussed in this introductory chapter, provide hope for a future global transformation in health, given how we are now in a new era. Since health disparities have been declared the civil rights issue of the twenty-first century, the global movement being driven by these thirteen contemporary forces constitutes a necessary response. The global transformation in health being sought requires the training and preparation of global leaders within this movement. This volume seeks to be a milestone, in both launching the field of equity in health and seeking to prepare such global leaders. In effect, this introductory chapter has underscored the validity of seeking to change the discourse in the United States within a major paradigm shift so we now speak of and focus upon the manifestation of equity in health as a new global approach to health disparities.

This introductory chapter has also begun to identify and weed out those destructive forces that must be removed in order to make way for new growth within a new field of equity in health. What should grow and come forth includes everything from new theories, new perspectives, new modes of research, new procedures, new policies, to entire new models of medical care and public health. It even requires new personal identities among those working on issues of health.

The remainder of this volume serves as a clearing in which the new field of equity in health may be further established. Each chapter suggests the parameters of the new field, including the kinds of new theories, perspectives, research, procedures, policies, and models evolving within the field of equity in health. The paradigm in which this field is rooted demands that a non-hierarchical equality guide us in all that we do, providing the hope that we are entering a new era, indeed.

REFERENCES

Airhihenbuwa, C. O. (2006). 2007 SOPHE presidential address: On being comfortable with being uncomfortable: Centering an Africanist vision in our gateway to global health. *Health Education and Behavior, 34*, 31–42. Retrieved December 15, 2006, from http://heb.sagepub.com/cgi/content/abstract/34/1/31

Airhihenbuwa, C. O. (2007). *Healing our differences: The global crisis of health and politics of identity.* Lanham, MD: Rowman & Littlefield.

Allen, C. E., & Easley, C. W. (2006). Racial and ethnic minorities. In B. S. Levy & V. W. Sidel (Eds.), *Social injustice and public health.* New York: Oxford University Press.

Ayeboafo, N. K. (2005). *Tigare speaks: Lessons for living in harmony.* Philadelphia: StarSpirit Press.

Bambas, A., & Casas, J. A. (2003). Accessing equity in health: Conceptual criteria. In R. Hofrichter (Ed.), *Health and social justice: Politics, ideology, and inequity in the distribution of disease.* San Francisco: Jossey-Bass.

Benzeval, M., Judge, K., & Whitehead, M. (1995). *Tackling inequalities in health.* London: King's Fund.

Betancourt, J. R., Green, A. R., Carrillo, J. R., & Park, E. R. (2005). Cultural competence and health care disparities: Key perspective and trends. *Health Affairs, 24*(2), 499–505.

Blendon, R. J. (2007). Why Americans don't trust the government and don't trust healthcare. In D. A. Shore (Ed.), *The trust crisis in healthcare: Causes, consequences, and cures.* New York: Oxford University Press.

Braveman, P. (2006). Health disparities and health equity: Concepts and measurement. *Annual Review of Public Health, 27*, 167–194.

Brownson, R. C., Baker, E. A., Leet, T. L., & Gillespie, K. N. (Eds.). (2003). *Evidence-based public health.* New York: Oxford University Press.

Carr-Chellman, A. A. (2006). *Global perspectives on e-learning: Rhetoric and reality.* Thousand Oaks, CA: Sage Publications.

Carter, R. T. (Ed.). (2005). *Handbook of racial-cultural psychology and counseling: Training and practice,* Vol. 2. New York: John Wiley & Sons.

Chen, L. C., & Berlinger, G. (2001). Health equity in a globalizing world. In T. Evans, M. Whitehead, F. Diderichsen, A. Bhuiya, & M. Wirth (Eds.), *Challenging inequities in health: From ethics to action* (pp. 34–47). New York: Oxford University Press.

Comas-Diaz, L., Lykes, M. B., & Alarcon, R. D. (1998). Ethnic conflict and the psychology of liberation in Guatemala, Peru, and Puerto Rico. *American Psychologist, 53*(7), 778–792.

Constantine, M. G., & Sue, D. W. (Eds.). (2005). *Strategies for building multicultural competence in mental health and educational settings*. New York: John Wiley & Sons.

Constantine, M. G., & Sue, D. W. (Eds.). (2006). *Addressing racism: Facilitating cultural competence in mental health and educational settings*. New York: John Wiley & Sons.

Diderichsen, F., Evans, T., & Whitehead, M. (2001). The social basis of disparities in health. In T. Evans, M. Whitehead, F. Diderichsen, A. Bhuiya, & M. Wirth (Eds.), *Challenging inequities in health: From ethics to action*. New York: Oxford University Press.

Drucker, E. M. (2006). Incarcerated people. In B. S. Levy & V. W. Sidel (Eds.), *Social injustice and public health*. New York: Oxford University Press.

Du Bois, W. E. B. (1899/1996). *The Philadelphia Negro, a social study*. Philadelphia: University of Pennsylvania Press.

Edelman, M. W. (2006). Foreword. In B. S. Levy & V. W. Sidel (Eds.), *Social injustice and public health*. New York: Oxford University Press.

Elder, J. P. (2001). *Behavior change and public health in the developing world*. Thousand Oaks, CA: Sage Publications.

Fielding, J. (2003). Preface. In R. C. Brownson, W. A. Baker, T. L. Leet, & K. N. Gillespie (Eds.). *Evidence-based public health*. New York: Oxford University Press.

Groce, N. E. (2006). People with disabilities. In B. S. Levy & V. W. Sidel (Eds.), *Social injustice and public health*. New York: Oxford University Press.

Hester, R. K., & Miller, W. R. (Eds.). (2003). *Handbook of alcoholism treatment approaches: Effective alternatives* (3rd ed.). Boston: Allyn and Bacon.

Hofrichter, R. (Ed.). (2006). *Health and social justice: Politics, ideology, and inequity in the distribution of disease*. San Francisco: Jossey-Bass.

House, J. S., & Williams, D. R. (2003). Understanding and reducing socioeconomic and racial/ethnic disparities in health. In R. Hofrichter (Ed.), *Health and social justice: Politics, ideology, and inequity in the distribution of disease*. San Francisco: Jossey-Bass.

Hu, W. (2007, April 9). To close gaps, schools focus on black boys. *The New York Times*, pp. A1, B5.

Institute of Medicine (IOM). (2001). *Crossing the quality chasm: A new health system for the 21st century*. Washington, DC: National Academies Press.

Kawachi, I., Daniels, N., & Robinson, D. E. (2005). Health disparities by race and class: Why both matter. *Health Affairs, 24*(2), 343–352.

Kawachi, I., & Wamala, S. (Eds.). (2007a). *Globalization and health*. New York: Oxford University Press.

Kawachi, I., & Wamala, S. (2007b). Globalization and health: Challenges and prospects. In I. Kawachi & S. Wamala (Eds.), *Globalization and health*. New York: Oxford University Press.

Kubzansky, L. D., Krieger, N., Kawachi, I., Rockhill, B., Steel, G. K., & Berkman, L. F. (2001). United States: Social inequality and the burden of poor health. In T. Evans, M. Whitehead, F. Diderichsen, A. Bhuiya, & M. Wirth (Eds.), *Challenging inequities in health: From ethics to action*. New York: Oxford University Press.

Kunitz, S. J. (2007). *The health of populations: General theories and particular realities*. New York: Oxford University Press.

LaVeist, T. A. (2005). *Minority populations and health: An introduction to health disparities in the United States*. San Francisco: Jossey-Bass.

Levine, R. S., Foster, J. E., Fullilove, R. E., Fullilove, M. T., Briggs, N. C., Hull, P. C., et al. (2001). Black-white inequalities in mortality and life expectancy, 1933–1999: Implications for Healthy People 2010. *Public Health Reports, 116*, 474–483.

Levy, B. S., & Sidel, V. W. (Eds.). (2006a). *Social injustice and public health*. New York: Oxford University Press.

Levy, B. S., & Sidel, V. W. (2006b). The nature of social injustice and its impact on public health. In B. S. Levy & V. W. Sidel (Eds.), *Social injustice and public health*. New York: Oxford University Press.

Lombardi, E., & Bettcher, T. (2006). Lesbian, gay, bisexual, and transgender/transsexual individuals. In B. S. Levy & V. W. Sidel (Eds.), *Social injustice and public health*. New York: Oxford University Press.

Mauer, M., & Chesney-Lind, M. (Eds.). (2002). *Invisible punishment: The collateral consequences of mass imprisonment*. New York: The New Press.

Merson, M. H., Black, R. E., & Mills, A. J. (Eds.). (2006). *International public health: Disease, programs, systems, and policies* (2nd ed.). Boston: Jones and Bartlett Publishers.

Miller, W. R., & Rollnick, S. (Eds.). (1991). *Motivational interviewing: Preparing people to change addictive behaviors* (1st ed.). New York: Guilford.

Miller, W. R., & Rollnick, S. (Eds.). (2002). *Motivational interviewing: Preparing people for change* (2nd ed.). New York: Guilford.

Mutaner, C., & Geiger-Brown, J. (2006). Mental health. In B. S. Levy & V. W. Sidel (Eds.), *Social injustice and public health*. New York: Oxford University Press.

Nairn, R., Pega, F., McCreanor, T., Rankine, J., & Barnes, A. (2006). Media, racism, and public health psychology. *Journal of Health Psychology, 11*(2), 183–196.

Núñez, A., & Robertson, C. (2006). Cultural competency. In D. Satcher & R. J. Pamies (Eds.), *Multicultural medicine and health disparities*. New York: McGraw-Hill.

Pedersen, P. (2006). Five antiracism strategies. In M. G. Constantine & D. W. Sue (Eds.), *Addressing racism: Facilitating cultural competence in mental health and educational settings*. New York: John Wiley & Sons.

Pedersen, P. B., Draguns, J. G., Conner, W. S., & Trimble, J. E. (2002). *Counseling across cultures* (5th ed.). Thousand Oaks, CA: Sage Publications.

Peter, F., & Evans, T. (2001). Ethical dimensions of health equity. In T. Evans, M. Whitehead, F. Diderichsen, A. Bhuiya, & M. Wirth (Eds.), *Challenging inequities in health: From ethics to action* (pp. 24–33). New York: Oxford University Press.

Prochaska, J. O., & DiClemente, C. C. (1983). Stages and processes of self-change of cigarette smoking: Toward an integrative model of change. *Journal of Consulting and Clinical Psychology, 51*, 390–395.

Prochaska, J. O., & DiClemente, C. C. (1992). Stages of change in the modification of problem behaviors. *Progress in Behavior Modification, 28*, 183–218.

Randall, V. R. (2006). *Dying while Black: An in-depth look at the crisis in the American healthcare system*. Dayton, OH: Seven Principles Press, Inc.

Restum, Z. G. (2005). Public health implications of substandard correctional care. *American Journal of Public Health, 95*(10), 1689–1691.

Sammons, M. T. (2001). Combined treatments for mental disorders: Clinical dilemmas. In M. T. Sammons & N. B. Schmidt (Eds.), *Combined treatments for mental disorders: A guide to psychological and pharmacological interventions* (pp. 11–32). Washington, DC: American Psychological Association.

Satcher, D. (2006). The role of government in minority health: A surgeon general's perspective. In D. Satcher & R. J. Pamies (Eds.), *Multicultural medicine and health disparities*. New York: McGraw-Hill.

Satcher, D., & Pamies, R. J. (2006). Preface. In D. Satcher & R. J. Pamies, (Eds.), *Multicultural medicine and health disparities*. New York: McGraw-Hill.

Shore, D. A. (Ed.). (2007a). *The trust crisis in healthcare: Causes, consequences, and cures*. New York: Oxford University Press.

Shore, D. A. (2007b). The (sorry) state of trust in the American healthcare enterprise. In D. A. Shore (Ed.), *The trust crisis in healthcare: Causes, consequences, and cures*. New York: Oxford University Press.

Sue, D. W. (2003). *Overcoming our racism: The journey to liberation*. New York: John Wiley & Sons.

Sue, D. W., & Sue, D. (2003). *Counseling the culturally diverse* (4th ed.). New York: John Wiley & Sons.

Sue, D. W., & Torino, G. C. (2005). Racial-cultural competence: Awareness, knowledge, and skills. In R. T. Carter (Ed.), *Handbook of racial-cultural psychology and counseling*, Vol. II (pp. 3–18). New York: John Wiley & Sons.

Taylor, C. (1994). The politics of recognition. In A. Gutman (Ed.), *Multiculturalism: Examining the politics of recognition*. Princeton, NJ: Princeton University Press.

van Ryn, M., & Burke, J. (2002). The effect of patient race and socioeconomic status on physicians' perceptions of patients. In T. A. LaVeist (Ed.). *Race, ethnicity, and health: A public health reader*. San Francisco: Jossey-Bass.

Vera, E. M., Buhin, L., & Shin, R. Q. (2006). The pursuit of social justice and the elimination of racism. In M. G. Constantine & D. W. Sue (Eds.), *Addressing racism: Facilitating cultural competence in mental health and educational settings*. New York: John Wiley & Sons.

Wallace, B. C. (1996). *Adult children of dysfunctional families: Prevention, intervention, and treatment for community mental health promotion*. Westport, CT: Praeger.

Wallace, B. C. (2000). A call for change in multicultural training at graduate schools of education: Educating to end oppression and for social justice. *Teachers College Record, 102*(6), 1086–1111.

Wallace, B. C. (2003). A multicultural approach to violence: Toward a psychology of oppression, liberation, and identity development. In B. C. Wallace & R. T. Carter (Eds.), *Understanding and dealing with violence: A multicultural approach* (pp. 3–39). Thousand Oaks, CA: Sage Publications.

Wallace, B. C. (2005a). A practical coping skills approach for racial-cultural training. In R. T. Carter (Ed.), *Handbook of racial-cultural psychology and counseling*, Vol. II. (pp. 97–119). New York: John Wiley & Sons.

Wallace, B. C. (2005b). *Making mandated addiction treatment work*. Lanham, MD: Jason Aronson/Rowman & Littlefield.

Wallace, B. C., Carter, R. T., Nanín, J. E., Keller, R., & Alleyne, V. (2003). Identity development for "diverse and different others": Integrating stages of change, motivational interviewing, and identity theories for race, people of color, sexual orientation, and disability. In B. C. Wallace & R. T. Carter (Eds.), *Understanding and dealing with violence: A multicultural approach* (pp. 41–91). Thousand Oaks, CA: Sage Publications.

Washington, H. A. (2007). *Medical apartheid: The dark history of medical experimentation on black Americans from colonial times*. New York: Random House.

Williams, D., & Jackson, P. B. (2005). Social sources of disparities in health. *Health Affairs*, 24(2), 325–334.

Zarcadoolas, C., Pleasant, A. F., & Greer, D. S. (2006). *Advancing health literacy: A framework for understanding and action*. San Francisco: Jossey-Bass.

1

New Theory, Paradigms, and Perspectives

Challenges in Eliminating Health Disparities

2

Bailus Walker, Jr.

Introduction

The U.S. Department of Health and Human Services (HHS) (HHS, 1985) Secretary's Task Force report on Black and Minority Health landed in 1985 with force. It was a landmark document with regards to minority health. The report was distinctive from a previous report in that it focused on all four minority groups in the United States as well as the White population, a perspective congruent with the increasing racial and ethnic diversity of the United States. The report also used the somewhat more dramatic statistical presentation of "excess deaths" rather than the usual comparison of death rates, bringing home the message that lives that were lost would not have been lost had minority death rates been the same as for the White population. The sheer weight of the report (approximately 3,000 pages), as well as its thoughtful analysis of the various causes of death, established a new high-water mark for academic rigor brought to bear on minority health issues. The report introduced more forcefully than ever the issue of health promotion/disease prevention into strategies about the health of these populations and as a result of the report, the Office of Minority Health was established within HHS, to advocate for and oversee the implementation of the report's recommendations (HHS, 1985).

Since the publication of the secretary's report, some progress has been made in focusing prevention efforts more tightly on the poor and minority populations. Keeping the issue high on the public health agenda, *Healthy People 2010*, the nation's policy on health promotion and disease prevention, includes as a goal the elimination of health disparities among different segments of the populations and illuminated ways in which health disparities can occur among various demographic groups in the United States. Numerous organizations and agencies continue to explore ways to reduce health status disparities, testing hypotheses, and experimenting with various health services constructs. Despite this progress, serious racial and ethnic health disparities exist, as report after report document that diseases do not affect the population equally. Moreover, the remaining problems are highly complex, and pose significant challenges for society as a whole, the focus of this review (HHS, 1998).

Challenges

In 1985, the Secretary's Task Force report identified a number of important categories of diseases that caused the overwhelming majority of excess death in minority populations: cancer, cardiovascular disease, chemical dependency (measured by death due to cirrhosis and liver disease), diabetes, infant mortality, and violence. Describing the situation in 2005, Zerhouni (Director of the National Institutes of Health) observes that despite signs of tremendous medical progress, minority racial and ethnic groups continue to experience an unequal burden of serious illnesses, premature death, and disability in the United States (Zerhouni, 2005).

The context of this continuation, which cannot be ignored, is somewhat different in complexity than it was when in 1985 the task force report was the centerpiece of public health discussion. For instance, communities today are undergoing profound transformations. Their contours can only be dimly perceived and their driving forces barely understood. The momentous consequences of these changes can hardly be imagined, although they may affect trends in health status disparities. In this context, it is evident that the landscape for eliminating health status disparities is changing as well. The dimensions of this change include increased population diversity, growth and shifts, vexing issues of poverty and its ramifications, globalism, energy, endocrine disruptors, pandemic disease, eco-affluence, anarchic violence, terrorism, and environmental ruin.

The demographics issues have attracted considerable debate as the population was expected to hit 300 million in 2006. Demographers and economists are talking about the impact of this swell in the U.S. population. They predict crowded cities and highways, new stresses on natural resources, and a widening gulf between society's haves and have-nots. As the population bounds toward 400 million, spurred by immigration, the United States faces yawning income and educational gaps, with more people who are poor and with limited access to health care. This may exacerbate efforts aimed at eliminating health status disparities (Kronholz, 2006; U.S. Census Bureau, 2005).

Also on the list are the long-standing social and economic problems associated with exposure to cigarette smoke, which have not been eradicated. This assertion is not to blur the important role played by media campaigns and community interventions in reducing smoking in the general population. But few public health specialists will dispute the current magnitude of this problem. The World Health Organization (WHO) estimates that 10 million people will be dying annually from cigarettes by the year 2020—a third of these in China. Cigarettes, which claimed about 100 million lives in the twentieth century, may well claim close to a billion in the present century (WHO, 2005).

Complex Diseases

The illnesses that make up the burden described by Zerhouni (2005) are "complex" or "multifactorial diseases," meaning that they cannot be ascribed to mutations in a single gene or to a single environmental factor. Rather they arise from combined actions of many genes, environmental risk factors, including socioeconomic factors and risk-conferring behaviors. Thus, efforts to address health status disparities are confronted with the challenge of sorting out how these factors interact and translating that information into effective strategies for disease prevention, diagnosis, and therapy (Merikangas & Risch, 2003).

Already, there is a great deal of research attention focused on the highly complex and poorly understood interaction between environmental exposure and genetic predisposition that appears to contribute to the onset of some diseases. But determining the interactions between genes and the environment during any disease process is a daunting task. At the same time evidence abounds that environmental factors contribute to disease, disability, and premature death in modern American society (National Institute of Environmental Health Sciences, 1999). The weight of evidence makes clear that unless environmental components of disease are considered, a complete epidemiology, or accurate diagnosis, cannot be achieved. Also, epidemiological and experimental studies repeatedly confirm that a genetic aberration may be necessary for a disease to occur, but the disease would not be manifested without an environmental risk factor. On another level, a complex convergence of multiple social, economic and political developments—our understanding of which is influenced by a broader acceptance of the global nature of environmental threats—has brought into stark relief environmental exposure that shapes persistent racial disparities in health outcomes. Although the full nature and extent of the health burden resulting from environmental exposure is not fully understood, it is evident that the environmental contribution to complex disease is significant (McMichael, Kjellstrom, & Smith, 2006). To be sure, numerous analyses have described disorders for which environmental exposure is a prerequisite, including cervical cancer and Type 1 diabetes. In this context the malleability of environmental risk factors is a particularly important consideration in determining priorities for public health and preventive medicine programs and services to eliminate health status disparities. Fixed factors, such as gender, birth cohort, and ethnicity may be important in characterizing risk, but cannot serve as the target of prevention.

Equally important in addressing the issues of health status disparities are the increasing volumes of information on the sensitivity of the fetus to environmental exposure. Here attention is on the effects of *in utero* exposure that cause functional changes. These alterations are not overtly or grossly teratogenic, but result in increasing susceptibility to disease/dysfunction later in life. While it has long been recognized that environmental triggers in the adult environment may result in disease, it is now evident that the fetus may be more sensitive to the same environmental insult. It is also clear that the effect of environmental exposure during fetal development may have far more detrimental effects on the etiopathology of the disease, both for the fetus as well as the adult in later life. A growing body of data indicates that subtle functional defects can lead to childhood–adult morbidity and/or mortality because of altered tissues, organs, and or systems during development. The basic mechanism of this development is unknown. Also unknown is the contribution of the fetal basis of childhood and adult disease to trends in health status disparities. But the advent of new technologies has opened avenues for more full exploration of these challenges (Drake & Walker, 2004; National Advisory Environmental Health Sciences Council, 2002).

Social and Behavioral

Another environmental consideration—in the broadest sense of the term "environment"—is social and behavioral determinants of disease and disability. In recent years a consistent theme across many health promotion/disease prevention papers is a call for more emphasis on the role of personal choices of health behavior in elevating or decreasing disease risks. These writings also emphasize the importance of understanding the role of social and economic policies that result in differential patterns of exposure of individuals and populations to risk factors and pathogenic environment. Central to such focus is an important role of economic, behavioral, and social factors whether manifested at the individual or population level. Social and behavioral scientists suggest that it is to these factors that we will largely have to look to develop a complete explanation of core epidemiologic observations concerning group and geographic differentials in the prevalence and incidence of disease. This suggestion is fueled by evidence that societal, behavioral, and economic factors work together to produce such problems as drug abuse, alcohol abuse, smoking, and obesity and other conditions directly or indirectly related to the health status disparities questions. In fact, many diseases historically considered in the purview of the biomedical sciences cannot be understood and treated without the benefit of social and behavioral research. However it is worth noting that the social and behavioral sciences are far more complex and variable than the biological/medical sciences as the focal point for a number of strategies in reducing health status disparities.

The challenge here has been identified by the Institute of Medicine and others. The institute notes that not only is there an almost uncountable number of factors affecting individual and social behavior, but these factors combine and interact in extremely complex and mutable ways. Partly for this reason and partly for historical and cultural reasons, research support and research training in these areas lag well behind those in other sciences. An important challenge is how best to increase this support to a level comparable to the need for this knowledge base. While the behavioral and social sciences have addressed fundamental health care questions, methods and tools developed in recent years have provided useful and effective answers to some of the most pressing problems besetting our society. This cannot be overlooked going forward on the health status disparities landscape (National Research Council, 2005).

Future Directions

It is often easier to delineate problems and challenges of health status disparities than to design and execute remedies, though the former is obviously an obligatory step.

Numerous studies have pointed to avenues of approach for reducing health status disparities. But like all good science these studies provoke more questions. This prompts the need to develop new theories pertinent at the intersections among a range of disciplines (i.e., health and biomedical sciences, social and behavioral sciences). When this theory building is coupled with long-term programmatic changes such as those that characterized the linkages between the health and social sciences, it is important to recognize the principles and concepts of transdisciplinary research. Applied in efforts to reduce health status disparities, transdisciplinary research provides a framework for the definition and analysis of the multiple factors that influence health and well-being. It implies the conception of research questions that transcend specialized knowledge bases or individual academic departments/institutes, typically because they are intended to solve research questions beyond the purview of the individual disciplines.

The National Institutes of Health (NIH) appears to be leading the way toward more transdisciplinary research that may have broad implication for addressing issues of health status disparities. The recently designed NIH Roadmap for Medical Research is aimed to identify and support research needs beyond the scope of any single NIH component and that would significantly enhance the individual mission of every NIH institute and center. Current Roadmap initiatives aim to bolster the development and availability of modern tools and information resources, foster novel methods of research collaboration, and markedly enhance the nation's clinical research enterprise. Growing out of inputs from national leaders in academia, industry, and the public, the NIH Roadmap also aims to reconfigure the scientific workforce by encouraging novel forms of collaboration, which are called for by the complexity of health status disparities. Even before the Roadmap, this approach was called for by a number of scientists (Zerhouni, 2005).

Willett (2002), for example, asserts that overly enthusiastic expectations regarding the benefits of genetic research for disease prevention have the potential to distort research priorities and spending for health. He suggests that future research should integrate genetic information into epidemiologic studies. Such integration can help clarify causal relation between both lifestyle (environmental) and genetic factors and risks of disease. Willett concludes that a balanced approach should provide the best data to make informed choices about the most effective means to prevent disease. Others argue that progress in understanding and preventing complex diseases will depend on additional branches of science such as cell biology, physics, computer science, mathematics, and quantitative biochemistry (Strohman, 2002). With these approaches in place, along with more proactive and coordinated health promotion and disease prevention strategies in both the private and public sectors, there is room for optimism that more progress will be made in understanding the multiple dimensions of health status disparities. After all this is a prerequisite for eliminating the century-old problem, and in the process enhance national vitality and significantly reduce preventable suffering and costs.

REFERENCES

Drake, A. J., & Walker, B. R. (2004). The intergenerational effects of fetal programming: Non-genomic mechanism for the inheritance of low birth and cardiovascular disease risk. *Journal of Endocrinology*, *180*, 1–16.

Kronholz, J. (2006). The coming crunch. *The Wall Street Journal*, Oct. 13, B1 col 2.

McMichael, A. J., Kjellstrom, T., & Smith, K. R. (2006). Environmental health. In M. H. Merson, R. E. Black, & A. J. Mills (Eds.), *International public health*. Gaithersburg, MD: Aspen Publishing.

Merikangas, K. R., & Risch, N. (2003). Genomic priorities and public health. *Science, 302*(5645), 599–602.

National Advisory Environmental Health Sciences Council. (2002). Fetal basis of childhood and adult disease: Role of the environment. *Environmental Health Perspectives, 110*(6), 150.

National Institute of Environmental Health Sciences. (1999). *Human health and the environment: Some research needs.* Bethesda, MD: U.S. Department of Health and Human Services, National Institutes of Health.

National Research Council. (2005). *Advancing the nation's health needs.* Washington, DC: National Academy Press.

Strohman, R. (2002). Maneuvering in the complex path from genotype to phenotype. *Science, 296*(5568), 701–703.

U.S. Census Bureau. (2005). *Population profile of the United States.* Washington, DC: U.S. Census Bureau.

U.S. Department of Health and Human Services (HHS). (1985). *Report of the Secretary's Task Force on Black and minority health*, Vol. 1. Washington, DC: HHS.

U.S. Department of Health and Human Services (HHS). (1998). *The initiative to eliminate racial and ethnic disparities in health.* Washington, DC: HHS.

World Health Organization (WHO). (2005). Fighting disease, fostering development. *The World Health Report.* WHO.

Willett, W. (2002) Balancing life-style and genomics research for disease prevention. *Science, 296*(5568), 695–698.

Zerhouni, E. A. (2005). US biomedical research: Basic, translational, and clinical sciences. *The Journal of the American Medical Association, 294*(11), 1352–1358.

Toward Evidence-Based and Culturally Appropriate Models for Reducing Global Health Disparities: An Africanist Perspective

3

Collins O. Airhihenbuwa and Titilayo A. Okoror

Introduction

Cultural identity is central to health education, health communication, and indeed all public health research and intervention. As a result, we believe that one must study and better understand the social cultural infrastructures in Africa if one is to understand values that are central to African identity and how identity influences decisions that are made about health and behavior. Social cultural infrastructure refers to nonmarket and nonphysical values that shape the moral and ethical codes by which relationships and expectations are defined, measured, and rewarded (Airhihenbuwa, 2007). One example is the debate over the most relevant frame for defining an African woman's agency as will be discussed later.

To understand the role of culture in health, we will describe the PEN-3 cultural model. PEN-3 is a cultural model that was developed in 1989 (Airhihenbuwa) to guide a cultural approach to HIV/AIDS in Africa. It has been used to study a range of health and behavioral issues and problems in the United States (Erwin, Spatz, Stotts, Hollenberg, & Deloney, 1996; Paskett et al., 1999; Walker, 2000) and Africa (Airhihenbuwa, 1993, 1995; Gwede & McDermott 1992; Webster, 2003). Others have also used PEN-3 to describe the planning, implementation, and evaluation of health interventions (Green & Kreuter, 1999; Huff & Kline, 1999). The model is composed of three

The Stigma research referenced in this paper is supported by funding from the National Institute of Mental Health NIMH Grant # 1 R24 MH068180.

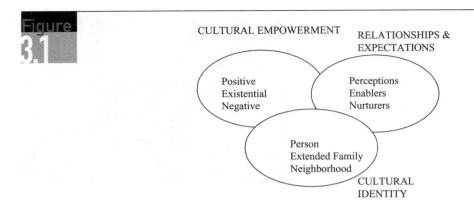

The PEN-3 model.

primary domains: Cultural Identity, Relationships and Expectations, and Cultural Empowerment. When a health issue is identified, such as HIV/AIDS related stigma, a 3 × 3 table is created to group the interaction between the domain of Relationships and Expectations with the domain of Cultural Empowerment. These two domains are discussed first, followed by a discussion of the third domain of Cultural Identity. The Cultural Identity domain is used to determine the point of intervention entry. Figure 3.1 shows the PEN-3 model. A discussion of the three domains of the PEN-3 follows.

Relationships and Expectations

The meanings of behavior are commonly framed in the context within which perception offers insights into behaviors related to health, the resources, and institutional forces that enable or disenable behavioral actions, and the influence of family, kin, and friends in nurturing the behavior. The three categories of Relationships and Expectations are perception, enablers, and nurturers.

Perception

The study of perception in health research typically focuses on factual information about disease etiology and nosology with little or no attention paid to the cultural, historical, and political contexts such as colonialism and imperialism. Scholars like Frantz Fanon (1958, 1968), Edward Said (1993), and Chinua Achebe (1988) have written extensively on varied roles and impact of colonization and imperialism on the conditions in Africa and elsewhere. For example, the impact of colonization produces experiences that fuse emotion with rational volition. The manifestation of behavior from such fusion of emotion and rationality are often overlooked in discourses that underscore emotionality while valorizing rationality as if it were free of emotion. Emotionality is central to how the impact of domination is expressed in the lives of the colonized as well as the colonizers. The representation of how events are perceived and shared is just as critical as documentation of the actual event even when it is different from what is perceived. Emotion is sometimes considered to be insignificant in the context of knowing in ways that confirms knowledge production as resulting only from volitional responses that can be elicited and obtained at will. Yet emotion is as critical to knowledge production as is rational volition. We know this to be true in cardiovascular health research where a heart attack suffered by a friend or kin could prompt initiation of risk reduction behavior such as leisure time physical activity and eating a more balanced meal. Emotion is also known to be central to initiation of HIV risk reduction activity as evident in persons who begin to use condoms during sex only after a friend or kin is known to have tested positive for HIV.

In the book entitled *A Pluralistic Universe*, the esteemed American philosopher William James (1909) concluded that scholarship that is devoid of emotion is bankrupt. Beyond affirming the role of emotion in behavior, the core issue of the social determinants of health centers around the centrality of emotionality in health behavior. The question of racism is as much an emotional production as it is a rational volitional one. It is the persistence of racism and structural discrimination that led W. E. B. Du Bois (1969) to conclude that the problem of the twentieth century is the problem of the color line. It is also the need to extend the question of inequity beyond race to account for gender differences that led Darlene Clark-Hines (1993) to deepen Du Bois's mantra by cautioning that instead of writing, "One ever feels his twoness," he would have mused about how one ever feels her "fiveness": Negro, American, woman, poor, Black woman. It is indeed the misrepresentation of truth as always universal in the production of knowledge that led Chinua Achebe (1988) to conclude that where one thing stands, something else must stand beside it. This is to say that the notion of a universal solution to health problems across geopolitical and cultural divides is a fallacy. Knowledge, beliefs, and values in decision making are products of culture. A central feature of such a cultural production is the degree to which emotion and rational volition enables or disenables our general health and well-being.

Enablers

Studies on enabling factors of health typically measure factors that enable or disenable health decisions on the basis of individual income and in many cases one's economic status. For example, condom use behavior has been measured by the affordability of condoms for use in preventing sexually transmitted infections like HIV. However, more fundamental contestations over enablers are the ways in which social scientists substitute lower social economic status for culture. Indeed the fascination of some anthropologists with African culture is in part influenced by the lower economic status of people in the villages. It is the experiences of folks in the villages that are approximated to represent Africa. Among African Americans, for example, low income is used as a proxy for identity in ways that sometimes demonize the identities of the very people for whom programs are designed to benefit. In the book entitled *YO' Mama's DisFunktional*, Robin Kelly (1997) critiques social scientists for representing behavior as both a synonym of culture as well as a determinant for class. For many social scientists, Kelly argues, negative behavior is a focus of study only when the population of interest is the "underclass" as though their income, their poverty level, or the kind of work they do are of no relevance to the health problems they manifest.

In the book entitled *Black Wealth and White Wealth*, Oliver and Shapiro (1997) argued that wealth is a more salient measure of health outcome than social economic factors. Social economic factors are typically defined and measured in the tripartite relations of income, education, and occupation (King & Williams, 1995). Of the three, income has assumed a dominant role. Oliver and Shapiro (1997) define income as "flow of dollars (salaries, wages, and payments periodically received as returns from an occupation, investment, or government transfer, etc.) over a set period, typically one year." Wealth on the other hand is defined as "the total extent, at a given moment, of an individual's accumulated assets and access to resources, and it refers to the net value of assets (e.g., ownership of stocks, money in the bank, real estate, business ownership, etc.) less debt held at one time" (p. 30).

As Airhihenbuwa describes in his new book, *Healing Our Differences* (2007), when one compares two individuals (one White and the other Black) who have the same income, occupation, and education, their generation-level in middle class status determines the directional flow of their income. The income of a first generation middle–class person typically flows downwards to support his or her kin who are probably mostly in the lower class and this middle-class person may likely need to obtain a bank loan to purchase a house. The income of a third or fourth generation middle-class person (who has the same income, occupation, and education as the first generation middle class) will likely remain and even be enlarged with support from financially privileged parents. This person may not need the bank for a down payment on a new house since they may be able to get the money from their parents with no interest. In the book *White-Washing Race* (2003) Michael Brown and his colleagues provide a comprehensive analysis of how one's legacy of accumulation or disaccumulation of wealth influences and dictates the direction and flow of resources.

This is even reinforced in the tax code in the United States as outlined by Oliver and Shapiro (1997). "The lower tax rates on capital gains and the deduction for home mortgages and real estate taxes, we argue, flow differentially to Blacks and Whites because of the fact that Blacks generally have fewer and different types of assets than whites with similar income" (p. 43). On the question of education, which is typically connected to occupation, the disparity in schools can be explained in part by the fact that schools are funded with property tax money. Schools in neighborhoods with higher property value and higher tax revenue are better resourced than lower property tax schools. The result is a disparity in the quality of education received by students, regardless of the students' socioeconomic status (SES) level, and is proportional with the property value of the neighborhood where the school is located. Such a systemic disparity tends to skew and sometimes undermine benefits that are gained from a nurturing family and friends.

Nurturers

Families and friends play major roles in health decisions and health behavior. Socialization is central to the idea of nurturing. Whether one is schooled or educated depends on the socialization in and out of school. We want to argue that not everyone that goes to school is educated just as there are many educated persons who did not go to school. The most famous among these are often referred to as organic intellectuals. While schooling offers training to acquire skills and hopefully some education, the process of education begins well before any exposure to school curriculum. For example, some African feminists, like Oyeronke Oyewumi (2003a) and Nkiru Nzegwu (2003), argue that motherhood should be understood as central to a woman's identity and agency. The cultural contexts in which many Africans are educated centralize motherhood as a most important status for the agency of an African woman. However, socialization that occurs in schools taught students to undermine motherhood as a woman's agency. Yet, many young students are introduced to motherhood in school through maternal mortality statistics and its associated language of subordination and marginalization that locates motherhood as a proxy for wifehood. Nurturing is very central to the question of motherhood as a defining identity for women than sisterhood. We believe that motherhood is central to our understanding of cultural empowerment.

Cultural Empowerment

Culture and Empowerment are two words that are almost never used as a coupling term because of the ways in which culture is often represented as a barrier and empowerment is represented as strength. The domain of Cultural Empowerment is thus an affirmation of the possibilities of culture, which ranges from positive to negative. Culture can be empowering in the sense that culture represents the continuum of good, indifferent, and bad (Airhihenbuwa & Webster, 2004). The Cultural Empowerment domain is thus composed of three categories, which are positive, existential, and negative.

Positive

The goal of cultural empowerment is to ensure that an intervention accentuates the positive rather than focusing only on the negative. This model insists that regardless of where or whom we focus on for intervention (the point of intervention entry), the positive cultural aspects of behavior and culture must be identified as the first priority, since every culture has something positive about it. We agree that an interventionist who fails to begin with positive aspects of the community and behavior must stay away from the community since a lack of such knowledge will lead to lack of trustworthiness whereby the interventionist becomes a part of the problem (Airhihenbuwa, 1999). An example is traditional healing modality that is grounded in cultural strategies for dealing with health promotion, disease prevention, and treatment. Some herbal remedies as prescribed by traditional healers have been found effective in curing common illnesses, such as malaria (Ajaiyeoba et al., 2004). Chewing a stick promotes dental health by reducing plaque and improving dental health (Aderinokun, Lawoyin, & Onyeaso, 1999; Al–Otaibi, Al–Harthy, Soder, Gustafsson, & Angmar-Mansson, 2003; Eid & Selim, 1994). Al–Otaibi (2004) reported that the use of a chewing stick resulted in significant reductions in plaque and gingival indices compared to tooth brushing. It is in the process of identifying positive cultural practices that some existential (unique) practices emerge.

Existential

There are many values and beliefs that are practiced in a culture but pose no threat to health. Interventionists should not blame these values for the failure of their interventions. An example is what Airhihenbuwa (1999) refers to as *language elasticity* in terms of the various codes and meanings of languages whereby language of flexible principles should not be judged with the rules of language of rigid principles. Even the same expression in a common language, such as English, that may be spoken in different parts of the world has different meanings that are culturally coded. Another existential quality is orature or orality in terms of interventions. We should ensure consistency between ways of communicating and ways of knowledge acquisition that are customary to learning in the culture. Ways of communication reflect patterns of relationships among a people who share a common language. In fact Makoni (2003) has been critical of linguists who study African languages but with little or no interest in the people who speak the language.

Indeed the language of scientific enquiring reflects certain existential values we place on a study population. Take for example the question of distrust and trustworthiness in researching African American populations. Evidence of years of medical atrocities visited on the Black bodies by physicians and other medical providers have led to understandably a sense of distrust among African Americans. The syphilis study conducted at Tuskegee is often cited as a culmination of such medical atrocities. Two issues remain a legacy of this study: (1) the name by which the study is associated and (2) the resulting distrust which has become a central concern for researchers. To address the first issue, Vanessa Northington Gamble (2005) has suggested that the syphilis study should be called the U.S. Public Health Services Syphilis Study. This correction in the name should properly align the owners of the study with its identity as traditionally done in research. In its present identity, the nefarious syphilis study, the community, and institution that was victimized are left to bear the burden of its name and legacy.

The second issue relates to the focus of intervention. When distrust results from an experience it begs the question as to whether the victims that have become distrustful should shoulder the responsibility for changing the relationship with the system that creates the distrust. Rather than focusing on African Americans to become trustworthy, we argue that we should focus instead on institutional trustworthiness (Crawley, 2001) or the lack thereof. It is the institution that has the responsibility to earn the trust of those they have wronged, and not the minorities that have been victimized (Wynia & Gamble, 2006). The need to earn the community and/or individual's trust is paramount when implementing an intervention designed to increase access to health services (Kumanyika, 2006). Health care providers' attitudes and perceptions about minorities have been reported as being either a barrier in or an enabler to access and utilization of health care services (Chandra & Paul, 2003). For example, increased use of cancer screening tests and blood pressure monitoring among low-income African American women was associated with higher levels of trust in their health care providers (O'Malley, Sheppard, Schwartz, & Mandelblatt, 2004).

This is similar to findings in a recent study on HIV counseling and testing among African American college students (Okoror, 2006). In this study, participants reported being more open and honest in sharing information about their behaviors due to the nonjudgmental and welcoming attitude of the counselor. It is safe to say that the fact that ethnic and racial minorities present themselves to receive care from an institution that has a history of discriminating against them is an indication of their (i.e., minorities) effort to trust (Goepp, 2006). Clearly, existential factors offer insights into certain negative behaviors to be understood in the community.

Negative

There are negative values and relationships that produce negative health outcomes. A number of these occur in the contexts of policy environment. Others may be the result of income and wealth of individuals, communities, and society. Yet others may be the position of women in society relative to decisions about sexuality or simply how a woman's agency is defined. In all these factors, how negative health issues are defined greatly impacts on how solutions are framed. With the emphasis on health gaps between the haves and have-nots, the language of these gaps has often defined approaches to studying the gaps. In the United States we focus on disparity. In Europe the emphasis tends to be on inequality while the global emphasis has been on inequity. Both disparity and inequality are quantitative languages that often focus on quantitative differences. Within such quantitative frames, what matters is the difference in the numbers of people who are sick or dead.

The language of equity is a qualitative value within which quantitative processes co-exist with other measures. Equity is not meant to eliminate all differences since certain differences, like gender and culture, are desirable and healthy. Equity in health focuses on eliminating unfair, unacceptable, and avoidable differences. In this language, it is the totality of the condition that is more important than how subgroups compare to one another. Excess deaths as a quantitative difference focus our attention on clinical intervention to prevent deaths, and rightly so. Unfortunately, this has become an exclusive focus that ignores qualitative assessment of the conditions of life that create and maintain certain levels of vulnerability that manifest in disease and death as outcomes.

It is this qualitative measure that Du Bois called for in the 1899 Philadelphia Negro Study, in which he concluded that we should focus on the overall living conditions of African Americans if we are to understand their state of vulnerability to disease and death rather than focusing almost exclusively on comparing them to Whites. There are healthy differences that should be encouraged and promoted. The question of identity is thus central to how we address negative health issues.

Assessment Phase in the Application of the PEN-3 Model

In the implementation of PEN-3 the researchers should engage the community to complete the assessment phase. The first step is to develop a 3 × 3 table to produce nine categories. This is done by crossing the components of the domain of Cultural Empowerment (i.e., positive, existential, negative) with the domain of Relationships and Expectations (i.e., perception, enabler, nurturer). The following is the description of the nine categories.

1. Positive Perception

A community dialogue should begin with the knowledge and openness that the views of the community are fully encouraged without distortions of the subject matter. A community dialogue should not begin with an a priori notion of the subject matter or what aspects of it should be addressed. Such a mind-set ends up silencing voices from the community.

2. Existential Perception

In a community dialogue or what we often refer to as a polylogue, attention must be paid to the language used, and the expressions for communications and meanings ascribed to what is being discussed. Words and meanings change as they cross cultural boundaries and their roles should be considered. In discussing condom use in Nigeria, for example, "raincoats"and "blo-blo" (meaning balloons) are a couple of the words used instead of the word "condom."

3. Negative Perception

History and politics are the shells for understanding personal behaviors. The impact of political history, such as apartheid in South Africa, should be addressed, in comprehending the disparities among the racial groups.

4. Positive Enablers

Systems and structures shape the way we behave. We cannot fully understand individual behavior unless we understand the structures and systems that shape individual behavior. The degree to which experiences are positive or negative depends to a high degree on the policy that shapes those experiences.

5. Existential Enablers

There are many aspects of a culture that are understood only from within. Traditional healing is an example of such a cultural system. Many people still seek traditional healing modalities, many at times in combination with western medicines: therefore their (traditional healers) roles should be addressed.

6. Negative Enablers

Recognize history, politics, and gender roles. The systemic inequities that differentially marginalize African women have left many to become dependent on men for economic support. Such a dependency results in increased vulnerability for their health. The level of vulnerability has occurred at multiple levels. There is vulnerability from engaging in sex with a partner who may be HIV positive. There is also the vulnerability that results from exposure to infection in a poorly resourced health clinic, since women are more likely than men to use health services.

7. Positive Nurturers

Developing an intervention should not always begin with importing an idea from the outside. Successful intervention can occur by looking within to understand how related issues have been addressed in the past. The role and composition of family becomes a very important example of looking within. Knowing what cultures have done to survive and thrive is central to developing a sustainable intervention.

8. Existential Nurturers

Nurturing is culturally produced and maintained. Breast-feeding represents a form of nurturance that is a cornerstone to the bonding that is established between a mother and her child. Contextualizing human relations and connectedness is central to establishing a sustainable intervention.

9. Negative Nurturers

No single person can address a pandemic that affects millions such as HIV and AIDS. Thus, multiple strategies should be explored by a team of multidisciplinary researchers. The fear of HIV typically results from the contexts of family and health care settings even when unintentional. Such stigma has led some families and communities to avoid sharing things with persons living with HIV and AIDS.

Having framed relevant socio–cultural issues into these nine categories, a collective decision must be made among the researchers and members of the community to prioritize the point of intervention entry. Such entry is based on what research results show about the context of prevention and the likelihood that this entry will lead to a significant change in controlling the epidemic. In the previous examples cited, a collective decision will be made based upon whether changes in any of the examples given will take place at the level of a person, the extended family, or the neighborhood/community. In a conventional model, we often begin the intervention by discussing the individuals. In the PEN-3 Model the identity component is the last component because it is the nature and context of the issues that drive which of the identity categories should be the focus of intervention.

Cultural Identity

In PEN-3, the question of identity is central to decisions made about where and when to begin an intervention. It is for this reason that this final domain is called the intervention phase. In the African context, gender has become a site where contestations over theorizing of identity clearly illuminate the differences in ways in which meanings of a woman's identity are far from being universal. The notion that sisterhood is global has been challenged for its manifestations in what has been referred to as "sisterarchy" whereby the white women are privileged and women of African descents are marginalized (Nzegwu, 2003; Oyewumi, 2003b). Sisterhood as a code that presupposes a global solidarity among women is typically framed as a counter-discourse to patriarchy. While patriarchy continues to exert a dominating force on women and young men, African feminist scholars argue that motherhood cannot be totally defined as a condition of being a victim as many scholarships on African women typically do. Moreover, motherhood as a victim of patriarchy is typically framed in the context of marriage whereby motherhood becomes a code for wifehood. The theorizing of the African woman's identity advanced by Oyewumi (1997, 2003b) and others denounces the limited representation of a woman in the role of wifehood and instead centralizes the woman's identity as a mother whose agency may or may not be located in a marriage. In fact, her physical location in a marriage does not limit her agency to the marital home. For one reason, family in Africa is a system of lineage which extends beyond the marital home.

The roles of men and women therefore are not limited to the marital enclaves but extends to their natal relations, which are predominantly stronger on one's mother lineage than one's father lineage. In fact the prophetic mantra of Mary McLeod Bethune (1933) in which she concluded that "the true worth of a race must be measured by the character of its womanhood" may very well be modified in a counterpoise which could read "the true worth of an African nation must be measured by the character of its motherhood." For Oyeronke Oyewumi (1997, 2003a, 2003b), Nkiru Nzegwu (2003), Amina Mama (2005), and other feminist scholars, motherhood is the most central defining factor of a woman's identity in Africa. Motherhood does not always mean giving birth even though it is a commonly used gold standard. The concept and practice of comothering clearly challenges any notion of birthright as the only precondition for motherhood.

As explained in *Healing Our Differences* (Airhihenbuwa, 2007), public endearment by which one defines a relationship between two friends but that have gone beyond the common bond of friendship is typically expressed in "my mother's child." The Edos will say *omwiyemwen*, Yoruba would say *Omoya*, and for Wolof in Senegal, it is *Domu Ndeye*. It is for this reason that we consider motherhood to be the *cultural womb* of the family and indeed a society. Without a cultural frame within which to understand identity, research or behavior will continue to advance a notion of African women only as victims. The absence of the centrality of cultural identity necessitates a reframing of new ways of addressing health issues in Africa (Airhihenbuwa, 2005). This is the motivation for advancing the PEN-3 model. The first two domains of PEN-3 are the assessment domains. This third domain is the intervention domain. Culture represents a shared pool of collective consciousness. It represents shared historical and political memories that position us to define the future from the possibilities of the present. Having completed the 3×3 table in the assessment phase, it is necessary to identify the point of intervention entry with the understanding that there could be multiple entry points for addressing the social contexts and behaviors that have been identified for promotion and/or change. This process removes the assumption that all interventions should focus only on a person. The three components of the domain of Cultural Identity are persons, extended family, and neighborhood.

Person

In many African cultures, a person is different from an individual. The Ghanaian philosopher Kwame Gyekye (1997) has argued that there is a difference between a person and an individual in African languages. An individual is the person whose behavior and values are considered unacceptable by the collective. For Gyekye, the community provides the context for creating and developing the identity of personhood. "A person comes to know who she is in the contexts of relationships with others, not as an isolated, lonely star in a social galaxy (p. 43)." Although personhood is earned, it is assumed that everyone is entitled to it until one abrogates certain principles and ethics that are believed to be minimal in sustaining the rights and privileges of personhood. To violate such principles and ethics is to be considered a nonperson.

As Airhihenbuwa discussed in *Healing Our Differences*, (2007) among the Edos of Nigeria, a person is referred to as '*omwan*.' The *omwan* who engages in action considered to be modeling a personality with high standards within the community principles and ethics is considered to be truly-*omwan* (truly a person). Conversely, the *omwan* who has violated what is considered to be minimal standards for a person in that community is often referred to as '*oni omwan*' (that one is not a person). Indeed, this representation of personhood is captured in pidgin English in Nigeria, when someone who is considered to have violated certain communal rules is dismissed as "dat one no bi person" (that one is not a person)—he is an individual since he is not a social being and thus not a part of the community. The critical lesson in this discourse on personhood is the role of the community and the larger society in defining and affirming identity at the level of the person. Thus intervention focusing on the behavior of the person is limited without a clear understanding of how the cultural community (or what Kwame Gyekye referred to as communocultural group) defines, shapes, and nurtures personhood. Beyond the contextualization of personhood, individualism is the African identity represented in health literature. African children's humanity is often reduced to bodies in need of Western intervention. The personhood of the image of children is hardly viewed.

Thanks to the African cultural production and transformative work of Dr. A. Olusegun Fayemi (www.fayemi.com) we are welcomed to images of Africans that are neither a romanticized nor diseased representation of children. What Fayemi offers us is simply images of children living the daily experience of being an African. In one of the pictures, the children are engaged in a cultural game, of six pairs of parallel holes, that nurtures and strengthens their analytical skills similar to skills development that is associated with building block commercially represented in the "Lego." The absence of *ogiuruise* (as it is called in Edo, Nigeria) in carved wood (in its potable from) did not prevent these children from recreating it on the ground to generate the same results. This is the same game and methods for analytical skill development and peer group support known to and used by their parents and forebears for generations.

Extended Family

Extended family is used here to problematize the notion of nuclear family as the point of family referent. As I argued in *Health and Culture: Beyond the Western Paradigm* (Airhihenbuwa, 1995), when African family is the point of referent, the western family could be considered a constricted family. As I indicated earlier, family in most African culture is a production of lineage rather than marriage. The cycles of decision making in many African families are quite expansive particularly since roles, responsibilities, and decision making are never weakened by marriage or the physical movement from one's natal home to the married home. This frame of family and language for transmitting meanings is central to the contestation over the identity of motherhood as we discussed earlier. Take the case of representation of mothers-in-law, for example. Two studies have shown that mothers-in-law in Senegalese and South African cultures discourage their pregnant daughters-in-law from using the available health care facilities. In an ethnographic study to understand this practice in Senegalese culture, Cheikh Niang (personal communication, October 2005) found that mothers-in-law saw themselves as totally responsible for the welfare of their pregnant daughters-in-law. As Airhihenbuwa (2007) discussed in *Healing Our Differences*, the value is so strong that these mothers would pray to God that rather than anything happening to their daughters-in-law, God should take their own lives instead. The strong belief in their responsibility and the related lack of confidence in the health centers led these mothers to discourage their daughters-in-law's use of such centers. In particular, the mothers have no control over and no confidence in the kind of care offered at these centers. Moreover, many of these centers are not connected to their communities or neighborhood.

Neighborhood

The framing of what constitutes a community or neighborhood is very central to the framing of a social cultural infrastructure. Geopolitical zones may define neighborhoods, family lineage often defines boundaries of decision about health. Whatever the boundary that constitutes neighborhood or community, it is the people that must help to define it. In addition, a community's capacity—that is, economic status and power structure (Airhihenbuwa & Webster, 2004)—is also important in the successful implementation and sustainability of a health program. As mentioned earlier, efforts should be made to use and effectively maximize available resources within the community, rather than introducing new resources that may be either unaffordable and/or inaccessible to community members once the program is over, thereby making such program unsustainable at the community level. For example, in implementing a program on proper methods of making water potable, introducing chemical purifiers to a community in which many members have low economic status could unintentionally create more problems than help. Rather, a sustainable effort may be to include a simple method, such as boiling water, as part of the program. This is a method community members are already used to, will find easy to implement, and would not necessarily involve additional monetary cost. It also increases the sustainability of the program.

Conclusion

Efforts have been directed in the last few decades on reducing global disparities, especially in many parts of Africa. However, such efforts have met with dismal results, and "victim-blaming" has ensued in which Africans have been on the receiving ends. Many of these programs have been ineffective and/or unsustainable largely because a number of them have been based on individualistic models that do not address the socio-cultural, historical, and political contexts that inform and influence health decisions and behaviors in African communities. The PEN-3 model is a cultural model that has been found effective in offering the community spaces for their voices to be heard in the development, implementation, and evaluation of programs. Rather than focusing solely on negative health behaviors, the model provides interventionists with the opportunity to access and address both the positive and existential behaviors within communities and, most importantly, build on the strengths located in the communities and the people who live in the community while working on changing the behavior of interest. First, we must always begin with the positive aspects of the culture and community within which personal behaviors are better understood.

REFERENCES

Achebe, C. (1988). Colonialists criticism. In *Hopes and impediments: Selected essays*. New York: Anchor Books.

Aderinokun, G. A., Lawoyin, J. O., & Onyeaso, C. O. (1999). Effect of two common Nigerian chewing sticks on gingival health and oral hygiene. *Odontostomatologie Tropicale, 22*(87), 13–18.

Airhihenbuwa, C. O. (1989). Perspectives on AIDS in Africa: Strategies for prevention and control. *AIDS Education and Prevention, 1*(1), 57–69.

Airhihenbuwa, C. O. (1993). Health promotion for child survival in Africa: Implications for cultural appropriateness. *International Journal of Health Education, 12*(3), 10–15.

Airhihenbuwa, C. O. (1995). *Health and culture: Beyond the western paradigm*. Thousand Oaks, CA: Sage Publications.

Airhihenbuwa, C. O. (1999). Of culture and multiverse: Renouncing 'the universal truth' in health. *Journal of Health Education, 30,* 267–273.

Airhihenbuwa, C. O. (2005). Theorizing cultural identity and behaviour in social science research. *CODESRIA Bulletin,* Nos. 3&4, 17–19.

Airhihenbuwa, C. O. (2007). *Healing our differences: The global crisis of health and politics of identity.* Lanham, MD: Roman & Littlefield.

Airhihenbuwa, C. O., & Webster, J. D. (2004). Culture and African contexts of HIV/AIDS prevention, care and support. *Journal of Social Aspects of HIV/AIDS Research Alliance, 1*(1), 4–13.

Ajaiyeoba, F. O., Falade, C. O., Fawole, O. I., Akinboye, D. O., Gbotosho, G. O., Bolaji, O. M., et al. (2004). Efficacy of herbal remedies used by herbalists in Oyo State Nigeria for treatment of *Plasmodium falciparum* infections—A survey and an observation. *African Journal of Medicine and Medical Sciences, 33*(2), 115–119.

Al-Otaibi, M. (2004). The miswak (chewing stick) and oral health. Studies on oral hygiene practices of urban Saudi Arabians. *Swedish Dental Journal,* (Suppl), *167,* 2–75.

Al-Otaibi, M., Al-Harthy, M., Soder, B., Gustafsson, A., & Angmar-Mansson, B. (2003). Comparative effect of chewing sticks and toothbrushing on plaque removal and gingival health. *Oral Health and Preventive Dentistry, 1*(4), 301–307.

Bethune, M. (1933, June 3). *A century of progress of Negro women*. Address presented at the Women Federation Conference, Chicago, IL.

Brown, M. K., Carnoy, M., Currie, E., Duster, T., Oppenheimer, D. B., Shultz, M. M., et al. (2003). *White-washing race: The myth of a color-blind society*. Berkeley, CA: University of California Press.

Chandra, A., & Paul, D. P. (2003). African American participation in clinical trials: Recruitment difficulties and potential remedies. *Hospital Topics, 81*(2), 33–38.

Clark-Hines, D. (1993). In the kingdom of culture: Black women and intersection of race, gender, and class. In G. Early (Ed.), *Lure and loathing: Essays on race, identity, and the ambivalence of assimilation*. New York: Penguin Press.

Crawley, L. M. (2001). African-American participation in clinical trials: Situating trust and trustworthiness. *Journal of the National Medical Association, 93*(12), (Suppl), 14s–17s.

Du Bois, W. E. B. (1899). *The Philadelphia Negro: A social study*. Philadelphia: University of Pennsylvania Press.

Du Bois, W. E. B. (1969). *The souls of Black folk: Essays and sketches.* 22nd ed. Greenwich, CT: Crest Books.

Eid, M. A., & Selim, H. A. (1994). A retrospective study on the relationship between miswak chewing stick and periodontal health. *Egyptian Dental Journal, 40*(1), 589–592.

Erwin, D. O., Spatz, T. S., Stotts, C., Hollenberg, J. A., & Deloney, L. A. (1996). Increasing mammography and breast self-examination in African American women using the Witness Project model. *Journal of Cancer Education, 11*(4), 210–215.

Fanon, F. (1958). *Black skin, white mask*. London: Penguin Press.

Fanon, F. (1968). *The wretched of the earth*. New York: Grove Press.

Gamble, V. N. (2005, November 14). *Health disparities, bioethics, and justice*. A public lecture. The Rock Ethics Institute. The Pennsylvania State University. University Park, PA.

Goepp, J. G. (2006). Reflections on trust and health services utilization. *Preventive Medicine, 42*(2), 81–82.

Green, L. W., & Kreuter, M. W. (1999). *Health promotion planning: An educational and ecological approach.* Mountain View, CA: Mayfield Publishing.

Gwede, C., & McDermott, R. J. (1992). AIDS in sub-Saharan Africa: Implications of health education. *AIDS Education and Prevention, 4*(4), 350–361.

Gyekye, K. (1997). *Tradition and modernity. Philosophical reflections on the African experience.* New York: Oxford University Press.

Huff, R. M., & Kline, M. V. (1999). *Promoting health in multicultural populations: A handbook for practitioners.* Thousand Oaks, CA: Sage Publications.

James, W. (1909). *A pluralistic universe.* New York: Longmans, Green and Company.

Kelly, R. D. G. (1997). *YO'mama's disfunktional! Fighting the culture wars in urban America.* Boston: Beacon Press.

King, G., & Williams, D. R. (1995). Race and health: A multidimensional approach to African American health. In B. C. Amick, S. Levine, A. R. Tarlov, & D. C. Walsh (Eds.), *Society and health.* Oxford: Oxford University Press.

Kumanyika, S. (2006). Trust in health care: Seeing it from the other side. *Preventive Medicine, 42,* 83–84.

Makoni, S. (2003). From misinvention to disinvention of language: Multilingualism and the South African constitution. In S. Makoni, G. Smitherman, A. Ball, & A. Spears (Eds.), *Black linguistics, language, society, and politics in Africa and the Americas.* London and New York: Routledge.

Mama, A. (2005). Gender studies for African's transformation. In T. Mkandiware (Ed.), *African intellectuals: Rethinking politics, language, gender and development.* Dakar, Senegal: CODESRIA Books and London: Zed Books.

Nzegwu, N. (2003). O Africa: Gender imperialism in academia. In O. Oyewumi (Ed.), *African women and feminism: Reflecting on the politics of sisterhood.* Trenton, NJ: Africa World Press.

Okoror, T. A. (2006). *Effect of enhanced HIV counseling and testing on students testing negative for HIV/AIDS.* Unpublished doctoral dissertation, Pennsylvania State University.

Oliver, M. L., & Shapiro, T. M. (1997). *Black wealth/white wealth: New perspectives on racial inequality.* New York: Routledge.

O'Malley, A. S., Sheppard, V. B., Schwartz, M., & Mandelblatt, J. (2004). The role of trust in use of preventive services among low-income African American women. *Preventive Medicine, 38*(6), 777–785.

Oyewumi, O. (1997). *The invention of women: Making an African sense of western gender discourses.* Minneapolis: University of Minnesota Press.

Oyewumi, O. (2003a). Abiyamo: Theorizing African motherhood. *JENDA: A Journal of Culture and African Women Studies.* Issue 4.

Oyewumi, O. (2003b). *African women and feminism: Reflecting on the politics of sisterhood.* Trenton, NJ: African World Press.

Paskett, E. D., Tatum, C. M., D'Agostino, R., Rushing, J., Velez, R., Michielutte, R., et al. (1999). Community-based interventions to improve breast and cervical cancer screening: Results of the Forsyth County Cancer Screening (FoCaS) Project. *Cancer Epidemiology, Biomarkers and Prevention, 8,* 453–459.

Said, E. W. (1993). *Culture and imperialism.* New York: Alfred A. Knopf.

Walker, C. (2000). An educational intervention of hypertension management in older African Americans. *Ethnicity and Diseases, 10,* 165–174.

Webster, J. D. (2003). *Using a cultural model to assess female condom use in Mpumalanga, South Africa.* Doctoral dissertation, Pennsylvania State University. Electronic Thesis and Dissertation #401.

Wynia, M. K., & Gamble, V. N. (2006). Mistrust among minorities and the trustworthiness of medicine. *PLoS Medicine, 3*(5), e244.

New Paradigms for Inclusive Health Care: Toward Individual Patient and Population Health

4

James O. Prochaska

For decades it has been known that behaviors are major causes of chronic disease and premature death. It is now known that behaviors, like alcohol abuse, depression, smoking, and stress, account for about 60% of total health care costs compared to only 15% of costs due to pharmaceuticals (Prochaska, 1996). But the dominant paradigms of research and practice result in interventions impacting on relatively small percentages of these health and mental health behaviors. Innovative approaches to research and practice can result in increases in behavioral health care services that can enhance health, reduce health care costs, and provide more inclusive care.

High Costs of Health and Mental Health Behaviors

Decades of research document that behaviors are major causes of chronic disease, disability, and premature death (U.S. Department of Health and Human Services [HHS], 2000). The most important costs are the distress, suffering, sickness, and diminished quality of life of patients struggling with chronic conditions caused by health and mental health behaviors. But families, friends, employers, communities, and health care systems suffer important costs as well. Unfortunately governments, employers, and health care systems often are most concerned with the financial costs of such conditions. Given that behaviors account for a majority of total health care costs, governments, employers, and health care systems have to be concerned that such costs can overwhelm health care.

There is no consensus on how much health care costs can be reduced by treating behaviors more inclusively. Some of the most compelling evidence is the longitudinal research of Dee Edington (2001) on changes in health care costs as a function of changes in the number of health and mental health behaviors such as smoking, inactivity, alcohol abuse, and stress. He found that if two health behavior risks were effectively reduced, health care costs were reduced by about $2,000 per year. If there was a reduction of four health behavior risks, costs were reduced by about $4,000. Edington also found that when there was an increase of two health behavior risks, costs increased by about $2,000 per year. And if there was an increase of four risks, costs increased by about $4,000. These data make a compelling case for treating health behavior risks that currently exist and preventing risks from occurring.

Low Impacts on Health and Mental Health Behaviors

In spite of the profound need for behavioral and psychological services, available treatments have relatively low population impacts. Low impacts have been due in part to the preoccupation of scientists and practitioners with the efficacy of treatments they research or provide; they are concerned with the percentage of participants who benefit from particular treatments. To date, impact has equaled efficacy times reach (Prochaska & Velicer, 2004). While treatment efficacy is important, there has been little attention paid to the percentage of at risk populations reached by these treatments. A treatment with significantly less efficacy but greater reach might have a much greater impact on a population's health.

For example, a smoking cessation program that produced 30% abstinence at long-term follow-up would have 50% greater efficacy than a treatment that produced 20% abstinence. Most evidence-based approaches would recommend the treatment that produces 30% abstinence. However, if the more efficacious treatment only reached 5% of smokers, perhaps because it is expensive, time demanding, or required specialized care, it would have only a 1.5% impact on the problem of smoking (30% efficacy × 5% reach = 1.5% impact). If the lesser treatment reached 75% of smokers, it would have a 15% impact (20% efficacy × 75% reach = 15% impact). So the treatment with 50% less efficacy would end up having 10 times greater impact on the most deadly of addictions.

Look at the low impacts current behavioral services have on some of the most important health and mental health behaviors. When health care systems offer smoking cessation clinics for free, removing cost as a barrier, the percentage of eligible smokers who participate nationally is about 1% (Lichtenstein & Hollis, 1992).

Identification of mental health problems in primary care has increased from about 25% to 50%. But only about 8% of these mental health patients reach appropriate psychological services (Cummings, 2003). This means that psychotherapies and behavior therapies are reaching only 4% of the populations in need of such treatments. If all we reach with behavioral and psychological treatments are 1% to 4% of populations, it is clear that our fields can have little impact on health and mental health behaviors.

In an invited meeting with medical directors from 30 of the nation's largest health care systems, we discussed the multiple consequences and high costs of behaviors. The medical directors were then asked, "Where does most primary care take place?" At first they guessed clinics, offices, or emergency rooms. Then they agreed it is at home. Next they were asked, "Who provides most primary care?" They agreed it was the patient. For children it is mothers and for elderly who are ill it is daughters.

Then the medical directors were asked: "What is the quantity and quality of behavior medicine that patients take home to either prevent or manage chronic diseases?" They quickly concluded that the quantity is usually zero and the quality is usually awful. Our health care systems are in trouble not because we spend too much on high-cost behaviors. They are in trouble because we spend too little on assessing and treating these high-risk behaviors.

Science's Low Impact on Health and Mental Health Behaviors

Health care systems suffer because too few resources are invested in research on high-impact treatments for high-risk behaviors. Historically less than 10% of the National Institutes of Health's (NIH's) total budgets were awarded to behavioral research. Behavior science shares some of the responsibility for this problem. The amount of grants a discipline receives is related to the amount of consensus in that discipline. Advocates for behavior research at National Cancer Institute (NCI) generated support for $50,000,000 for a Request for Applications (RFA) for six Centers of Excellence for Cancer Communications that would target primarily behavioral and psychosocial factors related to the prevention and management of cancer. Because the review group could not reach a consensus, not a dollar was awarded to any of the 20 or more proposals that were submitted. Fortunately on a second round of the RFA the money was awarded. But that is also predictable. The less consensus in a discipline the more revisions and resubmits are needed for grants and publications, the longer are the publication lags, the fewer citations there are, and lower are the status and salaries of such disciplines. Behavioral and social sciences pay a big price for not having greater consensus, and most of our disciplines are not even aware of the price we pay.

Unfortunately it can also become costly to hold on to a consensus that needs to be changed. In the science of behavioral and psychological therapies, there has been a consensus amongst researchers that efficacy studies utilizing Randomized Clinical Trials (RCTs) are the gold standard for evaluating interventions. As a result, the vast majority of NIH behavioral grants have been awarded for efficacy trials. The expectation was that over time such trials would accumulate a body of evidence supporting treatments that could have important impacts on health and mental health problems.

But examine the evidence with smoking cessation where the largest number of RCTs have been completed. In the first U.S. Public Health Services' Clinical Guidelines for Treating Tobacco about 3,000 studies were identified (Fiore et al., 1996). Meta-analyses were done on the 300 best studies and evidence-based recommendations were made for a relatively broad range of behavioral and pharmaceutical treatments. When this author was invited to comment on the guidelines, it was noted that only about 1% of the guidelines addressed the needs of smokers who were in the precontemplation and contemplation stages of change and who therefore were not prepared to quit in the next month (Prochaska, 1996). It was recommended that a second volume was needed since more than 80% of all smokers (Velicer et al., 1995) and more than 90% of daily smokers in the United States are not prepared to quit in the next month (Wewers, Stillman, Hartman, & Shopland, 2003).

A second volume of guidelines was published in 2000 in part because there were now more than 6,000 studies that could be used as evidence for updated guidelines (Fiore et al., 2000). In spite of 6,000 studies there still were no evidence-based guidelines for the vast majority of smokers who were not prepared to quit in the next month. The guidelines for these smokers were still based on the clinical judgment of the editor-clinicians.

How can a science not study large percentages of populations who have the very problem that the science is supposed to solve? By definition efficacy trials are designed to produce as much efficacy as possible rather than as much impact. To maximize efficacy these trials rely in part on selectivity (Glasgow, Lichtenstein, & Marcus, 2003). With pharmaceutical trials, for example, great resources are invested to select the most compliant patients. Patients with comorbidities are omitted in part because medication for other conditions may interfere with the efficacy of the trial's medication.

In most behavioral treatment trials, such as for smoking cessation, patients are screened for motivation or readiness to quit. The reason is that most behavioral treatments are action-oriented and are designed for people who are prepared to take action in the immediate future such as the next month, 2 weeks or even 7 days (Zhu et al., 1996). The result is that considerable evidence is produced for the relatively small percentage of smokers who are most motivated or prepared to quit. And until recently there was practically no evidence supporting treatments for the large majority of smokers.

Most smoking cessation trials also exclude people with comorbidities, such as anxiety, depression, and other addictions. The result is an inadequate evidence base for smokers with mental health problems. This is particularly problematic given that recent estimates are that 44% of all cigarettes are bought by smokers with mental illness (Laser et al., 2000).

Applied researchers often assume that research should drive practice. The fact is that the opposite is more often true, with practice driving research. To understand why so much of treatment research has been designed to maximize efficacy instead of impacts we need to explore how most practices are designed to treat health and mental health behaviors.

Practices' Low Impact on Health Behaviors

Most health care practices are designed to treat acute conditions, even though chronic diseases have been the cause of a majority of deaths in the United States since the 1920s. Few health care practices are designed to treat the majority of chronic health behaviors that are major causes of chronic diseases. Historically acute care practices followed a passive–reactive paradigm where health professionals passively waited for patients to reach them and then they reacted. Such practices can work relatively well when people are feeling acute distress, pain, or illness. The majority of such populations can be expected to reach out for help and the professionals can react with the best treatments they have available.

The problem with chronic health behaviors, like smoking, alcohol abuse, inactivity, and unhealthy diets, is that they don't usually cause acute distress, pain, or illness.

Consequently most people with health risk behaviors are not motivated to seek help. The relatively small minority who do are usually assumed to be motivated to take action now. Health professionals, therefore, are likely to believe that all they need are action–oriented treatments for patients who are prepared to take action. Treatment researchers are likely to assume that what will be most helpful to practitioners are therapies designed for people who are well-prepared or motivated to take immediate action. The result is science and practices that produce too little impact on the majority who are not prepared to take action.

For decades there was no apparent problem until health organizations began to recognize that these health behaviors were so damaging and costly that they needed to be intervened on proactively. These behaviors needed to be construed as "silent killers" the way hypertension is understood. Clinical guidelines require that practices be proactive in screening, diagnosing, and treating hypertension. Similarly, with health behaviors like smoking, clinical guidelines call on clinicians to be proactive and to reach out to patients to offer help rather than wait passively for such patients to ask for help.

Once health care shifts from a passive–reactive to proactive approach to practice it can become painfully clear that the majority of patients are not prepared to take immediate action. Clinical guidelines indicate that clinicians should proactively ask all patients if they smoke, chart smoking status, and advise them to quit smoking. The evidence indicates that such proactive practice will increase quit rates from 3% to 6%, which can have important public health impacts (Fiore et al., 1996, 2000). The problem is, can health care professionals differentiate between 3% and 6% success or will they perceive 94% failure? Will such results then reinforce the number one reason why most American physicians do not practice behavior medicine? Two-thirds of physicians have come to believe that their patients cannot change their behavior or will not change their behavior (Orleans, George, Houpt, & Brodie, 1985).

Health care professionals can become demoralized by practicing an action paradigm. Here is a real case of a 48-year-old man with problems with obesity, smoking, alcohol abuse, and stress. He was diagnosed as having Type 2 diabetes. His physician, with all good intentions, told him he had to test his blood glucose twice a day, take his medication twice a day, quit smoking, change his diet, lose weight, and lower his stress. This is an action-oriented prescription for producing a noncompliant patient and a demoralized physician.

Practice's Low Impact on Mental Health Behaviors

Why are only about 4% of mental health patients receiving appropriate psychological treatment and why have less than 25% ever received professional treatment (Veroff, Douvan, & Kulka, 1981). Here there are more complications. First, it should be noted that the more distressing and disabling the mental health condition, the more likely that individuals are receiving or have received professional mental health services. This is the case, for example, with psychotic conditions that can be distressing and disabling. But even here, help is often sought because a parent, partner, teacher, or employer has been proactive in recognizing a problem and has been proactive in helping such patients receive appropriate treatment.

For some conditions, individuals do not perceive their behaviors as high-risk or problematic. Some individuals with alcohol or drug abuse are not yet experiencing negative effects of abuse on their health and well-being. Others are using alcohol and drugs to self-medicate anxiety, depression, and distress that might otherwise motivate them to seek help. Still others are faced with alcoholism as the disease of denial and are not aware of the negative consequences of their behavior.

Of course there are other major barriers that can keep clients from seeking mental health services. Stigma, no insurance coverage, inadequate insurance, or a lack of services in deprived or rural communities are all too real. Clearly, these barriers need to be addressed by society and health care systems.

Because of barriers and because of the way that individuals perceive their problems, people may seek help but not for their mental health problems directly. It is well established that a majority of patients in primary care offices are suffering from symptoms related to anxiety, depression, stress, alcohol abuse, or other mental health problems. Unless the primary care practice is proactive in diagnosing mental health conditions, they are likely to go undiagnosed, misdiagnosed, untreated, or mistreated.

As indicated earlier, even in the 50% of cases where the mental health problem is identified, only 8% of patients follow through and show up for the recommended mental health service. This is reminiscent of Ken Howard's reports of the modal number of sessions for psychotherapy prior to managed care. It was minus one: call and no show.

Similar results occur even at times of life-threatening crises. With patients in the hospital for heart attacks who are prescribed life-saving cardiac rehabilitation available for free, the percentage who show up nationally is 20% to 30% (Beckie, 2001). Who shows up more, men or women? Most health professionals guess women, which is a good guess, but wrong. With most problems, women will seek help at about twice the rate of men. But according to data on 12 health related behaviors on nearly 30,000 HMO members, the only behavior where men were further along in the stages of change is exercise (Rossi, 1992). Cardiac rehabilitation is an action-oriented treatment that is heavily exercise-based. If cardiac patients are not prepared to start an exercise program, then why show up for cardiac rehabilitation?

Higher Impact Paradigms That Can Complement Current Paradigms of Research and Practice

Why do passive–reactive action-oriented programs reach small percentages of populations? Smoking has been the number one public health problem in the United States for 40 years, but only 20% of all smokers are prepared to quit (Velicer et al., 1995). About 40% in precontemplation are not intending to quit in the next 6 months and 40% in contemplation are intending to quit in the next 6 months, but not in the next month. These distributions do not mean that public health campaigns have had no impact. In countries like China and Germany, about 70% of all smokers are in precontemplation and 5% are prepared to quit (Etter, Perneger, & Ronchi, 1997). We cannot have the majority of our science be action-oriented and expect to impact on the health of nations. Action-oriented treatments need to be complemented by treatments that match patients' needs at each stage of change.

In an initial population trial, proactive telephone calls were used to reach a representative sample of 5,000 smokers to offer home-based treatments that would match the needs of those who were ready to quit, getting ready, or not ready. Approximately 80% were recruited (Prochaska et al., 2001a). With 4,500 smokers in an HMO, approximately 85% were proactively recruited (Prochaska et al., 2001b). With alcohol abusers on campus, over 70% were recruited, even though 70% were in precontemplation and 10% were prepared to take action (Laforge, 2007). The stage distributions were similar to smokers in China. In a national sample of people who were not managing stress effectively, approximately 70% were recruited by telephone (Evers, Johnson, Padula, Prochaska, & Prochaska, 2002). On a Centers for Disease Control and Prevention (CDC) measure of depression, this population had mean scores that would lead people to seek help for emotional problems.

What happens when only one high-impact principle is applied to reach populations with behavioral treatments? A proactive program was designed to dramatically increase the impact of free smoking cessation clinics that were reaching only 1% of smokers (Lichtenstein & Hollis, 1992). Physicians took time with every smoker to get them to sign up for the action-oriented clinics. If that didn't work, nurses took up to 12 minutes to get them to sign up. If that didn't work, health educators in the practice took up to 15 minutes. And if that didn't work, proactive counselors called the smokers at home to get them to sign up. This is the most intensive proactive recruitment protocol in the literature. With smokers in the precontemplation stage, the proactive practices were able to get 35% to sign up, but only 3% showed up, 2% finished up, and 0% ended up quitting. With a combined group of smokers in the contemplation and preparation stages, 65% signed up, 15% showed up, 11% finished up, and some unreported percentage ended up quitting.

Clinic Paradigm Complemented by Home-Based Paradigm

Besides proactively reaching out to populations to offer help that can match wherever they are at, a third principle is that services need to be easily accessible. As indicated earlier, most of primary care takes place at home. One of the major reasons that primary care relies so heavily on pharmaceuticals is that these treatments are home-based. They are prescribed by the health professional in the clinic, but they are applied at home by the patient. Of course, the patient has to be prepared to apply the treatment appropriately.

In the conflict in psychology over prescription rights, what has not been debated enough is the need to have home-based treatments with demonstrated efficacy. The most common technique applied across diverse therapies is homework (Norcross, Prochaska, & Gallagher, 1989). Unfortunately, most of these home-based services have not been systematically evaluated. But why is homework so widely prescribed? Even when people receive psychotherapy in clinics, they spend more than 99% of their waking week outside of therapy. What they do the rest of the week accounts for more of outcomes than the 10% of the outcome variance attributed to within therapy sessions (Lambert, 1992). Imagine physicians trying to increase efficacy by just focusing on their interventions in the physician's office. Most primary care treatment is provided by the pharmaceutical industry, which specializes in therapeutics delivered at home. These treatments have to have demonstrated efficacy in order to be approved by the FDA. Prescription rights would provide psychologists and their patients with home-based and evidence-based treatments that could complement evidence-based treatments received in the clinic or office.

There are other reasons to develop home-based treatments with demonstrated efficacy. They can reach many more people and therefore have much greater impact on populations. Consider, for example, the major epidemic of obesity and overweight in the United States that has about doubled in both adolescent and adult populations in just 20 years (Hedley et al., 2004). There have also been considerable increases in diabetes at younger years and in serious complications like loss of sight and limbs at younger ages (Thorpe, Florence, Howard, & Joski, 2004). The costs of weight-related conditions have already passed the costs of smoking. These costs threaten to be the straw that breaks the back of health care systems.

In spite of the alarms there has not been a corresponding increase in populations seeking professional services. But, these specialties are not prepared to meet the needs of most of the population. Market research has found that less than 5% of these populations in the United States want clinic-based or group-based services (personal communication, Jenny Craig, 2001). Over 50% of these populations want home-based services. When told these statistics, this author predicted that commercial programs probably reached about 1% of the at-need populations. When asked how this accurate prediction was made, the author simply multiplied 5% by 20% (the percentage ready to take action) and the estimate was 1%.

When medications to help manage weight came on the market, there were immediate demands for such home-based services. Even though some of the medications were clearly high-risk and had to be removed from the market, large numbers of people turned to such treatments.

At the 2004 annual meeting of the Society of Behavior Medicine, leaders from national organizations like the CDC and the Robert Wood Johnson Foundation called for interventions to reverse the overweight and obesity epidemic. They cited leading psychologists, like Kelly Brownell, who advocate social policies, like taxing high-fat foods and super-sized portions, as effective interventions. They cited other leading psychologists, like Jim Sallis, who advocate environmental reengineering, like driving bans in downtown districts, which would require consumers and employees to walk to their destinations.

In contrast, clinic-based treatments, like cognitive-behavior therapies, were not on the leaders' agendas. Why do national leaders often ignore such solutions? Social policies and environmental controls are population-based interventions; psychotherapies and behavior therapies have not been. If such treatments are to become core components of national initiatives for reducing overweight and obesity, they will need to become population-based, including home-based behavior medicines. Of course, they will also need to scientifically demonstrate significant impacts.

From Fragmented to an Integrated Health Care Paradigm

Just as a home-based paradigm can make treatments more easily accessible, so too can an integrated health care paradigm. As an innovative approach to population health, this alternative would integrate services across biological and behavioral disciplines. One major HMO is experimenting with a model that integrates professionals from medicine, psychology, and nursing as primary care physicians who are prepared to proactively serve primary-care patients and their problems. Once patients are proactively identified as having health or mental health behaviors that need treatment, the practices do not rely on referring such patients to professionals in other clinics or offices. Data indicate that only 8% of the patients will show up for such services.

Patients with such behavioral and psychological needs are proactively introduced to a primary care physician who is a psychologist. The psychologist immediately begins an assessment process to determine the appropriate treatment. This approach results in 80% of the patients entering treatment rather than 8%. Clearly this proactive and integrative practice provides the potential for much higher impacts.

Once we reach high percentages, will they complete treatment? A meta-analysis found that about 50% of participants discontinued treatment quickly (Wierzbicki & Pekarik, 1993). Across most medications, discontinuation is about 50% (Johnson et al., 2006). In the psychotherapy meta-analysis, education, minority status, and having an addiction were the best predictors but they accounted for a small amount of variance (Wierzbicki & Pekarik). In studies on mental health, heroin treatment, obesity, smoking, and exercise, the best predictors of drop out were stage of change and the pros and cons of changing (e.g., Brogan, Prochaska, & Prochaska, 1999). With mental health problems, we predicted over 90% of dropouts. The entire 40% who had terminated prematurely had a stage profile of patients in precontemplation. The 15% who terminated quickly but appropriately were in the action stage. With patients who recently quit an addiction, the clinical plan would be relapse prevention. But relapse prevention would not fit clients in precontemplation. The clinical strategy would be dropout prevention. By matching treatment to stage, people in precontemplation can complete treatment at the same rates as those in preparation (e.g., Prochaska, DiClemente, Velicer, & Rossi, 1993; Prochaska et al. 2001a, b).

In a review of the addiction literature, Connors, Walitzer, and Dermen (2002) found dropouts ranged from 50% to 75%. They compared two strategies to standard care: role-induction, which teaches patients about their treatment responsibilities, and Motivational Interviewing (MI) based on a stage paradigm. With a single MI session, completion of treatment doubled from 25% to 50%. The role induction had no significant effect.

High drop out rates occur when therapists have 50 minutes to establish a therapeutic relationship. What will happen if the integrative care model relies on 15-minute sessions like the protocol used in the HMO pilots? One prediction is that primary care psychologists will end up relying heavily on prescriptions for home-based medication, the way many psychiatry practices have done.

What will integrative care do when patients choose not to use medications? What will they do if there are no medications for behaviors like exercise? What will they do if behaviors like exercise and diet are the healthiest approaches to problems like obesity and overweight?

Clinician and Computer Paradigms

Evidence-based behavioral treatments delivered at home may require that a traditional clinician paradigm be complemented by computers. Computers can provide individualized and interactive interventions with expert systems that model expert clinicians. A growing consensus holds that computer-generated tailored communications are one of the most promising approaches for population-based assessments and interventions (Kreuter, Strecher, & Glassman, 1999).

In a population trial for alcohol abuse, primary care physicians were able to identify less than 1% of patients. An alcohol specialist was able to identify 6%. An interactive computer in the office identified 10%, which is about the base rate in primary care offices (Butler, Chiauzzi, Bromberg, Budman, & Buono, 2002). Such computers could start a process that could have 10 times the impact of primary care clinicians and almost twice the rate of an alcohol specialist.

Expert systems provide guidance on principles and processes of change needed to progress through the stages (Velicer et al., 1993). For example, from 40 questions, smokers receive reliable and valid feedback about their stage, whether they underestimate the benefits of quitting and overestimate the cons, and which of 10 change processes they are underutilizing, overutilizing or utilizing appropriately compared to peers in the same stage who progressed the most. In follow-up interactions, participants receive normative feedback compared to peers and ipsative feedback compared to their previous assessments. Participants learn what they are doing right, what mistakes they are making, and what they can concentrate on to progress the most.

Clinicians can receive similar feedback about their clients and how they can most help particular clients. Such feedback at the third session on stage of change, motivation, and the quality of the therapeutic relationship reduced deterioration rates by 50% and doubled positive outcomes (Whipple et al., 2003). Interactive technologies are likely to be to behavior treatments what pharmaceuticals are to biological treatments: the most cost-effective means of bringing optimal amounts of science to bear on major health and mental health problems in entire populations in relatively user-friendly ways but with no known side effects.

Clinician and Computer–Based Clinical Trials

In our first clinical trial with smoking cessation, we compared four treatments: (1) The American Lung Association's (ALA's) action and maintenance manuals; (2) Stage-matched manuals; (3) Stage-matched manuals and three computer-based expert system guides; (4) The manuals, guides, and four proactive counselor telephone calls over a 6-month period (Prochaska et al., 1993). A reactive sample of 753 smokers was randomly assigned by stage. At 18 months, computers alone were more than twice as effective as the ALA treatments (24% vs. 11% point prevalence abstinence). Computers alone compared to computers plus counselors were tied at 12 months, but at 18 months counselors plus computers produced 18% abstinence compared to 24% for computers alone.

Unlike computers, clinicians can learn from clinical experience. They changed protocols. With 4,500 smokers proactively recruited from an HMO, the computer plus counselors outperformed computers alone at 12 months (25.6% vs. 20.6%). At 18 months, the counselor condition declined, computers increased, and both were tied at 23.2% point prevalence abstinence (Prochaska et al., 2001b).

What went wrong? One hypothesis is that clients can become dependent on counselors the way individuals become dependent on substances like nicotine. Historically, therapy studies on addictions showed a pattern of rapid relapse when therapy terminated

(Hunt & Belspalec, 1974). Such relapse was attributed to addictions being resistant to change. Some of the relapse is due to termination of treatment and loss of the social support and social monitoring treatment provides.

With computer guides, populations keep progressing to increased abstinence rather than show rapid declines. Computers may enhance self-efficacy (Bandura, 1997). When intervention ends, people keep progressing from efforts based on self-change or self-reliance. If people become dependent on clinicians, then one strategy is to fade out therapy just as we fade out nicotine.

In population trials of alcohol abuse on campus, Laforge (2007) proactively recruited 70% of eligible students. Three full, Transtheoretical Model (TTM)-tailored, expert feedback reports produced significant reductions in alcohol problems in females but not males. Males relied more on processes of resistance (e.g., reactance and rationalization), which were the main suppressors of treatment effects. Future treatments have to reduce processes of resistance to help male populations progress to less risky drinking. Resistance is a key challenge clinicians also face when treating individuals with addictions (Miller & Rollnick, 2002).

From Standardized to Tailored Paradigms

Ironically, the individual patient paradigm has been moving to standardized treatments that are manual driven, while the population paradigm is moving toward individually tailored treatments that are algorithm driven. Historically, clinician–delivered therapies were viewed as most efficacious because they were individualized and interactive. The biggest drawback of these therapies is that they could not be delivered practically to entire populations, and therefore had limited impacts. As interactive and individualized technologies have been developed and widely disseminated, population–based interventions can be delivered with more consistent quality because they are based on scientific algorithms designed to provide expert guidance. At the same time, science became increasingly concerned about considerable variability in quality across individual clinicians. To control for such variability the evidence-based movement has striven to standardize therapies by making them manual driven. The unexpected consequence could be that individualized patients treated by clinicians could receive standardized therapies, while entire populations treated by computers could receive individually tailored therapies.

What are the most common causes of variability in psychology? Individual differences are what make this science and profession so unique, complex, and variable. Scientists are trained to believe that variance can best be reduced through external controls. Here psychology would model public health with the belief that professional policies can control clinicians who can then better control their clients and their outcomes. After 35 years of science and practice, I am convinced that psychology cannot control individuals' behaviors the way medicine and public health can control some of biology and society. I am convinced we can influence behavior most effectively when we have the opportunity to interact with individuals. As a student in the 1960s, I learned that the purpose of psychology was to understand, predict, and control behavior. As a scientist-practitioner, I teach that the purpose is to understand, predict, and influence behavior by interacting with individuals on a patient and population basis.

For now an innovative alternative to standardizing treatments by the use of mandatory manuals is to individualize treatments by the use of tailored interactions. In TTM tailored interventions, behavior change is construed as a process that unfolds over time and involves progress through a series of stages. At different stages, specific processes and principles of change are emphasized to maximize progress to the next stage. Considerable research with tens of thousands of participants demonstrates that there are great individual differences in how people change. Individuals differ, for example, in which stage they enter therapy, and they differ considerably on how much they are applying each principle and process of change. They also differ considerably on how quickly or slowly they progress through the stages and how far they regress back through the stages when they slip back rather than move ahead.

Given how dynamic change is and how individualized the process is, interventions are best tailored to the needs of the individual client (e.g., Velicer et al., 1993). The tailoring process requires reliable and valid assessments at any point in time and across time. The intervention process also needs to be dynamic and adjustable to the individual needs of each client at each therapeutic interaction. Rather than individual differences being treated as variability that must be controlled, such differences are seen as opportunities for tailoring treatment to the individual's current needs. Rather than trying to control individual differences as a threat to validity, tailored interventions can be driven by such differences as a foundation for external validity. Here psychology can build on its rich heritage of appreciating individual differences while treating entire populations.

Look at how these individualized interventions can help populations that often are perceived as not having enough ability to change. With teenage smokers, for example, the report to the Surgeon General on adolescent smoking from the U.S. Department of Health and Human Services (HHS; 1994) said to not bother with cessation programs for adolescent smokers. They wouldn't participate, and if they did, they wouldn't quit. Without tailored treatments and counseling, primary care practices in a Kaiser HMO reached out to all teens and recruited about 65% to participate. At long-term follow-up, 23.9% of the adolescent smokers had quit (Hollis et al., 2005), which is the same as the approximately 24% rate we find with representative populations of adult smokers (Prochaska et al., 2001a, b).

Remember that with smokers with mental illness there were no evidence-based treatments in the 2000 Clinical Guidelines (Fiore et al., 2000). Colleagues at the University of California at San Francisco reached out to smokers in their depression clinic and offered our tailored treatments plus counseling and Nicotine Replacement Therapy (NRT) and produced 24.9% abstinence (Hall et al., 2006). Across our population trials, we found that African American smokers and Hispanic-American smokers had somewhat higher quit rates than non-Hispanic Whites. The oldest smokers had the highest quit rates (Velicer, Redding, Sun, & Prochaska, 2007). Treatment stereotypes have suggested that certain populations, like younger, older, minority, or impaired individuals do not have the same ability to change. These results indicate that the problem is not inability to change: the problem is inaccessibility to quality change programs.

From Single to Multiple Behavior Change Paradigms

Attempts to enhance impacts by increasing efficacy or participation have failed. Proactive methods that recruit 80%+ have limited potential to increase. Increasing efficacy by doubling contacts (Velicer & Prochaska, 1999), adding counseling calls (Prochaska et al.,

1993; 2001b), adding handheld nicotine fading computers (Prochaska et al., 2001b), nicotine replacement patches or telecounseling with computers have been unsuccessful (Velicer et al., 2006). An alternative approach is to treat multiple rather than single behaviors to enhance population health and well-being.

Clinical trials have the luxury of treating one problem. With nicotine replacement therapy, for example, smokers with mental health problems were excluded. Yet, as noted, 44% of cigarettes in the United States are bought by populations with mental health problems (Laser et al., 2000). In practice, the majority of clients have multiple problems. The highest risk and highest cost people are those with multiple behavior problems.

In our first multiple behavior trial, we recruited 83.6% of parents ($N = 2360$) of teenagers. Using three full TTM tailored, expert system guides for each relevant behavior, we produced significant impacts at 24 months on smoking, diet, and sun exposure (Prochaska et al., 2004). From primary care, we recruited 5,500 patients and produced significant effects at 24 months on the same three behaviors and on maintenance of regular mammographies (Prochaska et al., 2005). Comparing treatments just for smoking to multiple behavior treatments that included smoking, the long-term abstinence rates were the same (22% to 25%). Analyses across studies found that smokers treated for multiple behaviors were just as effective in quitting smoking as smokers treated for their single risk of smoking (Prochaska, Velicer, Prochaska, Delucchi, & Hall, 2006). We can increase impacts by treating multiple behaviors without decreasing efficacy for a single addictive behavior like smoking. These results would lead to an update of the impact equation to include the number of behaviors changed: Impact = Reach × Efficacy × Number of Behaviors.

A multiple-behavior paradigm could benefit behavioral interventions in multiple ways. One is to have systematic treatments for impacting on multiple behavior problems. Another is to evaluate current treatments on their impacts on multiple behaviors or targets. Traditional efficacy trials have a primary target on which treatment efficacy is assessed.

These efficacy trials are based on medical and pharmaceutical models in which there is expected to be high biological specificity for both the cause and the cure of a condition. With acute conditions, for example, there is expected to be a specific germ, like bacteria, that causes a specific infectious disease. Then there are specific biological agents like antibiotics that can cure the specific infectious disease. So, randomized controlled trials (RCTs) are supposed to target single specific conditions with a single specific treatment to assess the specific efficacy of the treatment.

Behaviors and psychological treatments are not specific to specific conditions. Yet, the history of RCTs is that we evaluate them as if they are. In the classic National Institute of Mental Health (NIMH) comparative therapies trial for depression, cognitive therapies and interpersonal therapy were found to produce comparable outcomes to antidepressant medications (Elkin et al., 1989). What if these trials were evaluated on their impacts on multiple-behavior outcomes, such as depression, interpersonal relationships, cognitive functioning, affective expression, substance use and abuse, and/or weight? Would the outcomes still be comparable?

Similarly, in a recent depression treatment trial, exercise was found to produce outcomes on the Beck Inventory that paralleled outcomes with a leading antidepressant medication (Blumenthal et al., 1999). Exercise is known, however, to have at least 50 scientific benefits (Reed, Velicer, Prochaska, Rossi, & Marcus, 1997). How many scientific benefits are there from an antidepressant? If evaluated on multiple behavior changes, would exercise have greater impacts than antidepressants?

How many scientific benefits are there from psychotherapy? When asked that question, large audiences of therapists, counselors, and other psychologists do not know. Nor does this author know. It is remarkable that no one seems to know how many scientific benefits there are from one of behavior science's leading services. Pharmaceutical companies spend millions of dollars just to be able to make an additional valid claim for a specific medication. All of behavior science seems to have spent few resources to substantiate the many scientific benefits of psychotherapy.

High Specificity vs. High Generality

Psychology as a science and a profession is often seen as handicapped by the relatively low specificity of many of its most important variables. Science often places highest priority on high specificity and sensitivity of its most important variables. For example, an American Cancer Society Task Force was asked to predict the future of cancer prevention research and practice. About half the task force was genetically based and half were behaviorally based.

The genetically based scientists impressed the group with the specificity of their knowledge. Specific genes were found to produce one specific type of breast cancer. Other specific genes were found to produce a specific type of colon cancer. The implications for the future were clear: once medicine could re-engineer these genes, then specific types of breast cancer and colon cancer could be prevented.

How did the behaviorists respond? They asked what percentage of all breast cancers or colon cancers were caused by specific genes. The answer was 1% to 3%. The behaviorists could claim that about 30% of all cancer deaths are caused by a single behavior—smoking. And that's just cancer. The fundamental importance of such behaviors is that they have high generality rather than specificity. Such behaviors do not respect the boundaries of specific organs or specific diseases. These are broad-based variables that can have huge impacts on preventing and managing disease.

In modeling medicine and modeling biology, behavior science can seriously limit its impacts. A recent president of the American Psychological Association (APA) claimed that psychology's serious mistake was to model medicine rather than public health. Better still is the opportunity for psychology to develop a higher impact model for health and mental health.

Higher Impact Science and Service

Table 4.1 illustrates how in psychology we complement traditional paradigms of science and practice with emerging paradigms to increase impacts on health and mental health. Table 4.1 also illustrates how each of the ten paradigms cluster together as preferred approaches to science and practice of health and mental health. The acute care paradigms rely most often on a passive–reactive approach to practice, efficacy trials for science,

Table 4.1	**Two Clusters of Paradigms for Individual Patients and Populations**	
	Patient Health Complemented by	**Population Health**
	1. Individual Patients	1. Entire Populations
	2. Passive Reactive	2. Proactive
	3. Acute Conditions	3. Chronic Conditions
	4. Efficacy Trials	4. Effectiveness Trials
	5. Action Oriented	5. Stage-based
	6. Clinic-based	6. Home-based
	7. Clinician Delivered	7. Technology Delivered
	8. Standardized	8. Tailored
	9. Single Target Behavior	9. Multiple Target Behaviors
	10. Fragmented	10. Integrated

action-oriented treatments, standardized clinic based treatments delivered for single targets within individual patients. The emerging paradigms need to rely on proactive approaches to reaching entire populations to maximize impacts on multiple behaviors treated by tailored communications delivered primarily by patients using technologies at home. A more comprehensive approach to health and mental health behaviors would not substitute one particular paradigm for another, but rather would integrate traditional paradigms as special cases of higher impact approaches to science and practice. The passive–reactive paradigm, for example, is the special case for individual clients who reach out for treatment because of acute distress, pain, or illness. The proactive approach is the more general case designed to reach entire populations, including those in acute distress as well as those with chronic conditions not currently experiencing distress. Efficacy is integrated as part of a more general impact equation just as a multiple-behavior paradigm can include a single-behavior approach when select clients have only single conditions. The important point is we do not discard all of the outstanding knowledge and practices produced by past paradigms. Instead we can complement these approaches with more comprehensive paradigms that can produce science and practices that can have much greater impacts on health and mental health behaviors.

Lest some professionals become reactant by perceived risks from such paradigm enhancements, let us examine some of the anticipated consequences of such changes. First of all, current practices would not disappear. There is no discussion here of an either/or approach to science or treatment. In the history of transportation development, when trains were developed ships did not disappear. And when planes were developed, automobiles did not disappear. What is likely to disappear is our frustrating attempts of trying to treat health and mental health behaviors in health care systems that are essentially designed to deliver diagnoses and drugs. This is the treatment equivalent of trying to drive automobiles down railroad tracks. What is needed are scientific and practice paradigms that are designed to treat high-risk and high-cost behaviors seriously.

With more inclusive paradigms for research and practice, we can produce more inclusive approaches to care. Wouldn't it be wonderful if our highest-impact approaches to science and practice enhanced not only health, but also social justice?

REFERENCES

Bandura, A. (1997). *Self-efficacy: The exercise of control.* New York: W. H. Freeman and Company.

Beckie, J. (2001). *A womens' only cardiac rehabilitation program.* Grant funded by National Institute of Nursing Research (NINR).

Blumenthal, J. A., Babyak, M. A., Moore, K. A., Craighead, W. E., Herman, S., Khtri, P., et al. (1999). Effects of exercise training on older patients with major depression. *Archives of Internal Medicine, 159,* 2349–2356.

Brogan, M. M., Prochaska, J. O., & Prochaska, J. M. (1999). Predicting termination and continuation status in psychotherapy by using the transtheoretical model. *Psychotherapy, 36,* 105–113.

Butler, S. F., Chiauzzi, E., Bromberg, J. I., Budman, S. H., & Buono, D. P. (2002). Computer-assisted screening for alcohol problems in primary care. *Journal of Technology in Human Services, 2,* 1–19.

Connors, G., Walitzer, K., & Dermen, K. (2002). Preparing clients for alcoholism treatment: Effects on treatment participation and outcomes. *Journal of Consulting and Clinical Psychology 70,* 1161–1169.

Cummings, W. A. (2003, February). *The implosion of managed care.* Keynote address presented at the 14th Annual Art and Science Health Promotion Conference, Washington, DC.

Edington, D. W. (2001). Emerging research: A view from One Research Center. *American Journal of Health Promotion, 15,* 341–369.

Elkin, I., Shea, T., Watkins, J. T., Imber, S. D., Sotsky, S. M., Collins, J. F., et al. (1989). National Institute of Mental Health treatment of depression collaborative research program: General effectiveness of treatments. *Archives of General Psychiatry, 46,* 971–982.

Etter, J. F., Perneger, T. V., & Ronchi, A. (1997). Distributions of smokers by stage: International comparison and association with smoking prevalence. *Preventive Medicine, 25,* 480–585.

Evers, K. E., Johnson, J. L., Padula, J. A., Prochaska, J. M., & Prochaska, J. O. (2002). Stress management development for transtheoretical constructs of decisional balance and confidence. *Annals of Behavioral Medicine, S24.*

Fiore, M. C., Bailey, W. C., Cohen, S. J., Dorfman, S. F., Goldstein, M. G., Gritz E. R., et al. (1996). *Treating tobacco use and dependence: Clinical practice guideline.* Rockville, MD: U.S. Department of Health and Human Services, Public Health Service.

Fiore, M. C., Bailey, W. C., Cohen, S. J., Dorfman, S. F., Goldstein, M. G., Gritz, E. R., et al. (2000). *Treating tobacco use and dependence: Clinical practice guideline.* Rockville, MD: U.S. Department of Health and Human Services, Public Health Service.

Glasgow, R. E., Lichtenstein, E., & Marcus, A. C. (2003). Why don't we see more translation of health promotion research to practice? Rethinking the efficacy-to-effectiveness transition. *American Journal of Public Health, 93,* 1261–1267.

Hall, S. M., Tsoh, J., Prochaska, J., Eisendrath, S., Rossi, J. S., Redding, C. A., et al. (2006). Treatment of depressed mental health outpatients for cigarette smoking: A randomized clinical trial. *American Journal of Public Health, 96*(10), 1808–1814.

Hedley, A. A., Ogden, C. L., Johnson, C. L., Carroll, M. D., Curtain, L. R., & Flegal, K. M. (2004). Prevalence of overweight and obesity among US children, adolescents, and adults, 1999–2002. *The Journal of the American Medical Association, 29,* 2847–2850.

Hollis J. F., Polen, M. R., Whitlock, E. P., Lichtenstein, E., Mullooly, J., Velicer, W. F., et al. (2005). Teen REACH: Outcomes from a randomized controlled trial of a tobacco reduction program for teens seen in primary medical care. *Pediatrics, 115*(4), 981–989.

Hunt, W. A., & Bespalec, D. A. (1974). An evaluation of current methods of modifying smoking behavior. *Journal of Clinical Psychology, 30,* 431–438.

Johnson, S. S., Driskell, M. M., Johnson, J. L., Dyment, S. J., Prochaska, J. O., Prochaska, J. M., et al. (2006). Transtheoretical model intervention for adherence to lipid-lowering drugs. *Disease Management, 9*(2), 102–114.

Kreuter, M. K., Strecher, V. J., & Glassman, B. (1999). One size does not fit all: The case for tailoring cancer prevention materials. *Annals of Behavioral Medicine, 21,* 276–283.

Krishnan, K. R. (1999). Effects of exercise training on older patients with major depression. *Archives of Internal Medicine, 159,* 2349–2356.

Laforge, R. G. (2007). *A population based individualized alcohol harm reduction program feedback intervention.* Manuscript submitted for publication.

Lambert, M. J. (1992). Implications of outcome research for psychotherapy integration. In J. C. Norcross & M. R. Goldfried (Eds.), *Handbook of psychotherapy integration* (pp. 94–129). New York: Basic.

Laser, K., Boyd, J. W., Woolhandler, S., Himmelstein, D. U., McCormick, D., & Bor, D. H. (2000). Smoking and mental illness: A population-based prevalence study. *The Journal of the American Medical Association, 284,* 2606–2610.

Lichtenstein, E., & Hollis, J. (1992). Patient referral to a smoking cessation program: Who follows through? *Journal of Family Practice, 34,* 739–744.

Miller, W. R., & Rollnick, S. (2002). *Motivational interviewing* (2nd ed.). New York: Guilford Press.

Norcross, J. C., Prochaska, J. O., & Gallagher, K. (1989). Clinical psychologists in the 1980's: II. Theory, research and practice. *The Clinical Psychologist, 42,* 45–53.

Orleans, C. T., George, L. K., Houpt, J. L., & Brodie, H. K. H. (1985). Health promotion in primary care: A survey of U.S. family practitioners. *Preventive Medicine, 14,* 636–647.

Prochaska, J. J., Velicer, W. F., Prochaska, J. O., Delucchi, K., & Hall, S. M. (2006). Comparing intervention outcomes in smokers treated for single versus multiple behavioral risks. *Health Psychology, 25*(3), 380–388.

Prochaska, J. O. (1996). Guidelines for smoking cessation, Vol. 1: For the minority of smokers ready to quit. *Abstracts of Clinical Care Guidelines, 8*(6), 1–10.

Prochaska, J. O., DiClemente, C., Velicer, W., & Rossi, J. S. (1993). Standardized, individualized, interactive and personalized self-help programs for smoking cessation. *Health Psychology, 12,* 399–405.

Prochaska, J. O., & Velicer, W. F. (2004). Integrating population smoking cessation policies and programs. *Public Health Reports, Journal of the U.S. Public Health Service, 119,* 244–252.

Prochaska, J. O., Velicer, W. F., Fava, J. L., Rossi, J. S., & Tsoh, J. Y. (2001a). Evaluating a population-based recruitment approach and a stage-based expert system intervention for smoking cessation. *Addictive Behaviors, 26,* 583–602.

Prochaska, J. O., Velicer, W. F., Fava, J., Ruggiero, L., Laforge, R., & Rossi, J. R. (2001b). Counselor and stimulus control enhancements of a stage matched expert system for smokers in a managed care setting. *Preventive Medicine, 32,* 23–32.

Prochaska, J. O., Velicer, W. F., Redding, C. A., Rossi, J. S., Goldstein, M., DePue, J., et al. (2005). Stage-based expert systems to guide a population of primary care patients to quit smoking, eat healthier, prevent skin cancer and receive regular mammograms. *Preventive Medicine, 41,* 406–416.

Prochaska, J. O., Velicer, W. F., Rossi, J. S., Redding, C. A., Greene, G. W., Rossi, S. R., et al. (2004). Multiple risk expert systems interventions: Impact of simultaneous stage-matched expert system interventions for smoking, high-fat diet and sun exposure in a population of parents. *Health Psychology, 23,* 503–516.

Reed, G. R., Velicer, W., Prochaska, J. O., Rossi, J. S., & Marcus, B. (1997). What makes a good staging algorithm?: Examples from regular exercise. *American Journal of Health Promotion, 12,* 57–66.

Rossi, J. S. (1992). *Stages of change for 15 health risk behaviors in an HMO population.* Paper presented at the 13th Annual Meeting of the Society for Behavioral Medicine, New York, NY.

Thorpe, K. E., Florence, C. S., Howard, D. H., & Joski, P. (2004). The impact of obesity on rising medical spending. *Health Affairs, 4,* 480–486.

U.S. Department of Health and Human Services (HHS). (1994). *Preventing tobacco use among young people: A report to the Surgeon General.* HHS, Public Health Services, Centers for Disease Control and Prevention and Health Promotion, Atlanta, GA.

U.S. Department of Health and Human Services (HHS). (2000). *Healthy people 2010: Understanding and improving health* (2nd ed.). Washington, DC: U.S. Government Printing Office.

Velicer, W. F., Fava, J. L., Prochaska, J. O., Abrams, D. B., Emmons, K. M., & Pierce, J. (1995). Distribution of smokers by stage in three representative samples. *Preventive Medicine, 24,* 401–411.

Velicer, W. F., Friedman, R. H., Fava, J. L., Gulliver, S. B., Keller, S., Sun, X., et al. (2006). Evaluating nicotine replacement therapy and stage-based therapies in a population-based effectiveness trial. *Journal of Consulting and Clinical Psychology, 74*(6), 1162–1172.

Velicer, W. F., & Prochaska, J. O. (1999). An expert system intervention for smoking cessation. *Patient Education Counseling, 36,* 119–129.

Velicer, W. F., Prochaska, J. O., Bellis, J. M., DiClemente, C. C., Rossi, J. S., Fava, J. L., et al. (1993). An expert system intervention for smoking cessation. *Addictive Behaviors, 18,* 269–290.

Velicer, W. F., Redding, C. A., Sun, X., & Prochaska, J. O. (2007). Demographic variables, smoking variables, and outcome across five studies. *Health Psychology, 26*(3), 278–287.

Veroff, J., Douvan, E., & Kulka, R. A. (1981). *Mental health in America.* New York: Basic Books.

Wewers, M. E., Stillman, F. A., Hartman, A. M., & Shopland, D. R. (2003). Distribution of daily smokers by stage of change: Current population survey results. *Preventive Medicine, 36,* 710–720.

Whipple, J. L., Lambert, M. J., Vermeersch, D. A., Smart, D. W., Nielsen, S. L., & Hawkins, E. J. (2003). Improving the effects of psychotherapy: The use of early identification of treatment and problem-solving strategies in routine practice. *Journal of Counseling Psychology, 50,* 59–68.

Wierzbicki, M., & Pekarik, G. (1993). A meta-analysis of psychotherapy dropout. *Professional Psychology, 29,* 190–195.

Zhu, S. H., Stretch, V., Balabanis, M., Rosbrook, B., Sadler, G., & Pierce, J. P. (1996). Telephone counseling for smoking cessation: Effects of single-session and multiple-session interventions. *Journal of Consulting and Clinical Psychology, 64,* 202–11.

2

New Procedures and Policies—Implications for Funders, Researchers, and Policy Makers

What Types of Public Health Proposals Should Agencies Be Funding and What Types of Evidence Should Matter?: Scientific and Ethical Considerations

David R. Buchanan
and John P. Allegrante

Introduction

The national *Healthy People 2010* goal of eliminating health disparities has raised questions about the differences between individual medical interventions and community-wide public health interventions in terms of the best way to achieve this goal. When the focus of research shifts from investigating the efficacy of new experimental treatments on individuals to evaluating the effectiveness of community interventions in entire populations (also see Prochaska, chapter 4), however, at least two new major ethical considerations arise that deserve greater attention.

The first issue concerns the concept of and procedures for demonstrating respect for community autonomy. This topic is analogous to Beecher's (1966) original concept of individual informed consent and its primacy as an ethical component in research with human subjects. The second issue focuses on the demands of distributive justice and the ethical necessity of allocating scarce public resources fairly across different types of health research, in order to fulfill the National Institutes of Health (NIH) mission of uncovering "new knowledge that will lead to better health for everyone" (NIH, 2004). To address these concerns, this chapter delves into critical issues involved in finding an appropriate balance between scientific and ethical considerations in assessing the merits of community health intervention research, when the purpose of the research is to discover how health disparities can best be eliminated.

We begin this chapter with a description of the distinct characteristics of public health interventions, noting, in particular, how such interventions differ from clinical medical treatments. From there, we discuss the emerging challenges to the field posed by the recent call for "evidence-based" public health (Green, 2006). The main portion of the chapter addresses the need for achieving a sound balance among the demands for collecting the most rigorous scientific evidence possible, the intractable constraints faced in designing research on community interventions, and the rights of community members to be involved in the decisions about the goals and methods of community research, since such intervention research holds the potential to affect their lives in ways both intended and unintended. We then take up the question of ethical concerns regarding the fair allocation of public resources at NIH—a question of distributive justice. Based on the apparent disproportionate level of funding favoring clinical trials over community interventions, we argue that the skew toward individual interventions has resulted in an undue emphasis on individual behavior change as a common yet not necessarily warranted outcome measure in the hierarchy of funded research. In contrast, we present a proposal for broadening the types of evidence that should matter in assessing the potential value of community intervention studies. To address evident value conflicts between scientific promise and community responsiveness, the chapter concludes with a recommendation based on the work of Daniels and Sabin (1997) for using a fair procedure, called "accountability for reasonableness," for making decisions regarding the priority of different types of health research.

Public Health Interventions

In its landmark 1988 report, *The Future of Public Health*, the Institute of Medicine defined public health as follows: "Public health is what we, as a society, do collectively, to assure the conditions for people to be healthy" (Institute of Medicine, 1998, p. 19). The definition is notable for its emphasis on a collective social responsibility for the health of the population, and for its focus on fostering the ecological conditions necessary to protect and to promote the health of people living in communities. Drawing on this definition and other kindred reports (Institute of Medicine, 2002; Pew Health Commission, 1998), the two fundamental features that are now generally considered to distinguish public health from medicine are first, where medicine focuses on the individual patient, public health addresses the health of the population as a whole; and second, where medicine is mainly concerned with treating patients who are ill to restore health, public health concentrates primarily on the prevention of disease to help people maintain and promote their health. Based on these distinctions, public health interventions characteristically involve the enactment and dissemination of new policies and programs that create changes in the physical and social environments; these changes are designed to protect people and to enable preventive actions that promote the health of entire population groups.

It may be helpful to consider a couple of examples to illustrate the differences between medicine and public health. One topical example is syringe exchange programs and their effects on risk behavior and HIV prevention (Braine, Des Jarlais, Ahmad, Purchase, & Turner, 2004). Such programs create changes in both the physical and social environments that enable people at high risk to protect themselves from exposure to HIV. They are intended to prevent people from becoming infected with HIV, in contrast to medicine's principal obligation to treat people after they become infected. Another representative example is a program to reduce drunk-driving deaths developed by Holder and his colleagues (2000; 2002). This community-based intervention program had five major components: (1) community mobilization through media advocacy; (2) responsible beverage service training programs; (3) stepped up police roadblock sobriety checks; (4) crackdowns on alcohol sales to minors; and, (5) a reduction in the number of alcohol retail outlets. Clearly, this program involves a number of complex changes in the ecology of human behavior, changes that are intended to make drunk driving less likely. Illustrating the point, Hanson's chart of the "injury iceberg" (Figure 5.1) shows how public health programs characteristically seek to address a broad range of interpersonal, organizational, community, and societal level factors, whereas interventions that focus on the individual address only those biological, behavioral, and psychological causes of injury that are "above the waterline," while ignoring both physical and social environmental causes of injury that reside "below the waterline" (Hanson et al., 2005). These examples lay the foundation for understanding the unique challenges confronting efforts aimed at assessing the effectiveness of public health interventions in standard experimental research designs, demands that are increasingly being imposed on the field.

Challenges Facing Evidence-Based Public Health

In the wake of calls for "evidence-based" medicine (Evidence-Based Working Group, 1992), the field of public health now faces mounting pressures to gather evidence that public health programs and policies do, in fact, achieve their stated goals of decreasing morbidity and mortality rates and reducing health disparities (Green, 2006). Based on certain scientific standards for assessing the quality of research evidence, a hierarchy of research designs has by now become well established (see Table 5.1). At the pinnacle of this hierarchy is the randomized controlled trial (RCT), which is universally regarded as the "gold standard" of health research, because other research designs fail to control for various well-known threats to the validity of the research results (see Table 5.2). Unfortunately, due to their distinct goals and methods, public health interventions face a number of what we refer to as "structural impediments" that frequently make rigorous testing community interventions in RCTs virtually impossible. These structural impediments include practical, political, economic, and other constraints.

Practical Constraints

The first major challenge to designing and executing studies of community interventions is that, in contrast to well-controlled laboratory studies, communities are open and dynamic systems, with a virtually unlimited number of factors that may influence health outcomes. To improve the quality of community interventions, Flay (1986) has recommended testing the interventions under consideration in phases, from pilot tests, to prototype studies, to efficacy trials, and so on. But, due to the many variables operating at the community level, single discrete interventions have often been found to yield a null or minimal effect. Because it is impossible to control for the innumerable factors influencing community dynamics, public health interventions generally require tests of the cumulative impact of multiple interventions simultaneously, in order to achieve a "critical mass" to produce a detectable effect at the population level. Significantly, since it is often not possible to demonstrate the efficacy of the individual components

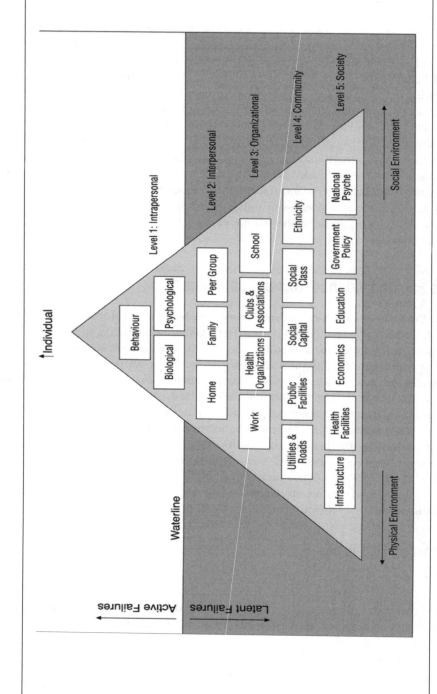

The "Injury Iceberg" ecological model, showing the relationship of the individual to the physical and social environment and levels of intervention. From "The Injury Iceberg: An Ecological Approach to Planning Sustainable Community Safety Interventions." by D. Hanson. J. Hanson. P. Vardon. K. McFarlane. J. Lloyd. R. Muller. et al. 2005. *Health Promotion Journal of Australia. 16*(1). 6. Copyright © 2005 by the *Health Promotion Journal of Australia.* Reprinted by permission.

Table 5.1	Hierarchy of Knowledge

- Randomized Controlled Trials
- Quasi-Experimental Research Designs
- Prospective Cohort Studies
- Cross-sectional Studies
- Retrospective Case-Control Studies
- Case Series & Registries
- Case Studies

Source: Evidence-Based Working Group. (1992). Evidenced-based medicine: A new approach to teaching the practice of medicine. *JAMA, 268*(17), 2420–2425.

first, community health intervention research faces a much greater burden in providing convincing preliminary evidence to demonstrate the plausibility of achieving positive results in a full-scale trial. Responsible beverage service training programs, for example, seem like a good idea, but it is difficult to demonstrate their impact on alcohol-involved traffic fatality rates when tested independently of other complementary efforts. On the other side of this same coin, plans for data analysis in community intervention research are necessarily much more complicated than clinical studies, which involve fewer confounding or uncontrolled factors that need to be taken into account (also see Prochaska, chapter 4). This problem imposes inextricable demands for even larger sample sizes in public health research.

The question of calculating adequate sample sizes for testing community interventions is controversial. Because such interventions are intended to produce effects at the community level (e.g., changes in a particular targeted morbidity or mortality rate for a geographic region), statisticians generally argue that the most appropriate unit of analysis is the community as a whole. Hence, the most rigorous research designs require randomly assigning communities, rather than individuals, to the different study conditions, in what are called group-randomized trials. When communities are the unit of analysis, however, studies of public health interventions are burdened with recruiting a large number of communities to participate in the research, a difficult, labor-intensive and time-consuming process (Luepker et al., 1994). Moreover, group-randomized trials are highly susceptible to selection biases, differential histories, and contamination due to the inherently small sample sizes (i.e., the number of communities) (Murray, 2001). That is, if the number of groups is less than 20, odds are that systematic differences between groups cannot be

Table 5.2	Common Well-Known Threats to Internal Validity

- History
- Maturation
- Testing
- Instrumentation
- Statistical regression
- Selection biases
- Attrition
- Hawthorne effect

overcome by standard randomization procedures. In such situations, the recommended course is to use matched stratification procedures, but matching can be implemented only if the most significant variables influencing community dynamics are known in advance, and then, if known, subsequently identifying communities that can be so matched. Even with such matching procedures, due to the relatively small numbers, it takes few unanticipated events that differentially affect the target communities (e.g., teens killed in a drunk-driving accident) to undermine the validity of the research results. In short, in terms of concrete practical considerations, community-wide intervention studies face major hurdles.

Political Constraints

In addition to practical constraints, one of the most significant challenges confronting research on community interventions is that public health interventions often involve policy changes, and randomly assigning communities to comparison conditions is frequently unacceptable for patent political reasons. For instance, it is reasonable to hypothesize that limiting the amount of added sugar in food products will reduce obesity rates, but politically, it is simply not feasible to randomly assign counties or states to treatment and comparison conditions to test this hypothesis. Similarly, many public health professionals are concerned about the impact of junk-food advertising on children's television, but demonstrating the positive impact of banning such ads in an RCT is politically impossible.

The feasibility of using RCTs becomes even more tenuous if there is speculation about potential unintended adverse effects. Syringe exchange programs, for example, have long been embroiled in arguments about whether their establishment condones drug use (Buchanan, Shaw, Ford, & Singer, 2003). Due to such moral and political compunctions, many public health interventions cannot be investigated in RCT research designs.

Economic Constraints

As noted above, the most robust research designs for testing the efficacy of public health interventions require large numbers of communities to be assigned to the intervention and comparison conditions. Such studies, however, are enormously expensive. A small number of group-randomized research designs have been conducted; the most well known is the COMMIT trial, in which 22 U.S. cities were randomly assigned to treatment and comparison conditions in an experiment designed to reduce smoking prevalence (Community Intervention Trial for Smoking Cessation [COMMIT], 1995a, 1995b). The cost of the COMMIT trial has been estimated at approximately $60 million, but unfortunately, as Murray (2001, p. 310) notes, "The disappointing results for several large trials have led some to question the value of group-randomized trials." Given their high cost and questionable track record, it appears unlikely that major group-randomized community intervention trials will be funded in the foreseeable future.

Other Constraints

On top of these many challenges, a lively debate has recently sprung up around questions of external validity and the degree to which local contextual factors may influence outcomes (Green & Glasgow, 2006). Green (1977), for example, has argued that achieving a balance between high internal validity, or "true efficacy" and high external validity, or "true effectiveness" in broader applications is one of the key dilemmas facing public health researchers when designing evaluative studies. Suffice to say, because communities are open, dynamic, and complex systems, an unresolved question is whether there are limits on the generalizability of community interventions, or conversely, the degree to which factors unique to the specific context (e.g., the particular political actors, the historical background, community composition, etc.) largely determine the success or failure of different efforts. A key point of contention, with little resolution in sight, is how much interventions can be adapted to suit local conditions before they should be considered a "different" or "new" program.

There are other technical issues that we could list, but the thrust of these concerns has been to underscore questions about the feasibility of conducting RCTs to determine the effectiveness of community interventions. If the combined impact of various structural impediments poses virtually insurmountable barriers to conducting the most rigorous research possible on public health interventions, then it is critically important to ask what a fair and equitable resolution of this state of affairs might be. Thus, the question is this: Should research on public health interventions simply be relegated to a lower status and lower priority in the allocation of limited research funding because such investigations will inevitably produce less rigorous, and more uncertain and debatable results? Or are there additional ethical considerations, beyond the rigor of the research, that merit further consideration in seeking a just resolution of these tensions?

Ethical Considerations in Community Intervention Research

In addition to the problems caused by the structural constraints described above, research on community interventions presents unique ethical challenges as well. In such public health research, one major concern is that the specification of an ethical process that is morally equivalent to the individual informed consent process used in clinical trials has not yet been formulated (Buchanan & Miller, 2006a). In clinical research, the process of gaining informed consent is straightforward; the purpose of the research, its methods, risks, and benefits (if any) are explained and the individual decides whether she wants to participate. But how is this procedure supposed to be extended to an entire community? If community members have a right to autonomy and it is ethically unwarranted for researchers to conduct health research without their agreement, then the critical ethical challenge is to lay out how respect for community autonomy should be secured.

In past practice, despite the fact that Institutional Review Boards (IRBs) are required to have at least one community representative, respect for community autonomy has generally been neglected. Based on IRB deliberations about whether the risks are sufficiently minimal that individual informed consent can be waived, IRB approval alone has been considered adequate to authorize community health intervention research. When an experimental intervention has been determined to pose minimal risks, IRBs have waived the consent requirement and permitted community intervention trials to proceed.

While IRB review for community health intervention research may be adequate in certain limited circumstances, it restricts the scope of investigations to relatively innocuous interventions (e.g., mass media campaigns), and thus, is not sufficient for the majority of public health work. Consider the aforementioned public health research question regarding the effect of police roadblocks to screen for impaired drivers, with the goal of identifying effective strategies to reduce traffic fatalities. At the individual level, is it fair to assume that the average social drinker would consider participating in the roadblock experiment in one's interest? At the community level, do community members have a right to question why their community was selected, whether they wish to participate, or whether alternative strategies should be considered? Would an IRB be justified in designating such research as posing only minimal risk?

To test more powerful community interventions, IRB approval alone cannot suffice. There must be a process that serves the same ethical function as individual informed consent, where the community as a whole can decide whether it is in their interests to participate. The dual needs for avoiding exploitation and affirming the community's right to autonomy have led researchers to try to address these concerns by establishing Community Advisory Boards (CABs), based on the model of oversight at federally-funded community health centers.

Stipulating an ethical standard that requires establishing a CAB is an important first step in addressing the ethical challenges posed by conducting public health research, but it is not enough. It immediately raises questions about representation: Who should sit on these boards? Who can legitimately speak on behalf of community interests? How should they be selected? What is an appropriate number of CAB members? What is the scope of their responsibilities? What sorts of decisions (e.g., research methods, budget allocations, personnel, etc.) should they be authorized to make?

Other researchers, particularly advocates of community-based participatory research, have recommended that additional processes should be required to insure the legitimacy of the consent process and to respect the community's right to self-determination. Recommended procedures include interviews with stakeholders and key informants, focus groups, community surveys, community forums, and partnerships with existing community associations (Buchanan, Miller, & Wallerstein, 2007; Israel et al., 2003; also see El-Bassel, Witte, & Gilbert, chapter 15). Likewise, Emanuel and his colleagues (2004) have recently articulated an ethical requirement for community collaboration in international health research; the requirement of community collaboration has been put forward as a necessary bulwark against the exploitation of vulnerable populations. They have identified seven indicators to gauge the degree to which this ethical requirement has been fulfilled (see Table 5.3). Moreover, the scope of researchers' duty to provide benefits to the community—in one form or another—is now being actively debated, a new development that portends even greater demands on public health researchers (Belsky & Richardson, 2004).

To address this concern, we recommend the following standard as one possible model: the more powerful the intervention and the greater the possibility of exploitation, the more demanding the process of gaining community participation should be in ratifying the decision to allow the research to be conducted in their community. The most powerful interventions must implement processes that aim at maximum feasible participation. Strategies in response to proposed research in Indian Country provide a model for broader community participation. Several tribes or tribal entities, most notably the Navajo Nation, have created their own separate Institutional Review Boards with stringent requirements of community support, evidence of community-wide benefit, and

Table 5.3	**Indicators of Community Collaboration**

- Developing partnerships between researchers, policy makers and the community;
- Involving community partners in sharing responsibilities for identifying important health problems;
- Involving community partners in assessing the value of the research;
- Involving community partners in planning, conducting, and overseeing research;
- Involving community partners in integrating research into the health care system;
- Respecting the community's values, culture, traditions, and social practices;
- Ensuring that the community members receive benefits from the conduct and results of the research.

Source: Emanuel, E. J., Wendler, D., Killen, J., and Grady. C. (2004). What makes clinical research in developing countries ethical? The benchmarks of ethical research. *The Journal of Infectious Diseases*, *189*(5), 930–937.

requirements to disseminate results to the appropriate tribal agencies and communities once the research is completed (American Indian Law Center, 1999).

For our purposes here, it is important to emphasize that (1) researchers have an obligation to respect the community's fundamental right to decide whether the goals of the research are valuable and the methods acceptable to them; and (2) such procedures entail exceptional efforts that make public health research more difficult than clinical trials. At a minimum, since the process of gaining community endorsement is much more complex and time-consuming than the process of gathering individual informed consent used in clinical trials, there need necessarily be a much longer start-up phase in conducting public health research, and consequently, additional funding at a level appropriate to the scientific and ethical requirements entailed in conducting public health research.

Based on the preceding analysis of the unique scientific and ethical considerations that arise when the focus of the research shifts from clinical to public health settings, we turn now to consider the implications for allocating federal health research funds.

Allocating Federal Health Research Funds Fairly

The question of allocating scarce public resources fairly is an issue of distributive justice. In fiscal year 2004, the budget for the U.S. National Institutes of Health (NIH) was approximately $28 billion. Because funding comes from taxpayer dollars, fairness in the allocation of these funds is imperative. The mission of the NIH is "to uncover new knowledge that will lead to better health for everyone" (NIH, 2004). The critical issue is what kinds of new knowledge are most likely to lead to success in achieving the nation's goals for better health for everyone.

Based on a long history of scientific research, there can be little question that RCTs enable researchers to rule out the greatest number of threats to the validity of the research results, and hence, provide the most rigorous research results possible. However, if one acknowledges that many factors make community intervention trials less feasible than clinical studies, then it raises the issue of how the potential social and scientific value of public health research can be fairly assessed. The National Institutes of Health are steeped in a culture of clinical trials, but the way that the NIH sets its research priorities has not gone unquestioned (Agres, 2004; Buchanan & Miller, 2006b; Dresser, 2001).

In response to a growing chorus of criticism, the NIH set out to make its decision-making processes more transparent in a 1998 report titled, *Setting Research Priorities at the National Institutes of Health* (Institute of Medicine, 1998). In this report, NIH officials identified five criteria that they said should guide the fulfillment of their fidu-ciary responsibilities to Congress and the American people: (1) public health needs, (2) scientific quality of the research, (3) potential for scientific progress, (4) portfolio diver-sification, and (5) adequate support of research infrastructure (Institute of Medicine, 1998). The report asserted that all of these criteria are pertinent to setting priorities, and conversely, giving precedence to any one of them alone could potentially lead to squandering valuable resources. Allocating funding strictly according to the number of deaths, for instance, would neglect chronic diseases such as mental illness and arthritis that produce long-term disability and high costs to society. Still, a number of concerns have been raised about both the adequacy and the implementation of these standards. Critics start by pointing out that the criteria are so broad that, in effect, NIH officials have almost total freedom in exercising their discretion over the use of these monies.

With respect to public health needs, for example, an initial intuition might be to assume that there should be a correlation between the distribution of disease burden and the allocation of research funds, with more funding going to those problems that cause a substantially greater burden of disease. But there are conflicting ways of measuring disease burden. Congressional representatives, for example, have complained that there appear to be widely disparate amounts of funding per afflicted person from one disease to the next, and they have pointedly asked why the NIH spends much more per death from HIV/AIDS than other causes of death, such as cancer, heart disease, or stroke, diseases whose prevalence rates are far greater than those for HIV/AIDS. The prominent bio-ethicist Daniel Callahan (2000), on the other hand, has argued that far too much money is spent on research on the diseases of old age, such as cancer, and that priority should instead be given to diseases that cause premature death (before the age of 65).

In the face of on-going controversies about which health problems should have high-est priority, an expedient resolution is simply to sidestep the question and fall back on the far less controversial standards of scientific promise in making funding decisions. With-out explicit directives mandating that community intervention research receive higher priority, the peer review process is designed and intended to rank proposals according to the quality of the scientific design. As a result, critics charge that decisions at NIH are driven more by rigor than relevance, with an undue emphasis on basic science over prac-tical application. Indeed, several commentators have lamented the overwhelming skew towards a biologically reductionistic emphasis on molecular and genetic determinants of health to the neglect and exclusion of research on social, behavioral, and environmental factors (McGinnis, Williams-Russo, & Knickman, 2002; Rees, 2004; Rogers, 2004).

There is another important consequence of the bias towards clinical medical trials in NIH funding decisions. It produces an unwarranted—indeed we argue potentially counterproductive—emphasis on seeking ever more powerful methods for effecting in-dividual behavior change. Two major factors have contributed to this state of affairs. Historically, Neubrauer and Pratt (1981) have shown how the public health focus on creating healthy living conditions shifted toward a focus on isolating the agent of disease, with the rise of the germ theory of disease and medical model around the turn of the 20th century. As infectious disease rates then fell over time, the primary focus of research attention shifted again, to an emphasis on the host—individual behaviors—most especially, with then-Assistant Surgeon General Michael McGinnis's and former CDC Director William Foege's widely-cited report on the "actual causes of death" (McGinnis & Foege, 1993).

The second major factor relates to the relative ease or difficulty in conducting clinical trials with individuals, versus public health interventions with whole population groups. If it is hard to conduct research on changing the social determinants of health, then conducting research on changing individual behaviors allows researchers to feel that they can still make worthwhile contributions to advancing public health goals. In combination, these two factors have created an atmosphere in which there is widespread acceptance of the idea that one of the most important outcomes of health research these days is demonstrating individual behavior change. To the extent that NIH funding priorities rise above the genetic and molecular level, there is now intense scientific interest in determining whether researchers can control human behavior in precisely the same way that they have learned to control the virulence of micro-organisms. What is missing from this research agenda is an appreciation of how social position structures the choices that people can and do make (MacIntyre, 1986; Marmot & Wilkinson, 1999; also see Lahiri & Pulungan, chapter 6).

From an epidemiological perspective, there is now overwhelming and irrefutable evidence that socioeconomic status is powerfully associated with health status (Marmot, 2003, 2004). That is to say, as far as we can tell, it is precisely those people in society who exercise the greatest degree of individual autonomy who also enjoy the best health. And conversely, those people who can exercise the least amount of autonomy—who have the least amount of control over their work conditions or other major life situations (e.g., marriage for women)—are those who have the poorest health. The conclusion that we draw from these data is that if researchers want to promote health, then they should focus on finding ways to promote individual autonomy, not restrict it. Public health research should focus on creating the conditions in which people can exercise the greatest degree of individual autonomy, and not trying to figure out how to develop new technologies for controlling their behavior (Buchanan, 2001, 2006a, 2006b).

As one further observation on this point, *Healthy People 2010* declared that one of the two principal goals for the nation is to improve quality of life (QOL) in this country. Little is actually said about what "quality of life" means in the document, but other scholars have illuminated the topic. The philosopher and bio-ethicist Dan Brock (1993, p. 105), for example, has defined quality of life as follows: "What is central to QOL is the capacity to exercise choice in forming and pursuing an integrated and coherent life plan." If the capacity for exercising choice is central to the meaning, and enjoyment, of quality of life, then research that aims to manipulate and control the choices people make is headed in the wrong direction, with potentially iatrogenic implications.

The thrust of these concerns has been to point out how demands for scientific rigor have resulted in shortchanging investment in community intervention research. The largely unquestioned mandate for upholding scientific standards serves to marginalize community intervention research, by relegating it to an inferior status not deserving priority in funding, due to perceived deficiencies in scientific design. In light of the many

Table 5.4	**Accountability for Reasonableness**

- Public rationale for decisions
- Reasonable understanding of how to meet needs of affected population, given resource constraints
- Mechanisms for challenging decisions and for revisiting decisions in light of counter-arguments
- Voluntary or public regulation of the process

structural impediments confronting community intervention studies, the invocation of "scientific promise" and the demand for "rigor in research" press towards individual clinical RCTs to the neglect of research on public health interventions. As a result, as the prospects for conducting research on the social determinants of health are diminished, so too is the likelihood of making a significant political commitment to eliminating health disparities.

Accountability for Reasonableness

The preceding section has shown how different value judgments are involved in assessing the relative merits of different types of health research. When faced with incompatible and seemingly irreconcilable value judgments, the demands of justice stipulate that groups ought to resort to fair procedures (e.g., democratic majority vote) to resolve their disagreements. Daniels and Sabin (1997) describe one such fair process for making controversial allocation decisions, a procedure they call "accountability for reasonableness." Daniels and Sabin developed their proposal to assist in setting priorities in medical care settings—specifically, insurers' decisions regarding coverage of particular medical interventions—but their recommendations are directly relevant to setting research priorities. They state that the decision-making process will be fair if the system has four features (see Table 5.4):

> One key feature is the provision of publicly accessible reasons, that is, a public rationale, for decisions. A second is that the rationale must constitute a reasonable construal of how to meet the [research] needs of a population under acceptable resource constraints. A third key feature is that there must be mechanisms for considering challenges to decisions that are made and for revisiting those decisions in light of counter-arguments. . . . [Fourth], there is voluntary or public regulation of the process to ensure that conditions 1–3 are met. (p. 307)

Regarding the fourth point, public regulation of the process, the NIH has acknowledged that its interactions with the public are "generally weak" and affirmed the need to more fully engage the public to redress concerns about the legitimacy and fairness of its distribution decisions (Institute of Medicine, 1998, p. 7). It is critically important at this time that community members and public health professionals vigorously advocate for oversight of the distribution of NIH funding by such public bodies. NIH officials and

Table 5.5	Hill's Criteria for Epidemiological Studies
	■ Temporal association ■ Strength ■ Dose-response relationship ■ Consistency ■ Biological plausibility ■ Alternative explanations ■ Specificity ■ Coherence

review groups are charged with evaluating proposals based on their prospects for uncovering new knowledge that will lead to better health for everyone. Their deliberations, however, must be reasonable with respect to the cogency of the rationales put forward regarding the prospects that the knowledge to be gained will result in improvements in population health. Justice demands that critical questions be posed and alternative criteria, beyond rigor in research, be judiciously considered.

What Types of Evidence Should Matter

If RCTs of community interventions are methodologically difficult and studies designed to influence individual behavior change possibly detrimental, then what types of evidence should matter in evaluating the merits of public health proposals? The future of public health research is largely dependent on our answer to this question.

First, public health needs to reclaim and honor its lineage. Historically, public health was founded on the science of epidemiology. Epidemiological research is based primarily on observational studies, retrospective case-control, and prospective cohort research designs. To certify the validity of these types of research, epidemiologists developed a set of "weight-of-evidence" standards, generally referred to as Hill's criteria, based on dimensions such as biological plausibility, consistency in association, and dose-response relationships (Hill, 1965; see Table 5.5). Despite the fact that many problems cannot be investigated in field experiments, public health researchers seem to have become almost apologetic about the quality of their research, rather passively seeming to accept the notion that epidemiology is a "second-rate" science relative to the clinical trial (Parascandola, 1998; Parascandola & Weed, 2001).

Fortunately, the recent Supreme Court ruling in *Daubert v. Merrell Dow Pharmaceuticals, Inc.* (in which the industry argued that claims, such as smoking causes cancer, that were not based on experimental research designs constituted "junk science") has served as a wake-up call for the field (Michaels & Monforton, 2005). The major national organization and public health professionals across the country have embarked on a major new initiative, the Project on Scientific Knowledge and Public Policy (SKAPP), to advance understanding of different criteria for assessing scientific validity (SKAPP, 2007). Thus, to advance research on community health interventions, a more articulate justification of valid scientific standards is crucial.

Second, for trials that recruit individual research participants, a number of readily identifiable alternative indicators can be derived from the concepts of individual autonomy and informed choice, and used instead of individual behavior change. For example, trials could propose outcome measures such as the following: (1) awareness of alternative courses of action; (2) ability to enumerate the advantages and disadvantages of the major alternatives; (3) greater self-understanding of one's reasons for choosing one course of action over another; (4) greater satisfaction with one's decision; and, (5) greater reassurance that one's decision better advances one's own life projects.

Third, the value of promoting autonomy can also be applied at the community level. When evaluating the merits of community interventions, a set of outcome measures similar to individual level outcomes can be imagined, including (1) the degree to which the community provides input and exercises control over research and community programs; (2) the degree to which community members feel their advice and suggestions are respected; (3) the degree to which participants see their concerns have been addressed; and (4) trust in the researchers.

Conclusion

In this chapter, we have argued that, for anyone interested in community intervention research, two key ethical concerns have yet to be resolved: (1) identifying an appropriate process for ensuring that the community members agree that the goals of the research are valuable and methods acceptable; and (2) deciding how to allocate scarce public resources designated for health research fairly. We have shown how there are evident tensions between scientific and ethical considerations, and claimed that a sound balance has yet to be achieved. As demonstrated here, RCTs may not be feasible in most community intervention research, and other standards will be needed to assess the merits of the proposed public health research. We have presented other types of evidence that should matter in trying to decide whether research on a proposed public health intervention is worthwhile. Due to the conflicting considerations between scientific promise and community responsiveness, we conclude that the NIH should establish fair procedures for resolving fundamental disagreements about the value of different types of research, a process embodied in the concept of "accountability for reasonableness."

REFERENCES

Agres, T. (2004). Questioning NIH priorities. *The Scientist, 5*(1), 2. Retrieved February 5, 2007, from http://www.the-scientist.com/article/display/22212/

American Indian Law Center. (1999). *Model tribal research code: With materials for tribal regulation for research and checklist for Indian health boards* (3rd ed.). Albuquerque, NM: American Indian Law Center, Inc. Retrieved October 2, 2005, from http://lawschool.unm.edu/ailc/publications.htm

Beecher, H. K. (1966). Ethics and clinical research. *New England Journal of Medicine, 274,* 1354–1360.

Belsky, L., & Richardson, H. S. (2004). Medical researchers' ancillary clinical care responsibilities. *British Medical Journal, 328*(7454), 1494–1496.

Braine, N., Des Jarlais, D. C., Ahmad, S., Purchase, D., & Turner, C. (2004). Long-term effects of syringe exchange on risk behavior and HIV prevention. *AIDS Education and Prevention, 16,* 264–275.

Brock, D. (1993). Quality of life measures in health care and medical ethics. In M. Nussbaum & A. Sen (Eds.), *The quality of life.* Oxford: Clarendon Press.

Buchanan, D. (2001). *An ethic for health promotion: Rethinking the sources of human well-being*. New York: Oxford University Press.

Buchanan, D. (2006a). Moral reasoning as a model for health promotion. *Social Science and Medicine*, *63*, 2715–2726.

Buchanan, D. (2006b). A new ethic for health promotion: Reflections on a philosophy of health education for the 21st century. *Health Education and Behavior*, *33*, 290–304.

Buchanan, D., & Miller, F. G. (2006a). A public health perspective on research ethics. *Journal of Medical Ethics*, *32*, 729–733.

Buchanan, D., & Miller, F. G. (2006b). Justice in research on human subjects. In R. Rhodes, L. Francis, & A. Silvers (Eds.), *The Blackwell guide to medical ethics*. New York: Blackwell.

Buchanan, D., Miller, F. G., & Wallerstein, N. (2007). Ethical issues in community based participatory research: Balancing rigorous research with community participation. *Progress in Community Health Partnerships 2*(1), 153–160.

Buchanan, D. R., Shaw, S., Ford, A., & Singer, M. (2003). Empirical science meets moral panic: An analysis of the politics of needle exchange. *Journal of Public Health Policy*, *24*(3–4), 427–444.

Callahan, D. (2000). Death and the research imperative. *New England Journal of Medicine*, *342*(9), 654–656.

Community Intervention Trial for Smoking Cessation (COMMIT). (1995a). I. Cohort results from a four-year community intervention. *American Journal of Public Health*, *85*(2), 183–192.

Community Intervention Trial for Smoking Cessation (COMMIT). (1995b). II. Changes in adult cigarette smoking prevalence. *American Journal of Public Health*, *85*(2), 193–200.

Daniels, N., & Sabin, J. (1997). Limits to health care: Fair procedures, democratic deliberation, and the legitimacy problem for insurers. *Philosophy and Public Affairs*, *26*, 303–350.

Dresser, R. (2001). *When science offers salvation: Patient advocacy and research ethics*. New York: Oxford University Press.

Emanuel, E. J., Wendler, D., Killen, J., & Grady, C. (2004). What makes clinical research in developing countries ethical? The benchmarks of ethical research. *Journal of Infectious Diseases*, *189*, 930–937.

Evidence-Based Working Group. (1992). Evidenced-based medicine: A new approach to teaching the practice of medicine. *Journal of the American Medical Association*, *268*(17), 2420–2425.

Flay, B. R. (1986). Efficacy and effectiveness trials (and other phases of research) in the development of health promotion programs. *Preventive Medicine*, *15*, 451–474.

Green, L. W. (1977). Evaluation and measurement: Some dilemmas for health education. *American Journal of Public Health*, *67*, 155–161.

Green, L. W. (2006). Public health asks of systems science: To advance our evidence-based practice, can you help us get more practice-based evidence? *American Journal of Public Health*, *96*, 406–409.

Green, L. W., & Glasgow, R. E. (2006). Evaluating the relevance, generalization, and applicability of research: Issues in external validation and translation methodology. *Evaluation and the Health Professions*, *29*, 26–53.

Hanson, D., Hanson, J., Vardon, P., McFarlane, K., Lloyd, J., Muller, R., et al. (2005). The injury iceberg: An ecological approach to planning sustainable community safety interventions. *Health Promotion Journal of Australia*, *16*(1), 5–10.

Hill, A. B. (1965). The environment and disease: Association or causation? *Proceedings of the Royal Society of Medicine*, *58*, 295–300.

Holder, H. D. (2000). Community prevention of alcohol problems. *Addictive Behaviors*, *25*, 843–859.

Holder, H. D. (2002). Prevention of alcohol and drug 'abuse' problems at the community level: What research tells us. *Substance Use & Misuse*, *37*(8–10), 901–921.

Institute of Medicine. (1988). *The future of public health*. Washington, DC: National Academies Press.

Institute of Medicine. (1998). *Scientific opportunities and public needs: Improving priority setting and public input at the National Institutes of Health*. Washington DC: National Academies Press.

Institute of Medicine. (2002). *Who will keep the public healthy? Educating public health professionals for the 21st century*. Washington, DC: National Academies Press.

Israel, B., Schulz, A. J., Parker, E. A., Becker, A. B., Allen, A. J., & Guzman, R. (2003). Critical issues in developing and following community based participatory research principles. In M. Minkler & N. Wallerstein (Eds.), *Community based participatory research for health*. San Francisco: Jossey-Bass.

Luepker, R. V., Murray, D. M., Jacobs, D. R., Jr., Mittelmark, M. B., Bracht, N., Carlaw, R., et al. (1994). Community education for cardiovascular disease prevention: Risk factor changes in the Minnesota Heart Health Program. *American Journal of Public Health, 84,* 1383–1393.

MacIntyre, S. (1986). The patterning of health by social position in contemporary Britain: Directions for sociological research. *Social Science & Medicine, 23*(4), 393–415.

Marmot, M. (2003). Understanding social inequalities in health. *Perspectives in Biology and Medicine, 46*(3), S9–23.

Marmot, M. (2004). Social causes of social inequalities in health. In S. Anand, F. Peter, & A. Sen (Eds.), *Public health, ethics, and equity.* Oxford: Oxford University Press.

Marmot, M., & Wilkinson, R. G. (1999). *Social determinants of health.* New York: Oxford University Press.

McGinnis, J. M., & Foege, W. H. (1993). Actual causes of death in the United States. *Journal of the American Medical Association, 270,* 2207–2212.

McGinnis, J. M, Williams-Russo, P., & Knickman, J. R. (2002). The case for more active policy attention to health promotion. *Health Affairs, 21,* 78–93.

Michaels, D., & Monforton, C. (2005). Manufacturing uncertainty: Contested science and the protection of the public's health and environment. *American Journal of Public Health, 95*(Suppl 1), S39–48.

Murray, D. (2001). Efficacy and effectiveness trials in health promotion and disease prevention: Design and analysis of group-randomized trials. In N. Schneiderman, M. A. Speers, J. M. Silva, H. Tomes, & J. H. Gentry (Eds.), *Integrating behavioral and social sciences with public health.* Washington, DC: American Psychological Association.

National Institutes of Health, Office of Extramural Research. (2004). *Policy on enhancing public access to archived publications resulting from NIH-funded research.* Retrieved February 5, 2007, from http://publicaccess.nih.gov/publicaccess_background.htm

Neubauer, D., & Pratt, R. (1981). The second public health revolution: A critical appraisal. *Journal of Health Politics, Policy and Law, 6*(2), 205–228.

Parascandola, M. (1998). Epidemiology: Second-rate science? *Public Health Reports, 113,* 312–320.

Parascandola, M., & Weed, D. L. (2001). Causation in epidemiology. *Journal of Epidemiology and Community Health, 55,* 905–912.

Pew Health Commission. (1998). *Recreating health professional practice for a new century.* Philadelphia: The Pew Charitable Trusts.

Project on Scientific Knowledge and Public Policy. (2007). *About us.* Retrieved January 26, 2007, from http://www.defendingscience.org/About-Us.cfm

Rees, J. (2004). The fundamentals of clinical discovery. *Perspectives in Biology and Medicine, 47*(4), 597–607.

Rogers, W. A. (2004). Evidence based medicine and justice: A framework for looking at the impact of EBM upon vulnerable or disadvantaged groups. *Journal of Medical Ethics, 30,* 141–145.

Income-Related Health Disparity and Its Determinants in New York State: Racial/Ethnic and Geographical Comparisons[1]

Kajal Lahiri
and Zulkarnain Pulungan

Introduction

Persistent health inequality in the United States along multiple dimensions has been put at the forefront by one of the challenging goals of *Healthy People 2010* (US-DHHS, 2000): to eliminate health disparities among all segments of the population, including differences that occur by gender, race, or ethnicity, education or income, disability, geographic location, and sexual orientation. In this chapter we study the quality of health and health inequality among racial/ethnic groups as well as across geographic areas of the State of New York. Even though certain aggregate indicators of health (e.g., life expectancy at birth, mortality rate, etc.) in New York have improved during last few decades (see NCHS, 2006), health disparities among racial/ethnic groups and among regions continue to exist. For example, as we will show below, the prevalence of diabetes is almost twice as high among Blacks compared to that among Whites; on the other hand, many New York City neighborhoods and unsuspecting areas of Upstate New York are characterized by extreme poor health. This is the first study to look at the health status and its disparity among New Yorkers along these dimensions.[1]

[1]This study has been supported by the Center for the Elimination of Minority Health Disparities, University at Albany, SUNY, and has benefited from presentations at the First Annual Health Disparities Conference, Columbia University (March 10–11, 2006), NIH Health Disparity Conference (October 23–24, 2006), and at a roundtable discussion at the Center for the Elimination of Minority Health Disparities, University at Albany. Comments and help from Richard Alba, Bill Jenkins, Richard Keller, Catherine Lawson, Louis McNutt, Thad Mirer, Jim Scanlan, Larry Schell, and Barbara Wallace are gratefully acknowledged. We, however, are responsible for all remaining errors and omissions.

A question arises as to what causes poor health and health disparities. A large number of studies have reported that socioeconomic status (SES) is a key factor affecting quality of health and health disparity (see for example, Adams, Hurd, McFadden, Merrill, & Ribeiro, 2003; Adler & Newman, 2002; Cutler, Deaton, & Lleras-Muney, 2006; Cutler & Lleras-Muney, 2006; Deaton, 2006). There are four broad pathways—health care, environmental exposure, health behavior, and chronic stress—through which SES affects health (Adler & Ostrove, 1999). Because SES is an important mediator for quality of health, studying health disparity cannot be separated from studying disparity in SES.

Rawls' First Principle of Justice (1971) requires that all individuals should have the same opportunity to achieve their potential health levels; see Bommier and Stecklov (2002). An egalitarian viewpoint of social justice requires that people in equal need of health care be treated equally, irrespective of characteristics such as income, place of residence, race, and so forth. Since discrimination in access to health care is likely to be based on income, we focus on income-related health inequality in this chapter. There seems to be broad consensus among health policy analysts that socioeconomic inequality in health is indeed inequitable and unjust, and is consistent with the Institute of Medicine (2002) definition of health disparity—any difference in health after adjusting for health care needs. This definition recognizes that factors such as income may be mediators of disparity in health care.[2] Numerous studies on measuring quality of health and health distributions have focused on mortality rates, prevalence of diseases/risk factors, psychological morbidity, quality of or access to health care services, and health care utilization rates.[3] In addition to looking at many of these factors, in this study we focus on a measure of health more generally, and calculate an index of health and health inequality based on self-assessed health (SAH) status. SAH is defined as the response to the survey question "Would you say that in general your health is: excellent, very good, good, fair, or poor" (Centers for Disease Control and Prevention [CDC], 1999–2004)?

SAH has been shown to be a good measure of overall health status. In their review, Idler and Benyamini (1997) show that SAH has strong predictive validity for mortality. Sickles and Taubman (1997) compiled results from worldwide studies on the association between self-assessed health and mortality, and reported that a lower level of SAH has higher mortality odds. Manor, Mathews, and Power (2001) found that SAH has a strong association with long-standing illness. Furthermore, Lahiri, Vaughn, and Wixon (1995) show that SAH is a useful predictor of the severity of diseases and disability. Humphries and van Doorslaer (2000) found that health inequality calculated on the basis of SAH status gives similar results to the results calculated based on a more objective health indicator (viz. McMaster Health Utility Index). More recently, Safaei (2006) finds SAH to be statistically more reliable than the binary chronic conditions as a measure of overall health.

In this chapter we generate a continuous measure of health by modeling the five-category SAH as an Ordered Probit Model (McKelvey & Zavoina, 1975) conditioned by several objective determinants including different diseases, behavioral risk factors, and socio-demographic characteristics. The estimated values from this model are used as a

---

[2]We found that between 40% and 50% of the total health inequality in our sample is due to income-related health inequality—an estimate that is much higher than 25% reported by Wagstaff and van Doorslaer (2004) for Canada.

[3]See, for instance, Williams and Collins (1995), Ayanian, Weissman, Chasan-Taber, and Epstein (1999), and Shishehbor, Litaker, Pothier, and Lauer (2006).

measure of individual health and income related health inequality using concentration index and concentration curve (Kakwani, Wagstaff, & van Doorslaer, 1997). Furthermore, to be useful for policy purposes, the income related health inequality is decomposed into its determinants (Wagstaff, van Doorslaer, & Watanabe, 2003) for the whole sample and specific sub-samples.

The chapter is organized as follows: The estimation procedures—the methods to calculate quality of health, income related health inequality and their determinants—are described; the data used in the empirical analysis is documented; results are then presented; and finally we summarize our conclusions.

Methods

In modeling SAH we follow the same procedures as Cutler and Richardson (1997, 1998) and Groot (2000). In the empirical modeling of the quality of health, three related concepts are distinguished: a true quality of health denoted as h^*, a vector of objective measures of health denoted as $\mathbf{h}^\circ$, and a subjective measure of health denoted as h^s. The true quality of health is a latent variable, which is unobservable. What we observe is a vector of objective indicators and a subjective measure of health. The true unobserved quality of health h^* is assumed to be a function of the vector of observed and objective measures of health, and a vector of individual characteristics denoted by $\mathbf{x}$. The subjective measure of health is measured on an ordinal scale with m self-assessed response categories. For the purpose of measuring health and health inequality we transform these ordinal responses into a cardinal measure. In this chapter we used an ordered response model to transform the order scale variable into a cardinal variable. To control for possible heterogeneity in self-assessed health, we estimate an Ordered Probit model with heteroskedasticity in errors. The model is formulated as follows:

$$h_i^* = \mathbf{h}_i^\circ \boldsymbol{\gamma} + \mathbf{x}_i \boldsymbol{\beta} + s(\mathbf{z}_i, \boldsymbol{\eta})\varepsilon_i \tag{1}$$
$$h_i^s = j \Leftrightarrow \mu_j \leq h_j^* \leq \mu_{j+1} \text{ for } j = 0, 1, \ldots, m - 1$$
$$\mu_0 = -\infty \text{ and } \mu_m = +\infty$$
$$i = 1, 2, \ldots, n$$

where $\boldsymbol{\gamma}$, $\boldsymbol{\beta}$, $\boldsymbol{\eta}$ are vectors of coefficients, $\boldsymbol{\mu} = (\mu_1, \ldots, \mu_{m-1})$ is an unknown vector of thresholds to be estimated together with the vectors of coefficients, ε_i is the error term and is assumed to be normally distributed, $s(\mathbf{z}_i, \boldsymbol{\eta}) = \sigma \sqrt{(1 + \exp(\mathbf{z}_i \boldsymbol{\eta}))}$ is a scale function to control for heteroskedasticity, and n is the number of observations. $\mathbf{z}_i$ is a vector of observed variables that affect the variance of the error term.[4]

The model is estimated using the maximum likelihood approach. The predicted quality of health, $\hat{h}_i^* = \mathbf{h}_i^\circ \hat{\boldsymbol{\gamma}} + \mathbf{x}_i \hat{\boldsymbol{\beta}}$, is used as a measure of individual health. The predicted health from the estimated Ordered Probit model will purge at least some part of the variation in SAH that is due to subjective idiosyncrasies of the respondents, not supported by objective health measures. Following van Doorslaer and Jones

---

[4]van Doorslaer and Jones (2003) have shown that this heteroskedastic model accommodates possible individual-specific heterogeneity in the subjective thresholds $\boldsymbol{\mu}$.

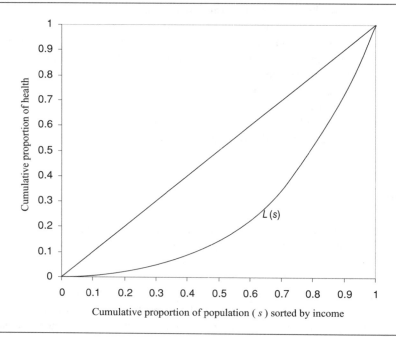

Concentration curve.

(2003), we rescale this prediction to be in the [0, 1] interval as $h_i = (\hat{h}_i^* - \hat{h}_{min}^*)/(\hat{h}_{max}^* - \hat{h}_{min}^*)$, where $\hat{h}_{max}^*$ and $\hat{h}_{min}^*$ are the maximum and the minimum of the predicted quality of health, respectively.

Using the estimated quality of health h_i, we measure income related health inequality using concentration curves and health concentration index (Wagstaff, Paci, & van Doorslaer, 1991).[5] A concentration curve plots the cumulative proportion of health $L(s)$ against the cumulative proportion of population s (starting with the lowest socioeconomic status and ending with the highest socioeconomic status), as shown in Figure 6.1. If the concentration curve $L(s)$ coincides with the diagonal, health is equally distributed over socioeconomic status. This means that there is no inequality in health across socioeconomic hierarchies in the population. The farther the concentration curve from the diagonal the larger is the degree of inequality. The area between concentration curve and the diagonal provides a measure of inequality. The concentration index is defined as twice the area between the concentration curve and the diagonal. The coefficient ranges from 0 (when across income everybody enjoys exactly the same health) to 1 (when all population's health is concentrated in the hands of the richest individual).

The concentration index can be calculated using equation (see Kakwani et al., 1997):

$$\hat{C} = \frac{2}{n\mu} \sum_{i=1}^{n} h_i R_i - 1 \tag{2}$$

where R_i is the ith individual fraction rank in socioeconomic status and μ is the mean of quality of health. The variance is estimated using the Huber–White procedure. The

---

[5]See also Lecluyse and Cleemput (2005) and Clarke and Ryan (2006).

disadvantage of the concentration index is its lack of straightforward interpretation in a natural unit, while its advantage is that it takes into account both coefficient variation of health and correlation between health and income rank (Milanovic, 1997). Koolman and van Doorslaer (2004) present a lucid interpretation of the concentration index.

Furthermore, to be more meaningful for policy purposes, income related health inequality is decomposed into its determinants as demonstrated by Wagstaff et al. (2003). Define a vector of explanatory variables as $\mathbf{w} = (\mathbf{h}° \ \mathbf{x})$. Given the relationship between health and explanatory variables as in equation (1), the concentration index can be written as

$$\hat{C} = \sum_{k=1}^{K} \left(\hat{\beta}_k \ \bar{w}_k / \bar{h} \right) C_k \tag{3}$$

where $\bar{h}$ is the mean of h, $\bar{w}_k$ is the mean of variable w_k from the vector of explanatory variables $\mathbf{w}$, and C_k is the concentration index of variable w_k.

Data, Descriptive Statistics, and Imputation

Data and Descriptive Statistics

The data used in this study are obtained from the New York State sample of the *Behavioral Risk Factor Surveillance System (BRFSS)* over 1999–2004, with a total of 22,083 sample observations.[6] Every year health departments of all states, with technical and methodological assistance from CDC, conduct monthly telephone interviews on randomly selected noninstitutional adults aged 18 years or older. The surveys are developed and conducted to monitor major behavioral risks among adults associated with premature morbidity and mortality. The number of observations is not the same for all variables. The differences can be attributed to (i) the absence of some questions in some years—for example, coronary heart disease was asked only in the interviews for the years of 1999, 2001, and 2003; and (ii) missing values due to "do not know," "not sure" responses, and refusals to answer. In addition, population socioeconomic characteristics are obtained from 2000 census information (U.S. Census Bureau, 2000).

Based on Census 2000 (U.S. Census Bureau, 2000), New York State population is 18,976,457 persons, which is 6.7% of the U.S. population. Sixty two percent of the population is non–Hispanic White, 15.9% is Black, 15.1% is Hispanic, 5.5% is Asian, and 0.4% is American Indian and Alaskan Native. As a comparison, the U.S. population consists of 69.1% non–Hispanic White, 12.3% Black, 12.5% Hispanic, 3.6% Asian, and 0.9% American Indian and Alaskan Native. So the percentage of minority population of New York State is higher than that of the United States.

In this chapter, we divide New York State into 17 geographic areas, which consist of 9 counties of Downstate and 8 economic development regions of Upstate. Upstate New York was divided into economic development regions due to small samples in individual counties. Racial/ethnic groups included in the comparison are non–Hispanic White (White), non–Hispanic Black (Black), Hispanic, Asian/Pacific Islander (Asian), and American Indian and Alaskan Native (AIAN).

---

[6]Sehili, Elbasha, Moriarty, and Zack (2005) have used these data source to study health inequality in the United States in terms of physically healthy days.

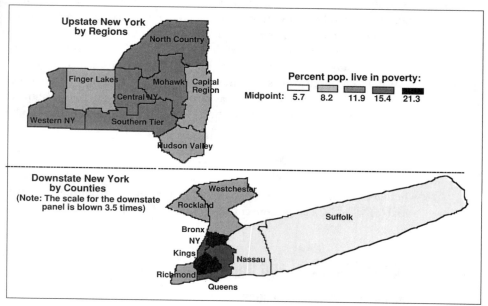

Percent population in poverty.

The population characteristics vary across New York State geographic areas, especially between Downstate and Upstate of New York. Sixty three percent of the New York State residents live in Downstate. Percentage of individuals who live in poverty in Downstate varies from 5% (Nassau County) to 25% (Bronx County), while in Upstate it varies from 9% (Putnam County) to 14% (Allegany County) as presented in Figure 6.2.[7] Income inequality, measured by Gini coefficient[8], varies across the areas from 0.33 (Nassau County) to 0.45 (Bronx County) for Downstate; and for Upstate, it varies from 0.36 (Hudson Valley) to 0.42 (North Country) (see Figure 6.3). In addition, the racial/ethnic composition of the population also varies considerably across the regions, where Downstate population is more diverse compared to Upstate population. For example 21% of Downstate population is Black compared to 7% of Upstate population. Figure 6.4 presents the percent Black population across the areas.

We follow the BRFSS guideline that the minimum number of observations to be meaningful for interpretation is 50. Specifically, the description of variables used in this study is as follows.

Socio-Demographic Variables. The average age of respondents in the sample is 45 years. Comparing racial/ethnic groups, White has the highest average age (48 years) and Asian has the lowest (39 years). Since age is an important determinant of health,

---

[7]All maps in this chapter were created using ArcView GIS (Environmental Systems Research Institute [ESRI], 2002). The breakpoints between classes are determined using a statistical formula (Jenk's optimization) that minimizes the variance within each class.

[8]Lorenz curve plots the cumulative proportion of income against the cumulative proportion of individuals ranked by income. The Gini coefficient is defined as twice the area between the Lorenz curve and the diagonal, and ranges from 0 to 1.

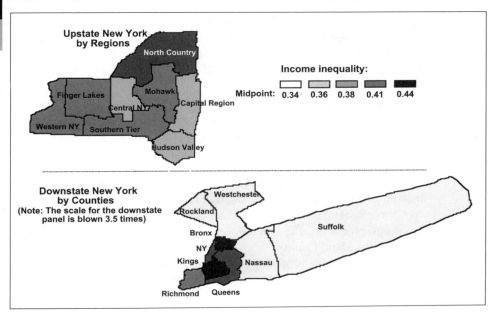

Income inequality.

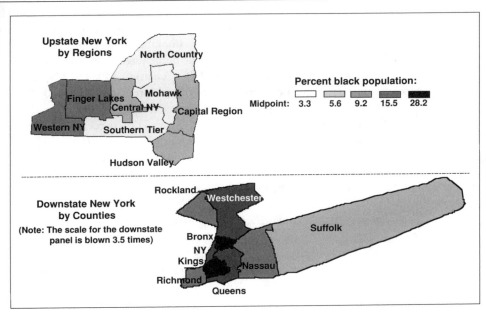

Percent black population.

we need to adjust for differing age distributions when comparing the prevalence of the diseases among racial/ethnic groups or areas. Across the geographic areas of New York State, the average age varies from 43 years (Queens County) to 49 years (Mohawk). Sixty percent of White respondents are married, compared to 37% of Black respondents. The percentage of married respondents in New York County is the lowest (35%) compared to other areas.

Education level varies considerably among racial/ethnic groups as well as across the areas. Only 13% of AIAN respondents have 4 years or more of college, compared to 61% of Asian respondents; across the areas, the percentage varies from 19% in Bronx County to 52% in New York County. The percentage of respondents who were unable to work varies from 1.6% (Asian) to 14% (AIAN), while the percentage across the areas varies from 1.3% (Westchester County) to 11.3% (North Country). Annual household income also varies considerably among racial/ethnic groups as well as across the areas. AIAN average annual household income is $34,390, compared to $62,470 of Asian. Across the geographic areas, the average varies considerably from $44,579 (Kings County) to $75,831 (Rockland County).

Eighty-six percent of the respondents have health insurance plans, but only 68% among Hispanics have health plans compared to 91% among Whites. Across the areas, the percentage varies from 77% (Queens County) to 92% (Western New York). The percentage of respondents who could not afford to see a doctor in the past 12 months also varies considerably among racial/ethnic groups, ranging from 8% (White) to 21% (Hispanic). Twenty percent of Rockland County respondents could not afford to see a doctor at least once, while in the Capital Region only 7% of the respondents had that experience.

The U.S. Surgeon General's Report (U.S. Department of Health and Human Services [HHS], 2004) has concluded that smoking is a source of many kinds of diseases and harms every organ of the body. Thus, smoking status could be a good explanatory variable to be included in equation (1). The percentage of smokers among racial/ethnic groups varies noticeably, ranging from 13% (Asian) to 34% (AIAN); the percentage of smokers across the area varies from 15% (Westchester County) to 28% (North Country) (see Figure 6.5). In addition to smoking, not exercising is categorized as a bad health habit that can result in several kinds of diseases. The percentage of respondents who participated in any sort of exercise in the past 30 days is 74%. Sixty-two percent of Hispanic respondents participated in any exercise in the past 30 days, compared to 79% for White respondents; across the areas, Bronx County has the lowest percentage (66%) and North Country has the highest (80%).

Self-Assessed Health Status. Figure 6.6 presents the distribution of SAH by racial/ethnic groups. Twenty-two percent of the respondents considered their health as "excellent," while only 4% considered their health as "poor." The distribution varies considerably among racial/ethnic groups. The percentage of "excellent" and "very good" health is significantly higher for Whites than for Blacks, Hispanics, or AIANs. In addition, the percentage of "fair" and "poor" health is lower for Whites than for Blacks, Hispanics, or AIANs. The percentage of "excellent" and "very good" health varies from 43% (Bronx County) to 62% (Capital District), and the percentage of "fair" and "poor" health varies noticeably from 10% (Finger Lakes) to 24% (Bronx County). Based on both criteria, Bronx County has the lowest quality of health compared to the other areas. It is noteworthy

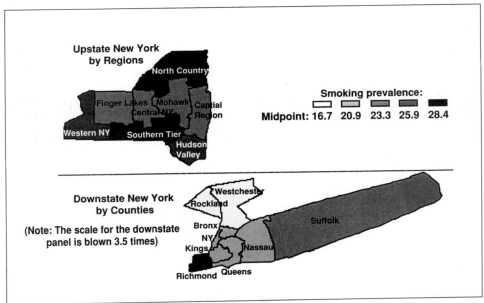

Prevalence of smoking.

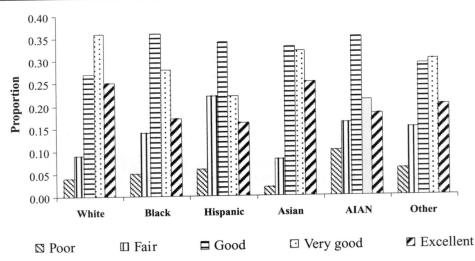

Distribution of self-assessed health by racial/ethnic groups.

that different cut points (criteria) can give different classifications. For example, if we use the percentage of "excellent" health as the criterion of quality of health then Westchester does the best.

Figure 6.7 presents the distribution of SAH by income groups. The figure indicates that as income increases the percentage of "excellent" health increases and the percentage

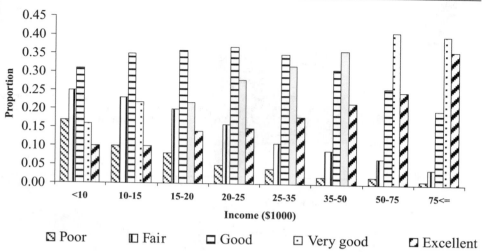

Distribution of self-assessed health by annual household income.

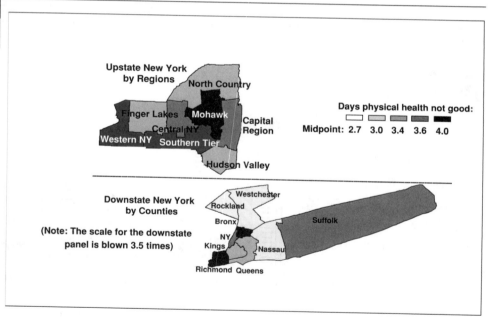

Number of days physical health not good.

of "poor" health decreases. This pattern indicates a strong association between income and quality of health—the so-called negative income health gradient.

Number of Days Physical and Mental Health not Good in the Past 30 Days. The pattern of number of days where physical health was not good is the same as the number of days where mental health was not good. Comparing racial/ethnic groups, Asian has the lowest

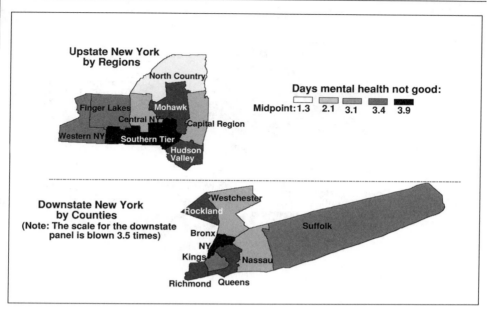

Number of days mental health not good.

average on both measures and AIAN has the highest. Across the areas the patterns of these two measures are different (see Figures 6.8 and 6.9). The lowest average number of days where physical health was not good is 2.6 days (Rockland County) and the highest average is 4.3 days (Mohawk). While the lowest average number of days where mental health was not good is 1.3 days (North Country), and the highest is 4.2 days (Bronx County).

Limited Activities Due to Health Problems. The overall prevalence of limited activities due to health problem is 16%. The prevalence varies substantially among racial/ethnic groups ranging from 6% (Asian) to 31% (AIAN). The prevalence varies from 12% (Queens County) to 22% (Rockland County).

Body Mass Index (BMI). Obesity—defined as BMI greater than 30 kg/m² —is the second leading cause of preventable death after smoking in the United States and is as a major cause of morbidity and disability (Must et al., 1999; Mokdad, Karks, Stroup, & Gerberding, 2004). Hence this variable is a good predictor of quality of health to be included in equation (1). Comparing racial/ethnic groups, the average BMI varies from 24 (Asian) to 28 (Black); across the areas it varies from 25 (New York County) to 28 (North Country). Figure 6.10 presents the prevalence of obesity across the geographic areas.

Asthma. The prevalence of asthma among respondents is 11.8%. Comparing racial/ethnic groups, the prevalence varies substantially from 5.9% (Asian) to 17.7% (AIAN). Across the areas, the prevalence varies from 8.5% (Westchester County) to 17.4% (North Country). Figure 6.11 presents the prevalence of asthma across the areas.

Figure
6.10

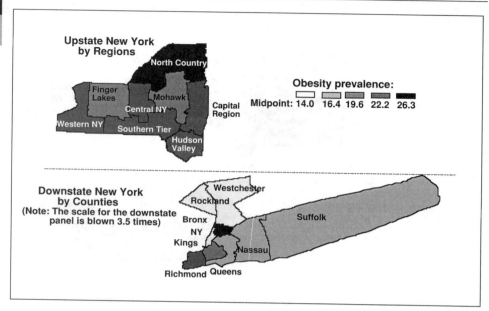

Prevalence of obesity.

Figure
6.11

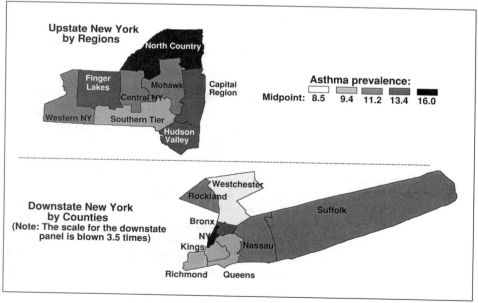

Prevalence of asthma.

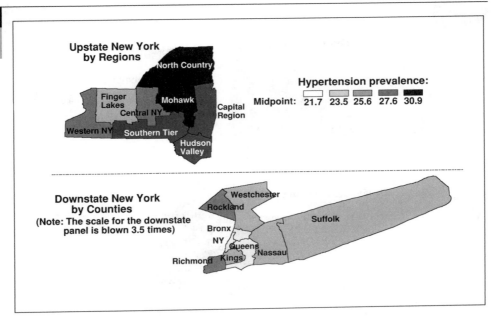

Prevalence of hypertension.

Hypertension (High Blood Pressure). The prevalence of high blood pressure among respondents is 24.3%. It is only 12.2% for Asians compared to 31.2% for AIANs. Across the areas the prevalence varies from 20.9% (New York County) to 33.5% (Mohawk). Figure 6.12 presents the prevalence of hypertension across the areas.

Coronary Heart Disease. Coronary heart disease prevalence is 4.2% in the pooled sample. The prevalence varies from 2% (Asian) to 7% (AIAN). Blacks, Hispanics, and Asians have lower prevalence than Whites. Across the regions, the prevalence varies from 3.3% (Richmond County) to 5.2% (Bronx County and Nassau County). North Country and Rockland County are excluded from the comparison for lack of sufficient observations.

Myocardial Infarction. The prevalence of myocardial infarction is 3.5%. Asians have the lowest prevalence (less than 0.1%) and AIANs have the highest (7.6%). Across the areas, the prevalence varies from 2.2% (Westchester County) to 5.3% (Central New York). North Country is excluded from the comparison for inadequate number of observations.

Stroke. The prevalence of stroke is 1.9%. Among racial/ethnic groups the prevalence varies considerably, ranging from 0.4% (Asian) to 6% (AIAN). The prevalence varies considerably across the areas, ranging from 1.5% (Hudson Valley) to 4.4% (Southern Tier). North Country and Rockland County are excluded from the comparison.

Diabetes. The overall prevalence of diabetes is 6.4%. It varies from 4.7% for Asians to 11.6% for AIANs. Across the areas, the prevalence varies from 5.0% (Suffolk County) to 14.1% (North Country). Figure 6.13 presents the prevalence across the areas.

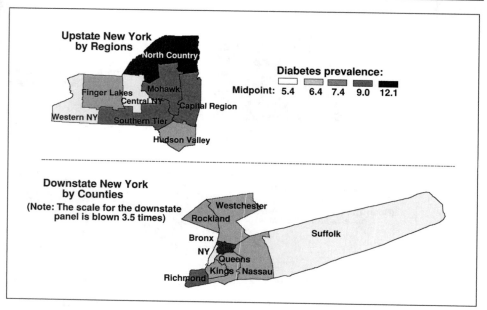

Prevalence of diabetes.

Arthritis. The prevalence of arthritis is 25.1% among the respondents. The prevalence varies substantially among racial/ethnic groups, ranging from 8.1% (Asian) to 35.1% (AIAN). Across the State, the prevalence varies from 18.2% (Bronx County) to 34.7% (North Country).

Pain, Aching, Stiffness, and Swelling in or Around a Joint. The prevalence of this medical condition is 38.3%. The prevalence varies considerably, ranging from 23.7% for Asians to 52.5% for AIANs. Across areas the prevalence varies from 29.0% (Kings County) to 46.7% (Western New York).

High Blood Cholesterol. The prevalence of high blood cholesterol is 31%. The prevalence varies from 24.5% for Hispanics to 48.3% for AIANs. Across the areas the prevalence varies from 25.5% (Southern Tier) to 41.6% (Rockland County).

Multiple Imputation

Information on some diseases and risk factors was not collected in some survey years. Table 6.1 presents the pattern of missing values attributed to the absence of questions in the survey questionnaires. For example, during 1999–2004, information on high blood pressure was collected only in 1999, 2001, and 2003 and not in 2000, 2002, and 2004.

In order to include all important diseases and risk factors as covariates in equation (1), we needed to fill in the missing values in our pooled sample. Otherwise, an omitted variable bias would result in the coefficient estimates of included variables. A currently accepted procedure to impute missing values is the multiple-imputation method of Rubin

Table 6.1	Missing Data Pattern in New York State BRFSS* Sample					
				Year		
Variable	1999	2000	2001	2002	2003	2004
Could not afford to see a doctor	✓	✓	.	.	✓	✓
Participate in any physical activities or exercises	.	✓	✓	✓	✓	✓
Fruit and vegetable servings per day	.	✓	.	✓	✓	.
Heavy drinking	✓	.	✓	✓	✓	✓
Activities limited due to health problem	.	✓	✓	.	✓	✓
Ever had asthma	.	✓	✓	✓	✓	✓
Ever told blood pressure high	✓	.	✓	.	✓	.
Ever told had coronary heart disease	✓	.	✓	.	✓	.
Ever told had myocardial infarction	✓	.	✓	.	✓	.
Ever told had stroke	✓	.	✓	.	✓	.
Ever told had arthritis	.	✓	✓	✓	✓	✓
Ever told blood cholesterol high	✓	.	✓	.	✓	.
Had pain, aching, stiffness, and swelling	.	✓	✓	.	.	.

Note: ✓ means the information was collected. *BRFSS = Behavioral Risk Factor Surveillance System

(1987) and Schafer (1997). The basic idea of multiple imputations is to create two or more completed datasets using the correlation structure of the available covariates, and then do analysis on each completed dataset. Subsequently, we make inferences based on both within and between variability of the estimates obtained from the completed datasets.

In this method, the missing values are filled in by drawing random samples from the conditional distribution of missing values given the observed values. Assuming the joint distribution of the variables is multivariate normal, and using the Markov Chain Monte Carlo (MCMC) method to obtain simulation-based estimates of the posterior parameters of the distribution, values from the conditional distribution for the missing values are drawn randomly given the observed values. It is noteworthy that most of our missing values are binary, rather than multivariate normal. However, Horton, Lipsitz, and Parzen (2003) show that the parameter estimates from the imputed dataset are unbiased as long as the imputed values are not rounded to binary (0, 1) values.

The performance of the multiple-imputation method can be seen in our case by comparing the descriptive statistics of the imputed variables before and after imputation, as presented in Table 6.2. The table shows that the mean and standard deviation of each variable before and after imputation are almost the same. Since the "missingness" does not depend on any variables in the dataset, the missing values are considered to be *missing completely at random* (MCAR). The MCAR characteristic of the missing values implies that the statistics obtained from incomplete data are unbiased. Since the statistics obtained from the imputed datasets are almost the same as those obtained from the incomplete (original) dataset, the statistics obtained from the imputed datasets are also unbiased.[9]

---

[9]In this study, we use SAS® to perform the multiple-imputation procedure and also all other calculations.

Table 6.2	Mean and Standard Deviation Based on Original and Imputed Datasets					
	Original Dataset		Imputed Dataset		Ratio	
Variable	Mean	Std. Dev.	Mean	Std. Dev.	Mean	Std. Dev.
Number of days physical health not good	3.562	8.002	3.578	8.011	1.004	1.001
Number of days mental health not good	3.317	7.501	3.322	7.501	1.001	1.000
Ever told had diabetes	0.070	0.256	0.070	0.256	1.000	1.000
Annual household Income ($1,000)	50.243	37.202	49.361	37.298	0.982	1.003
Could not afford to see doctor	0.113	0.316	0.113	0.316	1.000	1.000
Heavy drinking	0.133	0.340	0.134	0.340	1.005	1.000
Activities limited due to health problem	0.189	0.391	0.185	0.390	0.979	0.996
Ever had asthma	0.119	0.324	0.119	0.324	0.998	1.000
Ever told blood pressure high	0.276	0.447	0.280	0.447	1.013	1.001
Ever told had coronary heart disease	0.049	0.217	0.048	0.216	0.968	0.997
Ever told had myocardial infarction	0.043	0.204	0.042	0.203	0.959	0.997
Ever told had stroke	0.026	0.158	0.024	0.158	0.931	0.999
Ever told had arthritis	0.280	0.449	0.281	0.449	1.004	1.001
Ever told blood cholesterol high	0.324	0.468	0.304	0.469	0.937	1.001
Had pain, aching, stiffness or swelling	0.420	0.494	0.443	0.498	1.056	1.008
Participate in phys. activities or exercises	0.754	0.431	0.754	0.430	1.000	1.000
Fruit and vegetable servings per day	3.855	2.192	3.862	2.191	1.002	1.000

Results

Coefficient Estimates

Table 6.3 presents the coefficient estimates of equation (1). Since this study is based on pooled cross-sectional observational data without controlling for endogeneity, the coefficient estimates do not necessarily suggest any causality relationship—they merely reflect a measure of association between quality of health and the explanatory variables. So it is possible that the association reflects reverse causality. For example, good health may have a positive effect on income. However, the higher the coefficient's absolute value the stronger is the association between quality of health and the corresponding explanatory variable.

As the SAH ranges from "poor" (=1) to "excellent" (=5), a positive coefficient of an explanatory variable indicates that a higher value of the variable is associated with a higher quality of health, while a negative coefficient indicates that a higher value of the variable is associated with a lower quality of health. From Table 6.3, we can see that health status declines steadily as age increases. The negative coefficient estimate for gender indicates that females are healthier than males on average. All racial/ethnic dummies have negative coefficient estimates, implying that after controlling for objective health measures, the self-reported health of minority populations are lower than that of the White population. It may mean that there are omitted covariates in the regression

	Coefficient Estimate of the Ordered Probit Model		
Variable	**Coefficient Estimate**	**Standard Error**	**P-value**
Intercept	4.0997	0.1629	0.0000
Age 25–29	0.1848	0.0567	0.0011
Age 30–34	0.1662	0.0532	0.0018
Age 35–39	0.1028	0.0545	0.0593
Age 40–44	0.0531	0.0529	0.3148
Age 45–49	0.0814	0.0552	0.1404
Age 50–54	0.0088	0.0576	0.8784
Age 55–59	0.0532	0.0608	0.3811
Age 60–64	0.0130	0.0680	0.8478
Age 65–69	−0.1666	0.0739	0.0243
Age 70–74	−0.1162	0.0755	0.1236
Age 75–79	−0.3492	0.0842	0.0000
Age 80–84	−0.3112	0.0939	0.0009
Age >=85	−0.5571	0.1275	0.0000
Sex (male=1)	−0.0373	0.0239	0.1182
Black	−0.1423	0.0418	0.0007
Hispanic	−0.4037	0.0447	0.0000
Asian	−0.4191	0.0693	0.0000
AIAN	−0.1585	0.1451	0.2748
Other	−0.2822	0.0857	0.0010
Marital status	−0.0501	0.0240	0.0370
Body mass index/27	−0.6948	0.0614	0.0000
Grades 9–11 (Some high school)	0.3806	0.0843	0.0000
Grade 12 or GED (High school graduate)	0.5138	0.0762	0.0000
College 1 year to 3 years (Some college or technical school)	0.6270	0.0778	0.0000
College 4 years or more (College graduate)	0.7991	0.0793	0.0000
Self-employed	0.2432	0.0396	0.0000
Out of work	0.0186	0.0508	0.7136
A homemaker	−0.0158	0.0463	0.7335
A student	0.1424	0.0658	0.0306
Retired	−0.0979	0.0463	0.0343
Unable to work	−0.4573	0.0652	0.0000
Having health plan	0.1101	0.0399	0.0058
Annual Household Income ($1,000)	0.0048	0.0004	0.0000
Smoking	−0.2418	0.0275	0.0000
Participating in any physical activities or exercises	0.3076	0.0289	0.0000
Fruit and vegetable servings per day	0.0424	0.0072	0.0000
Number of days physical health not good	−0.0595	0.0025	0.0000
Number of days mental health not good	−0.0157	0.0016	0.0000
Ever told had diabetes	−0.7772	0.0543	0.0000
Could not afford to see doctor	−0.3063	0.0469	0.0000
Heavy drinking	0.0439	0.0338	0.1957

Table 6.3

Table
6.3

Coefficient Estimate of the Ordered Probit Model, Continued

Variable	Coefficient Estimate	Standard Error	P-value
Activities limited due to health problem	−0.6144	0.0392	0.0000
Ever had asthma	−0.2065	0.0348	0.0000
Ever told blood pressure high	−0.3967	0.0299	0.0000
Ever told had coronary heart disease	−0.4685	0.0721	0.0000
Ever told had myocardial infarction	−0.4392	0.0894	0.0001
Ever told had stroke	−0.3093	0.0838	0.0004
Ever told had arthritis	−0.1240	0.0319	0.0002
Ever told blood cholesterol high	−0.2090	0.0271	0.0000
Had pain, aching, stiffness or swelling in or around a joint	−0.2228	0.0386	0.0001
Dummy for NY City	−0.1934	0.0266	0.0000
Threshold 2	1.7705	0.0618	0.0000
Threshold 3	3.6140	0.1100	0.0000
Threshold 4	5.2001	0.1531	0.0000

McKelvey–Zavoina $R^2 = 0.60$

Note: Reference for Age group dummies is 18–24; for Education it is grade 8 or less; and for Employment status it is employed for wage.

(e.g., severity of diseases and risk factors, neighborhood effects, discrimination, etc.) that systematically affect the health of the minorities. Kobetz, Daniel, and Earp (2003) found that neighborhood poverty is associated with a greater likelihood of poor SAH.[10]

The negative coefficient of body mass index indicates that higher body mass index is associated with lower quality of health. With the dummy for elementary school or lower as the base, the coefficient estimates of all education levels are positive. These estimates tell us that higher education is associated with a better quality of health. The negative coefficient estimate of the dummy for living in New York City indicates that the conditional mean of quality of health of New York City population is lower than that of the rest of New York State population. It is noteworthy that the dummies for other cities such as Utica, Syracuse, Buffalo, Rochester, and Albany were not statistically significant and therefore were excluded from the equation. Respondents having a health insurance plan have better quality of health than respondents without a health plan, as expected. The coefficient estimate of annual household income is positive indicating that higher income is associated with better quality of health.

The coefficient estimate of smoking is negative which indicates smokers have lower quality of health than nonsmokers. Participating in physical activities or exercise has a positive association with the quality of health. Consuming more fruits and vegetables is associated with a better quality of health. This finding is consistent with the belief that dietary differences in fruits and vegetables contribute to differences in morbidity for

---

[10]It may also be due to relatively different thresholds used by White while reporting SAH; see Banks, Marmot, Oldfield, and Smith (2006). However, this explanation is less likely in our case because we allow for heteroskedastic errors where the race/ethnicity variables are statistically significant. See footnote 4.

chronic diseases (James & Nelson, 1997). A number of researchers have found that poor neighborhoods tend to have poor diets; certain aspects of disadvantaged neighborhoods act to hinder the procurement of healthy food; see Ecob and MacIntyre (2000) and Diez-Roux et al. (1999). Thus, the fruit and vegetable variable in our regression may be capturing certain omitted other neighborhood characteristics that affect health adversely.

All coefficient estimates of health variables (diseases and risk factors) are negative as expected, and almost all of them are statistically significant at the 5% level of significance. The relative magnitudes of the coefficient estimates are quite sensible. The diseases or risk factors generally considered serious such as diabetes, coronary heart disease, myocardial infarction, and stroke have relatively high coefficient estimates in absolute value. While the diseases or risk factors considered less serious have relatively low coefficient estimates in absolute value. These findings based on the New York State population are broadly consistent to the results obtained by Cutler and Richardson (1997, 1998) and Groot (2000) based on the U.S. population.

In many studies, it has been debated whether higher income inequality in a society is associated with poor average health. Van Ourti, van Doorslear, and Koolman (2006) show that when the relationship between income and health is concave, proportional income growth increases average health, and rising income inequality reduces average health. Wilkinson and Pickett (2006) compile results from 155 published peer review papers about the relationship between income inequality and population health. About seventy percent of the results suggest that health status is lower in societies where income is more unequal. The proponents of the association between income inequality and health are, for example, Wilkinson (1992), Kennedy, Kawachi, Glass, and Prothrow-Smith (1998), Soobader and LeClere (1999), and Subramanian and Kawachi (2003, 2004, 2006).

Studies on the relationship between income inequality and health have been conducted using various levels of data, from census track level to national level, and based on cross section and time series data. The measure of health outcome also varies including self-assessed health status, mortality rate, or life expectancy. For example, Subramanian and Kawachi (2003) test the association between income inequality and individual poor self-assessed health states in the United States.

Deaton and Lubotsky (2003) have, however, found that after controlling for the racial composition of population in a city, the effect of income inequality on health disappears. They argue that the higher is the percentage of minorities (e.g., Blacks) the higher the income inequality in the city.

In addition to the estimation results reported in Table 6.3, we also estimated equation (1) with three additional variables: county Gini coefficient (as a measure of income inequality), percent Black, and percent Hispanic. We found that the coefficients of all these variables were insignificant when the dummy for New York City area was included. Without the New York City dummy, however, the Gini coefficient was significant in this multilevel regression even when we controlled for percent Black and percent Hispanic, which is inconsistent to those found by Deaton and Lubotsky (2003). In our case, it can be explained by the fact that the patterns of income inequality and percent blacks across regions are quite different and, hence, are not collinear (see Figures 6.3 and 6.4). Since the New York City dummy is picking up the effect of the three variables and the effect of income inequality is weak, we decided to use the specification in Table 6.3 in subsequent analysis.

Table 6.4 presents the coefficient estimates of the scale function. These coefficient estimates indicate that the error in equation (1) is heteroskedastic and is a function of

Table 6.4

Coefficient Estimate of the Heteroskedasticity Scale Function			
Variable	Coefficient Estimate	Standard Error	P-value
Sex (male=1)	0.2084	0.0544	0.0002
Age 25–29	0.1109	0.1276	0.3851
Age 30–34	−0.0662	0.1386	0.6336
Age 35–39	−0.0365	0.1342	0.7861
Age 40–44	−0.0735	0.1342	0.5843
Age 45–49	0.0519	0.1251	0.6784
Age 50–54	0.1943	0.1236	0.1161
Age 55–59	0.2911	0.1230	0.0180
Age 60–64	0.4317	0.1208	0.0004
Age 65–69	0.2825	0.1471	0.0573
Age 70–74	0.2632	0.1429	0.0660
Age 75–79	0.4133	0.1461	0.0048
Age 80–84	0.2888	0.1809	0.1116
Age $\geq$ 85	0.8155	0.1737	0.0000
Black	0.3716	0.0818	0.0000
Hispanic	0.4014	0.0810	0.0000
Asian	0.3521	0.1505	0.0198
AIAN	0.6897	0.2313	0.0029
Annual household income ($1,000)	−0.0024	0.0009	0.0067
Having health plan	−0.2058	0.0794	0.0096
Education higher than high school	−0.1035	0.0574	0.0717
Sex (male=1)	0.2084	0.0544	0.0002

gender, age, race/ethnicity, annual household income, having health plan, and education. However, d'Uva, van Doorslaer, Lindeboom, O'Donnell, and Chatterji (2006) found that reporting heterogeneity of health status does not have a large quantitative impact on the measures of health inequality.

Estimates of Health Index

Quality of Health by Racial/Ethnic Groups

Table 6.5 presents the average estimated quality of health and health-adjusted life expectancy (HALE). Comparing racial/ethnic groups, Asian followed by White has the highest average estimated quality of health, while AIAN followed by Hispanic and Black have the lowest. The average age varies considerably among racial/ethnic groups from 38.6 years through 47.6 years. In addition, the average estimated quality of health of a group depends on age distribution in the group. A group with a higher proportion of young individuals, ceteris paribus, will have a better quality of health relative to groups with a lower proportion of young individuals. Comparing the average quality of health between groups in a population with different age distributions could be misleading.

Several methods can be used to control for the effects of age distribution. The simplest method is to compare the average estimated quality of health between groups of population by age groups. Another method is to incorporate the quality of health into

Table 6.5	Average Estimated Quality of Health and Health-Adjusted Life Expectancy (HALE)						
		All	White	Black	Hispanic	Asian	AIAN
Average quality of health		0.750	0.765	0.715	0.678	0.778	0.665
Age	Life expectancy			HALE (in year)			
20–24	58.23	43.05	44.24	40.23	36.81	43.75	37.52
25–29	53.50	39.35	40.44	36.62	33.40	40.05	33.74
30–34	48.74	35.52	36.48	32.90	29.87	36.19	30.33
35–39	44.00	31.68	32.51	29.22	26.35	32.33	26.73
40–44	39.33	27.97	28.69	25.66	23.02	28.65	23.28
45–49	34.78	24.41	25.02	22.30	19.90	25.11	20.23
50–54	30.36	20.99	21.48	19.15	16.99	21.68	17.82
55–59	26.09	17.76	18.16	16.17	14.28	18.48	15.27
60–64	22.01	14.74	15.05	13.47	11.85	15.30	12.77
65–69	18.19	11.96	12.16	10.95	9.68	12.58	10.17
70–74	14.69	9.56	9.68	8.77	7.87	10.61	8.11
75–79	11.54	7.39	7.48	6.75	6.07	8.38	6.13
80–84	8.79	5.63	5.70	5.22	4.69	6.34	4.86

the life table of the group. In other words, we combine morbidity and mortality data to obtain the estimates of Health-Adjusted Life Expectancy (HALE) (see Molla, Madans, Wagener, & Crimmins, 2003). The HALE measures the expected life (years) in perfect health condition. This measure is also called Healthy Life Expectancy (HLE). Since dependable life tables for different racial/ethnic groups are not available, in this study HALE is calculated based on the general U.S. population life table of 2002 (Arias, 2004). Thus, HALE estimated in this chapter is used to compare the quality of health among groups of populations by eliminating the effect of age distribution without differentiating the mortality rates among the groups. HALE for each racial/ethnic group by age groups is presented in Table 6.5.

The table shows that Whites in the youngest age group (20–24) have the highest HALE followed by Asian, and Hispanic has the lowest followed by AIAN. A 20-year old White individual is expected to live for 44.2 years in perfect health condition, while a Hispanic with the same age is expected to live for 36.8 years in perfect health condition. Thus, at age 20, a White individual is expected to live almost 7.5 years in perfect health longer than a Hispanic individual. It is clear from these results that by eliminating the effect of age distribution, Whites do better than Asian, while Hispanics do worse than AIAN. This is a remarkable result. Also note that if HALE for each racial/ethnic group is calculated based on its own life table, the disparity across racial/ethnic groups could be higher as quality of health is correlated with life expectancy (Mullahy, 2001).

Regional Disparity in Health

In this part, we do not compute HALE for each area for two reasons. First, the distributions of age across the areas are very similar so the effect of age distribution is negligible.

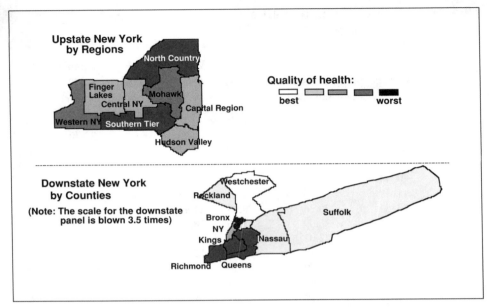

Average estimated quality of health by geographic areas.

Second, not all areas have enough observations required to compute HALE. The average quality of health by areas is presented in Figure 6.14. Nassau, Suffolk, Rockland, and Westchester Counties are the brightest areas reflecting the highest quality of health. In contrast, Bronx County is in the darkest area followed by Richmond County, North Country, Kings County, Queens County, and Southern Tier. None of the Upstate areas is in the brightest group, while Downstate areas vary from the brightest to the darkest, indicating that health disparity across Downstate areas is higher than that across Upstate areas. This finding is consistent with the socioeconomic variations across geographic areas presented in Figures 6.2, 6.3, and 6.4.

It is very common that quality of health is measured using dichotomized SAH; cf. CDC. For example, quality of health of a group may be defined as a percentage of individuals in "very good" and "excellent" health condition (e.g., Keppel, Pearcy, & Klein, 2004); or it may be defined as the complement of the percentage of individuals in "poor" and "fair" health condition. Unfortunately, this means that the health rank of a group depends on the chosen cut–off point in dichotomizing the SAH.

The procedure used in this chapter circumvents this problem of arbitrariness by utilizing all five categories of SAH.

Inequality

Similar to the case of the quality of health, we also compare income-related health inequality among racial/ethnic groups as well as across geographic areas of New York State. In addition, this section also presents the decomposition results for each racial/ethnic group and for different geographic areas.

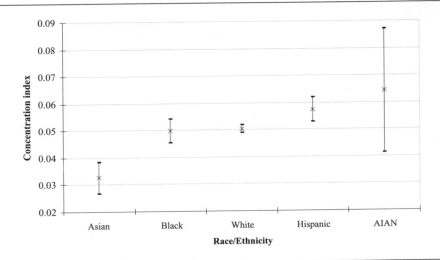

Concentration indices with 95%-confidence intervals by racial/ethnic groups.

Income–Related Health Inequality By Race/Ethnicity

Figure 6.15 presents the concentration index by racial/ethnic groups with corresponding 95%-confidence intervals. The standard errors of the concentration index are calculated using the Huber–White robust estimator. All indices are significantly greater than zero, indicating that health disparities between the rich and the poor exist in all groups. There is, however, substantial variation in the coefficients among groups. The highest inequality index is found within the AIAN group followed by Hispanics. The lowest inequality is found within the Asian group followed by Whites.

Another way to compare income–related health inequality between groups of populations is by comparing their concentration curves. Figure 6.16 presents the concentration curves expressed as the deviation of the concentration curve from the diagonal in order to amplify the differences between racial/ethnic groups. The figure provides more obvious evidence of the differences of income-related health inequalities between racial/ethnic groups. The Asian curve strictly dominates others, while the AIAN curve is dominated by others. These indicate that AIAN is the most unequal at all percentiles, while Asian is the least. Therefore, differences between racial/ethnic groups are not only in terms of the average quality of health but also in terms of health distribution itself over income among individuals within each group.

Regional Variation in Income Related Health Inequality

Concentration indices across the geographic areas are presented in Figure 6.17. North Country and Mohawk are in the darkest areas indicating the highest income related health inequality, while the brightest areas are represented by—from the lowest to the highest—Nassau, Westchester, Queens, and Suffolk County. Figures 6.14 and 6.17 show that areas with lower quality of health tend to have higher income related health inequality. These values have been plotted in Figure 6.18 for the 8 Upstate regions and 9 Downstate counties. The simple correlation coefficient between them is –0.67 and is statistically

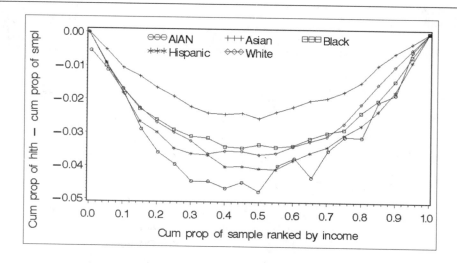

Concentration curve by racial/ethnic groups.

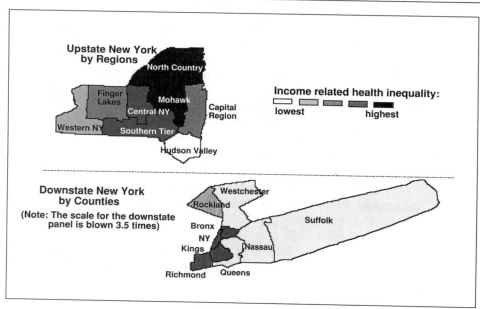

Income related health inequality by geographic areas.

significant. The worst two regions in terms of both health inequality and health are North Country (4) and Bronx County (9). It is interesting that both regions 4 and 9 report very high levels of medical risk factors like diabetes, obesity, and asthma, but the racial compositions of the two areas are diametrically opposite. On the other hand, two best counties are Nassau (11) and Westchester (17) where a very high average level of

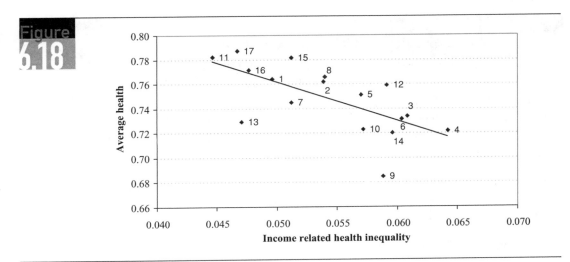

Average health *vs.* income related health inequality.

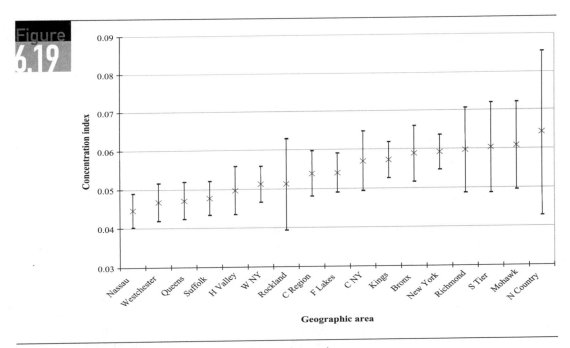

Regional concentration indices with 95%-confidence intervals.

health is achieved with very low health inequality. Interestingly, these two counties have a rather high percentage of African Americans in the population.

For more detailed information about the magnitude and significance of the concentration index across the areas, the corresponding 95%-confidence intervals by areas are presented in Figure 6.19. All coefficients are significantly different from zero, indicating that income-related health inequalities exist in all areas. The statistical significance of the

Table 6.6	Decomposition of Health Inequality by Racial/Ethnic Groups						
			Percentage Contribution of Each Factor to Health Inequality				
Race/Ethnicity	Age	Race/Ethnicity	Education	Employment	Income	Smoking	Could not afford to see doctor
All	7.00	5.71	18.63	18.99	41.19	2.48	7.34
White	13.07	–	16.86	18.17	45.40	2.99	6.31
Black	4.71	–	20.73	28.26	35.79	4.64	7.66
Hispanic	6.69	–	24.16	28.47	32.12	0.31	9.16
Asian	-1.96	–	17.45	8.71	63.19	1.35	12.31
AIAN	8.44	–	16.24	42.96	30.67	2.83	1.50

Note: Small contributors are not presented in this table.

difference in the concentration indices between geographic areas can be seen by comparing the confidence intervals. For instance, New York County has a significantly higher concentration index than those of Nassau, Westchester, Queens, and Suffolk Counties. But the concentration index of New York County is not significantly different from those of Kings and Bronx Counties.

An important public policy question is: what are the main factors that are contributing to the inequality? This can be answered by decomposing the inequality into its determinants, as presented in the next section.

Decomposition of Income Related Health Inequality

Decomposition analysis demonstrates the relative contribution of the different components of inequalities for different racial/ethnic groups as well as for different geographic areas. The analysis offers policy makers a starting point for geographical targeting to eliminate health disparity between the rich and the poor. The analysis does not provide unequivocal causal pathways between the determinants of health and income related health inequality. However, this method describes health inequality across income levels and provides explanations for the observed patterns for different groups of population.

In this chapter, we are interested in analyzing income-related health inequality attributable to socio-demographic factors including age, sex, race/ethnicity, marital status, education, employment status, health insurance, smoking status, and access to a doctor. Therefore, in the decomposition analysis, the explanatory variables included in equation (1) are only socio-demographic variables. The percent contribution of each component is calculated by racial/ethnic groups and also by geographic areas. Among all these factors, the contributions of the main variables by racial/ethnic groups are presented in Table 6.6.

For the overall New York State population, among the socio-demographic variables, three major factors contributing to income-related health inequality are household income, employment status, and education. Each of these three factors contributes at least 18% to the inequality. Our estimate of the contribution of income is similar to that in van Doorslaer and Jones (2003) who found that in Canada income contributes between 41%

| Table 6.7 | Decomposition of Health Inequality by Geographic Areas |

Percentage Contribution of Each Factor to Health Inequality (%)

Geographic Area	Age	Race/ Ethnicity	Education	Employment	Income	Smoking	Could not afford to see doctor
H Valley	11.723	2.898	14.400	20.680	43.801	1.540	7.715
C Area	11.425	2.729	17.185	18.509	41.877	3.617	6.735
Mohawk	11.509	1.980	17.181	22.284	35.310	3.728	10.032
N Country	2.343	-0.423	15.372	26.392	41.477	4.242	12.748
C NY	12.493	1.875	13.862	21.981	41.164	3.272	7.961
S Tier	8.061	2.046	17.799	26.207	34.958	4.643	8.578
W NY	12.135	3.085	15.937	23.205	39.463	2.891	6.031
F Lakes	7.440	4.098	18.908	15.137	44.668	4.314	7.844
Bronx	4.601	6.943	22.959	28.562	30.380	1.221	7.394
Kings	5.322	8.382	21.643	21.876	35.676	1.549	7.726
Nassau	12.651	3.603	16.421	14.401	47.478	1.680	5.509
New York	4.861	9.910	19.671	17.994	40.805	1.522	7.281
Queens	2.677	10.454	19.950	13.675	44.474	0.793	10.956
Richmond	10.606	3.828	11.995	23.479	41.043	1.586	8.990
Rockland	1.940	4.599	14.693	19.430	48.030	0.057	12.672
Suffolk	13.244	4.008	14.982	15.427	45.839	2.931	5.636
Westchester	7.353	6.875	19.880	13.252	46.472	1.854	6.365

Note: Small contributors are not presented in this table.

to 47% of income-related health inequality. However, we find that income is relatively less important for the disadvantaged minority groups (viz., Black, Hispanic, and AIAN). For Asian the corresponding percentage is very high (63%). If health status were distributed equally across income levels, employment status, and education levels, then the disparity between the rich and the poor in New York State population would be 79% lower.

After controlling for other factors, race/ethnicity contributes only 6% to the inequality. Race/ethnicity is highly intertwined with household income, employment status, and education—Blacks, Hispanics, and AIANs have lower household income, lower education levels, and lower employment rates compared to those of Whites. That is another reason why separate analysis for each group is necessary.

The pattern of the contributions of the socio-demographic variables varies considerably between racial/ethnic groups. Income has the largest contribution to the inequalities for all groups (except AIAN), indicating that income redistribution policy is the most effective policy to eliminate health disparity between the poor and the rich within these ethnic/racial groups. For AIANs, the most effective public policy is to ensure employment opportunities to all individuals. For Whites, the second largest contributor to income-related health inequality is employment status (18%) followed by education (16%); for Blacks the second largest is employment status (28%) followed by education (20%); for Hispanics the second largest is employment status (29%) followed by education (24%); for Asians the second largest is education (17%) followed by inability to see a doctor (12%). The differences in the patterns of the contributions indicate that different groups of population need different policies to eliminate health disparity between the rich and the poor.

Comparing across the geographic areas, the contribution of each factor to the inequality varies noticeably, too (see Table 6.7). Income is the largest contributor to the inequality for all areas, ranging from 30% (Bronx County) to 48% (Rockland County). In addition to income, employment status and education also contribute substantially to the inequality in all areas. The contribution of employment status varies considerably ranging from 13% (Westchester County) to 29% (Bronx County), while the contribution of education ranges from 12% (Richmond County) to 23% (Bronx County). Thus, in addition to income redistribution policy, ensuring employment opportunities and good educational access are also effective ways to eliminate health disparity between the rich and the poor in these areas. For Queens and New York Counties, race/ethnicity contributes to the inequality relatively high—10% and 10% respectively—compared to other areas. This indicates that providing good access to health care for minorities in these two counties is also an effective way to eliminate the disparity.

Conclusions

Following recent developments in measuring quality of health and health inequality, we use self-assessed health status conditioned by several objective determinants as a comprehensive measure of individual health. Among racial/ethnic groups, AIANs followed by Hispanics have the lowest average quality of health, while after adjusting for age distribution, Hispanics have the lowest average quality of health. Asians have the highest average followed by Whites, while after adjusting for age distribution, Whites have the best quality of health. These results highlight that when comparing quality of health between groups of populations, one needs to consider the age distribution within each group.

In Upstate New York, North Country and Southern Tier have the lowest average quality of health, whereas in Downstate Bronx, Richmond, Kings, and Queens Counties have the lowest. Comparing all regions of New York State, Nassau, Suffolk, Rockland, and Westchester Counties have very high levels of average health. However, quality of health is more unequal across Downstate areas than Upstate, as one would possibly expect.

We find statistically significant income-related health inequality within each racial/ethnic group and each geographic area of New York State. The highest inequality is found within the AIAN group followed by Hispanics, while the lowest inequality is found within the Asian group, followed by Whites. Across the 17 geographic areas, the highest income-related health inequality is found in North Country followed by Mohawk, while the lowest inequality is found in Nassau County followed by Westchester County. Areas with lower average quality of health have larger health disparity between the rich and the poor; the correlation is –0.67 and is statistically significant.

Decomposition analysis of income related health inequality presented in this chapter offers New York health policy makers certain guidelines to eliminate health disparity in the population. Three major factors generating the disparity are household income, employment status, and education. Contribution of each of these factors varies considerably between racial/ethnic groups as well as across the geographic areas suggesting different pathways from income to health. Income has the largest contribution to the disparity for all groups but AIANs and for all areas. This indicates that income redistribution policy is the most effective policy to eliminate the health disparity within each group (except AIAN), as well as within each area. The relative health status of AIAN in almost all recorded dimensions is disturbingly bad, and the most effective policy for this group was found to be the generation of employment opportunities. For Blacks and Hispanics, public policy that ensures employment opportunities is also an effective way to eliminate disparity.

Our results underscore the need for different public policy initiatives for different racial/ethnic groups and different geographic areas to eliminate health disparity between the rich and the poor. In the long run, policies that can ensure equality in income (e.g., income redistribution), employment opportunities, and educational access will have a substantial impact on improving the average quality of health and in eliminating health disparity.

REFERENCES

Adams, P., Hurd, M., McFadden, D., Merrill, A., & Ribeiro, T. (2003). Healthy, wealthy, and wise? Tests for direct causal between health and socioeconomic status. *Journal of Econometrics, 112*, 3–56.

Adler, N. E., & Newman, K. (2002). Socioeconomic disparities in health: Pathways and policies. *Health Affairs, 21*, 60–76.

Adler, N. E., & Ostrove, J. M. (1999). SES and health: What we know and what we don't. *Annals of the New York Academy of Sciences, 896*, 3–5.

Arias, E. (2004). *United States life tables, 2002*. National Vital Statistics Reports 53. Hyattsville, MD: National Center for Health Statistics.

Ayanian, J. Z., Weissman, J. S., Chasan-Taber, S., & Epstein, A. M. (1999). Quality of care by race and gender for congestive heart failure and pneumonia. *Medical Care, 37*, 1260–1269.

Banks, J. B., Marmot, M., Oldfield, Z., & Smith, J. P. (2006). *The SES health gradient on both sides of the Atlantic*. National Bureau of Economic Research working paper 12674. Cambridge, MA.

Bommier, A., & Stecklov, G. (2002). Defining health inequality: Why Rawls succeeds where social welfare theory fails. *Journal of Health Economics, 21*, 497–513.

Centers for Disease Control and Prevention (CDC). (1999–2004). *Behavioral Risk Factor Surveillance System Survey Data*. Atlanta, GA: U.S. Department of Health and Human Services, Centers for Disease Control and Prevention.

Clarke, P. M., & Ryan, C. (2006). Self-reported health: Reliability and consequences for health inequality measurement. *Health Economics, 15*, 645–652.

Cutler, D. M., Deaton, A., & Lleras-Muney, A. (2006). The determinants of mortality. *Journal of Economic Perspectives, 20*, 97–120.

Cutler, D. M., & Lleras-Muney, A. (2006). *Education and health: Evaluating theories and evidence*. National Bureau of Economic Research working paper 12352. Cambridge, MA.

Cutler, D. M., & Richardson, E. (1997). Measuring the health of the U.S. population. In M. N. Baily, P. C. Reiss, & C. Winston (Eds.), *Brookings papers on economic activity: Microeconomics* (pp. 217–271). Washington, DC: Brookings Institution.

Cutler, D. M., & Richardson, E. (1998). The value of health: 1970–1990. *American Economic Review, 88*, 97–100.

Deaton, A. (2006). Global pattern of income and health: Facts, interpretation, and policies. National Bureau of Economic Research working paper 12735. Cambridge, MA.

Deaton, A., & Lubotsky, D. (2003). Mortality, inequality and race in American cities and states. *Social Science & Medicine, 56*, 1139–1153.

Diez-Roux, A. V., Nieto, F. J., Caulfield, L., Tyroler, H. A., Watson, R. L., & Szklo, M. (1999). Neighborhood differences in diet: The Atherosclerosis Risk in Communities (ARIC) study. *Journal of Epidemiology and Community Health, 53*, 55–63.

d'Uva, T. B., van Doorslaer, E., Lindeboom, M., O'Donnell, O., & Chatterji, S. (2006). *Does reporting heterogeneity bias the measure of health disparity?* Timbergen Institute discussion paper, TI 2006-033/3.

Ecob, R., & MacIntyre, S. (2000). Small area variations in health related behaviors: Do these depend on the behavior itself, its measurement, or on personal characteristics? *Health & Place, 6*, 261–274.

Environmental Systems Research Institute (ESRI). (2002). *ArcView GIS.* Version 3.3. Redlands, CA: Author.

Groot, W. (2000). Adaptation and scale of reference bias in self-assessments of quality of life. *Journal of Health Economics, 19*, 403–420.

Horton, N. J., Lipsitz, S. R., & Parzen, M. (2003). A potential for bias when rounding in multiple imputation. *American Statistician, 57*, 229–232.

Humphries, K. H., & van Doorslaer, E. (2000). Income-related health inequality in Canada. *Social Science Medicine, 50*, 663–671.

Idler, E. L., & Benyamini, Y. (1997). Self-rated health and mortality: A review of twenty-seven community studies. *Journal of Health and Social Behavior, 38*, 21–37.

Institute of Medicine. (2002). *Unequal treatment: Controlling racial and ethnic disparities in health care.* Washington, DC: National Academies Press.

James, W., & Nelson, M. (1997). The contribution of nutrition to inequalities in health. *British Medical Journal, 314*, 1545–1550.

Kakwani, N., Wagstaff, A., & van Doorslaer, E. (1997). Socioeconomic inequalities in health: Measurement, computation, and statistical inference. *Journal of Econometrics, 77*, 59–103.

Kennedy, B. P., Kawachi, I., Glass, R., & Prothrow-Stith, D. (1998). Income distribution socioeconomic status, self-rated health in the United States: Multilevel analysis. *British Medical Journal, 317*, 917–921.

Keppel, K. G., Pearcy, J. N., & Klein, R. J. (2004). *Measuring progress in Healthy People 2010.* Statistical notes 25. Hyattsville, MD: National Center for Health Statistics.

Kobetz, E., Daniel, M., & Earp, J. A. (2003). Neighborhood poverty and self-reported health among low-income, rural women, 50 years and older. *Health & Place, 9*, 263–271.

Koolman, X., & van Doorslaer, E. (2004). On the interpretation of a concentration index of inequality. *Health Economics, 13*, 649–656.

Lahiri, K., Vaughan, D. R., & Wixon, B. (1995). Modeling SSA's sequential disability determination process using matched SIPP data. *Social Security Bulletin, 58*, 1–41.

Lecluyse, A., & Cleemput, I. (2005). Making health continuous: Implications of different methods on the measurement of inequality. *Health Economics, 15*, 99–104.

Manor, O., Matthews, S., & Power, C. (2001). Self-rated health and limiting longstanding illness: Inter-relationships with morbidity in early adulthood. *International Journal of Epidemiology, 30*, 600–607.

McKelvey, R., & Zavoina, W. (1975). A statistical model for the analysis of ordinal level dependent variables. *Journal of Mathematical Sociology, 4*, 103–120.

Milanovic, B. (1997). A simple way to calculate the Gini coefficient, and some implications. *Economics Letters, 56*, 45–49.

Mokdad, A. H., Marks, J. S., Stroup, D. F., & Gerberding, J. L. (2004). Actual causes of death in the United States, 2000. *Journal of the American Medical Association, 291*, 1238–1245.

Molla, M. T., Madans, J. H., Wagener, W. K., & Crimmins, E. M. (2003). *Summary measures of population health: Report of findings on methodologic and data issues.* Hyattsville, MD: National Center for Health Statistics.

Mullahy, J. (2001). Live long, live well: Quantifying the health of heterogeneous population. *Health Economics, 10*, 429–440.

Must, A., Spadano, J., Coakley, E. H., Field, A. E., Colditz, G., & Dietz, W. H. (1999). The disease burden associated with overweight and obesity. *Journal of the American Medical Association, 282*, 1523–1529.

National Center for Health Statistics (NCHS). (2006). *Health, United States, 2006: With chartbook on trends in the health of Americans.* Hyattsville, MD: Author.

Rawls, J. (1971). *A theory of justice.* Cambridge, MA: Harvard University Press.

Rubin, D. B. (1987). *Multiple imputation for nonresponse in surveys.* New York: John Wiley.

Safaei, J. (2006). Income and health inequality across Canadian provinces. *Health & Place, 9*, 3.

Schafer, J. L. (1997). *Analysis of incomplete multivariate data.* New York: Chapman and Hall.

Sehili, S., Elbasha, E. H., Moriarty, D. G., & Zack, M. M. (2005). Inequalities in self-reported physical health in the United States, 1993–1999. *Health Economics, 14*, 377–389.

Shishehbor, M. H., Litaker, D., Pothier, C. E., & Lauer, M. S. (2006). Association of socioeconomic status with functional capacity, heart rate recovery, and all-cause mortality. *Journal of the American Medical Association, 295*, 784–792.

Sickles, R. C., & Taubman, P. (1997). Mortality and morbidity among adults and elderly. In M. R. Rozenzweig & O. Stark (Eds.), *Handbook of population and family economics*. Amsterdam: North-Holland.

Soobader, M.-J., & LeClere, F. B. (1999). Aggregation and the measurement of income inequality: Effects on morbidity. *Social Science & Medicine, 48*, 733–744.

Subramanian, S. V., & Kawachi, I. (2003). The association between state income inequality and worse health is not confounded by race. *International Journal of Epidemiology, 32*, 1022–1028.

Subramanian, S. V., & Kawachi, I. (2004). Income inequality and health: What have we learned so far? *Epidemiologic Reviews, 26*, 78–91.

Subramanian, S. V., & Kawachi, I. (2006). Whose health is affected by income inequality? A multilevel interaction analysis of contemporaneous and lagged effects of state income inequality on individual self-rated health in the United States. *Health & Place, 12*, 141–156.

U.S. Census Bureau. (2000). *American FactFinder fact sheet*. Retrieved January 10, 2007, from http://factfinder.census.gov/

U.S. Department of Health and Human Services (US-DHHS). (2000). *Healthy People 2010: Understanding and improving health* (2nd ed.). Washington, DC: U.S. Government Printing Office.

U.S. Department of Health and Human Services (US-DHHS). (2004). *The health consequences of smoking: Surgeon General's report*. Washington, DC: U.S. Government Printing Office.

van Doorslaer, E., & Jones, A. M. (2003). Inequalities in self-reported health: Validation of a new approach to measurement. *Journal of Health Economics, 22*, 61–87.

Van Ourti, T., van Doorslaer, E., & Koolman, X. (2006). *The effect of growth and inequality in incomes on health inequality: Theory and empirical evidence from the European Panel*. Tinbergen Institute discussion paper, TI 2006-108/3. Rotterdam: Erasmus University.

Wagstaff, A., Paci, P., & van Doorslaer, E. (1991). On the measurement of inequalities in health. *Social Science & Medicine, 33*, 545–557.

Wagstaff, A., & van Doorslaer, E. (2004). Overall versus socioeconomic health inequality: A measurement framework and two empirical illustrations. *Health Economics, 13*, 297–301.

Wagstaff, A., van Doorslaer, E., & Watanabe, N. (2003). On decomposing the causes of health sector inequalities with an application to malnutrition inequalities in Vietnam. *Journal of Econometrics, 112*, 207–223.

Wilkinson, R. G. (1992). Income distribution and life expectancy. *British Medical Journal, 304*, 165–168.

Wilkinson, R. G., & Pickett, K. E. (2006). Income inequality and population health: A review and explanation of the evidence. *Social Science & Medicine, 62*, 1768–1784.

Williams, D. R., & Collins, C. (1995). US socioeconomic and racial differences in health: Patterns and explanations. *Annual Review of Sociology, 21*, 349–386.

7

Gbenga Ogedegbe, Antoinette Schoenthaler, and Senaida Fernandez

Introduction

The disproportionately high prevalence of hypertension (HTN) in African Americans compared to Whites is well documented. African Americans have the highest rate of HTN in the United States, affecting 40% compared to only 28% among Whites (Centers for Disease Control and Prevention [CDC], 2005). Despite the higher rates of treatment for HTN among African Americans, they have a lower rate of blood pressure (BP) control compared to Whites (30% versus 35% respectively) (Hertz, Unger, Cornell, & Saunders, 2005; Mensah, Mokdad, Ford, Greenlund, & Croft, 2005). Similarly, the prevalence of hypertension-related complications is much higher in African Americans compared to Whites. For instance, African Americans have a 1.8 times greater rate of fatal stroke, a 1.5 times greater rate of heart disease death, and a 4.2 times greater rate of hypertension-related end-stage kidney disease than Whites (Centers for Disease Control and Prevention, National Center for Health Statistics [CDC/NCHS], 2000; Giles, Kittner, Hebel, Losonczy, & Sherwin, 1995; Klag et al., 1997; Pavlik, Hyman, Vallbona, Toronjo, & Louis, 1997; Singh & Moore, 1996). More importantly, HTN is the second most common explanation of the mortality difference between African Americans and Whites (Wong, Shapiro, Boscardin, & Ettner, 2002). Despite the preponderance of evidence on the racial disparities in hypertension-related outcomes, there is little published data on potential mechanisms of the documented disparities in hypertension-related outcomes.

In 2003, the Institute of Medicine (IOM) published the seminal report, "Unequal Treatment: Confronting Racial and Ethnic Disparities in Health Care," outlining a framework to organize and identify the factors that contribute to racial disparities in health care (Smedley, 2003). According to this framework (illustrated in Figure 7.1), health disparities can be explained in one of three

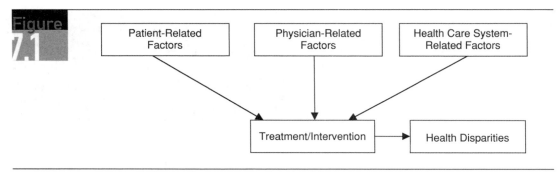

IOM framework of sources of health care disparities in the United States.

ways—patient–related factors such as preferences, beliefs, attitudes, socioeconomic status, and health literacy; physician–related factors such as bias, lack of cultural competence; and health–care systems–related factors such as access to care, insurance status,
and quality of care.

The report posits that patient-specific experiences, beliefs, and attitudes impact the
clinical encounter and treatment in both direct and indirect ways. Chief among these
factors are patient beliefs about acceptability of treatment recommendations, responses
to pharmacologic and nonpharmacologic interventions, mistrust of the medical system
(based on previous health care experiences and experiences with discrimination), and influence of distrust on patient preferences for treatment. In addition, health care provider
attitudes and beliefs, as well as constraints within the clinical interaction, may also impact treatment. The report describes specific pathways through which bias may enter
the clinical interaction and impact treatment, such as clinical uncertainty and provider
beliefs and stereotypes about patients. The necessity for providers to synthesize multiple
sources of information in a limited amount of time may lead to reliance on heuristics
(that may be influenced by bias) in order to arrive at treatment recommendations. Further, health care system-level factors may influence treatment and ultimately translate
into health disparities. These factors include: health care system response to language
barriers, quality of facilities and services accessible to minority patients, referral process
for accessing specialty services or care, and access to care and quality of care as a function
of insurance coverage limitations and insurance reimbursement policies.

In this chapter, we review the evidence to date from the hypertension literature that
addresses the three major components of the conceptual framework described in the
IOM report as an umbrella to frame the mechanisms for hypertension-related disparities
between African Americans and Whites. Relevant patient-related factors in the hypertension literature include poorer responsiveness to treatment (Chobanian et al., 2003);
poorer rates of adherence to prescribed antihypertensive medications (Bosworth et al.,
2006); and patient preferences and beliefs about HTN and its treatment (Ogedegbe,
Harrison, Robbins, Mancuso, & Allegrante, 2004). At the provider–level, disparities
may result from poor doctor-patient communication in the medical encounter due to a
racial/ethnic mismatch between the patient and physician (Cooper, 2004; Cooper-Patrick
et al., 1999; Johnson, Saha, Arbelaez, Beach, & Cooper, 2004); greater rates of clinical
inertia; differential rates of prescribing behavior; and stereotypic beliefs about African
American patients due to low levels of cultural competency. Problems at the level of

health care system include a lack of access to and quality of health care (Bach, Pham, Schrag, Tate, & Hargraves, 2004); and changes in the financing and delivery of health care services.

Patient-Level Barriers

Patient Preferences and Beliefs

Contrary to previous reports, recent data have revealed that hypertensive African Americans are more likely to be aware of their diagnosis, knowledgeable about its etiology and sequel, and receive treatment as compared to their White counterparts (Okonofua, Cutler, Lackland, & Egan, 2005). However, despite improvements in awareness and treatment, hypertensive African Americans are still less likely to exhibit adequate BP control (Sheats et al., 2005). To explain this disparity, Okonofua et al. assessed the racial/ethnic differences in beliefs about hypertension among a sample of older White, Hispanic, and African Americans and the relationship of responses to BP control (2005). Although no racial/ethnic differences emerged in the total number of correct responses, beliefs about the approaches to control BP varied significantly. For instance, African American and Hispanic respondents were more than twice as likely to believe that medications were the sole way to control high BP. Alternatively, White respondents were more likely to believe that lifestyle changes in tandem with medications would improve BP, which in fact was a significant predictor of higher BP control rates. Thus, the disparity in BP control rates between Whites and African Americans may not be due to a lack of knowledge about the disease and its consequences but rather a lack of awareness of the role of lifestyle modifications in managing hypertension (Okonofua et al., 2005).

Indeed, several studies have found that African Americans possess contradictory beliefs about the management and treatment of their HTN that may interfere with achieving adequate levels of BP control. In a qualitative study, assessing the treatment expectations of hypertensive African Americans, many of the participants expected to take an active role in their treatment; they expected their physicians to educate them about BP treatment, and they expect to take medications to lower their BP and prevent heart attack, stroke, and kidney failure. However, despite such appropriate expectations, a considerable proportion of patients had nonbiomedical expectations of their treatment. For instance, 38% expected a cure, 38% did not expect to take their medications for life, and 23% expected to take medications only when they have hypertension-related symptoms (Ogedegbe, Mancuso, & Allegrante, 2004). Such inappropriate expectations may be explained by belief systems that stem from cultural folklore or personal experience rather then current medical understanding. This in turn may contribute to poorer rates of medication adherence and BP control (Heurtin-Roberts & Reisin, 1992). In a quantitative study of urban African Americans, Wilson et al. (2002) found that 75% of the respondents equated the etiology of hypertension to nonmedical causes. These individuals instead defined high blood pressure (BP) in terms of episodic symptoms and personal experiences (i.e., their blood boiling when stressed) and not a specific sphygmomanometer reading.

In minority cultures, alternative medicines and home remedies often take precedence over traditional westernized practices (Brown & Segal, 1996). As such, being nonadherent to prescribed medications may not mean the participants are nonadherent in general; rather they may be actively utilizing an alternative treatment. This idea is supported by a study comparing the use of home remedies versus prescription medications in hypertensive African Americans. The researchers found that participants were likely to use home remedies when they believed such remedies were more beneficial than the prescribed medications and explained that "failure to comply with prescribed medication regimes does not mean the patient goes untreated" (Brown & Segal, p. 903). "It may be more likely that ethnic and racial minorities structure their medication adherence around the simultaneous use of informal treatments as well as the formal medical care system." Thus, it becomes important to examine the meaning one gives to hypertension and patients' cultural beliefs regarding treatment decisions.

Pathophysiology/Genetics

To date, there is no evidence that a unifying pathophysiologic theory can explain the disproportionately higher rates of HTN and blood pressure control among African Americans. Rather, the higher prevalence and consequences of hypertension in this population are due to a multitude of interrelated factors, which are not linked to race per se (Gadegbeku, Lea, & Jamerson, 2005). Genetic epidemiological studies have shown that the higher prevalence of HTN in African Americans may be due in part, to the quality of one's environment as opposed to a single genetic predisposition (Daniel & Rotimi, 2003). For instance, despite the higher proportion of African Americans that are considered salt sensitive, studies have failed to find a clear genetic mutation in the epithelial renal sodium transport. In addition, treatments that are designed to target sodium channel sodium reabsorption have not been as effective in lowering BP in African Americans as compared to Whites. Alternatively, a number of important behavioral factors including obesity, physical inactivity, excess dietary intake of sodium, and inadequate dietary intake of potassium, fruits, and vegetables in this population may contribute to the higher rates of salt-sensitivity and thus, increased rates of hypertension (Ferdinand & Saunders, 2006; Yancy, 2004).

Responsiveness to Nonpharmacologic Treatment

Though there are documented racial differences in the adoption of recommended therapeutic lifestyle behaviors such as increased physical activity and increased intake of fruits and vegetables, data from interventions targeted at therapeutic lifestyle behaviors indicate that African Americans benefit equally (if not more than Whites) in terms of BP compared to Whites. For instance, the degree of BP reduction secondary to a therapeutic lifestyle behavioral intervention plus a Dietary Approach to Systolic Hypertension (DASH) diet was comparable for both African Americans and Whites in the PREMIER trial (Appel et al., 2003). A subanalysis of the data did not reveal any racial difference in the benefits of the intervention; White women and men had an average drop in BP by 4.2 and 5.7 mmHg respectively, compared to a 2.1 and 4.6 mmHg drop in African American men and women (Svetkey et al., 2005). In the DASH trial, African Americans derived the greatest benefit from the intervention in reducing systolic BP as compared to Whites and other ethnic groups (Appel et al., 2001). This difference was even more pronounced among the hypertensive African Americans, who exhibited a reduction in BP by 13.2/6.1 mmHg as opposed to a 6.3/4.4 mmHg BP reduction in hypertensive Whites (Svetkey et al., 2005). Other trials have demonstrated similar benefits, thus suggesting that responsiveness to therapy may not explain the difference noted among hypertensive African Americans and Whites. Limitations of prior studies of nonpharmacologic approaches include the lack of data in primary care settings as well as community-based settings where the majority of patients receive their care.

Responsiveness to Pharmacologic Treatment

It is well documented that African Americans are less likely to respond to beta-blockers and ACE inhibitors as monotherapy compared to Whites. This assumption is based on the low rennin levels noted in African Americans compared to Whites (Flack, Peters, Mehra, & Nasser, 2002). In a meta-analysis of the effects of different classes of antihypertensive medications in African Americans conducted by Brewster, van Montfrans, & Kleijnen (2004), the rates of BP reduction due to treatment with ACE inhibitors were not significantly different from those not on treatment (Brewster et al., 2004). Moreover, of the 23% hypertensive patients that reached the diastolic blood pressure (DBP) goals, only 10% were taking ACE inhibitors. However, because BP control often entails treatment with more than one antihypertensive medication, the use of ACE inhibitors and beta-blockers in hypertensive African Americans may be irrelevant in explaining racial disparities in BP control between African Americans and Whites. Several studies have shown that when a combination of agents is prescribed, there are few racial differences in rates of treatment-to-goal outcomes for Whites versus African Americans (Chobanian et al., 2003).

Medication Adherence

Rates of nonadherence among hypertensive patients vary widely. It has been estimated that only 50%–70% of hypertensive patients report being adherent to their prescribed medical treatment (World Health Organization, 2003). As compared to their White counterparts, hypertensive African Americans have poorer rates of medication adherence, which may account for the poorer BP control rates in them (Bosworth et al., 2006). In the Systolic Hypertension in the Elderly Pilot Study, African Americans were reported to have lower adherence than their White counterparts (Furberg & Black, 1988). Similar findings were noted in the Hypertension Detection and Follow-up Program (HDFP) where adherence (measured as taking at least 80% of prescribed pills) was reported to be 60% at 1 year among Whites compared to 48% among African Americans (Shulman et al., 1982). The only data in African Americans in a large clinical trial about adherence to antihypertensive medications using objective electronic monitors as adherence measure came out of the African American Study of Kidney Disease and Hypertension trial (Lee et al., 1996). Using Pill counts 34% of patients had poor adherence, while Medication Event Monitoring System (MEMS) classified almost half of the population as nonadherent (47%). This lack of adherence may explain the worse outcomes seen in African Americans compared to Whites in inner-city populations, which comprise increasingly minority populations. In studies by Shea, Misra, Ehrlich, Field, and Francis conducted with predominately African American and Latino patients in New York City, 85%–98% of patients who presented to the emergency room with severe forms of HTN were previously diagnosed and treated for HTN in outpatient clinics (1992a, 1992b). Thus, poor adherence to a treatment regimen rather than failure to diagnose or initiate treatment for HTN was a major predisposing factor of poor BP control in the predominantly African American patient population studied.

Despite evidence documenting the poorer rates of adherence among African Americans, the reasons for the racial disparities remain inconclusive. To identify possible mechanisms, Bosworth et al. (2006) assessed the role of 20 variables related to BP control in a sample of hypertensive African American and White Veteran Affairs (VA) patients. Despite having equal access to care and medications, African American patients were more likely to have inadequate BP control and report being nonadherent to their anti-hypertensive medications. In multivariate analysis, poor adherence to medication, greater perceived seriousness of hypertension, and increased frequency of urination were the only significant predictors of poor BP control in African Americans. Although not assessed in this study, the researchers speculate that factors related to trust in the patient–physician relationship may be contributing to the racial differences in BP control (Bosworth et al.).

Patient Satisfaction With Care and Health Literacy

Satisfaction with health care services is also emerging as an important determinant of adherence to prescribed regimes. Individuals' overall satisfaction with relationships within the health care system is positively correlated with medication adherence. Interestingly, low overall satisfaction with care is also related to increased number of symptoms related to anti-hypertensive medications (Harris, Luft, Rudy, & Tierney, 1995). In a study of African American men, patients modified their treatment regime as a means of asserting control when they were dissatisfied with part of their medication plans (Rose, Kim, Dennison, & Hill, 2000). Researchers Cooper-Patrick et al. (1999) have emphasized the importance of teaching physicians to understand a patient's perception, as individual beliefs influence medication behaviors. With regards to health literacy, although there is abundant evidence of its relationship to health outcomes, there is no published information on its impact on BP control or noted racial disparities in hypertension-related outcomes.

Physician-Level Barriers

Poor Doctor–Patient Communication

The patient–physician relationship is at the heart of an effective interaction between physicians and patients in primary care practices. Within the medical setting, interpersonal processes are characterized by the social–psychological aspect of the patient–physician interaction. An essential component of this definition is the ability to communicate with the patient in a sensitive and caring manner (Cleary & McNeil, 1988). To date, researchers have found that differences in communication styles increase the probability that conflicting perspectives will lead to lowered participation and satisfaction within the medical visit (Cooper-Patrick et al., 1999; Doescher, Saver, Franks, & Fiscella, 2000; Roter et al., 1997). For instance, in the work done by Cooper-Patrick et al. (1999), patients in race/ethnic–concordant relationship visits had higher ratings of positive affect; they were longer in length and rated as more participatory, as well as satisfying, as compared to those in race/ethnic–discordant relationships (Cooper-Patrick et al.; Johnson et al., 2004; Roter et al.). African American patients, in particular, participate significantly less and are least satisfied with the technical and interpersonal aspects of care when they have a White physician (Cooper-Patrick et al.; Tucker et al., 2003). The quality of the patient–physician relationship plays an important role in improving health outcomes (Kaplan, Greenfield, Gandek, Rogers, & Ware, 1996)

To understand the type and quality of information exchanged during the patient–physician encounter, several researchers have used coding schemes to analyze audiotaped recordings of medical visits (Kaplan et al., 1996; Orth, Stiles, Scherwitz, Hennrikus, & Vallbona, 1987; Stewart, Napoles-Springer, & Perez-Stable, 1999). Although, the race/ethnicity of the patient versus physician was not examined, it has been found that medical visits characterized by more information giving and less physician control in the form of dominant talk and interruptions were associated with lower BP levels among hypertensive patients (Kaplan et al.; Orth et al.). To date, only one study tested the relationship between physician communication styles and adherence to anti-hypertensive medication. Specifically, Konrad, Howard, Edwards, Ivanova, & Carey (2005) examined the effects of patient–physician racial concordance and continuity of care in elderly hypertensive patients. Using data from the 1986–1987 Piedmont Health Survey of the Elderly, the researchers found that hypertensive African American patients that identified public clinics as their usual source of care and had an African American physician were significantly more likely to be taking their anti-hypertensive medications compared to those in race-discordant relationships. Alternatively, African American patients without regular source of primary care received fewer HTN diagnoses, and if diagnosed, were less likely to report taking his or her anti-hypertensive medications (Konrad et al.). Finally, African Americans patients that switched physicians during the study period were more likely to use their anti-hypertensive medication if the new physician was White (Konrad et al.). Although the authors do not speculate why this is so, the finding may be an artifact of the years of data collection. That is, large majorities of practicing physicians during the 1980s were White and further, patients surveyed in this trial were assigned their new physicians rather than given a choice (American Medical Association, 2005).

Treatment Intensity

It has been speculated that when treating minority patients, physicians are less likely to aggressively intensify antihypertensive therapies, ultimately resulting in a higher rate of uncontrolled BP in these patient populations. Assessing physicians' adherence to the recent publication of the seventh Report of the Joint National Committee on Prevention, Detection, Evaluation and Treatment of HTN (JNC-7) treatment guidelines provides a test of this hypothesis. Through a review of electronic medical records, Hicks et al. (2004) compared rates of adherence to the JNC-7 guidelines, BP control, and intensification of treatment to patient characteristics of an ethnically diverse sample. In multivariate analysis, JNC-adherent visits were significantly more frequent among African American and Latino patients than among Whites. Despite lower levels of JNC-adherence, White patients were more likely to have their BP controlled as compared to African Americans and Latinos (Hicks et al., 2004). To identify the potential variables underlying racial differences in BP control, Hicks et al. further examined the impact of patient and provider characteristics on treatment intensity rates in a subset of patients with a minimum of two hypertension-related outpatient visits. As in the previous study, Latinos were significantly less likely to have their medication intensified as compared to both the Whites and African Americans. However, after adjusting for demographic factors and level of physician experience the racial/ethnic difference in rates of intensification was not significant. Rather, frequency of patient clinic visits and the presence of diabetes predicted a less aggressive treatment (Hicks, Shaykevich, Bates, & Ayanian, 2005).

System-Level Barriers

Although systems-level barriers (lack of access, medication costs, high copayments) adversely affect HTN control (Bone et al., 2000; Douglas, Ferdinand, Bakris, & Sowers, 2002; Shea et al., 1992b), there is evidence that most cases of uncontrolled HTN occur in patients with good access to care (Hyman & Pavlik, 2001; Knight et al., 2001; Kotchen et al., 1998; Stockwell, Madhavan, Cohen, Gibson, & Alderman, 1994). Thus, the NHANES data suggest that most persons with uncontrolled HTN have access to care, and have seen a physician on an average of at least 3 times in the prior year (Hyman & Pavlik, 2001). This may be more prevalent in African Americans, who in one survey were found to have uncontrolled HTN in 75% of VA patients despite free access to care, free medications and regular follow-ups (Berlowitz et al., 1998).

Lack of Access to Care

There have been several studies that have related lack of access to care as a reason for poor health outcomes, especially in minority populations (IOM, 2003). Independent of health insurance coverage, the availability of health care services within a neighborhood can also impact the course of illness and the chance for recovery. Racial/ethnic minorities are more likely to reside in neighborhoods that have an inadequate number of pharmacies, receive care from physicians less prepared to counsel diverse patients, and less likely to have clinics with the medical technology needed for appropriate care (Sorensen et al., 2003; Weissman, Campbell, Gokhale, & Blumenthal, 2001). For instance, in a study by Shea et al. (1992b) among predominantly Latino and African American hypertensive patients who presented to the emergency department of an urban teaching hospital with uncontrolled hypertension, the majority of them had no primary care physician and their level of adherence to prescribed medications was related to their lack of primary care providers. What is not certain is whether this factor is true only for minority patients. A recent study by Rehman, Hutchison, Hendrix, Okonofua, & Egan (2005) addressed this issue by comparing BP control rates between African Americans and their White counterparts who receive care in Veterans Affairs hospital systems and non-VA hospital systems to see if access to care could explain the racial disparities in

BP control. The ethnic disparity in BP control between African Americans and Whites was approximately 40% less at VA than at non–VA health care sites. The authors conclude that ensuring access to health care could constitute one constructive component of a national initiative to reduce ethnic disparities in BP control and cardiovascular risk (Rehman et al.).

Quality of Care

Although lack of medical insurance adversely affects BP, there is evidence that among equally insured patients the quality of care is significantly different across the health care setting. For instance, minority patients are less likely to have access to the higher quality of care associated with private, teaching, and high-volume clinics (IOM, 2003). Rather, they are more likely to receive care in public hospital emergency rooms and have less stable relationships with private physicians even when insured at the same level as Whites (IOM, 2003). Data from NHANES suggest that most patients with uncontrolled HTN have access to care, and have seen a physician on an average of at least three times in the prior year (Hyman & Pavlik, 2001). However, despite having access, the rates of uncontrolled HTN are more prevalent in minorities than Whites. In a survey of a Veterans Administration ambulatory practice, 75% of hypertensive African Americans were found to have uncontrolled HTN despite free access to care, free medications, and regular follow-up visits to their physicians (Berlowitz et al., 1998). This discrepancy may be due in part to the quality of physician care available to the minority patient. That is, as compared to Whites, minority patients are more likely to be treated by physicians that differ in regard to their clinical qualifications and resources (Bach et al., 2004). Thus, even when equally insured, minorities face additional barriers to care, including a relative scarcity of minority health care providers that are board certified (Bach et al.).

Summary

While it is clear that there are racial disparities in hypertension-related outcomes and blood pressure control between African Americans and Whites, some data are now emerging shedding light on the mechanisms that may explain these hypertension-related disparities. In the IOM framework, these can be categorized into physician-level factors and health care system factors. While most data at the current time are based on patient-level factors such past patient preferences for care, beliefs, and socioeconomic status, this cannot be said of physician-level factors where data have emerged only for patient-physician communication, race-discordance issues, and treatment intensity for hypertensive patients. Similarly, there are very little data suggesting that preferential treatment once in the health care system can explain hypertension-related disparities. Future research should definitely focus on other potential mechanisms such as health literacy, cultural competence and, more importantly, studies that will take into account not just one aspect of the framework but a comprehensive approach. Our ability to develop meaningful interventions will depend on the nature of the mechanisms that can be identified.

REFERENCES

American Medical Association. (2005, December 19). *Race and the AMA: A chronology*. Retrieved March 27, 2006, from http://www.amaassn.org/ama/pub/category/9496.html

Appel, L. J., Champagne, C. M., Harsha, D. W., Cooper, L. S., Obarzanek, E., Elmer, P. J., et al. (2003). Effects of comprehensive lifestyle modification on blood pressure control: Main results of the PREMIER clinical trial. *Journal of the American Medical Association, 289*(16), 2083–2093.

Appel, L. J., Espeland, M. A., Easter, L., Wilson, A. C., Folmar, S., & Lacy, C. R. (2001). Effects of reduced sodium intake on hypertension control in older individuals: Results from the Trial of Nonpharmacologic Interventions in the Elderly (TONE). *Archives of Internal Medicine, 161*(5), 685–693.

Bach, P. B., Pham, H. H., Schrag, D., Tate, R. C., & Hargraves, J. L. (2004). Primary care physicians who treat blacks and whites. *New England Journal of Medicine, 351*(6), 575–584.

Berlowitz, D. R., Ash, A. S., Hickey, E. C., Friedman, R. H., Glickman, M., Kader, B., et al. (1998). Inadequate management of blood pressure in a hypertensive population. *New England Journal of Medicine, 339*(27), 1957–1963.

Bone, L. R., Hill, M. N., Stallings, R., Gelber, A. C., Barker, A., Baylor, I., et al. (2000). Community health survey in an urban African–American neighborhood: Distribution and correlates of elevated blood pressure. *Ethnicity & Disease, 10*(1), 87–95.

Bosworth, H. B., Dudley, T., Olsen, M. K., Voils, C. I., Powers, B., Goldstein, M. K., et al. (2006). Racial differences in blood pressure control: Potential explanatory factors. *American Journal of Medicine, 119*(1), 70.e9–15.

Brewster, L. M., van Montfrans, G. A., & Kleijnen, J. (2004). Systematic review: Antihypertensive drug therapy in black patients. *Annals of Internal Medicine, 141*(8), 614–627.

Brown, C. M., & Segal, R. (1996). The effects of health and treatment perceptions on the use of prescribed medication and home remedies among African American and White American hypertensives. *Social Science & Medicine, 43*(6), 903–917.

Centers for Disease Control and Prevention (CDC). (2005). Racial/ethnic disparities in prevalence, treatment, and control of hypertension—United States, 1999–2002. *Morbidity and Mortality Weekly Report, 54*(1), 7–9.

Centers for Disease Control and Prevention, National Center for Health Statistics (CDC/NCHS). (2000). *NHANES III [1988–94]*. Hyattsville, MD: Author.

Chobanian, A. V., Bakris, G. L., Black, H. R., Cushman, W. C., Green, L. A., Izzo, J. L., Jr., et al. (2003). Seventh report of the Joint National Committee on Prevention, Detection, Evaluation, and Treatment of High Blood Pressure. *Hypertension, 42*(6), 1206–1252.

Cleary, P. D., & McNeil, B. J. (1988). Patient satisfaction as an indicator of quality care. *Inquiry, 25*(1), 25–36.

Cooper, L. A. (2004). Health disparities. Toward a better understanding of primary care patient–physician relationships. *Journal of General Internal Medicine, 19*(9), 985–986.

Cooper-Patrick, L., Gallo, J. J., Gonzales, J. J., Vu, H. T., Powe, N. R., Nelson, C., et al. (1999). Race, gender, and partnership in the patient-physician relationship. *Journal of the American Medical Association, 282*(6), 583–589.

Daniel, H. I., & Rotimi, C. N. (2003). Genetic epidemiology of hypertension: An update on the African diaspora. *Ethnicity & Disease, 13*(2 Suppl 2), S53–66.

Doescher, M. P., Saver, B. G., Franks, P., & Fiscella, K. (2000). Racial and ethnic disparities in perceptions of physician style and trust. *Archives of Family Medicine, 9*(10), 1156–1163.

Douglas, J. G., Ferdinand, K. C., Bakris, G. L., & Sowers, J. R. (2002). Barriers to blood pressure control in African Americans. Overcoming obstacles is challenging, but target goals can be attained. *Postgraduate Medicine, 112*(4), 51–70.

Ferdinand, K. C., & Saunders, E. (2006). Hypertension-related morbidity and mortality in African Americans—Why we need to do better. *Journal of Clinical Hypertension (Greenwich), 8*(1 Suppl 1), 21–30.

Flack, J. M., Peters, R., Mehra, V. C., & Nasser, S. A. (2002). Hypertension in special populations. *Cardiology Clinics, 20*(2), 303–319, vii.

Furberg, C. D., & Black, D. M. (1988). The systolic hypertension in the elderly pilot program: Methodological issues. *European Heart Journal, 9*(2), 223–227.

Gadegbeku, C. A., Lea, J. P., & Jamerson, K. A. (2005). Update on disparities in the pathophysiology and management of hypertension: Focus on African Americans. *Medical Clinics of North America, 89*(5), 921–933, 930.

Giles, W. H., Kittner, S. J., Hebel, J. R., Losonczy, K. G., & Sherwin, R. W. (1995). Determinants of Black–White differences in the risk of cerebral infarction. The National Health and Nutrition Examination Survey Epidemiologic Follow-up Study. *Archives of Internal Medicine, 155*(12), 1319–1324.

Harris, L. E., Luft, F. C., Rudy, D. W., & Tierney, W. M. (1995). Correlates of health care satisfaction in inner-city patients with hypertension and chronic renal insufficiency. *Social Science & Medicine, 41*(12), 1639–1645.

Hertz, R. P., Unger, A. N., Cornell, J. A., & Saunders, E. (2005). Racial disparities in hypertension prevalence, awareness, and management. *Archives of Internal Medicine, 165*(18), 2098–2104.

Heurtin-Roberts, S., & Reisin, E. (1992). The relation of culturally influenced lay models of hypertension to compliance with treatment. *American Journal of Hypertension, 5*(11), 787–792.

Hicks, L. S., Fairchild, D. G., Horng, M. S., Orav, E. J., Bates, D. W., & Ayanian, J. Z. (2004). Determinants of JNC VI guideline adherence, intensity of drug therapy, and blood pressure control by race and ethnicity. *Hypertension, 44*(4), 429–434.

Hicks, L. S., Shaykevich, S., Bates, D. W., & Ayanian, J. Z. (2005). Determinants of racial/ethnic differences in blood pressure management among hypertensive patients. *BMC Cardiovascular Disorders, 5*(1), 16.

Hyman, D. J., & Pavlik, V. N. (2001). Characteristics of patients with uncontrolled hypertension in the United States. *New England Journal of Medicine, 345*(7), 479–486.

Institute of Medicine. (2003). *Unequal treatment: Confronting racial and ethnic disparities in health care.* Washington, DC: National Academies Press.

Johnson, R. L., Saha, S., Arbelaez, J. J., Beach, M. C., & Cooper, L. A. (2004). Racial and ethnic differences in patient perceptions of bias and cultural competence in health care. *Journal of General Internal Medicine, 19*(2), 101–110.

Kaplan, S. H., Greenfield, S., Gandek, B., Rogers, W. H., & Ware, J. E., Jr. (1996). Characteristics of physicians with participatory decision-making styles. *Annals of Internal Medicine, 124*(5), 497–504.

Klag, M. J., Whelton, P. K., Randall, B. L., Neaton, J. D., Brancati, F. L., & Stamler, J. (1997). End-stage renal disease in African–American and white men. 16-year MRFIT findings. *Journal of the American Medical Association, 277*(16), 1293–1298.

Knight, E. L., Bohn, R. L., Wang, P. S., Glynn, R. J., Mogun, H., & Avorn, J. (2001). Predictors of uncontrolled hypertension in ambulatory patients. *Hypertension, 38*(4), 809–814.

Konrad, T. R., Howard, D. L., Edwards, L. J., Ivanova, A., & Carey, T. S. (2005). Physician–patient racial concordance, continuity of care, and patterns of care for hypertension. *American Journal of Public Health, 95*(12), 2186–2190.

Kotchen, J. M., Shakoor-Abdullah, B., Walker, W. E., Chelius, T. H., Hoffmann, R. G., & Kotchen, T. A. (1998). Hypertension control and access to medical care in the inner city. *American Journal of Public Health, 88*(11), 1696–1699.

Lee, J. Y., Greene, P. G., Douglas, M., Grim, C., Kirk, K. A., Kusek, J. W., et al. (1996). Appointment attendance, pill counts, and achievement of goal blood pressure in the African American Study of Kidney Disease and Hypertension Pilot Study. *Controlled Clinical Trials, 17*(4 Suppl), 34S–39S.

Mensah, G. A., Mokdad, A. H., Ford, E. S., Greenlund, K. J., & Croft, J. B. (2005). State of disparities in cardiovascular health in the United States. *Circulation, 111*(10), 1233–1241.

Ogedegbe, G., Harrison, M., Robbins, L., Mancuso, C. A., & Allegrante, J. P. (2004). Reasons patients do or do not take their blood pressure medications. *Ethnicity & Disease, 14*(1), 158.

Ogedegbe, G., Mancuso, C. A., & Allegrante, J. P. (2004). Expectations of blood pressure management in hypertensive African–American patients: A qualitative study. *Journal of the National Medical Association, 96*(4), 442–449.

Okonofua, E. C., Cutler, N. E., Lackland, D. T., & Egan, B. M. (2005). Ethnic differences in older Americans: Awareness, knowledge, and beliefs about hypertension. *American Journal of Hypertension, 18*(7), 972–979.

Orth, J. E., Stiles, W. B., Scherwitz, L., Hennrikus, D., & Vallbona, C. (1987). Patient exposition and provider explanation in routine interviews and hypertensive patients' blood pressure control. *Health Psychology, 6*(1), 29–42.

Pavlik, V. N., Hyman, D. J., Vallbona, C., Toronjo, C., & Louis, K. (1997). Hypertension awareness and control in an inner-city African–American sample. *Journal of Human Hypertension, 11*(5), 277–283.

Rehman, S. U., Hutchison, F. N., Hendrix, K., Okonofua, E. C., & Egan, B. M. (2005). Ethnic differences in blood pressure control among men at Veterans Affairs clinics and other health care sites. *Archives of Internal Medicine, 165*(9), 1041–1047.

Rose, L. E., Kim, M. T., Dennison, C. R., & Hill, M. N. (2000). The contexts of adherence for African Americans with high blood pressure. *Journal of Advanced Nursing, 32*(3), 587–594.

Roter, D. L., Stewart, M., Putnam, S. M., Lipkin, M., Jr., Stiles, W., & Inui, T. S. (1997). Communication patterns of primary care physicians. *Journal of the American Medical Association, 277*(4), 350–356.

Shea, S., Misra, D., Ehrlich, M. H., Field, L., & Francis, C. K. (1992a). Correlates of nonadherence to hypertension treatment in an inner-city minority population. *American Journal of Public Health, 82*(12), 1607–1612.

Shea, S., Misra, D., Ehrlich, M. H., Field, L., & Francis, C. K. (1992b). Predisposing factors for severe, uncontrolled hypertension in an inner-city minority population. *New England Journal of Medicine, 327*(11), 776–781.

Sheats, N., Lin, Y., Zhao, W., Cheek, D. E., Lackland, D. T., & Egan, B. M. (2005). Prevalence, treatment, and control of hypertension among African Americans and Caucasians at primary care sites for medically under-served patients. *Ethnicity & Disease, 15*(1), 25–32.

Shulman, N., Cutter, G., Daugherty, R., Sexton, M., Pauk, G., Taylor, M. J., et al. (1982). Correlates of attendance and compliance in the hypertension detection and follow-up program. *Controlled Clinical Trials, 3*(1), 13–27.

Singh, G. K., & Moore, M. A. (1996). Advance report of final mortality statistics. *Monthly Vital Statistics Report, 45*(3), 1–76.

Smedley, B. (2003). Assessing potential sources of racial and ethnic disparities in care: Patient-and-system-level factors. In Institute of Medicine (Ed.), *Unequal treatment: Confronting racial and ethnic disparities in health care*. Washington, DC: National Academies Press.

Sorensen, G., Emmons, K., Hunt, M. K., Barbeau, E., Goldman, R., Peterson, K., et al. (2003). Model for incorporating social context in health behavior interventions: Applications for cancer prevention for working-class, multiethnic populations. *Preventive Medicine, 37*(3), 188–197.

Stewart, A. L., Napoles-Springer, A., & Perez-Stable, E. J. (1999). Interpersonal processes of care in diverse populations. *Milbank Quarterly, 77*(3), 274, 305–339.

Stockwell, D. H., Madhavan, S., Cohen, H., Gibson, G., & Alderman, M. H. (1994). The determinants of hypertension awareness, treatment, and control in an insured population. *American Journal of Public Health, 84*(11), 1768–1774.

Svetkey, L. P., Erlinger, T. P., Vollmer, W. M., Feldstein, A., Cooper, L. S., Appel, L. J., et al. (2005). Effect of lifestyle modifications on blood pressure by race, sex, hypertension status, and age. *Journal of Human Hypertension, 19*(1), 21–31.

Tucker, C. M., Herman, K. C., Pedersen, T. R., Higley, B., Montrichard, M., & Ivery, P. (2003). Cultural sensitivity in physician–patient relationships: Perspectives of an ethnically diverse sample of low-income primary care patients. *Medical Care, 41*(7), 859–870.

Weissman, J. S., Campbell, E. G., Gokhale, M., & Blumenthal, D. (2001). Residents' preferences and preparation for caring for underserved populations. *Journal of Urban Health, 78*(3), 535–549.

Wilson, R. P., Freeman, A., Kazda, M. J., Andrews, T. C., Berry, L., Vaeth, P. A., et al. (2002). Lay beliefs about high blood pressure in a low- to middle-income urban African–American community: An opportunity for improving hypertension control. *American Journal of Medicine, 112*(1), 26–30.

Wong, M. D., Shapiro, M. F., Boscardin, W. J., & Ettner, S. L. (2002). Contribution of major diseases to disparities in mortality. *New England Journal of Medicine, 347*(20), 1585–1592.

World Health Organization. (2003). *Adherence to long-term therapies: Evidence for action*. Geneva, Switzerland: World Health Organization.

Yancy, C. W. (2004). The prevention of heart failure in minority communities and discrepancies in health care delivery systems. *Medical Clinics of North America, 88*(5), xii–xiii, 1347–1368.

Incessant Displacement and Health Disparities

8

Mindy Thompson Fullilove

Introduction

My studies of cities are rooted in the study of the U.S. AIDS epidemic. I started conducting research on AIDS in 1986. Almost immediately, leaders of minority communities pointed out to our research group that the crack epidemic was destabilizing neighborhoods and required our attention. Initially, we focused on the ways in which crack use and sales shaped individual behavior. But gradually we realized that it was the changing neighborhoods that demanded our attention.

Critical to the shift in our thinking was a paper by Rodrick Wallace, "A Synergism of Plagues: 'Planned Shrinkage,' Contagious Housing Destruction, and AIDS in the South Bronx," that outlined the ecological argument for a link between the destruction of housing in the South Bronx as a result a policy called "planned shrinkage" and the high rates and spatial distribution of the epidemic in that borough (Wallace, 1988). Under this policy, fire stations were closed in selected poor minority neighborhoods. In the absence of adequate fire protection, the rate of fires soared and apartment buildings were destroyed. Within a 5-year period, some health areas in the Bronx lost as much as 80% of their existing housing. This housing loss was accompanied by massive displacement of people leading to a fundamental restructuring of the geography of the South Bronx. HIV was already present in the South Bronx at the time the policy of planned shrinkage was implemented. It showed up, several years later, in a shotgun pattern that closely followed the dissemination of the displaced population.

The Wallaces have continued to examine the connection between the destruction of housing and the dissemination of HIV in the United States. In their seminal book, *A Plague on Your Houses* (Wallace & Wallace, 1998) they describe the larger implications of the destruction of housing in the South Bronx and other New York City neighborhoods. Specifically, the massive destruction of housing caused by planned shrinkage escalated the size and spread of the AIDS epidemic through geographic linkages, both at the regional and national scale.

As we began to study neighborhoods, we realized that the policy of planned shrinkage was neither the first nor the last program that led to forced displacement of populations (Fullilove, 2004). A more complete list includes urban renewal under the Housing Act of 1949; planned shrinkage, or more generically, catastrophic disinvestment; the demolition of public housing under the 1992 HOPE VI program; gentrification, which has been promoted by a number of policies and programs; and mass incarceration of poor and minority people. These policies created a scenario of incessant displacement, which has fallen most heavily on poor people of color, forced to live in segregated neighborhoods and deprived of equal investment opportunity at least as early as 1937, when the redlining policy of the federal Homeowners Loan Corporation was instituted.

All of these policies have destroyed older buildings in poor neighborhoods, thereby creating a nationwide deficit of low-income housing. For example, the urban renewal program carried out under the Housing Act of 1949 had, by 1967, destroyed 400,000 units but created only 10,000 low-income units (Weiss, 1985). Thus, the situation of incessant displacement has been complicated by a situation of "musical chairs" in which some poor people must be homeless at any given time (Sclar, 1990). But the cumulative effects of incessant displacement and insecure housing go far beyond housing to affect community life at every level. In this chapter, I will use interviews and observations collected as part of a study of urban renewal to suggest that these seemingly discrete policies have interacted to create a set of disadvantages that contribute to the spread of AIDS and as well as other health and social problems. The proposal here is that incessant displacement is at the root of America's health disparities. Indeed, what is proposed is that a series of policies of displacement and disinvestment have acted synergistically to create the social conditions for ill health in the United States.

Methods

Case Studies of Urban Renewal

The data for this paper are drawn from a study of urban renewal conducted under the federal Housing Act of 1949 (see Fullilove, 2004, for more details). The study examined urban renewal in five sites: Newark, NJ; Roanoke, VA; St. Louis, MO; Pittsburgh, PA; and San Francisco, CA. The project employed situation analysis, a theoretically-derived qualitative research method, to complete five case studies (Green, Hernández-Cordero, Schmitz, & Fullilove, in press; Mitchell, 1983; Sullivan & Fullilove, 2003). Three kinds of data were collected. First, interviews were conducted with people in each city selected because they had one of three key relationships to the urban renewal story: they were responsible for planning and carrying out urban renewal, were themselves displaced, or were observers and/or advocates watching the process. A total of 65 people were interviewed for the five–city study. Second, maps and photographs depicting the areas before, during, and after urban renewal were collected. Third, local literature on urban renewal, including newspaper articles, documentaries, and monographs, were collected. Members of the study team made multiple visits to each site in order to accomplish these tasks. The first phase of fieldwork was conducted between April 2001 and December 2002; additional fieldwork was carried out in Newark, New Jersey in 2004.

For purposes of this chapter, interviews were analyzed for comments specific to the policies of segregation, redlining, urban renewal, planned shrinkage/catastrophic disinvestment, gentrification, HOPE VI, and mass incarceration. In addition, using methods from population, community, and ecosystem ecology and quantitative geography, our team examined the movement of populations over time in the Newark, NJ area.

Human Subjects

We obtained two kinds of consent during this project. We obtained consent from each participant to tape and transcribe the interview and to cite his/her remarks with his/her name attached. These procedures were approved by the Institutional Review Board at New York State Psychiatric Institute. We also sought permission to deposit tapes and transcripts in the Columbia University Oral History Collection. Toward that end, each participant was given a transcript of his/her interview to edit as he or she wished and was asked to give written consent to deposit the interview in the archive. The consent process for the deposit of an oral history tape and transcript was governed by the interviewee rather than an institutional review board.

Limitations

This qualitative study of five cities does not provide a full documentation of the impact of these disparate policies in all African American communities. Furthermore, we have fuller documentation of the more recent and more visible policies, such as HOPE VI, and less documentation of the older, more secretive policies such as redlining.

Results

Segregation

The neighborhoods we examined were all segregated neighborhoods, that is to say, places in which blacks had to settle because of formal and/or informal policies and practices that blocked their living in other parts of the city. The stories of how these neighborhoods came into being varied. African Americans had lived in the Hill District in Pittsburgh since the 1800s. By contrast, black settlement in the Fillmore District in San Francisco occurred in the 1940s, spurred by war-time employment and made possible by the internment of the Japanese people who had been earlier settlers in the area. These histories of restricted settlement were entwined with the development of social, economic, political, and cultural organizations interior to the segregated area.

Frank Bolden, celebrated reporter for the African American newspaper, *The Pittsburgh Courier*, described in some detail the long struggle by blacks to win political control of their neighborhoods, including the Hill District. This political power allowed them to fight for better services and to improve neighborhood life. At the same time, black residents of the Hill also fought to develop cultural institutions, ranging from symphony orchestras to book clubs, economic institutions, including hotels, beauty shops, pharmacies, and jazz clubs, and recreation for children, such as that provided by the Irene Kaufman Settlement House. Among the many comments about life in such a highly developed, albeit segregated, neighborhood, Lois Cain, also of Pittsburgh, noted:

> All the resources we needed, my mother, my grandfather, my grandmother, my father, all got it right here [in the Hill]. I am amazed at that, because now you have to kind of shop around. If you want to turn your dollar over with your people, you've got to get a list and a map. But you could stay right here, and never leave it, and get everything you needed, from party-time to church. This is my memories of the Hill, was that families stayed together.

Redlining

Redlining was introduced in 1937 by the Homeowners Loan Corporation (HOLC). It was intended to protect investment by indicating which areas offered the best opportunities. According to the HOLC algorithm, new buildings with white inhabitants merited an "A" rating, while old buildings with non-white inhabitants received a "D." Redlining imposed serious hardship on ghetto neighborhoods because it made it difficult to get money for investment. As pointed out by people who lived in the Central Ward of Newark, NJ, redlining made it difficult to get insurance or to borrow for repairs and remodeling (Booth, 2004). Richard Cammarieri, a resident of the Central Ward of Newark, pointed out that "stick-built" housing[1] needed regular maintenance; absent regular investment, it deteriorated more rapidly than it might have otherwise. Because the presence of any number of minority people led an area to be downgraded on redlining maps, all segregated areas were treated as relatively risky sites for investment.

Urban Renewal

The under-investment in ghetto areas was linked to urban renewal because lack of maintenance increased the likelihood that redlined areas would show the greatest wear and tear and be at highest risk for a declaration of "blight." At the heart of setting up an urban renewal plan was a city's declaration that an area was blighted. Urbanist Dennis Gale explained:

> Part of the idea behind urban renewal is that the officials in Washington realized that you would never get private capital to invest back in the city, to build new office buildings, build shops, housing, et cetera—you could never encourage them to do that as long as there were these significant numbers of minorities and low-income people in the cities.... So the idea was, the only way that we can hope to get private capital back into the cities, because we can't do it alone without federal money, the only way to do it is to get rid of all the slums and deterioration. You label it as bad, you clear it all out. You

---

[1]"Stick-built" housing is built on site, piece by piece.

have a featureless plane, and call it urban renewal. There is no longer any bad, there is nothing. And then you build from scratch.

In Pittsburgh's Lower Hill District, where 4,000 people had lived, worked, and shopped, a new arena was erected, directed at providing entertainment for middle-class white people of the area. Planner Robert Pease, who helped to develop the urban renewal strategy of Pittsburgh, was involved in assessing the Hill District's need for renewal. He remembered:

There was a family there [in the Hill] who had a son the same age as my son. But I could look at the walls and see outside through the walls. And it was bitter cold.... Well, the conditions in the Hill, not every family lived that way, because there was some pretty decent housing there, not expensive but decent, with indoor plumbing and all the good things. But there were a lot of slums that were overcrowded and really needed to be cleared.

Sala Udin—who grew up in the section of the Hill District Pease was describing and served as its city councilman at the time of our fieldwork—commented:

I think that the sense of community and the buildings are related within an old area. The buildings were old, the streets were cobblestone and old, there many small alleyways and people lived in those alleyways. The houses were very close together. There were small walkways that ran in between the alleyways that was really a playground. So, the physical condition of the buildings helped to create a sense of community. We all lived in similar conditions and had similar complaints about the wind whipping through the gaps between the frame and the window, and the hole in the walls and the leaking fixtures, the toilet fixtures that work sometimes and don't work sometimes. But that kind of common condition bound us together.

Despite the existence of a sense of community and the mix of buildings in varying conditions, the neighborhoods were obliterated, creating the "featureless plane" that Dennis Gale described. This "new land" was used for many different purposes, ranging from low-income housing projects to cultural centers. The people who had lived in the neighborhoods were dispersed. The new places in which they settled tended to be heavily black and less integrated by class than the old neighborhoods had been. Dense high-rise housing projects, such as those erected in the Central Ward of Newark, typified the extreme isolation of the very poor black people from others unlike themselves. Those with more resources settled in nearby neighborhoods, often close to where they had lived prior to urban renewal, what might be called "next-over" or "circumjacent" neighborhoods.

Catastrophic Disinvestment

The continuation of segregation—and in some cases its intensification—meant that redlining practices continued to affect areas of black settlement. While not necessarily achieving the status of stated policy, as did the planned shrinkage policy in New York, disinvestment reached similarly catastrophic levels in many of the next-over neighborhoods we visited. One such neighborhood was Gainsborough, a section of Roanoke, Virginia, which was marked for urban renewal, but never cleared. The declaration of urban renewal effectively blocked investment in the area. Slowly, the area deteriorated and the housing stock fell apart. Fires destroyed the buildings, and forced the population out. As people left, the businesses and other institutions suffered. As Evelyn Bethel, a resident of the area, pointed out,

> The small businesses that we had where people were self-sufficient to a degree, no matter how much or how little they made, they were self-sufficient, and they had a core of ready-made customers. When the people were forced out, your business could no longer survive, so it was a devastating loss to the residents as well as the business owners.

Dr. Walter Claytor, whose family lost substantial holdings in the area as a result of this catastrophic disinvestment, took the city of Roanoke to court. He won a settlement based on making the link between the declaration of the area as a site for urban renewal and the loss of use of the family's property (Chittum, 2005).

During our fieldwork, we examined the patterns of population movement, with a particular focus on Newark. We used census data from 1950 to 2000 and photographs along an ecological transect from the center of Newark to a wealthy suburb 8 miles away. We were able to discern a pattern of a moving front of catastrophic disinvestment that was moving away from the center of Newark, slowly destroying the neighborhoods—indeed, the cities—in its path. This wave of disinvestment was also pushing the black population from the center of Newark toward cities to the west. As the poor population was pushed west, some of the city's problems spilled over, destabilizing the circumjacent towns of Irvington, Elizabeth, and East Orange, New Jersey. An examination of FBI Uniform Crime statistics for 2001 showed that crime rates for Irvington, located in the first ring of cities around Newark, were higher than those in Newark to the east or Union and other suburbs that lay to the west (see Figure 8.1). The steady movement of population from east to west over the decades 1950 to 2000 suggested that Newark's western suburbs lay in the path of a slow-moving glacier of urban troubles.

Gentrification

Investment was evident at the back of the moving front of disinvestment—which is to say, near the origins of destabilization by the urban renewal area—in several cities we visited, including Roanoke, Newark, and Pittsburgh. Crawford Square, next to the Civic Arena, was such a site of new investment. Carlos Peterson, a resident of the Lower Hill prior to urban renewal, had watched as disinvestment caused this next-over neighborhood to sag and disappear. He commented:

> I think the city government and urban developers waited twenty years for this area to kind of like, decline on its own, to make it easier for them to come in and redevelop the property. And I think some of the buildings could have been saved. It could have been more of what it was, but upgraded in terms of people, property, and so forth. Right now, I think that what they've developed in terms of Crawford Square, they basically

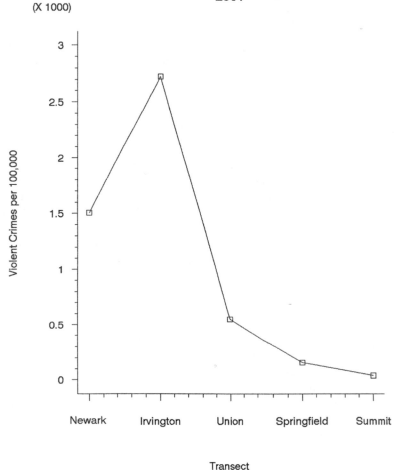

Violent Crime Rate-Springfield Transect
2001

Springfield Avenue, which runs west from the center of Newark through the towns of Irvington, Union, Springfield, and Summit, served as a transect for studying urban decay in the area adjacent to urban renewal. The FBI Uniform Crime Statistics for 2001 were highest in Irvington, consistent with movement of urban decay in a westward direction out from the site of urban renewal in the Central Ward of Newark.

razed everything. They just took everything down. And I used to call it the carcass of the Hill. You looked at the Hill and there was this carcass up there. I thought that if they could have saved the structures, because there was so much character. Now it's like looking at some sort of cul-de-sac from suburbia, you know? People don't look out their windows, they don't sit on their porches, they don't barbecue and work on their cars. You know, it's just not black folks.

Frank Bolden, who spoke about Crawford Square at some length, concluded:

> Now even today, they still haven't done anything to beautify the Hill, except they put up the Civic Arena, and they put up Crawford Village, which has homes that are too expensive for the poor people to buy or rent. Now there are a few down there but I am talking about masses of the Negroes. Now they want to continue, they want to still beautify the Hill. They are hoping to bring white people back to the city to work, because those people living in Crawford Village and so forth now, do not patronize anything in the Hill District. They patronize downtown. They are no use to us.

Hope VI

Federal housing projects linked into this process in a number of ways. First, housing projects were an important social reform when first introduced in the 1930s. They offered clean, decent housing for poor and working families. Indeed, housing projects developed in that era were often models of design. However, because housing projects were segregated, they were part of the creation of segregated neighborhoods. Second, many people displaced by urban renewal settled in housing projects, often finding that the housing projects offered great improvements over the housing in urban renewal areas.

In addition to segregation, housing projects created isolation by class, geography, and function. This last point is worth comment, because it is clear that people in poor neighborhoods used their housing for shelter and enterprise. Furthermore, houses were mixed with businesses of many kinds. Housing projects, by contrast, were strictly residential and were often located on campuses far from commercial or industrial districts. Housing projects in Pittsburgh and San Francisco—located at some distance from the original urban renewal areas and strikingly barren as urban sites—were examples of all four kinds of isolation operating at the same time. Muhandes Salaam Allah, in Roanoke, said, with some bitterness:

> I don't know whether the ultimate goal was to impoverish these black communities, but certainly anybody who has any understanding knows that if you spend thirty years in the project and you are not able to build equity, you are not going to be able to pass anything on to your children. And when you destroy a neighborhood where people own their own home, and replace it with a project, where people don't own nothing, then what is going to be the consequences in a thirty or forty year period? It's going to be that these people are going to be an impoverished group of people. And they are not participating in the American Dream. They are participating in the Housing Authority nightmare.

In St. Louis, the ill-conceived Pruitt-Igoe Housing Project—to which some people displaced from the Mill Valley urban renewal project moved—was the first in the nation to be demolished because of its failure as a housing community. Though it was demolished in 1972, ground it had occupied was still vacant at time of our fieldwork in 2001. In the 1990s many housing projects were deemed "distressed communities," a label that was applied rather broadly to an array of building types and conditions, reminiscent of urban renewal and the appellation of "blight." These "distressed housing communities" were slated for destruction and replacement with new housing for a mix of income groups. At the time of our fieldwork in Pittsburgh and Newark, HOPE VI projects were changing the face of public housing.

Though HOPE VI was described as an amelioration of distressed housing communities, it had a high cost in terms of social stability. By reconfiguring housing projects, HOPE VI lowered the number of slots of public housing and excluded some people from getting a new apartment because of negative factors in their history. Furthermore, people were displaced before the new housing was built. They often relocated at some distance from the old projects and lost contact with their former homes. By the time it was possible for them to return, it was no longer feasible. For example, in Pittsburgh, people moved to former steel towns along the Monongehela River.

Aware of these possible outcomes, residents of one Pittsburgh housing complex, Bedford Dwellings, took up the fight against displacement (Murphy, 2005). They targeted the fact that the housing projects were slated for destruction prior to the erection of new housing. They were able to alter the construction plan so that the first phase of work was the construction of new housing erected across the street from the existing public housing. This allowed people to move from the housing project to new homes. This preserved, and even strengthened, the existing social fabric, while avoiding the social and economic costs of dispersing people while erecting new buildings.

Mass Criminalization

In 1986, in response to a dramatic rise in the sales of crack cocaine, the U.S. government launched a "war on drugs," which accelerated rates of incarceration, especially among African Americans. By 2004, 2.13 million were incarcerated, 41% of them African American (Golembeski & Fullilove, 2005). These high levels of incarceration undermined community life in many ways: destabilizing families, increasing levels of infectious diseases, and creating a class of people who had lost their civil rights, including the right to vote.

People interviewed in our study described in great detail the ways in which deindustrialization and the collapse of neighborhood social controls shifted social functioning away from the tight control that Sala Udin described. In the small alleyways of the Hill District, or the tight streets of Northeast Roanoke, adults were constantly watching the activities of the children. Furthermore, people had legitimate jobs, which brought money into the neighborhood where it was shared among networks of neighbors and friends. When these factors shifted, the whole culture changed and crime and violence flourished.

Viewing Policies in Space

We mapped the spatial patterns created by these policies for the five cities in our study. These policies are national in scope and substantially similar in their impact relating to the spatial connections between segregation/redlining, urban renewal, catastrophic disinvestment, gentrification, and HOPE VI. The Hill District, as we have noted, was a black segregated area by 1930 (Darden, 1973). Urban renewal was implemented in the Lower Hill, clear-cutting the habitat and severing convenient pedestrian connections to downtown by putting in major roadways.

The section of the Hill adjacent to the clearance area—referred to in local parlance as the "Middle Hill"—suffered from catastrophic disinvestment, which spread north and west from the area of urban renewal. Carlos Peterson, who watched the slow deterioration of the buildings, called this the "Carcass of the Hill," as depicted in one of his drawings of the process. During this process, the population of the Hill fell by half.

Gentrification began with clearance of the deteriorating homes and stores at the edge of the Civic Arena and the building of Crawford Square. HOPE VI, which is replacing two housing projects, started demolition in 1999. Gentrification at Crawford Square, at the HOPE VI sites, and elsewhere will increase the population of the Hill, but few of those displaced are expected to return. This is largely attributed to the costs of the new housing.

These policies have each contributed to specific trials and tribulations, as noted by the commentators quoted above, but they also have had a cumulative impact of intensifying—relative to the rest of U.S. society—Black impoverishment, political disenfranchisement, and social disconnection.

Discussion

The complex urban settings within which people are able to maximize their well-being require stability and a relatively constant replenishment of resources. The policies that we have described here—segregation, redlining, urban renewal, catastrophic disinvestment, gentrification, HOPE VI, and mass criminalization—undermined the functioning of African Americans by the denial of resources and the imposition of repeated displacement. The policies, because they were temporally and spatially related, have acted synergistically to maximize the deleterious effects on social, cultural, and economic functioning. In such a context, a new behavioral language of survival emerges, carrying with it greatly increased risk for violence, mother and infant mortality, sexually transmitted disease, and drug addiction (Wallace, Fullilove, & Flisher, 1996). Policy makers and public health professionals who work in the field of health disparities must understand how much the history of disinvestment, abandonment, and displacement have created the landscape of health disparities that we see in 2007. HIV/AIDS is not always the most visible, obvious outcome of these forces. Rather, it is one of a host of public health conditions from asthma to obesity that have been affected by the inability of minority communities—most notably African American communities—to create stable, sustainable neighborhoods for which adequate housing is a necessary, albeit not sufficient, condition.

Psychological studies have demonstrated that a number of fundamental psychological processes govern the individual's relationship to place. These include: orientation to place (Seamon & Mugerauer, 1985), attachment to place (Fried, 1966), and ascription of identity from place (Proshansky, 1983). The rupture of the individual's relationship with place is a profoundly disturbing experience that can lead to serious and prolonged mental distress (Fullilove, 1996). Dispossession triggers this painful process for each of the individuals involved. In addition, destruction of neighborhoods destroys collective assets, such as political organization, culture, social networks, and social norms.

But perhaps the most striking finding to emerge from our studies is the observation that, in the five cities we studied, population dispersal that started in the 1950s was still in motion as of the writing of this chapter, without any signs of slowing or stopping. Thus, the larger ecological system of those metropolitan areas was affected by the arc of policies that undermined habitat and forced people to relocate. On-going population displacement has consequences even more severe than those that result from a single episode of displacement, effectively preventing the displaced people from reorganizing their networks and re-establishing healthy ways of living in a given place.

Neither AIDS nor violence can be controlled or contained among the young in communities subject to public policies of recurrent forced displacement (Wallace & Wallace, 1995). However, it is also clear that deterioration in public health and public order caused by such policies cannot and will not be contained within the populations directly subject to them, but will poison the well for all, by a great variety of mechanisms of spatial and social diffusion. The wealthy suburbs surrounding Newark, Roanoke, St. Louis, San Francisco, and Pittsburgh are deeply implicated in the fate of the poor, wherever they reside.

The incessant displacement of the past 50 years, and the accompanying housing destruction that has been a hallmark of the policies that led to forced relocation, has created the social context of the U.S. AIDS epidemic. A serious effort to stop on-going displacement is essential to the fight against the spread of the epidemic. To that end, Rodrick Wallace (2006) proposed seven tasks that should be added to the nation's AIDS prevention agenda, as well as its fight against health disparities in general: (1) help every family be strong; (2) end forced displacement of minority communities; (3) bring manufacturing jobs back to the United States; (4) rebuild community networks in devastated neighborhoods; (5) rebuild low-income housing; (6) end mass criminalization of minority and poor people; and (7) enforce anti-discrimination laws.

REFERENCES

Booth, S. (Director). (2004). *Urban renewal is people removal* [Film]. (Available from LaBooth Production.)

Chittum, M. (2005, November 17). A long time coming: The Claytor family wins compensation for property seized by city of Roanoke. *The Roanoke Times*, pp. 1, 13.

Darden, J. T. (1973). *Afro-Americans in Pittsburgh: The residential segregation of a people*. Lexington, MA: D.C. Health and Company.

Fried, M. (1966). Grieving for a lost home: Psychological costs of relocation. In J. Q. Wilson (Ed.), *Urban renewal: The record and the controversy* (pp. 359–379). Cambridge, MA: The M.I.T. Press.

Fullilove, M. T. (1996). Psychiatric implications of displacement: Contributions from the psychology of place. *American Journal of Psychiatry, 153*(12), 1516–1523.

Fullilove, M. T. (2004). *Root shock: How tearing up city neighborhoods hurts America and what we can do about it*. New York: Ballantine Books.

Golembeski, C., & Fullilove, R. E. (2005). Criminian (In)justice in the city and its associated health consequences. *American Journal of Public Health, 95*, 1701–1706.

Green, L., Hernández-Cordero, L., Schmitz, K., & Fullilove, M. (in press). "We have a situation here!": Using situation analysis for health and social research. In R. Miller (Ed.), *Qualitative methods for social work research*. New York: Columbia University Press.

Mitchell, J. C. (1983). Case and situation analysis. *Sociological Review, 31*, 187–211.

Murphy, P. (2004). The housing that community built. *Shelterforce Online, November/December* (138). Retrieved on August 16, 2007, from http://www.nhi.org/online/issues/138/bedford.html

Proshansky, H. M. (1983). Prospects and dilemmas of environmental psychology. In N. R. Feimer & E. S. Geller (Eds.), *Environmental psychology: Directions and perspectives* (pp. 5–23). New York: Praeger.

Sclar, E. D. (1990). Homelessness and housing policy: A game of musical chairs. *American Journal of Public Health, 80*, 1049–1052.

Seamon, D., & Mugerauer, R. (Eds.). (1985). *Dwelling, place, & environment: Towards a phenomenology of person and world*. New York: Columbia University Press.

Sullivan, M. A., & Fullilove, M. T. (2003). Case study methodology and the study of rare events of extreme youth violence: A multilevel framework for discovery. In M. H. Moore, C. A. Petrie, A. A. Bragga, & B. L. McLaughlin (Eds.), *Deadly lessons: Understanding lethal school violence* (pp. 351–363). Washington, DC: National Academies Press.

Wallace, D., & Wallace, R. (1998). *A plague on your houses: How New York was burned down and national public health crumbled*. London: Verso.

Wallace, R. (1988). A synergism of plagues: "Planned shrinkage," contagious housing destruction, and AIDS in the Bronx. *Environmental Research, 47,* 1–33.

Wallace, R. (2006). *How to overcome neighborhood marginalization*. New York Stop AIDS Conference Workbook. New York: Community Research Group.

Wallace, R., Fullilove, M. T., & Flisher, A. J. (1996). AIDS, violence and behavioral coding: Information theory, risk behavior and dynamic process on core-group sociogeographic networks. *Social Science & Medicine, 43,* 339–352.

Wallace, R., & Wallace, D. (1995). U.S. apartheid and spread of AIDS to the suburbs: A multi-city analysis of the political economy of spatial epidemic threshold. *Social Science & Medicine, 41*(3), 333–345.

Weiss, M. A. (1985). The origins and legacy of urban renewal. In J. P. Mitchell (Ed.), *Federal housing policy and programs: Past and present* (pp. 253–276). New Brunswick, NJ: Rutgers University.

3

The Legacy and Role of Racism—Implications and Recommendations for Research and Practice

Strategies for Reducing Disparities in African Americans' Receipt and Use of Mental Health Services

9

Madonna G. Constantine,
Mai M. Kindaichi,
Sheila V. Graham,
and Nicole L. Watkins

Nearly 13% of the national population of the United States identifies as African American. Historically, there has been ambiguity about the terms "African American" (which refers to ethnicity) and "Black" (which refers to race and includes individuals of diverse ethnic origins), because Caribbean and African immigrants oftentimes are included in national estimates of the population of African Americans (U.S. Department of Health and Human Services [HHS], 2001). Scholarly attention toward the psychological experiences of people of African descent has grown steadily over the past 40 years, and continued research on the complex psychological experiences of African American individuals is mandated as our national population becomes increasingly diverse (Constantine, 2007; Constantine & Sue, 2005). However, despite advances in psychological care and research concerning African Americans, there are continued disparities in mental health service use, access to and quality of mental health services, and research regarding the mental health needs of diverse African Americans (Dixon & Vaz, 2005; Wallace & Constantine, 2005).

In the past decade, increased attention has been drawn to evidence of physical and mental health disparities between African Americans and White Americans in particular. Notable and startling physical health disparities experienced by the African American community include rates of diabetes that are at least three times as high as those of Whites; infant mortality rates that are twice as high than those of Whites; high incidences of breast and prostate cancer among African Americans; and dramatic increases in the incidence of HIV/AIDS among African Americans, particularly African American women, such that AIDS has become one of the 10 leading causes of mortality among Black people (National Center for Health Statistics, 2006b; HHS, 2001). Additionally, prevalence rates of asthma among African Americans are 25% greater than those of Whites, and African

Americans are 20% more likely than Whites to be diagnosed with asthma during the course of their lives (National Center for Health Statistics, 2006a). Moreover, African Americans' exposure to racism and discrimination has been linked in the literature with physical conditions such as cardiovascular and psychological reactivity, elevated levels of blood pressure, and overall elevated levels of psychological stress (e.g., Williams & Neighbors, 2001; Williams & Williams-Morris, 2000). In addition to the psychological stress that may be experienced in the course of contending with severe and chronic illnesses at rates disproportionate to other segments of the American population, African Americans' mental health concerns may be compounded by psychosocial experiences related to interpersonal, cultural, and institutional racism (Constantine, 2006).

Reported rates of mental illness and mental health concerns among African Americans are not consistent in the literature. Although the rates of mental illness among African Americans are believed to be similar to those of White Americans (HHS, 2001), such statistics are questionable because African Americans tend to be overrepresented in high-need populations and among those that may not be included in large-scale catchment studies, or because specific experiences of subgroups (e.g., children and older adults) may not be researched comprehensively. The Epidemiologic Catchment Area study (Robins & Regier, 1991) found that African Americans reported lower lifetime rates of Major Depression and Dysthymic Disorder and higher rates of phobic disorders and somatization symptoms than did Whites. As a problem that originally affected more Whites than Blacks, suicide is now the third leading cause of death among African American youth between the ages of 15 and 24 years (Kochanek, Murphy, Anderson, & Scott, 2004), and rates of suicide among African American males have been found to peak between the age cohorts of 20–24 to 30–34 and then 70 years old and older (Joe, 2006). Among older African Americans, rates of anxiety disorders, personality disorders, and alcohol abuse have not been reported to differ from the rates for older Whites, and depression and suicide rates tend to be lower among African American elders than Whites (Robins & Regier).

Disparities exist among segments of the African American community with respect to the receipt and use of mental health services. For example, among high-risk youth aged 6–18 years who received public care (i.e., substance use treatment, child welfare, adjudication in juvenile justice, mental health services, and public school services for serious emotional disturbance), 47.7% of African American youth were reported not to receive specialty services compared with 30.7% of non-Latino White youth (Yeh, McCabe, Hough, Dupuis, & Hazen, 2003). In a related study (Garland et al., 2005), African American youth were approximately one-half as likely to receive mental health services compared with non-Latino White youth. Among individuals with identified co-occurring mental health and substance abuse disorders, White clients received mental health services more often than Black clients; conversely, Black clients were more likely than White clients to receive specific drug treatment and detoxification services (Alvidrez & Havassy, 2005). In terms of help-seeking behavior, researchers (e.g., Richardson, Anderson, Flaherty, & Bell, 2003; Snowden & Pingitore, 2002) have reported that African Americans are more likely than their White counterparts to seek mental health care through primary physicians rather than psychiatrists. Thus, there appear to be differences not only in the passive receipt of mental health services, but also in the active pursuit of formal mental health services (Dixon & Vaz, 2005).

Explanations for mental health disparities experienced by African Americans consist of compounding factors including interpersonal and institutional racism, biases in assessed mental health needs, access to mental health services, variations in treatment qualities, and differences in patient preferences and beliefs about mental health (e.g., Constantine, 2006, 2007; HHS, 2001; Snowden, 2001; Williams & Williams-Morris, 2000). For example, because African Americans tend to be more visible in discrete populations that are characterized by high stress and limited resources than their White counterparts, they may experience unequal access to adequate treatment and commensurate care (e.g., Kuno & Rothbard, 2005). Ronzio, Guagliardo, & Persaud (2006) found that low-income, predominantly African American areas of a major urban city had lower proportions of mental health providers (i.e., psychiatrists, psychologists, and mental health counselors) than did higher-income, predominantly White areas. In addition to inequality in access to mental health care, there are distinct psychosocial stressors and disparities experienced by low-income African American individuals (Chow, Jaffee, & Snowden, 2003).

The intersections of race and socioeconomic class (i.e., social location characterized by wealth, income, education, and job/career status) for African Americans may contextualize mental health disparities to the extent that African Americans are overrepresented in low-income brackets, are susceptible to greater environmental stressors, and may have less financial and geographic access to mental health service facilities (Chow et al., 2003; HHS, 2006; Ronzio et al., 2006). According to the 2000 U.S. Census the median income of African Americans was slightly over $29,000, compared with the median for the total national population, which was over $41,000; in other words, the median income for African American families was only 70% of the total national population. Further, compared with 12% of the national population, 23.5% of African Americans in the United States live at or below the poverty level. In the context of mental health concerns, the National Center for Health Statistics (2005) reported that, without accounting for socioeconomic class, African American individuals over the age of 18 reported psychological distress at a slightly higher percentage (3.4) than did White Americans (3.0) in 2002–2003; among African American individuals living below the poverty level, the percentage of individuals who reported psychological distress was 7.3. It appears that the influence of financial strain and the multifaceted psychosocial conditions that can accompany poverty can take a distinct toll on the psychological well-being of African Americans (Constantine, 2006).

In the service of addressing mental health care disparities and promoting social justice (Vera & Speight, 2003), mental health professionals must consider the extent to which the services they provide to African Americans are congruent with their cultural values or ways of being. Unfortunately, the values of Western models of psychotherapy and counseling reflect Eurocentric worldview orientations and may be limited in their application to African Americans (Wallace & Constantine, 2005). For example, Eurocentric values that are arguably embedded in many U.S. mental health care models include an intrapsychic locus of psychopathology and treatment, biological models of mental illness, autonomy as the equivalence of developmental maturation, and individualism (Constantine, Myers, Kindaichi, & Moore, 2004). In contrast, Africentric cultural values highlight the importance of faith, unity, collective work and responsibility, purpose, creativity, self-determination, and cooperative economics (Karenga, 1965, 1988). Some theorists and researchers have included values of harmony control, balance with others and nature, collectivism, communalism, spirituality, orality and oral traditions, orientation to time as a function of social interaction, rhythm, and improvisation in conceptualizations of Africentric cultural values (e.g., Constantine, Gainor, Ahluwalia, & Berkel, 2003; Myers, 1993; Wallace & Constantine, 2005). Because values and traditions linked intrinsically with African cultural values often are manifested in current African American cultural practices (e.g., Constantine, Lewis, Conner, & Sanchez, 2000), it may be that some African Americans may not seek or feel assisted by counseling and psychotherapy because the services provided and lens through which distresses are understood are culturally *incongruent* with their ways of being.

The complex constellation of mental health disparities experienced by African Americans has been discussed in studies and scholarly papers (e.g., HHS, 2001). Structural factors, such as geographic, financial, and temporal access to formal mental health services, provide only partial explanations for service use discrepancies. Disparities in mental health care treatment also may be evidenced in therapeutic processes such as assessment, diagnosis, duration of treatment, and treatment modality (APA, 2003; Neighbors, Trierweiler, Ford, & Muroff, 2003; Ridley, 2005). In addition, mental health care disparities may be perpetuated by mental health professionals' biases such as assumptions of the homogeneity of Black cultural experiences, which minimize within-group differences influenced by acculturation status, gender, socio-economic status, racial identity attitudes, age, and so forth (Dana, 2002). Furthermore, African Americans may experience various barriers to mental health care treatment including culturally based beliefs in the use and efficacy of mental health care services (e.g., Sanders Thompson, Bazile, & Akbar, 2004; Terrell & Terrell, 1981).

In accordance with professional calls and guidelines that underscore multicultural initiatives (i.e., APA, 2003; Sue, Arredondo, & McDavis, 1992), mental health professionals play a critical role in enforcing social justice in mental health care service. In this chapter, the authors discuss various characteristics of and attitudes about mental health services that may serve as barriers to parity in mental health service delivery and services among African Americans. This discussion is followed by strategies for mental health providers and systems in addressing these service delivery disparities.

Barriers to Equitable Mental Health Treatment

The African American community has been documented extensively as a population underserved by the health system and the mental health field in particular (Copeland, 2005; Sanders Thompson, 2006; Snowden, 2001). Although other populations of color have been found to receive less than adequate mental health services (Shin, Chow, Camacho-Gonsalves, Levy, & Allen, 2005), the experience of people of African decent in the United States is unique given nearly 250 years of slavery, the subsequent century of legal segregation, and continued individual, cultural, and institutionalized racism (Jones, 1997). As mentioned, structural barriers related to the lack of access to health services (e.g., monetary, geographic access, and time constraints), as well as characteristics of mental health services (e.g., biases in diagnosis and treatment), and attitudes regarding mental health informed by racial-cultural experiences (e.g., cultural mistrust, stigmas and perceived racism) all have been presented as possible barriers contributing to this disparity (Copeland, 2005; Corrigan, 2004; Fischer & Shaw, 1999; Ronzio et al., 2006; Sanders

Thompson et al., 2004; Williams & Williams-Morris, 2000). Although the summary below serves as a springboard for future research and inquiry, the aforementioned barriers are discussed and considered in the context of mental health disparities experienced within the African American community.

Structural Barriers

Snowden (2001) reported that although differences in mental health service use between Blacks and Whites have decreased substantially over the past 30 years, several barriers to equity in mental health care still remain. The overrepresentation of African Americans living in poverty or near poverty indicates that socioeconomic class might be partially responsible for the underrepresentation of this same community in the population receiving mental health services. When compared to Whites, African Americans tend to have lower incomes, are less likely to receive a college education, are more likely to be unemployed, and are less likely to hold white-collar jobs (e.g., executive, managerial, professional, sales, clerical, administrative and technical positions) (Williams & Williams-Morris, 2000). Perhaps more alarming to the mental health community is the inverse relationship between income and rates of psychiatric diagnosis; more specifically, individuals in lower-income brackets have been found to be twice as likely to be diagnosed with major psychiatric disorders, such as types of schizophrenia, than those from higher income brackets (Williams & Williams-Morris).

Financial barriers, more specifically the lack of insurance and low income, may compromise access to mental health service and serve as major obstacles in seeking and continuing professional mental health care (Mansfield, Addis, & Courtenay, 2005). Although poverty and lack of financial resources contribute largely to the existing disparities in mental health treatment experienced by African Americans, race appears to magnify that disparity. For example, after accounting for differences in education level, Blacks continue to be underpaid when working in jobs similar to their White counterparts (Williams & Williams-Morris, 2000). Furthermore, Snowden and Thomas (2000) found that African Americans who have privatized medical insurance were less likely to receive mental health services on par with their White counterparts, whereas African Americans and Whites who have public health insurance (i.e., Medicaid) did not experience disparities in receiving outpatient care.

Geographic accessibility to mental health services also must be considered when attempting to understand the phenomenon at hand. In a nation where residential segregation is connected directly to the unequal distribution of resources available to those populations (e.g., educational, commercial, and environmental), access to mental health care is confounded by location. Ronzio et al. (2006) tracked the location of mental health providers (i.e., psychologists, psychiatrists, and mental health counselors) in the Washington, DC area and calculated the ratio of mental health services to neighborhood demographic characteristics. Not surprisingly, the presence of mental health providers was negatively correlated with indicators of poverty and concentration of African American neighborhoods. Municipal tracts were either very poorly served by mental health services, correlating with the visibility of African Americans and low-income individuals, or very well served, correlating with the visibility of higher-income individuals. In addition to decreased access to formal mental health services, African Americans living in underserved neighborhoods are exposed to higher levels of crime, population turnover, violence, noise, and crowding, all of which may compound mental health concerns for residents in these communities (Williams & Williams-Morris, 2000).

Perceived Negative Characteristics of Mental Health Services

Ridley (2005) noted that clients of color are more likely to have less favorable experiences than their White counterparts in the following areas of mental health service: underdiagnosis of mental health concerns, which may lead to ineffective care or harm; assignment to less experienced mental health professionals; and overrepresentation in public mental health facilities that provide lesser quality care. Although Black individuals tend to have less access to mental health care than do their White counterparts (e.g., HHS, 2001; Snowden, 2001), when this access is granted or allowed based on circumstance, it is more likely to be in poor quality or in emergency settings. Historically, African Americans who encountered the mental health system had been institutionalized prematurely (Snowden, 2001). Terrell and Terrell (1984) discussed the differential diagnostic assumptions that White clinicians make about Black clients. Despite similar symptom presentation, Blacks were diagnosed with paranoid schizophrenia at higher levels than their White and Latino counterparts. White clinicians also recommended Blacks for involuntary admission to mental hospitals at disproportionate rates. Such experiences and expectations of interactions with mental health systems may engender and heighten mistrust. As a result, African Americans may delay interacting with mental health service providers when symptoms or distress are experienced less severely. This may lead many African Americans to seek emergency mental health services in emergency departments when their levels of distress become too marked (Kunen, Niederhauser, Smith, Morris, & Marx, 2005). In effect, this phenomenon may feed into the common perception among African Americans that mental health services are utilized in psychiatric emergencies (e.g., chronic depression, psychotic break) and during times of crisis, as opposed to preventive therapy or on-going treatment (Morris, 2001). Moreover, members of the Black community may associate mental health care services exclusively with psychopharmacology and severe psychological and psychiatric concerns (Dana, 2002).

Unfavorable Attitudes and Beliefs About Mental Health Services

Considering the history of disparity in mental health service provision, the mistrust exhibited by African Americans toward mental health systems may be adaptive. According to the cultural mistrust paradigm, Blacks are critical of White clinicians' biased diagnostic and treatment methods. Ridley (1995) found support for the idea of cultural paranoia—that many Blacks are highly suspicious and guarded in cross-cultural exchanges with White counselors. Moreover, Thompson, Worthington, and Atkinson (1994) reported that Black women carry feelings of cultural mistrust and guardedness in therapeutic situations. Cultural mistrust also has been found to successfully predict premature termination among Black clients (Terrell & Terrell, 1984).

Sanders Thompson et al. (2004) addressed the impact of attitudes, beliefs, and expectations held by many African Americans toward the mental health field. They conducted a qualitative study with a sample of 201 African Americans, revealing that

African Americans tended to perceive therapy to be a resource necessitated by severe mental illness (e.g., schizophrenia, severe depression, and suicidal ideation), as compared to daily life distress or mood-related concerns. Some identified cultural barriers to seeking mental health services included the need to resolve concerns within the familial system and a desire to demonstrate strength, as opposed to weakness, the latter of which is associated with the desire to seek psychotherapy.

The mistrust of institutionalized health care by the African American community goes beyond clinical issues. The historical exploitation of Black Americans in research studies has been linked to the current underrepresentation of this population in some facets of clinical research (Freimuth et al., 2001) and may contribute to a distrust of all health care systems of which mental health is a part. In the well-documented 40-year Tuskegee Syphilis Study, over 400 Black male sharecroppers suffering from the illness were deprived the knowledge of their diagnosis of syphilis and available treatment, allowing clinicians to observe its eventually fatal symptoms (Corbie-Smith, 1999). Freimuth et al. (2001) conducted a qualitative study with 60 focus groups across the nation exploring the recruitment of African American research subjects. In their study, distrust of White researchers emerged as a common barrier to involvement in the medical community, including participation in research, treatment, and preventive services. It also is possible that racial biases in the overdiagnosis of schizophrenia among African Americans (Snowden, 2001) may contextualize stigmas toward mental health as well as Black clients' mistrust in therapeutic processes. Furthermore, individuals who have limited familiarity with mental health services, including the purposes and expectations of different forms of treatment, may have considerable uncertainty, apprehension, and fear about psychological services. As a result, it seems reasonable not to pursue or sustain formal mental health services as a viable means of help (Kearny, Draper, & Barón, 2005).

Beliefs and knowledge about mental health services also may serve as barriers to accessing psychological care in the African American community. In particular, stigma, lack of knowledge of symptoms related to mental illnesses, and the use of alternative resources (e.g., prayer and attending church) have been identified as reasons some African Americans have not sought mental health services (Constantine et al., 2000; Corrigan, 2004). People of African descent may endorse stigmas related to counseling and mental health service, including the association of mental health service with extreme illness and being "crazy" (Wallace & Constantine, 2005).

Clients' impressions of their counselors and mental health practitioners also may have implications for their engagement in counseling processes and their initial approach to mental health services (Constantine, 2002; Constantine et al., 2002). As mentioned previously, African American clients may exhibit normative mistrust of members of the mental health community (e.g., Terrell & Terrell, 1981), which may contribute to apprehension in approaching counselors and therapists. This phenomenon has been studied through the lens of racial matching between therapists and clients. However, a meta-analysis on racial matching studies revealed no overall effects of client–clinician racial–ethnic matching on service retention, number of sessions attended, or post-treatment functioning (Shin et al., 2005). More important than the race of their counselor, African American clients have been found to want empathy and symptom alleviation from mental health providers (Constantine, 2002; Gillispie, Williams, & Gillispie, 2005). A study of 121 African American inpatient mental health consumers found that higher levels of perceived therapist empathy and subjective improvement in quality of life were predictive of service satisfaction (Gillispie et al., 2005). Among college students of color, Constantine (2002) found that attitudes toward counseling contributed significantly to general satisfaction with counseling. Perception of counselors' multicultural competence also was found to partially mediate the relationship between general counseling competence and satisfaction with counseling. These results suggested that multicultural competence is an important mechanism for mental health providers in increasing their ability to work effectively with this population.

Choosing Culturally-Sanctioned Ways of Coping With Problems or Issues

The underutilization of traditional mental health services (e.g., individual or group psychotherapy and counseling) by many African Americans also may reflect the use of alternate coping strategies among Blacks to address psychological and environmental stressors. That African Americans are less likely to seek help from these traditional forms of service may not imply a lack of resources. Formal mental health services, including individual and group therapy, may be viewed in the Black community as secondary to community-based supports, such as family, friends, and relationships built through religious activities (Lewis-Coles & Constantine, 2006). In fact, Snowden (1998) reported that African Americans tended to use assistance from friends, family members, or participating in conjunction with formal mental health services. Similarly, older African Americans were found to seek help more regularly than older White Americans in a variety of ways, including engaging members of the clergy, medical professionals, friends or family members, or participating in a life-skills lecture; they were less than one-third as likely to seek professional mental health treatment and over two times more likely to seek a religious authority (Dupree, Watson, & Schneider, 2005).

Several researchers and scholars (Atkinson, Thompson, & Grant, 1993; Constantine et al., 2002; Morris, 2001) have encouraged mental health professionals to adopt flexible roles, including those of advocate and social change agent, in response to addressing the needs of people of color. Nontraditional forms of treatment may be required in order to successfully penetrate the above-mentioned barriers and meet the mental health needs of African Americans. Brody et al. (2006) presented a model of such a treatment strategy in which a family-centered preventive intervention program (i.e., the Strong African American Families Program) operates from a "competence-promoting perspective" by assuming family members possess the required skills and competencies to raise children. In a sample of 332 rural African American families with children around 11 years of age, significant increases in targeted parenting behaviors, and regulated, communicative parenting, as well as a decrease in high-risk behavior among youths were observed. Liddle, Jackson-Gilfort, and Marvel (2006) offered a similar model adopted from Multidimensional Family Therapy, namely the *cultural theme engagement module*. Clinical guidelines for an intervention aimed at effective treatment engagement of African American adolescent males were comprised of strategies including the assessment of multiple systems, use of popular culture of interest to Black adolescents, and discussion and acknowledgement of salient cultural themes (e.g., cultural mistrust, anger/rage, alienation, spirituality, racial socialization, and racism).

In light of the ample disparities experienced by African Americans on the individual, cultural, and institutional levels, it is essential that mental health providers working with this community develop the skills, knowledge, and awareness that can increase their effectiveness and improve the quality of services available to all African Americans. In the following section, we discuss strategies for decreasing disparities in African Americans' access to and receipt of formal mental health services.

Strategies

We highlight below several strategies to (1) improve the quality of mental health services for African American clients, (2) minimize structural barriers in the receipt of mental health care among African Americans, and (3) decrease the stigma associated with counseling use among African Americans and promote more favorable help-seeking attitudes among African Americans.

1. Mental health professionals need to feel comfortable bringing up and discussing issues of race with African American clients (Morris, 2001), while considering the racial identity development and racial–cultural values that emphasize group affiliation and family networks among these clients.
2. Race represents one aspect of individuals' various social locations and it informs their experience. However, the extent to which clients identify more saliently as Black or African American more than other reference groups (e.g., sexual orientation, gender, social class, etc.) can shape their subjective understanding of their concerns and can inform therapeutic interventions. The complex nature of the intersections of multiple identities warrants consideration when conducting assessment and employing therapeutic modes of intervention.
3. In the spirit of cultural self-awareness, mental health practitioners should exercise mindfulness about the cultural limitations of some approaches, techniques, and instruments used in the practice of assessment, counseling, and psychotherapy. For example, psychological evaluations are not comprehensive without information regarding clients' multiple contexts and social locations. For African American clients in particular, clinicians need to be mindful of the power of psychological assessment in the classification of Black people and the ripple effects that such tests may engender. Mental health practitioners are highly encouraged to be aware of the cultural validity of the psychological instruments they use, along with possible cross-cultural differences in test interpretation (APA, 2003).
4. Atkinson et al. (1993) highlighted various functions that mental health practitioners might assume in working with clients of color, such as advisor, advocate, social or environmental change agent, facilitator of indigenous support systems (e.g., incorporating shamanistic rituals into therapy sessions), consultant, ombudsperson, and facilitator of self-help resources. These unconventional roles offer alternate methods to traditional counseling in addressing the individual, cultural, and systemic problems with which many African American clients may present.
5. Trust, or rather its absence, is one of the biggest barriers to the effective mental health treatment of African American clients. African Americans have adaptively been socialized to be distrustful of institutional systems in general, including mental health care. It is important for mental health professionals to demystify the

therapeutic process. Purposeful methods of outreach are fundamental in fostering trust and psychoeducation in African American communities.

6. Mental health practitioners should integrate a social justice orientation in their work and actively minimize the oppressive stances that may be unknowingly enacted in therapy and the society at large. One intentional method includes working within the mental health field to promote cultural competence by continual self-examination, training initiatives, research agendas, and so on. Vera and Speight (2003) contended that a commitment to social justice means applying influence beyond the mental health field to take steps in advocacy, prevention, and outreach for underserved populations. Sue (1995) recommended that, in conjunction with addressing the mental health outcomes of oppression in therapy with clients from marginalized groups, mental health professionals must adopt a proactive and preventive stance in combating social inequalities.

7. Clients "assess" the level of safety and comfort in the environment as soon as they walk in the door (Ward, 2005). Increasing the visibility of mental health professionals of color or "changing the face" of mental health in the Black community may foster clients' experiences of safety in a mental health setting.

Conclusion

In the United States, traditional forms of mental health care reflect Western European epistemologies of psychological well being and pathology. Because therapy has been characterized as "the handmaiden of the status quo" (Halleck, 1971), mental health practitioners may unknowingly devalue culturally congruent ways of being for African Americans that contrast with Western norms. The therapeutic environment is a microcosm of the larger society (Sue & Sue, 2003); consequently, mental health care practitioners are not immune to perpetuating oppression and other forms of discrimination. Because of multiple factors that contribute to disparities in mental health services accessed and received by African Americans, it behooves mental health practitioners to modify their approaches to meet the needs of this population. Mental health professionals should work at the individual, community, and institutional levels to address external barriers, differential quality of care, and beliefs that African Americans may bring into their interactions with mental health systems. These professionals should challenge themselves to amend their conceptualizations of helping to respond to the diverse socio-cultural histories, values, and mental health needs of African American clients to eradicate current mental health disparities.

REFERENCES

Alvidrez, J., & Havassy, B. E. (2005). Racial distribution of dual-diagnosis clients in public sector mental health and drug treatment settings. *Journal of Health Care for the Poor and Underserved*, *16*, 53–62.

American Psychological Association. (2003). Guidelines on multicultural education, training, research, practice, and organizational change for psychologists. *American Psychologist*, *58*, 377–402.

Atkinson, D. R., Thompson, C. E., & Grant, S. K. (1993). A three-dimensional model for counseling racial/ethnic minorities. *The Counseling Psychologist*, *21*, 257–277.

Brody, G. H., Murray, V. M., Gerrard, M., Gibbons, F. X., McNair, L., Brown, A. C., et al. (2006). The strong African American families program: Prevention of youth's high-risk behavior and a test of a model of change. *Journal of Family Psychology, 20,* 1–11.

Chow, J. C., Jaffe, K., & Snowden, L. (2003). Racial/ethnic disparities in the use of mental health services in poverty areas. *American Journal of Public Health, 93,* 792–797.

Constantine, M. G. (2002). Predictors of satisfaction with counseling: Racial and ethnic minority clients' attitudes toward counseling and ratings of their counselors' general and multicultural counseling competence. *Journal of Counseling Psychology, 49,* 255–263.

Constantine, M. G. (2006). Institutional racism against African Americans: Physical and mental health implications. In M. G. Constantine & D. W. Sue (Eds.), *Addressing racism: Facilitating cultural competence in mental health and educational settings* (pp. 33–41). Hoboken, NJ: Wiley.

Constantine, M. G. (2007). Racial microaggressions against African American clients in cross-racial counseling relationships. *Journal of Counseling Psychology, 54,* 1–16.

Constantine, M. G., Gainor, K. A., Ahluwalia, M. K., & Berkel, L. A. (2003). Independent and interdependent self-construals, individualism, collectivism, and harmony control in African Americans. *Journal of Black Psychology, 29,* 87–101.

Constantine, M. G., Kindaichi, M. M., Arorash, T. J., Donnelly, P. C., & Jung, K-S. K. (2002). Clients' perceptions of multicultural counseling competence: Current status and future directions. *The Counseling Psychologist, 30,* 407–416.

Constantine, M. G., Lewis, E. L., Conner, L. C., & Sanchez, D. A. (2000). Addressing spiritual and religious issues in counseling African Americans: Implications for counselor training and practice. *Counseling and Values, 45,* 28–38.

Constantine, M. G., Myers, L. J., Kindaichi, M., & Moore, J. L. (2004). Exploring indigenous mental health practices: The roles of healers and helpers in promoting well-being in people of color. *Counseling and Values, 48,* 110–125.

Constantine, M. G., & Sue, D. W. (2005). *Strategies for building multicultural competence in mental health and educational settings.* Hoboken, NJ: Wiley.

Copeland, V. C. (2005). African Americans: Disparities in health care access and utilization. *Health & Social Work, 30,* 265–269.

Corbie-Smith, G. (1999). The continuing legacy of the Tuskegee Syphilis Study: Considerations for clinical investigation. *American Journal of the Medical Sciences, 317,* 5–8.

Corrigan, P. (2004). How stigma interferes with mental health care. *American Psychologist, 59,* 614–625.

Dana, R. H. (2002). Mental health services for African Americans: A cultural/racial perspective. *Cultural Diversity and Ethnic Minority Psychology, 8,* 3–18.

Dixon, C. G., & Vaz, K. (2005). Perceptions of African Americans regarding mental health counseling. In D. A. Harley & J. M. Dillard (Eds.), *Contemporary mental health issues among African Americans* (pp. 163–174). Alexandria, VA: American Counseling Association.

Dupree, L. W., Watson, M. A., & Schneider, M. G. (2005). Preferences for mental health care: A comparison of older African Americans and older Caucasians. *Journal of Applied Gerontology, 24,* 196–210.

Fischer, A. R., & Shaw, C. M. (1999). African Americans' mental health and perceptions of racist discrimination: The moderating effects of racial socialization experiences and self-esteem. *Journal of Counseling Psychology, 46,* 395–407.

Freimuth, V. S., Quinn, S. C., Thomas, S. B., Cole, G., Zook, E., & Duncan, T. (2001). African Americans' views on research and the Tuskegee Syphilis Study. *Social Science and Medicine, 52,* 797–801.

Garland, A. F., Lau, A. S., Yeh, M., McCabe, K. M., Hough, R. L., & Landsverk, J. A. (2005). Racial and ethnic differences in utilization of mental health services among high-risk youths. *American Journal of Psychiatry, 162,* 1336–1343.

Gillispie, R., Williams, E., & Gillispie, C. (2005). Hospitalized African American mental health consumers: Some antecedents to service satisfaction and intent to comply with aftercare. *American Journal of Orthopsychiatry 75,* 254–261.

Halleck, S. L. (1971). Therapy is the handmaiden of the status quo. *Psychology Today, 4,* 30–34, 98.

Joe, S. (2006). Explaining changes in the patterns of Black suicide in the United States from 1981 to 2002: An age, cohort, and period analysis. *Journal of Black Psychology, 32,* 262–284.

Jones, J. M. (1997). *Prejudice and racism* (2nd ed.). New York: McGraw-Hill.

Karenga, M. R. (1965). *Nguzo Saba.* San Diego, CA: Kawaida.

Karenga, M. R. (1988). *The African American holiday of Kwanzaa*. Los Angeles: University of Sankore Press.

Kearney, L. K., Draper, M., & Barón, A. (2005). Counseling utilization by ethnic minority college students. *Cultural Diversity & Ethnic Minority Psychology, 11*, 272–285.

Kochanek, K. D., Murphy, S. L., Anderson, R. N., & Scott, C. (2004). *Deaths: Final data for 2002. National Vital Statistics Reports*. Retrieved from http://www.cdc.gov/nchs/data/nvsr/nvsr53/nvsr53˙05.pdf

Kunen, S., Niederhauser, R., Smith, P. O., Morris, J. A., & Marx, B. D. (2005). Race disparities in psychiatric rates in emergency departments. *Journal of Consulting and Clinical Psychology, 73*, 116–126.

Kuno, E., & Rothbard, A. B. (2005). The effect of income and race on quality of psychiatric care in community mental health centers. *Community Mental Health Journal, 41*, 613–622.

Lewis-Coles, M. E., & Constantine, M. G. (2006). Racism-related stress, Africultural coping, and religious problem-solving among African Americans. *Cultural Diversity and Ethnic Minority Psychology, 3*, 433–443.

Liddle, H. A., Jackson-Gilfort, A., & Marvel, F. A. (2006). An empirically supported and culturally specific engagement and intervention strategy for African American adolescent males. *American Journal of Orthopsychiatry, 75*, 215–225.

Mansfield, A. K., Addis, M. E., & Courtenay, W. (2005). Measurement of men's help seeking: Development and evaluation of the Barriers to Help Seeking Scale. *Psychology of Men & Masculinity, 6*, 95–108.

Morris, E. F. (2001). Clinical practices with African Americans: Juxtaposition of standard clinical practices and Africentricism. *Professional Psychology: Research and Practice, 32*, 563–572.

Myers, L. J. (1993). *Understanding an Afrocentric worldview: Introduction to an optimal psychology* (2nd ed.). Dubuque, IA: Kendall/Hunt.

National Center for Health Statistics. (2005). *Health, United States 2005, with chart book on trends in the health of Americans*. Retrieved December 10, 2006, from http://www.cdc.gov/nchs/data/hus/hus05.pdf#061

National Center for Health Statistics. (2006a). *Asthma prevalence, health care use and mortality: United States, 2003–05*. Retrieved December 11, 2006, from http://www.cdc.gov/nchs/products/pubs/pubd/hestats/ashtma03-05/asthma03-05.htm

National Center for Health Statistics. (2006b). *Death: Leading causes for 2003*. Retrieved December 11, 2006, from http://www.cdc.gov/nchs/products/pubs/pubd/hestats/leadingdeaths03/leadingdeaths03.htm

Neighbors, H. W., Trierweiler, S. J., Ford, B. C., & Muroff, J. R. (2003). Racial differences in DSM diagnosis using a semi-structured instrument: The importance of clinical judgment in the diagnosis of African Americans. *Journal of Health and Social Behavior, 43*, 237–256.

Richardson, J., Anderson, T., Flaherty, J., & Bell, C. (2003). The quality of mental health care for African Americans. *Culture, Medicine, and Psychiatry, 27*, 487–498.

Ridley, C. (1995). *Overcoming unintentional racism in counseling and therapy: A practitioner's guide to intentional intervention*. Thousand Oaks, CA: Sage.

Ridley, C. R. (2005). *Overcoming intentional racism in counseling and therapy: A practitioner's guide to intentional intervention* (2nd ed.). Thousand Oaks, CA: Sage.

Robins, L. N., & Regier, D. A. (Eds.). (1991). *Psychiatric disorders in America: The epidemiologic catchment area study*. Washington, DC: American Psychiatric Press.

Ronzio, C. R., Guagliardo, M. F., & Persaud, N. (2006). Disparity in location of urban mental service providers. *American Journal of Orthopsychiatry, 76*, 37–43.

Sanders Thompson, V. L. (2006). Therapists' race and African American client's reactions to therapy. *Psychotherapy: Theory, Research, Practice, Training, 43*, 99–110.

Sanders Thompson, V. L., Bazile, A., & Akbar, M., (2004). African Americans' perceptions of psychotherapy and psychotherapists. *Professional Psychology: Research and Practice, 35*, 19–26.

Shin, S., Chow, C., Camacho-Gonsalves, T., Levy, R., & Allen, I. E. (2005). A meta-analytic review of racial-ethnic matching for African American and Caucasian American clients and clinicians. *Journal of Counseling Psychology, 52*, 45–56.

Snowden, L. R. (1998). Racial differences in informal help seeking for mental health problems. *Journal of Community Psychology, 26*, 429–438.

Snowden, L. R. (2001). Barriers to effective mental health services for African Americans. *Mental Health Services Research, 3*, 181–187.

Snowden, L. R., & Pingitore, D. (2002). Frequency and scope of mental health service delivery to African Americans in primary care. *Mental Health Services Research, 4*, 123–130.

Snowden, L. R., & Thomas, K. (2000). Medicaid and African American outpatient mental health treatment. *Mental Health Services Research, 2*, 115–120.

Sue, D. W. (1995). Multicultural organizational development: Implications for the counseling profession. In J. G. Ponterotto, J. M. Casas, L. A. Suzuki, & C. M. Alexander (Eds.), *Handbook of multicultural counseling* (pp. 474–492). Thousand Oaks, CA: Sage.

Sue, D. W., Arredondo, P., & McDavis, R. J. (1992). Multicultural counseling competencies and standards: A call to the profession. *Journal of Counseling and Development, 70*, 477–483.

Sue, D. W., & Sue, D. (2003). *Counseling the culturally diverse* (4th ed.). Hoboken, NJ: Wiley.

Terrell, F., & Terrell, S. L. (1981). An inventory to measure cultural mistrust among Blacks. *Western Journal of African American Studies, 5*, 180–184.

Terrell, F., & Terrell, S. (1984). Race of counselor, client sex, cultural mistrust level, and premature termination from counseling among Black clients. *Journal of Counseling Psychology, 31*, 371–375.

Thompson, C. E., Worthington, R., & Atkinson, D. R. (1994). Counselor content orientation, counselor race, and Black women's cultural mistrust and self-disclosures. *Journal of Counseling Psychology, 41*, 155–161.

U.S. Department of Health and Human Services. (2001). *Mental health: Culture, race and ethnicity—A supplement to mental health: A report of the Surgeon General*. Rockville, MD: U.S. Department of Health and Human Services, Public Health Office, Office of the Surgeon General.

Vera, E. M., & Speight, S. L. (2003). Multicultural competencies, social justice, and counseling psychology: Expanding our roles. *The Counseling Psychologist, 31*, 253–272.

Wallace, B. C., & Constantine, M. G. (2005). Africentric cultural values, psychological help-seeking attitudes, and self-concealment in African American college students. *Journal of Black Psychology, 31*, 369–385.

Ward, E. C. (2005). Keeping it real: A grounded theory study of African American clients engaging in counseling at a community mental health agency. *Journal of Counseling Psychology, 52*, 471–481.

Williams, D. R., & Neighbors, H. (2001). Racism, discrimination, and hypertension: Evidence and needed research. *Ethnicity and Disease, 11*, 800–816.

Williams, D. R., & Williams-Morris, R. (2000). Racism and mental health: The African American experience. *Ethnicity and Health, 5*, 243–267.

Yeh, M., McCabe, K., Hough, R. L., Dupuis, D., & Hazen, A. (2003). Racial/ethnic differences in parental endorsement of barriers to mental health services for youth. *Mental Health Services Research, 5*, 65–77.

Genetics or Social Forces? Racial Disparities in Infant Mortality

Richard J. David and James W. Collins, Jr.

Introduction

Information on molecular genetics has exploded in recent decades. From the description of the double helix by Watson and Crick in 1953 to the sequencing of the human genome in 2003 and the beginnings of genomic medicine, scientific knowledge has accumulated at a breathtaking pace. Over the same decades, the United States, the world leader in newborn intensive care, fell from 6th to 27th in its international standing for infant mortality rate. Meanwhile the racial gap for infant mortality has widened. The rate of death in the first year of life for African American infants increased from 1.6 times to 2.3 times the rate of White infants (David & Collins, 1991; Martin, Kochanek, Strobino, Guyer, & MacDorman, 2005). The worsened national statistics for infant mortality are not just the result of including the poor outcomes for African Americans. In 2001 the infant mortality rate for White infants born in the United States was 5.7 per 1,000 live births, which would give that subgroup a rank of 23rd in the world, not much better than 27th. That U.S. White rate was more than twice as high as the country with the best record in the world, Singapore at 2.4 deaths per 1,000 live births (Martin et al., 2005).

Observing these trends should give pause to those who are tempted to approach public health problems with strictly technological solutions, of which genomic medicine is the latest example. The widening racial disparity during the era of molecular genetics would also prompt skepticism that genetic research holds the key to understanding and eliminating African American–White disparities in infant mortality, a worthy goal of the Healthy People 2010 objectives (U.S. Department of Health

A version of this chapter appeared in the *Journal of the American Public Health Association* under a different title. This material is reprinted with permission from the American Public Health Association.

and Human Services, 2005). Indeed, it has been argued by anthropologists for years that "race" has little or no meaning as a genetic category, but rather derives all its usefulness from its very clear social, political, cultural, and historical meaning (Marks, 1995; Montagu, 1974). These social meanings of race have clear public health implications (Cooper, 1984; Cooper & David, 1986; Cooper, Steinhauer, Miller, David, & Schatzkin, 1981; David & Collins, 1991). In this chapter we will attempt to evaluate the expected utility of two approaches to racial disparities, one based on race as a social construct and the other based on race as a proxy for geographic ancestry and genetics.

"Race," Geographic Ancestry, and Health

"Race" in its traditional genetic conceptualization has been undermined by a wealth of information from molecular biology over the past 30 years. Most human variation (90–95%) is found within the population of any continent, with only an additional 5–10% accounted for by differences between populations (Marks, 1995; Rosenberg et al., 2002). Patterns of human variation reflect our evolutionary history as a young species (anatomically modern *Homo sapiens*), originating in Africa roughly 200,000 years ago. For more than half of the intervening time, all modern humans lived in Africa, with smaller founding populations arriving in Asia and Europe within the past 80,000 to 50,000 years (Marks, 1995; Tishkoff, & Kidd, 2004).

When hundreds of variable sites in the genome are sampled, geographical structure of diversity can be discerned, roughly corresponding to continental barriers to ancient migrations. These statistical clusters do not fit into the traditional, essentialist concept of "races." Attempts to conflate such constructs with traditional racial classification impede a more sophisticated understanding of genomic diversity (Bamshad, Wooding, Salisbury, & Stephens, 2004; Foster & Sharp, 2004). Geographical structuring is inferred from multiple neutrally varying sites. In contrast, medically relevant loci are often subject to strong natural selection or to genetic drift of rare alleles following population bottlenecks, and the populations of interest do not necessarily coincide with those based on continent of origin (Foster & Sharp, 2004; Jorde & Wooding, 2004).

Differences in allele frequencies between geographic populations have well-known effects in the incidence of uncommon diseases like cystic fibrosis and sickle cell (Drayna, 2005). Whether they will turn out to have parallels in common complex diseases remains to be demonstrated (Colhoun, McKeigue, & Davey-Smith, 2003; Cooper, Kaufman, & Ward, 2003; Farral & Morris, 2005). There is as yet no complex disease for which the genetic components are completely or even largely understood, but the popular genetic conception of "race" in medical research in this country takes genetic difference between Whites and African Americans as a starting point.

Now to the list of such complex conditions as heart disease, hypertension, and diabetes researchers have suggested adding preterm birth (Dizon-Townson, 2001; Varner & Esplin, 2005). The hunt is on for "preterm birth genes" that can explain the disparity in prematurity and infant mortality between African Americans and Whites. The March of Dimes Research Agenda on Prematurity lists "Genetic factors" as the second rubric under the category "Racial/ethnic disparities" (Green et al., 2005). A typical rationale for the genetic approach is that "African American women suffer twice the rate of preterm

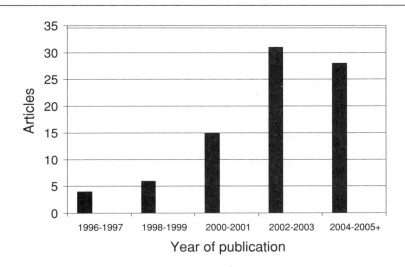

Reports describing polymorphisms putatively implicated in the risk of preterm birth or other adverse birth outcomes. All articles before 2003 and 45 of 59 from 2003 onward cited in table in Fiscella (2005). Remaining 14 articles (23–36) from PubMed search in February 2006.

birth compared to Caucasians even when confounding social and economic variables are controlled for" (Dizon-Townson, 2001). Can all or even most of the multifaceted social, economic, political, and historical effects of racial discrimination be adequately "controlled" with the variables commonly measured (David & Collins, 1991; Krieger, Rowley, Herman, Avery, & Phillips, 1993)? Clearly some investigators believe they can.

Reports of polymorphisms associated with adverse birth outcomes appear to be growing exponentially at this time (Figure 10.1). Fiscella (2005) reviewed this literature extensively and published his findings in late 2005. He tabulated 70 reports describing 32 different genetic variants putatively implicated in the risk of preterm birth along with racial differences in gene frequency. A PubMed search in February 2006, identified 14 additional reports (Amory et al., 2004; Doh et al., 2004; Engel et al., 2005; Erichsen, Engel, Eck, Welch, & Yeager, 2006; Hartel et al., 2005; Kalish, Vardhana, Gupta, Perni, & Witkin, 2004; Kalish et al., 2005; Kalish, Vardhana, Normand, Gupta, & Witkin, 2006; Nukui, Day, Sims, Ness, & Romkes, 2004; Perni et al., 2004; Resch et al., 2004; Valdez et al., 2004; Wang et al., 2004; Witkin et al., 2003). Of the combined total of 84 articles, 59 have been published since 2002. Does existing population health evidence support this increasingly intense pursuit of a genetic basis for racial disparities in birth outcomes?

From the New Deal to BiDil

It can be argued that social and economic forces, rather than scientific evidence, drive this research trend. Current social and political discourse in this country favors individual-level and technology-based solutions over extensions (or even maintenance) of the social contract implicit in American politics since the New Deal. More and more, a business

Causes of Infant Death	Total	White	African American	RR
All causes	688.9	571.2	1347.7	2.4
Congenital malformations (Q00–Q99)	141.8	138.5	167	1.2
Disorders related to short gestation (P07)	108.4	74.7	293.6	3.9
Sudden infant death syndrome (R95)	62.1	51.8	122.1	2.4
Maternal pregnancy complications (P01)	34.3	26.1	80.5	3.1
Complications of placenta, cord, membranes (P02)	25.7	22.3	45.6	2.0

Table 10.1 Cause-Specific Infant Death Rates, United States, 2000 — Death Rate (Per 100,000 Live Births)

RR – Rate ratio (African American/White)
Source: National Vital Statistics Reports (2002).

model dominates medical research, with over 20% of the genes in the human genome now under patent (Jensen & Murray, 2005). In 2005 the first "ethnic drug," BiDil, was approved by the FDA for treatment of heart failure specifically in African Americans (Kahn, 2003, 2005). The licensing of this product is seen by many as the first of many pharmaceuticals that will be tailored to different physiology in different people—genomic medicine. And of course people belonging to different "races" will be assumed to differ at the genome level, providing distinct niche markets. Sociologist Troy Duster predicts that because "race is such a dominant category" such endeavors in biomedicine "can leave [their] own indelible mark once given the temporary imprimatur of scientific legitimacy by molecular genetics" (Duster, 2005). Given the risk of wasting large amounts of scientific effort and reinforcing popular misperceptions of "race," do the existing population data justify this quest?

Race and Mortality

An overview of racial disparities in birth outcomes will help to put the current research agenda into perspective. The five leading causes of death in the first year of life in the United States for African American and White infants (Centers for Disease Control and Prevention [CDC], 2002) are shown in Table 10.1. The table also shows the ratios of African American to White infant death rates (RR) for each of the major causes. These ratios range from a high of 3.9 for "disorders related to short gestation" to a low of 1.2 for "congenital malformations." It is noteworthy that the mortality disadvantage of African Americans is observed across all of the major categories of infant death. A similar pattern is seen in adults. Of the ten leading causes of death, African Americans have lower death rates for only two: chronic lung disease and Alzheimer's disease (CDC, 2006). It is highly unlikely for any given population to have concentrated multiple deleterious mutations in such a way that they are at higher risk for almost all of the common complex disorders on a genetic basis. Social, economic, and cultural processes, on the other hand, could reasonably be hypothesized to cause adverse impacts on historically disadvantaged groups in a multifaceted and many-layered manner (Cooper & David, 1986; Cooper et al., 1981; David & Collins, 1991; Krieger et al., 1993). Indeed, social class gradients have been demonstrated for a variety of diseases in all age groups since the classic studies of the 19th century (Ackerknecht, 1953, pp. 44, 109, 123–137; Engels, 1968, p. 109). A contemporary report from the United Kingdom reveals that the same pattern persists today: a significant social class mortality gradient, as well as significant gradients for 15 of the 17 specific causes of child morbidity (Petrou, Kupek, Hockley, & Goldacre, 2006).

Birth Weight and Ancestry

Birth weight, a commonly used proxy for gestational maturity, is the most important determinant of infant mortality differences between Whites and African Americans. Most of the African American–White gap in first-year mortality is attributable to their three-fold higher rate of infants born at very low birth weight (less than 1,500 grams), essentially all of whom are preterm (Iyasu, Becerra, Rowley, & Hogue, 1992). Short gestation is tightly linked with low birth weight, but is more difficult to measure, especially at the population level (David, 1980, 2001). Researchers point out the persistence of a racial birth weight disparity after controlling for various social or environmental risk factors (Dizon-Townson, 2001; Hoffman & Ward, 1999). Do population patterns of birth weight support a genetic basis?

One feature of population patterns of preterm or low birth weight births that is at odds with genetic explanations of population differences is secular change. Average birth weights have risen in populations native to Japan, Pakistan, and Southeast Asia, among others, either following economic changes within the country of origin or immigration to more affluent societies (Clarson, Barker, Marshall, & Wharton, 1982; Gruenwald, 1968; Li, Ni, Schwartz, & Daling, 1990). Similarly, birth weights in the state of Illinois—within both white and African American families—increased from 33 to 74 grams over the generation from the 1960s to the 1990s (Chike-Obi, David, Coutinho, & Wu, 1996). More recently the National Center for Health Statistics reported that the rates of singleton preterm births changed significantly between 1989 and 1996 for both Whites and African Americans (CDC, 1999). Population changes in phenotype caused by genetic drift or natural selection occur over tens of thousands of years, not over decades. Clearly these changes over brief periods of time must have an environmental, not a genetic basis.

Perhaps the most direct test of the hypothesized linkage between continent of ancestry ("race") and birth weight was a comparison of birth weights among three groups of women delivering in Illinois over a 15-year period: U.S.-born White women, U.S.-born African American women, and African-born women (David & Collins, 1997). Earlier research had shown that African American individuals have significant European genetic admixture. If birth weight differences between African Americans and Whites in North America were determined by different frequencies of alleles responsible for low birth weight and these "low birth weight genes" were derived from African populations, then they should be most in evidence in African women, less so in African Americans, and least in women with largely European ancestry, so-called "Whites." What we found was quite different. The overall birth weight distributions for infants of U.S.-born White

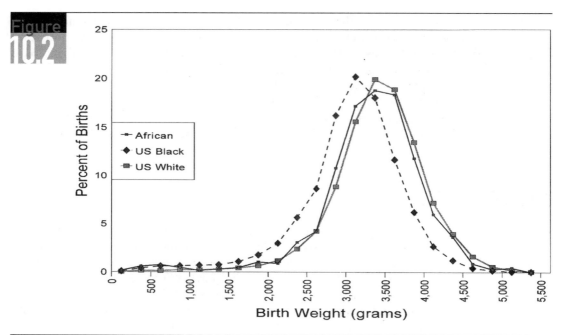

Birth weight distributions of three Illinois sub-populations. (From *New England Journal of Medicine* (1997). *337*:1211. Reprinted with permission.)

women and African-born women were almost identical, with U.S.-born African American women's infants describing a distinctly different population, weighing hundreds of grams less (Figure 10.2). U.S.-born African American women also experience higher rates of very low birth weight than either the White or African-born women once appropriate confounders were controlled (David & Collins, 1997).

We performed a similar analysis of births to Afro-Caribbean women immigrating to the United States and again found that those women gave birth to infants hundreds of grams heavier than the infants of U.S.-born African American women (Pallotto, Collins, & David, 2000). A recent report from Portugal (Harding, Santana, Cruickshank, & Boroujerdi, 2006) showed similar findings, except that the birth weights of the infants of African-born women in Portugal were actually somewhat higher than the weights of both groups of Portuguese-born women, those of African and of European ancestry.

Healthy Immigrants or Unhealthy Society?

The possibility exists that the phenomenon observed in these groups of women migrating from majority Black countries in Africa and the Caribbean represents a "healthy immigrant" effect, as described for other populations (Marmot, Adelstein, & Bulusu, 1984). We explored this hypothesis in a study of the birth weight patterns emerging in the generation after women migrated from African or Caribbean countries to the United States. Our findings again contradicted predictions based on genetic race. We analyzed the intergenerational birth weight patterns among the descendants of U.S.-born and foreign-born White and Black women (Collins, Wu, & David, 2002). European immigrants to the United States gave birth to daughters of similar birth weight to the girls born into established European American families and these girls grew up to have daughters whose average birth weight was higher than their own. This is the same pattern of rising birth weights over a generation that we had described previously in Illinois (Chike-Obi et al., 1996). On the other hand, African and Caribbean immigrants gave birth to daughters who were heavier than the girls born into established African American families. Most striking, these first generation African American girls grew up in the United States and went on to have daughters whose birth weights were lower on average than their own weights had been at birth. This generational trend is opposite to that seen in the non-immigrant population and opposite to the trend in European immigrant families (Collins et al., 2002). It is possible that a "healthy immigrant" effect could exist for Africans and not for Europeans, given the more stringent visa requirements for African immigrants (Brandon, 1997), but if such immigration selection were in some way related to genetics, the pattern should persist into the next generation. That is not what we observed. Our findings are not readily explained by any genetic mechanism but rather suggest cumulative negative effects of minority status through the life course from fetus to childbearing woman.

So an overview of the pattern of racial disparities in birth outcomes in the United States can be summarized as follows. Like health disparities in U.S. adults, the disadvantage in cause-specific death rates for African American infants compared to White infants is distributed across nearly all causes. Racial disparity in infant deaths is highest for deaths related to prematurity and lowest for birth defects and chromosomal disorders. The pattern of low birth weight and prematurity in the population is not static but shows significant secular change over a generation or less. The low birth weights typical for black infants in the United States or Portugal are not seen among infants born to recent immigrants from Africa or the Caribbean. After a generation of minority status, however, the birth weights in these families approximate those in the established Black minority population of the respective country.

Disparity Research Grounded in a Social Conception of Race

As suggested at the outset, the epidemiologic evidence suggests that public health planners look to social and environmental rather than genetic differences between African American and White women in the campaign to eliminate health disparities. As Rudolph Virchow (1985) put it when considering mass diseases affecting German society in the 1870s, these conditions "indicate disturbances rooted in our social and governmental institutions, hence preventable." Even as biotechnology firms were applying for gene patents and molecular biologists were formulating their first studies in pursuit of a "preterm birth gene" in Black women, another strategy was being formulated. This approach to racial disparities research turned away from "race" to "racism." Stimulated by a series of conferences convened by the CDC under the leadership of Diane Rowley and Carol Hogue in the early 1990s (Blackmore et al., 1993; Rowley et al., 1993), a new picture of African American–White differences began to emerge. Race as a social category is associated with a complex array of disparities in life experience in our highly racialized society.

Geronimus (1986, 1992), who was first to point out the deterioration of birth outcomes of African American women as they age from their teens into their 20s, the so-called "weathering" phenomenon, noted the elevated and rising levels of lead in the blood of African American women living in polluted neighborhoods. We described adverse birth outcomes for African American women exposed to neighborhood violence (Collins & David, 1997), other unsatisfactory aspects of their residential environments, and stressful life events (Collins et al., 1998). The subjective reports of increased levels of life stress described by African American women compared to White women fit with published statistics. To take two striking examples, African Americans—both women of childbearing age and their partners—are more than twice as likely to be in the Army (Grieco & Cassidy, 2005; U.S. Census Bureau, 2001) and seven times as likely to be incarcerated (Grieco & Cassidy; U.S. Department of Justice, 1998) as Whites. In our case-controlled study of African American women giving birth in two Chicago hospitals, fully 16% reported incarceration of their partner during the pregnancy (Lespinasse, David, Collins, Handler, & Wall, 2004). In addition to these examples of community and institutional level effects of racism, recent studies by our group (Collins, David, Handler, Wall, & Andes, 2004) and others (Dole et al., 2004; Mustillo et al., 2004; Stancil, Hertz-Picciotto, Schramm, & Watt-Morse, 2000) demonstrate similar deleterious effects on the interpersonal level. These studies showed an adverse impact of perceived racial discrimination on the birth outcome for African American women.

Importance of Eliminating Racial Disparities for Reducing White Infant Mortality

The importance of this direction of investigation extends beyond its potential benefits for African Americans. As noted, White Americans also fare poorly compared to other countries, despite the world's largest per-capita expenditure on medical care (Reinhardt, Hussey, & Anderson, 2004). The U.S. racial gap in infant mortality and the gap between the United States and the world's leader in infant mortality reduction have increased in tandem over the past half-century (David & Collins, 1991). Is there a causal pathway that could explain this tight temporal correlation? The missing concept to formulate this pathway is social class. Health statistics in the United States record categories of ethnicity but not social class (Cooper, Kaufman, & Ward, 2003). However, an extensive literature documents the impact of social class in other wealthy, industrialized societies, including infant mortality (Arntzen & Nybo Andersen, 2004; Devlieger, Martens, & Bekaert, 2005; Dyer, 2005; Shaw, Blakely, Atkinson, & Crampton, 2005). In a recent cross-sectional study of 16 wealthy OECD countries, Muntaner et al. (2002) analyzed the impact of national level politics on birth outcomes. The authors reported their findings as follows: "In summary, the rates of low birth weight and infant deaths from all causes were lower in those countries with more voter turnout, more left votes, more left members of parliament, more women in government, a stronger social pact and various aspects of the welfare state, and low income inequality, as measured in a variety of ways."

Understanding health outcomes for the majority population in the United States requires a model that incorporates both race (as a social construct) and social class. We would propose a model that links the two by the mechanism of class power. That is, the political influence exercised by an economic class depends on its political unity in pursuing its class agenda. To the extent that racial identity inhibits class identity, class unity and thus class political power would be reduced. We speculate that the unique history of race in the United States has led to a situation in which political unity and influence of the working classes—ordinary wage earners—are relatively low, as indicated by the international comparison reported by Muntaner et al. (2002) in the previous paragraph.

Race, Class, and History: Implications for Health Disparities

Our national history includes decimating the population of one ethnic group and enslaving another. Unlike the exploitation of the populations of distant colonies by European empires, African Americans labored alongside people of other ethnic backgrounds right here, necessitating a set of ideological justifications and supporting institutions. African Americans contributed disproportionately to the country's wealth and acquired disproportionately little of it, a situation that began in the 16th century and continues today (Bennett, 1982; Farley, 1984). No other modern nation shares our unique history. This past has led to the "peculiar institutions" of present-day American politics. As virtually the only industrialized country that has no labor party and no universal health care, our politics is indeed unusual. The speculation that our nation's history of race relations has led to our lack of class-based political institutions derives from the fact that popular culture and consciousness revolve around racial identity in the United States. Although racial ideologies have had (Müller-Hill, 1984; Peukert, 1987)—and continue to have (Dickey, 2004)—their own ugly history in Europe and elsewhere, there is no other industrialized nation where racial politics have been so dominant and consistent over time as in the United States (Black, 2003, p. 21 ff.).

To be understood, the renewed interest in "race" as a genetic concept must be viewed in this context. Scientific discovery and technologic advancement proceed according to their own dynamic of discovery, but scientists are part of society and subject to its political and cultural influences. The yearning for simple solutions to irreconcilable contradictions within a class-stratified society such as the United States has led to the recurrent reinvention of the concept of genetic "race" (Chase, 1980; Leroi, 2005; Muntaner, Nieto, & O'Campo, 1996) despite abundant scientific evidence against it. It would almost appear that the idea is essential to the maintenance of class society as we know it.

Where does this point us in the ongoing effort to eliminate the glaring and shameful health disparities—racial and otherwise—that afflict our population? We can take encouragement from two observations. First, poor health outcomes for African Americans are inextricably connected to poor health of the U.S. majority population relative to other affluent countries. This may seem like more bad news, but viewed from a different perspective it means that the objective basis exists for broad political unity to change the status quo. Second, despite the cultural influences that promote racial identity (Kleinfeld, 2001), popular attitudes have shown movement toward breaking down racial separation (Sack & Elder, 2001), with the number of mixed marriages increasing ten-fold since 1960, now accounting for 4% of couples (Fletcher, 1998). Thus, social class unity—across racial lines—could develop over time, making possible deep political change.

Researchers, especially those in public health and epidemiology, can help guide reform efforts. To provide effective progressive leadership, we must acknowledge that being a good scientist is not enough. History and culture influence the questions we ask. Scholars and health professionals must be willing to make detailed comparisons between the United States and other countries in the attempt to reduce adverse infant outcomes (Thompson, Goodman, & Little, 2002). Studies that link health outcomes to explicit social, economic, and political processes (Cooper et al., 2001; Daniels, Kennedy, & Kawachi, 2000) are an essential area for future work. The evidence presented earlier in this chapter suggests that a redirection of disparities research will come as part of a more profound change involving the whole society. Within that context and as a part of the process of social change, researchers will learn to strive for objectivity at the same time that they struggle for social justice.

REFERENCES

Ackerknecht, E. H. (1953). *Rudolph Virchow, doctor, statesman, anthropologist.* Madison: University of Wisconsin Press.

Amory, J. H., Adams, K. M., Lin, M. T., Hansen, J. A., Eschenbach, D. A., & Hitti, J. (2004). Adverse outcomes after preterm labor are associated with tumor necrosis factor-alpha polymorphism –863, but not –308, in mother–infant pairs. *American Journal of Obstetrics and Gynecology, 191,* 1362–1367.

Arntzen, A., & Nybo Andersen, A. M. (2004). Social inequality in infant mortality: An overview of Nordic epidemiological studies, 1980–2001. *Scandinavian Journal of Public Health, 32,* 381–389.

Bamshad, M., Wooding, S., Salisbury, B. A., & Stephens, J. C. (2004). Deconstructing the relationship between genetics and race. *Nature Reviews Genetics, 5,* 598–609.

Bennett, L. (1982). *Before the Mayflower: A history of Black America.* Chicago: Johnson.

Black, E. (2003). *War against the weak: Eugenics and America's campaign to create a master race.* New York/London: Four Walls Eight Windows.

Blackmore, C. A., Ferre, C. D., Rowley, D. L., Hogue, C. J., Gaiter, J., & Atrash, H. (1993). Is race a risk factor or a risk marker for preterm delivery? *Ethnicity & Disease, Fall 3,* 372–377.

Brandon, G. (1997). Yoruba. In D. Levinson & M. Ember (Eds.), *American immigrant cultures: Builders of a nation* (Vol. 2). New York: MacMillan.

Centers for Disease Control and Prevention. (1999). Preterm singleton births—United States, 1989–1996. *Morbidity and Mortality Weekly Report, 48,* 185–189. Retrieved from http://www.cdc.gov/mmwr/preview/mmwrhtml/00056645.htm

Centers for Disease Control and Prevention. (2002). Table 7. *National Vital Statistics Report, 50*(12), 21. Retrieved March 18, 2005, from http://www.cdc.gov/nchs/data/nvsr/nvsr50/50_12t7.pdf

Centers for Disease Control and Prevention. (2006). Table 2. Percentage of total deaths, death rates, age-adjusted death rates for 2003. Retrieved February 19, 2006, from http://www.cdc.gov/nchs/data/hestat/finaldeaths03_tables.pdf#2

Chase, A. (1980). *The legacy of Malthus: The social costs of the new scientific racism.* Chicago: University of Illinois Press.

Chike-Obi, U., David, R. J., Coutinho, R., & Wu, S. Y. (1996). Birth weight has increased over a generation. *American Journal of Epidemiology, 144,* 563–569.

Clarson, C. L., Barker, M. J., Marshall, T., & Wharton, B. A. (1982). Secular change in birthweight of Asian babies born in Birmingham. *Archives of Disease in Childhood, 57,* 867–871.

Colhoun, H. M., McKeigue, P. M., & Davey-Smith, G. (2003). Problems of reporting genetic associations with complex outcomes. *Lancet, 361,* 865–872.

Collins, J. W., & David, R. J. (1997). Urban violence and African-American pregnancy outcome: An ecologic study. *Ethnicity & Disease, 7*, 184–190.

Collins, J. W., David, R. J., Handler, A., Wall, S., & Andes, S. (2004). Very low birth weight in African–American infants: The role of maternal exposure to interpersonal racial discrimination. *American Journal of Public Health, 94*, 2132–2138.

Collins, J. W., David, R. J., Symons, R., Handler, A., Wall, S. N., & Andes, S. (1998). African-American mother's perception of their residential environment, stressful life events, and very low birth weight. *Epidemiology, 9*, 286–289.

Collins, J. W., Wu, S., & David, R. J. (2002). Differing intergenerational birth weights among the descendants of US-born and foreign-born Whites and African-Americans in Illinois. *American Journal of Epidemiology, 155*, 210–216.

Cooper, R. S. (1984). A note on the biologic concept of race and its application in epidemiologic research. *American Heart Journal, 108*, 715–723.

Cooper, R. S., & David, R. J. (1986). The biological concept of race and its application to public health and epidemiology. *Journal of Health Politics, Policy and Law, 11*, 97–116.

Cooper, R. S., Kaufman, J. S., & Ward, R. (2003). Race and genomics. *New England Journal of Medicine, 348*, 1166–1170.

Cooper, R. S., Kennelly, J. F., Durazo-Arvizu, R., Oh, H. J., Kaplan, G., & Lynch, J. (2001). Relationship between premature mortality and socioeconomic factors in black and white populations of US metropolitan areas. *Public Health Reports, 116*(5), 464–473.

Cooper, R. S., Steinhauer, M., Miller, W., David, R., & Schatzkin, A. (1981). Racism, society and disease: An exploration of the social and biological mechanisms of differential mortality. *International Journal of Health Services, 11*, 389–414.

Daniels, N., Kennedy, B., & Kawachi, I. (2000). *Is inequality bad for our health?* Boston: Beacon Press.

David, R. J. (1980). The quality and completeness of birthweight and gestational age data in computerized birth files. *American Journal of Public Health, 70*, 964–973.

David, R. J. (2001). Commentary: Birthweights and bell curves. *International Journal of Epidemiology, 31*, 1241–1243.

David, R. J., & Collins, J. W. (1991). Bad outcomes in Black babies: Race or racism? *Ethnicity & Disease, 1*, 236–244.

David, R. D., & Collins, J. W. (1997). Differing birth weight among infants of U.S.-born blacks, African-born blacks, and U.S.-born whites. *New England Journal of Medicine, 337*, 1209–1214.

Devlieger, H., Martens, G., & Bekaert, A. (2005). Social inequalities in perinatal and infant mortality in the northern region of Belgium (the Flanders). *European Journal of Public Health, 15*, 15–19.

Dickey, C. (2004, August 22). Racism's rising tide. *Newsweek International Edition*. Retrieved March 25, 2005, from http://www.msnbc.msn.com/id/5709026/site/newsweek/

Dizon-Townson, D. S. (2001). Preterm labour and delivery: A genetic predisposition. *Paediatric and Perinatal Epidemiology, 15*(Suppl. 2), 57–62.

Doh, K., Sziller, I., Vardhana, S., Kovacs, E., Papp, Z., & Witkin, S. S. (2004). Beta2-adrenergic receptor gene polymorphisms and pregnancy outcome. *Journal of Perinatal Medicine, 32*, 413–417.

Dole, N., Savitz, D. A., Siega-Riz, A. M., Hertz-Picciotto, I., McMahon, M. J., & Buekens, P. (2004). Psychosocial factors and preterm birth among African American and White women in central North Carolina. *American Journal of Public Health, 94*, 1358–1365.

Drayna, D. (2005). Founder mutations. *Scientific American, 293*, 78–85.

Duster, T. (2005). Medicine, race and reification in science. *Science, 307*, 1050–1051.

Dyer, O. (2005). Disparities in health widen between rich and poor in England. *BMJ, 331*, 419.

Engel, S. A., Erichsen, H. C., Savitz, D. A., Thorp, J., Chanock, S. J., & Olshan, A. F. (2005). Risk of spontaneous preterm birth is associated with common proinflammatory cytokine polymorphisms. *Epidemiology, 16*, 469–477.

Engels, F. (1968). *The condition of the working class in England*. Stanford, CA: Stanford University Press. (Originally published as Die Lage der Arbeitenden Klasse in England, Leipzig, 1845.)

Erichsen, H. C., Engel, S. A., Eck, P. K., Welch, R., & Yeager, M. (2006). Genetic variation in the sodium-dependent vitamin C transporters, SLC23A1, and SLC23A2 and risk for preterm delivery. *American Journal of Epidemiology, 163*, 245–254.

Farley, R. (1984). *Blacks and Whites: Narrowing the gap?* Cambridge, MA: Harvard University Press.

Farrall, M., & Morris, A. P. (2005). Gearing up for genome-wide gene-association studies. *Human Molecular Genetics, 14*, Spec No. 2:R157–162.

Fiscella, K. (2005). Race, genes and preterm delivery. *Journal of the National Medical Association*, *97*, 1516–1526.

Fletcher, M. A. (1998, December 28). America's racial and ethnic divides: Interracial marriages eroding barriers. *Washington Post*, p. A1. Retrieved March 26, 2005, from http://www.washingtonpost. com/wp-srv/national/daily/dec98/melt29.htm

Foster, M. W., & Sharp, R. R. (2004). Beyond race: Towards a whole-genome perspective on human populations and genetic variation. *Nature Reviews Genetics*, *5*, 790–796.

Geronimus, A. T. (1986). The effects of race, residence, and prenatal care on the relationship of maternal age to neonatal mortality. *American Journal of Public Health*, *76*, 1416–1421.

Geronimus, A. T. (1992). The weathering hypothesis and the health of African-American women and infants: Evidence and speculations. *Ethnicity & Disease*, *2*, 207–221.

Green, N. S., Damus, K., Simpson, J. L., Iams, J., Reece, E. A., Hobel, C. J., et al. (2005). Research agenda for preterm birth: Recommendations from the March of Dimes. *American Journal of Obstetrics and Gynecology*, *193*, 626–635.

Grieco, E. M., & Cassidy, R. C. (2005). Overview of race and Hispanic origin, Census 2000 Brief, U.S. Census Bureau. Retrieved March 19, 2005, from http://www.census.gov/prod/2001pubs/ c2kbr01-1.pdf

Gruenwald, P. (1968). Fetal growth as an indicator of socioeconomic change. *Public Health Reports*, *83*, 867–872.

Harding, S., Santana, P., Cruickshank, J. K., & Boroujerdi, M. (2006). Birth weights of black African babies of migrant and nonmigrant mothers compared with those of babies of European mothers in Portugal. *Annals of Epidemiology*, *Feb 3*, [Epub ahead of print].

Hartel, C., von Otte, S., Koch, J., Ahrens, P., Kattner, E., Segerer, H., et al. (2005). Polymorphisms of haemostasis genes as risk factors for preterm delivery. *Thrombosis and Haemostasis*, *94*, 88–92.

Hoffman, J. D., & Ward, K. (1999). Genetic factors in preterm delivery. *Obstetrical & Gynecological Survey*, *54*, 203–210.

Iyasu, S., Becerra, J., Rowley, D., & Hogue, C. J. (1992). Impact of very low birthweight on the African American–White infant mortality gap. *American Journal of Preventive Medicine*, *8*, 1333–1347.

Jensen, K., & Murray, F. (2005). Enhanced intellectual property landscape of the human genome. *Science*, *310*, 239–240.

Jorde, L. B., & Wooding, S. P. (2004). Genetic variation, classification and 'race.' *Nature Genetics*, *36*(Suppl), S28–33.

Kahn, J. (2003). Getting the numbers right: Statistical mischief and racial profiling in heart failure research. *Perspectives in Biology and Medicine*, *46*, 473–483.

Kahn, J. (2005). *Perspective: Ethnic drugs*. Hastings Center Reports. Retrieved March 16, 2005, from http://www.thehastingscenter.org/pf/news/ethnicdrugspf.htm

Kalish, R. B., Nguyen, D. P., Vardhana, S., Gupta, M., Perni, S. C., & Witkin, S. S. (2005). A single nucleotide A > G polymorphism at position -670 in the *Fas* gene promoter: Relationship to preterm premature rupture of fetal membranes in multifetal pregnancies. *American Journal of Obstetrics and Gynecology*, *192*, 208–212.

Kalish, R. B., Vardhana, S., Gupta, M., Perni, S. C., & Witkin, S. S. (2004). Interleukin-4 and -10 gene polymorphisms and spontaneous preterm birth in multifetal gestations. *American Journal of Obstetrics and Gynecology*, *190*, 702–706.

Kalish, R. B., Vardhana, S., Normand, N. J., Gupta, M., & Witkin, S. S. (2006). Association of a maternal CD14 -159 gene polymorphism with preterm premature rupture of membranes and spontaneous preterm birth in multi-fetal pregnancies. *Journal of Reproductive Immunology*. [Epub ahead of print; accessed 2-17-06]

Kleinfield, N. R. (2001). Guarding the borders of the hip-hop nation. In Correspondents of the *New York Times* & J. Lelyveld, *How race is lived in America: Pulling together, pulling apart*. New York: Henry Holt.

Krieger, N., Rowley, D. L., Herman, A. A., Avery, B., & Phillips, M. T. (1993). Racism, sexism, and social class: Implications for studies of health, disease, and well-being. *American Journal of Preventive Medicine*, *9*(6 Suppl), 82–122.

Leroi, A. L. (2005, March 14). A family tree in every gene. *New York Times*.

Lespinasse, A. A., David, R. J., Collins, J. W., Handler, A., & Wall, S. (2004). Maternal support in the delivery room and birthweight among African American women. *Journal of the National Medical Association*, *96*, 187–195.

Li, D. K., Ni, H. Y., Schwartz, S. M., & Daling, J. R. (1990). Secular change in birthweight among southeast Asian immigrants to the United States. *American Journal of Public Health, 80,* 685–688.

Marks, J. (1995). *Human biodiversity: Genes, race, and history.* New York: Aldine De Gruyter.

Marmot, M. G., Adelstein, A. M., & Bulusu, L. (1984). Lessons from the study of immigrant mortality. *Lancet, 1*(8392), 1455–1457.

Martin, J. A., Kochanek, K. D., Strobino, D. M., Guyer, B., & MacDorman, M. F. (2005). Annual summary of vital statistics—2003. *Pediatrics, 115,* 619–634.

Montagu, A. (1974). *Man's most dangerous myth: The fallacy of race* (5th ed.). New York: Oxford University Press.

Müller-Hill, B. (1984). Tödlishe Wissenschaft: Die Aussonderung von Juden, Zigeunern und Geisteskranken, 1933–1945 [Murderous science: Elimination by scientific selection of Jews, Gypsies, and others in Germany, 1933–1945]. Hamburg: Rowolt Taschenbuch Verlag.

Muntaner, C., Lynch, J. W., Hillemeier, M., Lee, J. H., David, R., Benach, J., et al. (2002). Economic inequality, working-class power, social capital, and cause-specific mortality in wealthy countries. *International Journal of Health Services, 32,* 629–656.

Muntaner, C., Nieto, F. J., & O'Campo, P. (1996). The bell curve: On race, social class, and epidemiologic research. *American Journal of Epidemiology, 144,* 531–536.

Mustillo, S., Krieger, N., Gunderson, E. P., Sidney, S., McCreath, H., & Kiefe, C. I. (2004). Self-reported experiences of racial discrimination and Black–White differences in preterm and low-birthweight deliveries: The CARDIA study. *American Journal of Public Health, 94,* 2125–2131.

Nukui, T., Day, R. D., Sims, C. S., Ness, R. B., & Romkes, M. (2004). Maternal/newborn GSTT1 null genotype contributes to risk of preterm, low birthweight infants. *Pharmacogenetics, 14,* 569–576.

Pallotto, E. K., Collins, J. W., & David, R. J. (2000). The enigma of maternal race and infant birth weight: A population-based study of U.S.-born Black and Caribbean-born Black women. *American Journal of Epidemiology, 151,* 1080–1085.

Perni, S. C., Vardhana, S., Tuttle, S. L., Kalish, R. B., Chasen, S. T., & Witkin, S. S. (2004). Fetal interleukin-1 receptor antagonist gene polymorphism, intra-amniotic interleukin-1beta levels, and history of spontaneous abortion. *American Journal of Obstetrics and Gynecology, 191,* 1318–1323.

Petrou, S., Kupek, E., Hockley, C., & Goldacre, M. (2006). Social class inequalities in childhood mortality and morbidity in an English population. *Paediatric and Perinatal Epidemiology, 20,* 14–23.

Peukert, D. J. K. (1987). *Inside Nazi Germany: Conformity, opposition, and racism in everyday life.* New Haven, CT: Yale University Press.

Reinhardt, U. E., Hussey, P. S., & Anderson, G. F. (2004). U.S. health care spending in an international context. *Health Affairs (Millwood), 23,* 10–25.

Resch, B., Gallistl, S., Kutschera, J., Mannhalter, C., Muntean, W., & Mueller, W. D. (2004). Thrombophilic polymorphisms—Factor V Leiden, prothrombin G20210A, and methylenetetrahydrofolate reductase C677T mutations—and preterm birth. *Wien Klin Wochenschr, 116,* 622–626.

Rosenberg, N. A., Pritchard, J. K., Weber, J. L., Cann, H. M., Kidd, K. K., Zhivotovsky, L. A., et al. (2002). Genetic structure of human populations. *Science, 298,* 2381–2385.

Rowley, D. L., Hogue, C. J., Blackmore, C. A., Ferre, C. D., Hatfield-Timajchy, K., Branch, P., et al. (1993). Preterm delivery among African–American women: A research strategy. *American Journal of Preventive Medicine, 9*(6 Suppl) 1–6.

Sack, K., & Elder, J. (2001). The New York Times poll on race: Optimistic outlook but enduring racial division. In Correspondents of the *New York Times* & J. Lelyveld, *How race is lived in America: Pulling together, pulling apart.* New York: Henry Holt.

Shaw, C., Blakely, T., Atkinson, J., & Crampton, P. (2005). Do social and economic reforms change socioeconomic inequalities in child mortality? A case study: New Zealand 1981–1999. *Journal of Epidemiology and Community Health, 59,* 638–644.

Stancil, T., Hertz-Picciotto, I., Schramm, M., & Watt-Morse, M. (2000). Stress and pregnancy among African–American women. *Paediatric and Perinatal Epidemiology, 14,* 127–135.

Thompson, L. A., Goodman, D. C., & Little, G. A. (2002). Is more neonatal intensive care always better? Insights from a cross-national comparison of reproductive care. *Pediatrics, 109,* 1036–1043.

Tishkoff, S. A., & Kidd, K. K. (2004). Implications of biogeography of human populations for 'race' and medicine. *Nature Genetics, 36*(Suppl). S21–27.

U.S. Census Bureau. (2001). *Statistical Abstract of the United States: Section 10: Annual National Defense and Veteran Affairs, Table No. 500: Department of Defense Manpower: 1950 to 2000.* Retrieved March 19, 2005, from http://www.census.gov/prod/2002pubs/01statab/defense.pdf

U.S. Department of Health and Human Services. (2005). *Healthy People 2010 Web site.* Retrieved March 18, 2005, from http://www.healthypeople.gov/About/goals.htm

U.S. Department of Justice, Bureau of Justice Statistics. (1998). *Correctional populations in the United States.* Retrieved March 19, 2005, from http://www.ojp.usdoj.gov/bjs/pub/pdf/cpus98.pdf

Valdez, L. L., Quintero, A., Garcia, E., Olivares, N., Celis, A., Rivas, F., Jr., et al. (2004). Thrombophilic polymorphisms in preterm delivery. *Blood Cells, Molecules and Diseases, 33,* 51–56.

Varner, M. W., & Esplin, M. S. (2005). Current understanding of genetic factors in preterm birth. *BJOG, 112*(Suppl. 1), 28–31.

Virchow, R. (1985). Collected essays on public health and epidemiology. *Science History Publications, USA, 2,* 5. (Originally published as *Gesammelte Abhandlungen aus dem Gebiete der öffentlichen Medicin und der Seuchenlehre.* Berlin: August Hirschwald Verlag, 1879.)

Wang, H., Parry, S., Macones, G., Sammel, M. D., Ferrand, P. E., Kuivaniemi, H., et al. (2004). Functionally significant SNP MMP8 promoter haplotypes and preterm premature rupture of membranes (PPROM). *Human Molecular Genetics, 13,* 2659–2669.

Witkin, S. S., Vardhana, S., Yih, M., Doh, K., Bongiovanni, A. M., & Gerber, S. (2003). Polymorphism in intron 2 of the fetal interleukin-1 receptor antagonist genotype influences midtrimester amniotic fluid concentrations of interleukin-1beta and interleukin-1 receptor antagonist and pregnancy outcome. *American Journal of Obstetrics and Gynecology, 189,* 1413–1417.

A Psychosocial Model of Resilience Theory and Research: A Recommended Paradigm for Studying African Americans' Beliefs and Practices Toward Colon Cancer Screening

Anderson J. Franklin,
Sweene Oscar,
Monique Guishard,
Shameka Faulkner,
and Ann Zauber

Colorectal cancer is the third most common cancer diagnosis and the second highest cause of cancer death in the United States (Greenlee, Hill-Harmon, Murray, & Thun, 2001; Winawer, Fletcher, Miller, Godlee, & Stolar, 1997; Winawer et al., 2003). Although colorectal cancer incidence and mortality rates have decreased by 11% and 25% respectively for whites since 1973, the rates for blacks have increased by 12% and 8% respectively over the same period (Ries et al., 2001). Also the colorectal cancer death rates have grown more disparate; currently the colorectal cancer death rates are 16.4 per 100,000 for whites and 22.5 per 100,000 for blacks (Brawley & Freeman, 1999).

African Americans have a high morbidity and mortality from colorectal cancer. In a special article of the *American Journal of Gastroenterology* a number of recommendations were made to reduce this trend including lowering the suggested age for beginning colorectal cancer screening (CRC) for African Americans to the age of 45 years than 50 years (Agrawal et al., 2005). There are a number of reasons for these higher rates of colorectal cancer in African Americans, but not getting CRC screening in a timely fashion is one of them (James, Campbell, & Hudson, 2002; Winawer et al., 1997; Winawer et al., 2003).

Source of Support: This project was supported by a grant from the National Cancer Institute, grant No. NCI 5U56CA096299.

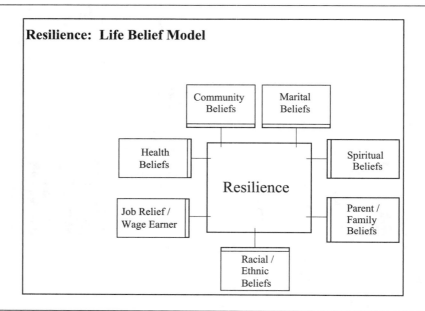

Conceptual model of resilience and life beliefs.

We propose that one means to understand the health practices of African Americans is through the lens of a psychosocial model of resilience theory and research. This chapter presents the results of a study exploring the utility of resilience theory in guiding understanding of the beliefs and practices of African Americans toward colon cancer screening.

Resilience Theory

We began with the assumption that African Americans who have survived to senior years and have demonstrated successful navigation of a multiplicity of risk factors including poverty, discrimination, and racism are resilient. Beliefs and strategies to manage everyday conditions are a product of an interactive process (see Figure 11.1). The conceptual model of resilience and life beliefs shown in Figure 11.1 illustrates a number of proposed links. These include the relationship between resilience and the following: parent/family beliefs, spiritual beliefs, marital beliefs, community beliefs, health beliefs, job-related beliefs, and racial/ethnic beliefs. These beliefs are important cognitive schemas with behavior patterns that develop over the life span.

As a result of processes of survival, African Americans have evolved specific ways of coping and developing cognitive schemas about how to conduct themselves in the world while preserving dignity and self-respect (Franklin, 1999, 2004; Franklin & Boyd-Franklin, 2000). We define resilience as successful adaptation despite challenging or threatening circumstances (Masten, Best, & Garmezy, 1990).

The history of African Americans adapting and surviving in the face of challenging and threatening circumstances goes back to their enslavement and subsequent experiences of segregation, discrimination, and racism up to the present day. More specifically, the challenging and threatening experiences African Americans have faced include encounters with physicians and the medical establishment, justifying Washington's (2007) reference to medical apartheid, which also notes the dark history of medical experimentation on this group, going back to colonial times in America. Randall (2006) similarly details the history of medical experimentation on Blacks from slavery through to contemporary prison and military experimentation or "abuse." Randall (2006, p. 124) concludes that while "many Blacks may not know all of the details of the experimentation and abuse, these episodes are a part of the collective Black consciousness that influence Blacks' attitudes toward the health care system." Washington (2007) feels it is essential to detail this history in order to contextualize what has resulted: a deep distrust of the whole medical establishment on the part of African Americans, which must partly inform any meaningful analysis of issues of public health and health-seeking behavior. At the same time, we contend that no meaningful analysis of how African Americans have survived and successfully adapted to a host of challenging and threatening circumstances can occur without a discussion of resilience. It is the rationale for our proposing a central role for the psychosocial model of resilience theory and research.

While African American health-seeking behavior has been extensively researched, rarely are internal cognitive schemas based on cultural, social, and familial traditions that are employed for coping across the life span systematically included in these analyses—in particular, as they are linked to the schema of resilient behavior implicit in our model (see Figure 11.1).

We propose that resilience theory will provide a framework for understanding where health-prevention and related behaviors fit in the overall life schemas of persons at risk. This involves considering the multiple dimensions of beliefs drawn upon by people that guide their approach to living and determine how they implement choices within a variety of life risks, including health risks. Following this orientation, we propose that persons incorporate in their personal resilience strategy a prioritization of life tasks by domains of importance (e.g., family, work, religion). This may help to further explain the behavior of non-adherent African Americans, as they at times cannot afford to believe that they are at risk for cancer absent symptoms, given other more immediate life priorities (Lipkus et al., 1996; Lipkus, Lyna, & Rimer, 2000). We will also use resilience theory to understand the processes that would lead to better access to and actual use of colorectal cancer screening in minority populations. These research findings have potential to guide the development of a targeted intervention to encourage colorectal cancer screening among minority individuals.

Research Aims

The research is guided by the following aims:

1. To assess the culturally-specific colorectal cancer knowledge, risk perceptions, and attitudes among African Americans living in New York City in order to better understand barriers to CRC screening.
2. To investigate how resilience theory/strategies within an ethno-cultural perspective may illuminate and foster understanding of factors that impede or facilitate

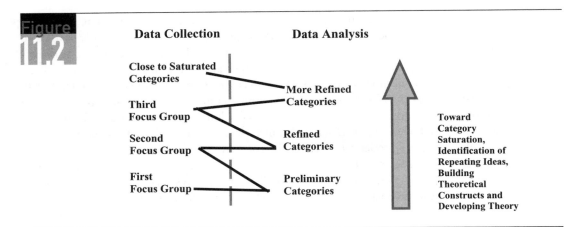

Zig-zag data collection and analysis to achieve saturation of categories.

participation in such preventive behavior as CRC cancer screening among African-Americans.

3. To apply findings in order to develop culturally tailored community outreach and other medical resources in order to more effectively conduct colorectal cancer screening programs for this population.

Materials and Methods

Our participants were 37 African American women between the ages of 50 and 88 years old with an average age of 69. Participants were seen divided across five focus groups. All were informed and consented to participate in the study according to the Institutional Review Board Guidelines for both The City College of New York and Memorial Sloan Kettering Cancer Center. Each focus group was conducted by a female interviewer in the same age cohort as the subjects and trained in the interview process utilizing a semi-structured interview protocol (Kreuger, 1994; Morgan, 1997). The interview protocol had questions that addressed three areas: knowledge of colorectal cancer screening, health beliefs and practices, and resilient behavior. All focus group interviews were audio recorded.

Each focus group interview was transcribed and verified for accuracy by members of the research team. Focus group interviews were read for themes employing qualitative techniques in which responses to all questions were first read as a collective narrative irrespective of individual questions. This involved several levels of analyses consistent with grounded theory methodology in which prevalent themes arising in the narrative prioritizes the focus and interpretation of the groups' views (Auerbach & Silverstein, 2003). The procedure follows a "zig zag" process as depicted in Figure 11.2 in which the first focus group provides preliminary categories with analysis of subsequent groups adding to the refinement of categorical grouping of key themes into a family of codes (Kelsey, 2004).

Results

We hypothesized that resilience plays an important role in African Americans' health beliefs and practices. More specifically we posited that African Americans have developed capacities to assess and manage adverse life circumstances, and that these mechanisms of survival and thriving at times deprioritize health and place emphasis on navigating activities of daily living (Franklin, 2004; Franklin & Boyd-Franklin, 2000). As a result of adopting this life orientation, seeking help for an illness often occurs after becoming overly symptomatic. In order to test our hypothesis the focus group transcripts were analyzed for community and personal health beliefs and practices.

Our Guiding Research Questions

Within this context, we are focusing upon our findings with regard to two key research questions:

1. What role does the acquisition of health knowledge play in health seeking behavior?
2. Can resilience theory explain variation in screening behavior over and above what is explained by other theories?

Results By Research Question and Emergent Themes

In representing the typical thematic response to questions some of the coded categories are formed by using "in vivo" codes utilizing actual words or phrases of respondents to best capture the category as well as sentiments of the focus group. What follows are our key questions with thematic outcomes for each.

Summation of Results for (1) What Role Does the Acquisition of Health Knowledge Play in Health-Seeking Behavior?

Our participants revealed a myriad of issues that contributed to a lack of health-seeking behavior despite exposure to health information in various forms (e.g., pamphlets, radio, and TV PSAs). The five themes that emerged from this analysis were as follows: (1) We don't read health information and don't want to know; (2) I'm too young to think about it and too old to bother; (3) We keep hoping it will be better tomorrow; (4) If it doesn't bother you, don't bother it; and (5) Skepticism about cancer risks information targeted to and disseminated in the Black community.

Summation of Results for (2) Can Resilience Theory Explain Variation in Screening Behavior Over and Above What Is Explained by Other Theories?

Respondents' narratives provided support for our hypothesis that resilient strategies utilized over the life span can potentially interfere with perceiving risk for and obtaining CRC screening. The four themes that emerged from this analysis were: (1) Culture gets in the way; (2) I diagnose and treat myself before going to the doctor; (3) I put it off because there are no symptoms; and (4) I will only go for screening if my doctor recommends it.

Theoretical Narrative. When we asked our participants whether and if they utilized health information in various forms (pamphlets, radio and TV PSAs) we anticipated there would be a pervasive "lack of use" discourse. We also expected that they would deny susceptibility to disease, procrastinate seeking health screening, and have fatalistic beliefs. Our data revealed that participants indeed neither read health information nor did they want to know about the possible existence of illness. Denial, procrastination were manifested in different ways.

Participants' sample quotes illustrating each of the four themes that emerged through our analysis with regard to our research question number one are shown below:

Theme #1 (Emerged for research question #1): We don't read health information and don't want to know: "[B]ecause people don't read the information, they don't want to read it . . . they don't read it in its entirety . . . they may read the first . . . caption but then they'll put it aside. . . . Sometimes medical terms are . . . not clear, they use medical terms and not ah language that we can understand . . . that's another reason."

Theme #2 (Emerged for research question #1): I'm too young to think about it and too old to bother: ". . . I have no other comment than to just agree that um age factor may have a lot to do with it. Some people feel that they are too young to even start thinking about this. They decide that they don't need to read it because it's not going to happen to them. Their age may be a factor in them not even wanting to pay attention to the information."

"Then there are some people who don't want to know . . . they say whatever I have whatever condition my body is in I'm going to die with it. Sometimes you think I'm seventy years old. I'm eighty years old. I've lived long enough anyway I have too many problems so if that problem take me away well then so be it."

Theme #3 (Emerged for research question #1): We keep hoping it will be better tomorrow: "I think procrastination has a lot to do with it. We . . . are very busy . . . sometimes doing nothing, other times we have a reason for being busy. . . . Ah . . . you think you have a lot of time. First of all you in denial, you think this couldn't happen to you, it can happen to everybody else and you say I know I should go to the doctor. I should know that I should be screened against certain ah diseases or disorders or whatever ah but you say well I'll go next week. I'll go when I have my vacation or I'll go when I have less appointments and you keep putting it off."

Theme #4 (Emerged for research question #1): Skepticism about cancer risks information targeted to and disseminated in the Black community: "I don't believe that this information has been that well disseminated because I've never heard about colon cancer until recently or until I know someone who had it. But it never really registered with me. I never really had any brochures or even paid attention if it was advertised on TV. It hasn't been, have you seen it on TV?"

Specific Examples of Results for (2) Can Resilience Theory Explain Variation in Screening Behavior Over and Above What Is Explained by Other Theories?

Theoretical Narrative. Respondents' narratives provided support for our hypothesis that resilient strategies utilized over the life span can potentially interfere with perceiving risk for and obtaining CRC screening.

The following are participants' sample quotes illustrating each of the four themes that emerged through our analysis with regard to our research question number two:

Theme #1 (Emerged for research question #2): Culture gets in the way: "Also I think you have to consider the cultural . . . a person's cultural background and including that sometimes their religious beliefs. . . . I mean that plays a very big part especially if you come. I'm a southerner so I can say this people who come out of the south ah certain things you ah just might not believe in going to the doctor for. . . . You may not want the doctor to look up certain areas on your body and that kind of thing and also what you sort of inherited in many cases from your parents."

"Not only that we are a proud people. And we figure I'm not going to do that sometimes. . . . Those White people go to everything. We have to stop being that way, when we work and have put your money . . . they know that they are taught from the cradle. . . . We don't know until we are older that's been another problem. Not that we don't read or listen to the right thing. . . . We gotta stop that mentality and focus on what we are entitled to. . . . "

Theme #2 (Emerged for research question #2): I diagnose and treat myself before going to doctor: "I try to listen to my body. 'Cause I'm really focused on what's happening with me. Ah I know how I feel when I wake up. I think if what I feel is not normal and it goes on about a week or two I'm gonna have it checked out . . . and I make notes on everything. . . . "

Theme #3 (Emerged for research question #2): I put it off because there are no symptoms: "That's the one thing that you will put off, because there is no symptom there is no feeling there is nothing that tells you that there is a polyp inside of your body and its needs to come out or it needs to be addressed. If you have something on your hand or something on you can see you'll run to the doctor. This is something that is hidden so you keep putting it off. . . . "

Theme #4 (Emerged for research question #2): I will only go for screening if my doctor recommends it: "If the doctor recommends it. When you go to your regular primary physician then you be concerned about it. Then you go and do it."

Discussion

The use of qualitative research to get at the narrative voice of subjects on any given topic is being utilized more because of its hypothesis-generating ability derived directly from the personal stories of people (Bernard, 1994; Franklin & Boyd-Franklin, 2000; Marshall & Rossman, 1999; Rubin & Rubin, 1995). It is another methodology that can be used to complement quantitative techniques. This study is a first step to explore personal views of key representatives of the African American community, female elders, with regard to CRC screening via focus groups as well as in-depth individual interviews with the goal of assembling from this methodological strategy deep insights about potential barriers and facilitators to health practices. Our research had specific aims to learn about health beliefs and practices toward CRC screening as well as to see if internal cognitive schemas or beliefs acquired across the life span seemed to inform health-seeking behavior, consistent with our guiding psychosocial model of resilience. Specifically, we sought to understand whether African American community ethnocultural beliefs shaped participants' views and approaches to getting CRC screening.

One question raised from the results is about the common public health and medical practice of utilizing brochures and any other informational documents to communicate information about CRC screening. The general opinion amongst participants was that they were not effective because few people read them. Given the strength of that sentiment it not only emerged as representing a shared feeling amongst our study participants, arising as a key theme, but also suggested a collective attitude that has evolved in the community about this form of communication having much less effectiveness. This finding may reflect issues of literacy, especially as the direct quotes of the elder women suggested something other than the level of discourse common to the college educated. In support of this interpretation, Kreps, Alibek, Neuhouser, Rowan and Sparks (2005, p. 253) note that "most health related materials typically require high school, college, or graduate reading levels." Furthermore, "risk communication often involves complex vocabularies that are not familiar to the average person" and "literacy barriers affect those vulnerable populations that are most in need of good communication" (Kreps et al., 2005, p. 235)

There was also what we called a "Tuskegee legacy" innuendo amongst participants on this point—meaning that public service announcements coming into the community cannot always be trusted. Just how widespread this notion is within the African American community is worthy of further study, particularly as we weigh such considerations within our help-seeking paradigms. In support of this finding of distrust, the work of many others is pertinent.

For example, the research of LaVeist (2005) locates lower rates of health care use by racial and ethnic minorities in issues of level of trust of health care institutions. Also, citing the research of van Ryn and Burke (2002), African Americans endorsed at twice the rate of Whites items indicating that hospitals often seek more personal information than needed, and that "hospitals have sometimes done harmful experiments on patients without their knowledge" (LaVeist, p. 117). Also, nearly three times as many African Americans perceived, when compared to Whites, that racial discrimination in a doctor's office is common (p. 117). Meanwhile, other evidence reveals good reasons for distrust, given how physicians "consistently reported more negative attitudes toward African American patients than toward White patients" (p. 120). More specifically, this included perceptions that African Americans were more likely to abuse alcohol or drugs, be noncompliant with medications. Whites were perceived as more likely to strongly desire a physically active lifestyle and as having adequate social support; White patients were more likely to be the "kind of person" the physician could see being friends with (p. 120). Other negative perceptions of African Americans held by physicians included being less likely to see them as very intelligent, or at least somewhat educated; meanwhile, Whites were more likely to be viewed as very pleasant and very rational (LaVeist).

As another source of support for our finding of distrust, Washington's work (2007) on medical apartheid may be cited. We may have found evidence of the same lingering effects of medical experimentation in America discussed by Washington—constituting the deep distrust pinpointed as a central part of the lasting legacy. Further support for this finding comes from the work of Randall (2006) as to what may still be lingering in the collective Black consciousness as result of the legacy of medical experimentation on Blacks in America, including up to the present. It is also worth noting that our sample of elder African American women may also be influenced by recent history. Randall (2006, p. 123) cites: "[M]any women of color have been sterilized without their informed consent so that medical residents could practice performing tubal ligation and hysterectomies," while other experiments as recently as 1972 involved giving out experimental contraceptive devices that led to uncontrolled bleeding and complete hysterectomy. Thus, our findings of distrust reflect other analyses in the literature.

Moreover, this finding of distrust may also relate to our prior finding about not reading health communications literature, as an alternative to a low literacy interpretation, or as an interpretation in addition to it. There may be a possible common orientation to public health communications that has been acquired and perhaps supported by a community mythology around appraising and therefore distrusting information and medical services given to the Black community.

Related to the finding of a self-reliance orientation, what emerged was a practice of people tending to depend upon their own perceptions of indicators of the time to seek screening for colon cancer or any other health condition. Many in this cohort relied upon self-diagnosis and home remedies, with the manifestation and development of clear symptoms being necessary before seeking help. In addition, the relationship to the provider was represented as equally important with participants feeling they would be more likely to get CRC screening if their doctor advised it. This finding is important and provides the hope that doctors can play an important role in facilitating CRC screening behavior among African American patients. In order to understand this finding of a willingness to trust and follow through with medical advice, against a backdrop of historical and collective mistrust because of the legacy of experimentation and abuse of Blacks in America, LaVeist (2005) may provide some insight. LaVeist discussed the significance of research findings where patients who were race concordant with their physicians rated their visits with physicians as more participatory compared to those who were race discordant; and that African American patients who were race concordant with their physicians rated them as excellent and reported receiving needed medical care and preventive care; and those patients reporting the highest level of satisfaction were race concordant with their health care provider (pp. 121–124). Hence, African Americans such as those in our study who seem open and receptive to the recommendations of a doctor may benefit most by experiencing race concordant dyads with their physicians so that they have a participatory experience that includes dialogue about needed screenings, such as for CRC.

The overall implications of our study findings are pertinent to our third research aim: To apply findings in order to develop culturally tailored community outreach and other medical resources in order to more effectively conduct colorectal cancer screening programs for this population. In this regard, culturally tailored interventions for the African American community need to acknowledge the legacy of distrust, yet avoid this becoming a prophecy which might become fulfilled. However, trust can be built via access to physicians, medical personnel, peer educators and community outreach/health workers who all create positive, engaging, participatory experiences for African Americans and are free of negative attitudes toward them. This means that training in cultural competence is key for all of those representing the value of accessing medical services and health screenings. What may also be acknowledged is how systemic interventions are also needed so that more physicians of color are trained and available to correct the current imbalance preventing African Americans from enjoying race concordance with their physicians—and potentially receiving care that could be rated as excellent, just as a majority of Whites and Asians enjoy (see LaVeist, 2005). For the training of all physicians and medical personnel, regardless of race or ethnicity, the IOM (2001) report must be followed, which recognizes the importance of cultural sensitivity, cultural appropriateness, or cultural competence as factors related to good quality health care.

Finally, with regard to our study's themes, there is a personal dimension that infers dependence not only upon individual beliefs and practices but also beliefs that have evolved from an intergenerational community orientation to health. Yet, as a common thread running through all of the themes that emerged in our study there is a supra-ordinate theme of resilience—an adaptation to life circumstances that many African Americans have acquired and come to know as a way of doing things; it may also reflect historical ways of adapting to challenges and threats, including those going back to the days of enslavement. A person or group's adaptation to their life conditions, and how it evolves patterns of behavior over time, are important to study. We offer that this dimension of the psychosocial context is another important factor in the equation for understanding the barriers and facilitators to CRC screening. Moreover, we support and recommend the adoption of qualitative research methodology as a tool in this endeavor to adequately capture this psychosocial dimension best expressed in the voices of participants in focus groups and interviews. Most importantly, we recommend the psychosocial model of resilience theory and research as a valuable paradigm for use in guiding the work of other researchers and practitioners seeking to understand and investigate the health beliefs and related practices of African Americans, as well as when developing culturally appropriate interventions. The psychosocial model of resilience will also serve as an important model and compelling new paradigm to which physicians and other medical personnel need to be exposed to, so that their training results in their attaining a sufficient level of cultural sensitivity and competence. It may only be as a consequence of such training of practitioners and researchers that we can realistically aspire to first reduce and ultimately eliminate health disparities.

REFERENCES

Agrawal, S., Bhupinderjit, A., Bhutani, M., Boardman, L., Nguyen, C., Romero, Y., et al. (2005). Colorectal cancer in African Americans. *American Journal of Gastroenterology*, 100, 515–523.

Auerbach, C. F., & Silverstein, L. B. (2003). *Qualitative data: An introduction to coding and analysis.* New York: New York University Press.

Bernard, H. R. (1994). *Research methods in anthropology: Qualitative and quantitative approaches.* Thousand Oaks, CA: Sage Publications.

Brawley, O. W., & Freeman, H. P. (1999). Race and outcomes: Is this the end of the beginning for minority health research? *Journal of National Cancer Institute, 9*, 1908–1909.

Franklin, A. J. (1999). Invisibility syndrome and racial identity development in psychotherapy and counseling African American men. *The Counseling Psychologist, 27*(6), 761–793.

Franklin, A. J. (2004). *From brotherhood to manhood: How Black men rescue their relationships and dreams from the invisibility syndrome.* New York: John Wiley & Sons.

Franklin, A. J., & Boyd-Franklin, N. (2000). Invisibility syndrome: A clinical model towards understanding the effects of racism upon African American males. *American Journal of Orthopsychiatry, 70*(1), 33–41.

Greenlee, R. T., Hill-Harmon, M. B., Murray, T., & Thun, M. (2001). Cancer statistics, 2001. *A Cancer Journal for Clinicians, 51*, 15–36.

Institute of Medicine. (2001). *Crossing the quality chasm: A new health system for the 21st century.* Washington, DC: National Academies Press.

James, A. S., Campbell, M. K., & Hudson, M. A. (2002). Perceived barriers and benefits to colon cancer screening among African Americans in North Carolina: How does perception relate to screening behavior? *Cancer, Epidemiology, Biomarkers and Prevention, 11*, 529–534.

Kelsey, K. (2004). *Grounded theory designs.* Retrieved December 14, 2004, from http://www.okstate.edu/ag/agedcm4h/academic/aged5980/power/598314.ppt

Kreps, G. L., Alibek, K., Neuhauser, L., Rowan, K. E., & Sparks, L. (2005). Emergency/risk communication to promote public health and to respond to biological threats. In M. Haider (Ed.), *Global public health communication: Challenges, perspectives, and strategies.* Boston: Jones and Bartlett Publishers.

Kreuger, R. A. (1994). *Focus groups: A practical guide for applied research.* Thousand Oaks, CA: Sage Publications.

LaVeist, T. A. (2005). *Minority populations and health: An introduction to health disparities in the United States.* San Francisco: Jossey-Bass.

Lipkus, I. M., Lyna, P. R., & Rimer, B. K. (2000). Colorectal cancer risk perceptions and screening intentions in a minority population. *Journal of the National Medical Association, 92*(10), 492–500.

Lipkus, I. M., Rimer, B. K., Lyna, P. R., Pradhan, A. A., Conaway, M., & Woods-Powell, C. T. (1996). Colorectal screening patterns and perceptions of risk among African-American users of a community health center. *Journal of Community Health, 21*(6), 409–427.

Marshall, C., & Rossman, G. (1999). *Designing qualitative research.* Thousand Oaks, CA: Sage Publications.

Masten, A. S., Best, K., & Garmezy, N. (1990). Resilience in development: Implications of the study of successful adaptation for developmental psychopathology. In D. Cicchetti (Ed.), *The emergence of a discipline: The Rochester symposium on developmental psychopathology: I.* Hillsdale, NJ: Erlbaum.

Morgan, D. L. (1997). *Planning focus groups.* Thousand Oaks, CA: Sage Publications.

Randall, V. R. (2006). *Dying while Black: An in-depth look at the crisis in the American healthcare system,* Dayton, OH: Seven Principles Press, Inc.

Ries, L. A. G., Eisner, M. P., Kosary, C. L., Hankey, B., Miller, B. A., Clegg, L., & Edwards, B. K. (2001). *SEER Cancer Statistics Review, 1973–1998.* Bethesda, MD: National Cancer Institute.

Rubin, H. J., & Rubin, I. S. (1995). *Qualitative interviewing: The art of hearing data.* Thousand Oaks, CA: Sage Publications.

van Ryn, M., & Burke, J. (2002). The effect of patient race and socioeconomic status on physicians' perceptions of patients. In T. A. LaVeist (Ed.), *Race, ethnicity, and health: A public health reader.* San Francisco: Jossey-Bass.

Washington, H. A. (2007). *Medical apartheid: The dark history of medical experimentation on black Americans from colonial times.* New York: Random House.

Winawer, S. J., Fletcher, R., Miller, L., Godlee, F. & Stolar, M. (1997). Colorectal cancer screening: Clinical guidelines and rationale. *Gastroenterology, 112*, 594–642.

Winawer, S. J., Fletcher, R., Rex, D., Bond, J., Burt, R., Ferrucci, J., et al. (2003). Colorectal cancer screening and surveillance: Clinical guidelines and rationale—Update based on new evidence. *Gastroenterology, 124*, 544–560.

4

Collaborations, Partnerships, and Community-Based Participatory Research

Eliminating Disparities in Health and Disease Outcomes: A Call for Interdisciplinary Collaboration

Of all the forms of inequality, injustice in healthcare is the most shocking and inhumane. Dr. Martin Luther King, Jr.

Jamila R. Rashid,
Shaffdeen A. Amuwo,
Elizabeth L. Skillen,
Cindi Melanson, and
Robin M. Wagner

ealthy People 2010, a comprehensive, national health promotion and disease prevention agenda developed by the U.S. Department of Health and Human Services (HHS), identified eliminating health disparities as a national goal (HHS, 2000). An initiative to eliminate health disparities, now three decades old, had been launched in follow-up to *Healthy People: The Surgeon General's Report on Health Promotion and Disease Prevention*, which had been published in 1979 (HHS, 1979). Since then, progress toward achieving the *Healthy People 2010* national goals has been tracked, and demonstrates that the nation has not met many of the measurable objectives for which tracking data are available (HHS, 2006). For example, of the 281 *Healthy People 2010* objectives for which tracking data were available, only 10% had met the target, 49% had moved toward the target, 26% had either remained unchanged or moved away from the target, and 14% had demonstrated mixed progress. This failure to achieve more of the measurable objectives may be due to inadequate focus on the social and environmental determinants of health and health disparities (Williams, 2005, chapter 8) and suggests an urgent need for collaborative research to accelerate progress on these long-standing problems.

In this chapter on the elimination of health disparities through research, we will (1) provide a historical perspective on the condition of health disparities in the United States; (2) define health disparities and describe some of the contributors in the United States; (3) describe a framework for health disparities research; (4) summarize some of the critical health disparities that should be addressed through research; (5) describe efforts to develop health disparities research priorities; (6) propose a framework for establishing research priorities related to health disparities; and (7) suggest an approach for engaging in collaborative, interdisciplinary research and next steps.

Historical Perspective

Overall health status has improved significantly in the United States since the turn of the century. For example, over the course of the 20th century (1900 to 2000), life expectancy in the United States increased dramatically, from 47.6 to 77.7 years for Whites (30.1% increase) and from 33.0 to 72.2 years among Blacks (39.2% increase). However, even with this marked improvement, Black people are still experiencing lower life expectancies than whites (HHS, 2005a). For example, Satcher and colleagues examined trends in Black–White standardized mortality ratios (SMRs) for each age–sex group, from 1960 to 2000, and found that in that period, the Black–White gap measured by the SMRs changed very little, and it actually worsened for infants and for Black men age 45 to 64 (Satcher et al., 2005). Given the complexity of overall health status or quality of life, life expectancy alone is not sufficient to measure health improvement, partly because longevity as a measure of quality of life can be compromised by disabling physical, mental, social, or psychological conditions, as well as by social isolation and financial limitations that can occur with aging (HHS, 2006). How these conditions could be measured across race and ethnicity to show that the differential in health remains a major challenge.

Evidence of health disparities has been documented for more than a century. In 1906, sparked by the assertion that Negroes were an inferior race, W. E. B. Du Bois used census and disease data from the late 1800s to document widespread disparities in heart disease, infant deaths, maternal deaths, tuberculosis, and syphilis. From this landmark examination, Du Bois asserted that such health disparities had nothing to do with inferiority and were strongly associated with multiple factors, including poverty, lack of education, and social factors (Du Bois, 1906). Since Du Bois' efforts over 100 years ago, health disparities have received limited attention. The role of research in understanding disparities, what contributes to them, and how to solve them has been limited (Gamble & Stone, 2006).

Since multiple complex factors and conditions contribute to disparities, eliminating disparities in health will require transdisciplinary and interdisciplinary strategies with partners in and outside of government. A collaborative, interdisciplinary, coordinated approach will accelerate discovery of the causes of health disparities. By pooling scientific and programmatic expertise and resources across disciplines, and by identifying, supporting, and implementing common elements of research plans and priorities through joint research initiatives, collaborating researchers could more quickly and effectively develop remedies and accelerate the application of those remedies.

At a minimum, five overarching areas of research are needed:

1. Measurement or estimation of disease burden (Centers for Disease Control and Prevention [CDC], 2006a; Gerberding, 2006).

2. Surveillance and studies to measure progress, elicit causes, or identify determinants of health and health disparities (CDC, 2006a; Satcher & Rust, 2006; Williams, 2005, chapter 8).
3. Development, testing, and evaluation of solutions designed to
   - reduce disease, injury, and disability (CDC, 2006a) and
   - prepare for threats at individual, community, and population levels (National Institutes of Health [NIH], 2001).
4. Enhancement of workforce, systems, and infrastructure needed to promote public health practice (Baquet, Hammond, Commiskey, Brooks, & Mullins, 2002; Gerberding, 2006; HHS, 2005b; Satcher et al., 2005).
5. Translation and dissemination of research (Baquet et al., 2002; Gerberding, 2006; Satcher & Rust, 2006).

Research in some of the areas described above has been conducted. However, to achieve greater impact and change more of the intervening factors that mediate the effects of socioeconomic status (SES) on health, this research must also be supplemented with a coordinated, interdisciplinary approach that includes greater focus on the social, economic, and environmental factors of disparities (Williams, 2005). Such research should be explored at the community and sub population level and should elucidate the contributions of policy, practice, and interventions that are needed to achieve health equity and eliminate disparities.

Overall, too little focus has been placed on interdisciplinary research. When conducted, efforts to assess the efficacy or effectiveness of interdisciplinary approaches have been minimal (Stokols et al., 2003). Without clearly and collectively identifying the necessary research priorities as described, critical steps toward improving health for the nation might become even more challenging. Research improves programs through the increase in the number of evidence-based, public health interventions available to public health professionals (Thacker et al., 2005). Increasing the understanding of the social and environmental determinants of health and health disparities, and the knowledge of effective population-based interventions, will provide a key step in the elimination of health disparities (Brownson, Gurney, & Land, 1999).

Defining Health Disparities and Their Contributors

Dictated by the complexity and array of contributing factors, there are a variety of definitions of disparity (Last, 2006). We have chosen the definition found in the *Dictionary of Public Health* to inform us. In that source, *health disparities* are:

> Differing levels of health indicators like life expectancy, infant and perinatal mortality rates, that are observed among segments of a population, discernible in the size of the health gap between the highest and the lowest segment of the population, that often correlate with economic indicators, educational level, employment and housing conditions (Last, 2006).

Such disparities can be observed across a wide variety of health conditions and tend to arise among populations with varying exposures to healthy factors in a variety of social contexts, including family, neighborhood, work, and the social environment, and these factors are linked to race, education, poverty, and other socioeconomic characteristics (Williams, 2005). These characteristics and the associated factors contribute to the experience of disparities among populations. Furthermore, a number of studies have informed us of the most frequently identified causes of disparities (Baquet et al., 2002; CDC, 2006a; Satcher & Rust, 2006; Williams, 2005). Contributing factors to health disparities, including individual factors (behavioral and personal), structural or system factors, and institutional factors are described below.

   1. Individual (behavioral and personal) factors. Behavioral factors are primarily those factors and conditions that come into play when making decisions to engage in healthy behaviors, such as not smoking or engaging in adequate physical exercise. Personal factors include age, education, employment status, poverty status, and availability of personal resources (Baquet et al., 2002; Satcher & Rush, 2006). The fact that a person's educational attainment and poverty status is associated with poorer health outcomes for some diseases is well known and recent findings of *Healthy People 2010* midcourse review further support this fact (HHS, 2006).

   2. Structural factors. Structural factors are the social, environmental, and neighborhood conditions that can support or impede one's ability to practice healthy behaviors, or receive needed health services. Such factors can be outside one's locus of control and include the availability of neighborhood resources such as healthy food choices and the availability of facilities for exercise and walking (Angel & Angel, 2006). Such factors can interfere with one's ability to practice good behavioral choices, or complicate attempts to access health care.

   3. Institutional factors. Institutional factors constitute the policies and institutional characteristics that influence access, availability, and effectiveness of care. These factors were well articulated in the seminal Institute of Medicine (IOM) report, *Unequal Treatment* (2003) and include unfair or unequal treatment when seeking care, lack of cultural sensitivity, and lack of specialty services or professionals with cultural and linguistic expertise (Baquet et al., 2002), long wait times, racial bias (inferior or inadequate care due to one's race), and discrimination (Satcher & Rust, 2006).

A Framework for Health Disparities Research

In enumerating contributors to disparities in cancer, Baquet et al. (2002) described four broad categories of contributors that included risk factors and exposure; knowledge, attitudes and practices; access, use, and delivery of services; and biologic/genetic differences. Likewise, Satcher and Rust (2006), building on an IOM framework (IOM, 2003), identified three levels of contributors for lung cancer: individual, provider, and system or institutional.

   The work of Satcher, Baquet, and others (Baquet et al., 2002; Gerberding, 2006; Satcher & Rust, 2006; Stokols et al., 2003) provides a starting point for research proposed earlier in this discussion. The individual, structural, and system contributors to health disparities described are outlined in Figure 12.1. This suggested framework is provided as a tool for organizing and examining collaborative research priority setting efforts.

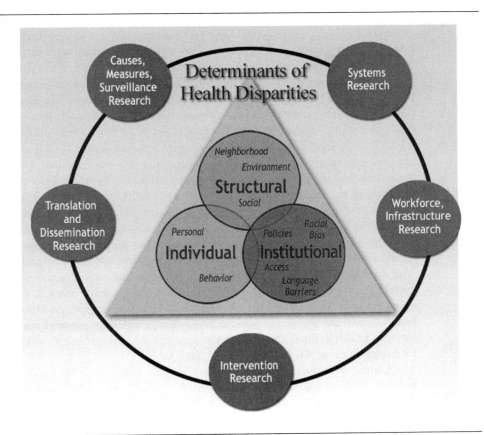

Research framework for the elimination of health disparities.

In order to provide a succinct description of the framework, proposed research will need to include several broad, interdisciplinary research categories. These categories are indicated by the five outer circles of Figure 12.1: causes, measures, and surveillance research; systems research; workforce, infrastructure research; intervention research; and translation and dissemination research. These research categories support and encompass the primary contributors to health disparities that research needs to address. The overlapping circles inside the triangle indicate the complexity of the contributors to health disparities and imply a need to consider the relationship within and among each group of factors.

Critical Health Disparities That Research Should Address

Health disparities can be observed across many subpopulations and conditions, can occur by race, ethnicity, age, gender, geography, or disability status, and tend to occur as a result of exposures to certain risks, opportunities, and resources (CDC, 2006a; Williams, 2005, chapter 8). Despite three decades of interventions to reduce and ultimately eliminate them (HHS, 1979, 1991, 2000), health disparities continue to plague the public health system. The tenacity of this problem would be problematic under any circumstances, but extensive demographic changes are occurring across the United States, with rapid and challenging growth in the subpopulations who are likely to experience more of the individual, structural, and institutional factors that contribute to disparities. Table 12.1 illustrates health disparities in years of potential life lost (YPLL) that are observed across different racial and ethnic population groups for selected causes of death (HHS, 2005a). The YPLL is an estimate of the average time a person would have lived had he or she not died prematurely and emphasizes deaths that occur early in life. Blacks or African Americans had the greatest years of potential life lost from all causes of death. This may be partially due to their much higher rates of YPLL from homicide and HIV which tend to occur among younger age groups. Asian or Pacific Islanders had the least years of potential life lost from all causes.

The health of the United States has improved in many aspects, but the health of racial and ethnic groups for some causes of death continues to lag behind (HHS, 2005a). The demographic changes in the U.S. population due to increasing racial and ethnic diversity and people living longer (HHS, 2006), along with other factors such as the rising costs of health care and emerging new diseases, compound efforts to eliminate health disparities. These phenomena may perhaps widen the gap and worsen the current status of health in the United States and possibly the United States' ranking in the world for health systems (HHS, 2006; WHO, 2000).

Adding impetus to the case for more focused research on health disparities are the recently released findings of the *Healthy People 2010* midcourse review (HHS, 2006). The midcourse review is an assessment of the Nation's progress toward increasing quality of years of healthy life and elimination of health disparities for all Americans. In the midcourse review, disparities are measured as the percent difference between the best group rate and other related group rates. "Best" or most favorable group rate is used to indicate a reference point and refers to the most favorable rate among the groups associated with a particular characteristic (HHS, 2006). The *Healthy People 2010* midcourse review (HHS, 2006) notes that although we have experienced significant overall improvements in many of the leading health indicators, a number of disparities still exist. For example, the rate of congestive heart failure hospitalizations in Black non–Hispanic aged 64–75 years was more than twice the rate of that for White non–Hispanics of the same age group. Stroke death rates[1] increased between 10 and 49 percentage points for Asian or Pacific Islander, Black non–Hispanic, and White non–Hispanic populations, compared with American Indian or Alaskan Natives. Although death rates for coronary heart disease (CHD) declined between 1999 and 2002, the difference in death rates for CHD between Black non–Hispanic and Asian or Pacific Islanders increased between 10 and 49 percentage points (HHS, 2006).

Even more alarming are the disparities in HIV infections and AIDS. The rate of new cases of AIDS[2] in the Black non–Hispanic population was 15 times higher than

---

[1]"Death rate" refers to "age-adjusted death rate" except when age specific rates are indicated.
[2]The case rate is defined here as new cases of AIDS between 1998 and 2003 (HHS, 2006).

| Table 12.1 | Years of Potential Life Lost[1] Before Age 75 for Selected Causes of Death, According to Race and Hispanic Origin: United States, 2002 (adapted from Health, United States, HHS, 2005a) |

	Race and Hispanic Origin, Age Adjusted Rates[3], 2002					
Cause of Death[2]	White[4]	Black or African American[4]	American Indian or Alaska Native[4]	Asian or Pacific Islander[4]	Hispanic or Latino[4]	White, not Hispanic or Latino
All causes	6,936.6	12,401.0	8,278.0	3,635.5	5,865.9	6,997.9
Diseases of the heart	1,111.8	2,212.8	959.9	539.4	796.9	1,143.8
Ischemic heart disease	759.5	1,218.7	648.4	352.0	540.1	781.3
Cerebrovascular diseases	173.5	474.1	201.7	186.5	193.4	169.4
Malignant neoplasms	1,582.8	2,196.6	1,066.0	990.3	1,052.9	1,629.7
Trachea, bronchus and lung	418.5	561.9	226.3	173.8	150.5	443.7
Colorectal	134.0	213.7	115.7	92.8	96.7	137.6
Prostate[5]	51.3	160.3	36.3	20.8	44.1	51.7
Breast[6]	297.5	495.9	187.1	188.4	205.1	305.9
Chronic lower respiratory diseases	183.5	222.8	137.0	44.8	69.0	193.3
Influenza and pneumonia	75.1	146.7	100.9	38.0	65.5	75.8
Chronic liver disease and cirrhosis	162.9	161.3	495.8	40.0	237.9	152.1
Diabetes mellitus	160.3	396.7	344.7	76.4	207.1	155.8
Human immodeficiency virus (HIV)	84.7	720.6	79.9	24.8	179.1	67.8
Unintentional injuries	1,101.6	1,129.3	1,764.6	431.1	958.1	1,117.4
Motor vehicle-related injuries	604.0	558.5	1,089.3	269.7	569.6	603.3
Suicide	380.1	196.5	420.8	162.7	185.6	413.9
Homicide	159.7	962.2	366.5	127.5	330.2	114.8

[1] The concept of years of potential life lost (YPLL) involves estimating the average time a person would have lived had he or she not died prematurely. This measure is used to help quantify social and economic loss owing to premature death, and it has been promoted to emphasize specific causes of death affecting younger age groups. YPLL inherently incorporates age at death, and its calculation mathematically weights the total deaths by applying values to death at each age. The method of calculating YPLL varies from author to author, each producing different rankings of leading causes of premature death. One can choose between heart disease, cancer, or accidents as the leading cause of premature death, depending on which method is used. "Years of Potential Life Lost (YPLL)—What Does it Measure?" by J. W. Gardner and J. S. Sanborn (1990). *Epidemiology, 1*(4), pp. 322–329.

[2] Underlying cause of death code numbers are based on the applicable revision of the International Classification of Diseases (ICD) for data years shown.

[3] Age-adjusted rates are calculated using the year 2000 standard population.

[4] The race groups, White, Black Asian or Pacific Islander, and American Indian or Alaska Native, include persons of Hispanic and non-Hispanic origin. Persons of Hispanic origin may be of any race. Death rates for the American Indian or Alaska Native and Asian or Pacific Islander populations are known to be underestimated.

[5] Rate for male population only.

[6] Rate for female population only.

the rate among Asian or Pacific Islanders (best rate) in 2003. The rate for the Hispanic population was more than five times the best rate, and the rate for the American Indian or Alaska Native population was twice the best rate.

Injury, violence, and homicides are yet other areas where disparities continue to occur. The disparities between the Black non-Hispanic population and the Asian or Pacific Islander for firearm-related deaths has increased by more than 100 percentage points since the beginning of the decade. For motor vehicle crash death rates[3], the American Indian or Alaska Native population had the highest rate of death, at three times the rate for the Asian or Pacific Islander population, and Black non-Hispanic and White non-Hispanic populations both had rates 50 to 99 percent higher than the Asian or Pacific Islander population. Motor vehicle crash death rates were more than twice as high in males as in females (HHS, 2006). The Black non-Hispanic population had an especially high level of homicide death rates—more than seven times that of the White non-Hispanic population in 2002. The American Indian or Alaska Native and Hispanic populations had death rates that were three times the rate for the White non-Hispanic population. In addition, between 1999 and 2002, the difference in rates of homicide between Black non-Hispanic and White non-Hispanic populations increased by over 50 percentage points (HHS, 2006).

Poor mental health and substance abuse are concerns for people in all stages of life, but these disproportionately affect certain populations. For instance, persons who live in inner city and rural settings, the homeless, and other persons who receive basic medical care in emergency departments often do not receive treatment for mental health and substance abuse (HHS, 1999).

These disparities, the limited progress so far, and the demographic and so-cial trends that are exacerbating health disparities support a call for collaboration across federal and nonfederal partners and for the public to identify, fund, imple-ment, and evaluate interdisciplinary research approaches for the elimination of health disparities.

Efforts to Develop Health Disparities Research Priorities

Research priorities have been developed recently by individual federal and nonfederal agencies and institutions (CDC, 2006a; NIH, 2001), but most were developed through categorical, focused efforts (Gerberding, 2006) rather than more interdisciplinary and collaborative approaches. In some cases where interdisciplinary approaches were used, as noted in the Institute of Medicine (IOM) March 2006 Report Brief on health disparities, the impact has been "mitigated by a lack of coordination and limited strategic plan-ning" (IOM, 2006, p. 1). This IOM report showed that an integrated interdisciplinary approach is sorely needed (IOM, 2006). It also identified planning, coordination, com-prehensiveness, and funding as areas "still ripe for improvement"; suggested a ten-point recommendation for planning, implementing, coordinating, and funding; and recognized

---

[3]Between 1999 and 2002 (HHS, 2006).

a need for "an aggressive research agenda" as a core effort for eliminating disparities (IOM, 2006, p. 1). Several coordinated efforts across agencies and disciplines have been recently attempted. In 2000, in response to Public Law 106–525, the Minority Health and Health Disparities Research and Education Act of 2000, the National Institutes of Health (NIH) engaged in a highly collaborative process for establishing strategic research initiatives within each of its Institutes and Centers. With its National Center for Minority Health and Health Disparities leading the effort, NIH drafted a 5-year trans-NIH strategic plan for addressing minority health and health disparities (NIH, 2001). NIH's intent was twofold: (1) to chart its course, including defining its role and responsibility, for improving the health of the Nation; and (2) to identify gaps and opportunities in health disparities research that could not be addressed by any single institute, yet must be addressed to have the greatest impact. The NIH strategic plan (NIH, 2001) focuses on three areas of research: measures, infrastructure, and community information and outreach (see Table 12.2).

Another federal effort to develop national research recommendations for public health, including health disparities, was launched in January 2005 at CDC. This effort closely followed recommendations of three different CDC workgroups that met to deliberate the best options for developing a CDC-wide research agenda. It culminated in the publication of *Advancing the Nation's Health: A Guide to Public Health Research Needs, 2006–2015* (hereafter referred to as the *Research Guide* [CDC, 2006a]). This document was developed as a comprehensive long-range vision of national and global public health research needs, and is intended as a tool to help identify knowledge gaps that must be addressed to implement CDC's new Health Protection Goals (CDC, 2006b). It also describes which research is most needed to supply critical evidence to improve public health programs and interventions, and serves as platform for collaborations with federal partners to address the most pressing current and future public health problems (CDC, 2006a).

Similar to the NIH's effort, the *Research Guide* (CDC, 2006a) was developed by CDC through extensive external and internal partner collaboration. Particular attention was given to addressing health disparities throughout the process. To ensure that special attention would be paid to health disparities research, CDC established a special workgroup comprised of leading health equity champions. Members of this workgroup were invited to serve as expert health disparity advisors to the entire process, providing input into where disparities should be addressed attentively. In addition, other leading health disparities experts were identified and invited to participate in other phases of the public engagement process.

To further ensure that health disparities were addressed throughout the *Research Guide*, every research theme or idea submitted for initial inclusion was evaluated for relevance to reducing health disparities. As an additional step to ensure the inclusion of innovative, interdisciplinary research to address the complex nature of disparities, including social determinants and environmental factors, a special section on health disparities prevention and elimination appears in the crosscutting research chapter (chapter IX). This health disparities section in the *Research Guide* addresses four fundamental research domains: surveillance, measures, translation, and community-based participatory research. The following table (Table 12.3) lists key research in the *Research Guide* (CDC, 2006a). Most research on health disparities can be found in the chapter on crosscutting

Table 12.2	**NIH Strategic Plan for Health Disparities Research**	
Research objectives	■ Advance understanding of the development and progression of diseases and disabilities that contribute to health disparities.	
	■ Develop new or improved approaches for detecting or diagnosing the onset or progression of diseases and disabilities that contribute to health disparities.	
	■ Develop new or improved approaches for preventing or delaying the onset or progression of diseases and disabilities that contribute to health disparities.	
	■ Develop new or improved approaches for treating diseases and disabilities that contribute to health disparities.	
Research infrastructure objectives	■ Increase the number of participants in clinical trials from minority and ethnic populations and other special populations experiencing health disparities.	
	■ Expand opportunities in research training and career development for, and provide research supplements to, research investigators from minority and other populations experiencing health disparities.	
	■ Increase funding support for construction and renovation of research facilities across the nation, aimed at enhancing the ability of these institutions to conduct health disparities research.	
	■ Provide increased funding at institutions across the country for resources, new equipment, and shared equipment programs for use in health disparities research.	
	■ Increase representation in peer review from minority and ethnic populations and other populations experiencing health disparities.	
Outreach objectives	■ Provide the latest research-based information to health care providers to enhance the care provided to individuals within populations experiencing health disparities.	
	■ Facilitate the incorporation of science-based information into the curricula of medical and allied health professions schools, and into continuing education activities of health professionals.	
	■ Maintain ongoing communication linkages and dialogue with minority, ethnic, and other populations, including the underserved, who experience health disparities.	
	■ Develop computer databases and internet resources to disseminate current information about scientific research, and discoveries and other activities regarding health disparities.	
	■ Develop targeted public health education programs focused on particular disease areas, in order to reach those individuals within minority, ethnic, and other populations who experience health disparities within these disease areas.	

Source: National Institutes of Health. (2001). *Strategic research plan and budget to reduce and ultimately eliminate health disparities*, Volume 1: Fiscal years 2002–2006, p. 9.

Table 12.3	Examples of Priority Research on Health Disparities From Advancing the Nation's Health, A Guide to Public Health Research Needs, 2006–2015

Location in Guide	Proposed Research
Promote Crosscutting Public Health Research (Chapter IX)	■ Develop new methods to estimate the burden of preventable disease to ensure the appropriate allocation of resources to the most effective public health interventions (p. 101). ■ Develop assessment tools that enable determination of the impact of social determinants of health and health disparities that can be used to inform new policies and programs (p. 101). ■ Assess and increase the effectiveness, prevalence of use, opportunities for optimal use, strategies to increase use, and cost effectiveness associated with interventions to prevent and control leading causes of premature death, illness, and disability in disadvantaged populations (p. 101). ■ Evaluate the structures, policies, practices, and norms that differentially force different populations into various contexts (e.g., the mechanisms of institutionalized racism) (p. 101). ■ Examine role of historical urban renewal efforts in current disparities (p. 102). ■ Determine long-term spatial reorganization on overall community health (p. 102). ■ Determine the economic and social benefits associated with reducing disparities (and the societal cost of continued health disparities) (p. 102).

Source: Centers for Disease Control and Prevention (CDC). (2006a). *Advancing the nation's health: A guide to public health research needs, 2006–2015.*

research; however, other chapters also include proposed areas for health disparities research (see Table 12.4).

Federal agencies are not the only experts working to identify important research to eliminate disparities. In 2005, the Society for Public Health Education (SOPHE) embarked on creating its first research agenda on health disparities, 10 years after its first research agenda on health education. Leaders of SOPHE brought together over 85 stakeholders to determine how a health education research agenda could help address health disparities. The premise of the 2005 summit was, "If community participation is central to the mission of health education and eliminating health disparities, then how can we engage the community in the dissemination and implementation of research?" (Gambescia et al., 2006). At the end of the summit, participants reached consensus on the ten most important health education research questions to be addressed in the next decade to eliminate disparities (see Table 12.5). SOPHE is disseminating these research questions and beginning dialogue around these issues through a variety of venues.

For many research questions, the single effort of any one agency would yield greater benefit if collaborative interdisciplinary approaches of many federal departments and their partners were taken. Thus, coming together to find synergy and commonality will

Table 12.4	Health Disparities Research in Other Research Guide Chapters	
Prevent and Control Infectious Diseases (Chapter III)	■ Develop programs that reduce health disparities in vaccine coverage. (p. 25)	
Promote Preparedness to Protect Health (Chapter IV)	■ Develop reliable, valid tools and strategies to profile the vulnerability of communities along multiple sociocultural and community dimensions, including mechanisms responsible for health disparities. (p. 36)	
Promote Health to Reduce Chronic Diseases and Disability (Chapter V)	■ Identify and understand the causal factors (e.g., health behaviors, literacy, education, socioeconomic status, insurance coverage, access to health care, quality of care, self-care and preventive-care practices, and health systems structure) that contribute to the significant disparity in chronic disease burden experienced by various populations (e.g., groups characterized by race/ethnicity, gender, sexual orientation, disability, and socioeconomic status). (p. 49)	
Create Safer and Healthier Places (Chapter VI)	■ Identify risk factors associated with interpersonal violence and suicidal behavior, particularly among adolescents and other vulnerable populations at increased risk for injury resulting from such behaviors. (p. 66)	
Work Together to Build a Healthy World (Chapter VII)	■ Describe associations between different socioeconomic indicators of [global] health (e.g., education, income, social status, race/ethnicity) within a system framework and across different stages of life. (p. 78)	
Manage and Market Health Information (Chapter VIII)	■ Develop approaches and strategies to identify and segment populations with health disparities to customize health marketing campaigns. (p. 94)	

Source: Centers for Disease Control and Prevention (CDC). (2006a). *Advancing the nation's health: A guide to public health research needs, 2006–2015.* Atlanta, GA: Author.

be a key determinant of success. Bringing together the important research priorities of NIH, as described in its 5-year trans-research initiative (NIH, 2001), with research priorities of CDC and other federal departments and other HHS agencies would be more effective and efficient. Linked with efforts of other nonfederal partners, this collaboration would help build an interdisciplinary research agenda, amass the resources, and create the will needed to achieve success.

Proposed Framework for Collaboration on Health Disparities Research

To address health disparities meaningfully, research priorities that are interdisciplinary, identified, supported, and conducted in collaboration with other federal and nonfederal

Table 12.5	Society for Public Health Education Research Agenda for Health Disparities

- How do economics and the built environment such as the availability of housing and sidewalks affect health, and how we can encourage the urban design and planning of communities to eliminate health disparities?
- How does power operate in different social contexts to create and maintain disparities?
- What factors exist in certain populations that protect them from major health issues? For example, what can we learn from African-American female teens who experience less drug abuse than other teens? How can health educators and society promote such protective factors?
- What is the impact of health literacy on health status, and how can we improve message tailoring to reach different groups?
- How can we culturally tailor interventions to influence access to health services?
- How do we engage and partner with policy makers in diffusing relevant research?
- What information are consumers getting on health, and how does this information differ by race, ethnicity, socioeconomic, and cultural group?
- Does engagement in community-based participatory research alter engagement in community structures, processes, and other attributes?
- How can we develop more evaluation instruments that assess dynamic, changing, and social conditions such as social event history analysis?
- How can we improve the measurement of both intended and unintended effects and outcomes in evaluation studies?

Source: Gambescia, S. F., Woodhouse, L. D., Auld, M. E., Green, B. L., Quinn, S.C., & Airhihenbuwa, C.O. (2006), 534–535.

partners are needed to address critical knowledge gaps. The collaborative development of these priorities would showcase the role research plays in improving health generally and would accelerate achievement of our *Healthy People 2010* specific goal of eliminating disparities. To achieve a coordinated research approach that fully engages federal government, academia, partners, and the public, a framework is needed, and it must draw from all who have a strong stake in the content and outcome.

The four domains of health disparities elimination research identified in the *Research Guide*, the trans-research priorities of NIH, and health education priorities of SOPHE provide a starting place to build upon and form a more comprehensive and widely endorsed framework for establishment of national research priorities for the elimination of health disparities. Steps used by NIH, CDC, and SOPHE have been effective. Development of coordinated national research priorities for the elimination of health disparities should follow a similar approach. This proposed approach would also benefit from recent applications of a "systems" thinking approach to solving public health problems (Jones et al., 2006). According to Peter Senge and Colleen Lannon-Kim (1991), "Systems thinking is a discipline for seeing wholes, recognizing patterns and interrelationships, and learning how to structure those interrelationships in more effective, efficient ways." A systems thinking approach to setting coordinated priorities for elimination of disparities through collaboration would involve a series of steps that include

1. Utilizing a systems thinking approach to design and prepare others for engagement.
2. Identifying and continuously engaging participants with diverse and interdisciplinary expertise in health disparities or primary disease areas with significant disparities.
3. Setting an effective and efficient interdisciplinary structure that considers diversity of roles and responsibilities.
4. Building support for the proposed framework.
5. Working collaboratively to draft starter research priorities.
6. Expanding and engaging a broad base of partners and the public to help refine research priorities.
7. Forming cross-agency implementation workgroups.
8. Refining research priorities through formal internal and external review, tracking, and assessment.
9. Conducting analysis and dissemination of collaboration activities, research initiatives, and other outcomes.

To ensure greater success, interdisciplinary approaches must be carried out collaboratively with all partner sectors, including federal, state, and local partners; tribal health systems and organizations; academic, national, professional, and national minority organizations; community-based organizations; faith-based institutions; and a broad spectrum of the public.

Collaboration, Interdisciplinary Approaches, and Next Steps

Given the complexity and magnitude of the task, a comprehensive, government-wide, interdisciplinary approach is essential. Knowing that the elimination of disparities will impact health for all, several federal departments and their respective agencies are already working to facilitate steps toward interdisciplinary collaboration across federal agencies. From these initial efforts, an expanded list of research directions that can benefit from interdisciplinary collaboration have been identified (CDC & HHS, 2007). This recent effort to collaborate across federal agencies on interdisciplinary research approaches to eliminate health disparities has already yielded some value. For example, federal agencies have remained engaged in the collaboration, continued to work within their agencies to promote research priorities that emerged from this process, and have remained committed to working across agencies to find support for sustaining the collaboration.

NIH's minority health and health disparities 5-year trans-research initiative, the most recent effort of CDC to include a category on social determinants of health and health disparities in the *Research Guide*, and SOPHE's recent effort to develop a health disparities agenda for health education represent the most recent, broadly disseminated efforts to develop research agendas on health disparities. To our knowledge, no literature describes the creation of a successful collaboration across multiple federal departments and disciplines on specific areas of health disparities research.

The elimination of disparities in health has proven to be difficult, and to some may seem an impossible task; however, the reasons for this difficulty are not clear to many. Part of the difficulty may be a failure to examine the complex nature of the social determinants of health and health disparities. There have also been challenges to successfully targeting the *right* determinants. Finally, a major challenge has been to effectively implement, evaluate, and rapidly translate evidence-based research findings to practice.

Conclusion

While identifying the key areas for research is a critical step to eliminating health disparities, there is much work yet to be done. Collaboration across federal agencies and other partner groups is needed to draw on existing leadership and expertise in this area of research. The process and guidelines for building the collaboration will evolve as the collaboration is developed. Agreement on a process for selecting priorities and developing the collaborative research priorities must also be articulated. Minimally, it should be based on fundamental criteria for successful collaboration (CDC & HHS, 2007). In addition, as the IOM report showed from the NIH experience, the availability of resources and infrastructure to sustain the effort over time will have to be identified.

As the need for collaboration on research priorities is further articulated, communication among academic, state, and urban health partners; foundations; advocacy groups; and community, national, and tribal organizations will be essential. Such collaborative efforts should promote interested agencies to reach consensus on common areas of interest that would benefit from the pooling of expertise and resources needed to implement the identified research priorities. Once research is funded to support the proposed collaborative health disparities research priorities, the knowledge gained should help inform and influence public health policy and practice in several areas, including the development of more streamlined policies to ease and promote trans-agency support for funded initiatives and memoranda of understanding; development of, and greater support and appreciation for, improved approaches and policies for engaging public partners; reduction in the level of complexity involved in working across federal and nonfederal agencies to jointly fund initiatives; and improvement in efforts to build community capacity and infrastructures needed to carry out research initiatives. In addition, the success of these efforts could greatly contribute to the science of collaboration and change how we do business for years to come.

REFERENCES

Angel, J., & Angel, R. (2006). Minority group status and healthful aging: Social structure still matters. *American Journal of Public Health, 96*, 1152–1159.

Baquet, C. R., Hammond, C., Commiskey, P., Brooks, S., & Mullins, D. (2002). Health disparities research: A model for conducting research on cancer disparities: Characterization and reduction. *Journal of the Association for Academic Minority Physicians, 13*, 33–40.

Brownson, R. C., Gurney, J. G., & Land, G. H. (1999). Evidence-based decision making in public health. *Journal of Public Health Management Practice, 5*, 86–97.

Centers for Disease Control and Prevention (CDC). (2006a). *Advancing the nation's health: A guide to public health research needs, 2006–2015*. Retrieved April 26, 2007, from http://www.cdc.gov/od/science/PHResearch/cdcra/index.htm

Centers for Disease Control and Prevention. (2006b). *Health protection goals*. Retrieved April 26, 2007, from http://www.cdc.gov/about/goals.htm

Centers for Disease Control and Prevention & U.S. Department of Health and Human Services. (2007). December 5–6th Federal Partners Meeting, *Accelerating Collaboration on Health Disparities Research*. Meeting Summary Report, Unpublished.

Du Bois, W. E. B. (Ed.). (1906, May 29). *The health and physique of the Negro American: Report of a social study made under the direction of Atlanta University; together with the proceedings of the eleventh conference for the study of the Negro problems*. Atlanta, GA: Atlanta University Press.

Gambescia, S. F., Woodhouse, L. D., Auld, M. E., Green, B. L., Quinn, S. C., & Airhihenbuwa, C. O. (2006). Framing a transdiciplinary research agenda in health education to address health disparities and social inequities: A road map for SOPHE action. *Health Education and Behavior, 33*, 532–537.

Gamble, V., & Stone, D. (2006). U.S. policy on health inequities: The interplay of politics and research. *Journal of Health Politics, Policy and Law, 31*, 93–126.

Gardner, J. W., & Sanborn, J. S. (1990). Years of potential life lost (YPLL)—What does it measure? *Epidemiology, 1*(4), 322–329.

Gerberding, J. L. (2006). Protecting health—The new research imperative. *Journal of the American Medical Association, 294*, 1403–1406.

Institute of Medicine. (2003). Assessing potential sources of racial and ethnic disparities in care. In B. D. Smedley, A. Y. Stith, & A. R. Nelson (Eds.), *Unequal treatment: Confronting racial and ethnic disparities in health care*. Washington, DC: National Academies Press.

Institute of Medicine. (2006). *Examining the health disparities research plan of the National Institutes of Health: Unfinished business*. Washington, DC: National Academies Press.

Jones, A. P., Homer, J. B., Murphy, D. L., Essien, J. D. K., Milstein, B., & Seville, D. A. (2006). Understanding diabetes population dynamics through simulation modeling and experimentation. *American Journal of Public Health, 96*, 488–94.

Last, J. M. (2006). *A dictionary of public health*. Oxford, New York: Oxford University Press.

National Institutes of Health. (2001). *Strategic research plan and budget to reduce and ultimately eliminate health disparities, Volume 1: Fiscal years 2002–2006*. Retrieved April 26, 2007, from http://ncmhd.nih.gov/our_programs/strategic/pubs/VolumeI_031003EDrev.pdf

Satcher, D., Fryer, G. E., McCann, J., Troutman, A., Woolf, S. H., & Rust, G. (2005). What if we were equal? A comparison of the black–white mortality gap in 1960 and 2000. *Health Affairs, 24*, 459–464.

Satcher, D., & Rust, G. (2006). A three-dimensional approach to the elimination of racial–ethnic disparities in lung health. *Clinics in Chest Medicine, 27*, 535–542.

Senge, P., & Lannon-Kim, C. (1991). *The Systems Thinker Newsletter, 2*. Cambridge, MA: Pegasus Publications.

Stokols, D., Fuqua, J., Gress, J., Harvey, R., Phillips, K., Baezconde-Garbanati, L., et al. (2003). Evaluating transdisciplinary science. *Nicotine & Tobacco Research, 5*, S21–S39.

Thacker, S., Ikeda, R., Gieseker, K., Mendelsohn, A., Saydah, S., Curry, C., et al. (2005). The evidence base for public health: Informing policy at the Centers for Disease Control and Prevention. *American Journal of Preventive Medicine, 28*, 227–223.

U.S. Department of Health and Human Services. (1979). *Healthy people: The surgeon general's report on health promotion and disease prevention* (U.S. Department of Health, Education, and Welfare Publication No. 79-55071). Washington, DC: U.S. Government Printing Service. Retrieved April 26, 2007, from http://profiles.nlm.nih.gov/NN/B/B/G/K/_/nnbbgk.pdf

U.S. Department of Health and Human Services. (1991). *Healthy people 2000: National health promotion and disease prevention objectives*. Retrieved April 26, 2007, from http://odphp.osophs.HHS.gov/pubs/hp2000/

U.S. Department of Health and Human Services. (1999). *Mental health: A report of the surgeon general—Executive summary*. Rockville, MD: U.S. Department of Health and Human Services, Substance Abuse and Mental Health Services Administration, Center for Mental Health Services, National Institutes of Health, National Institute of Mental Health.

U.S. Department of Health and Human Services. (2000). *Healthy People 2010: Understanding and improving health*. Retrieved April 26, 2007, from http://www.healthypeople.gov/Document/tableofcontents.htm#under

U.S. Department of Health and Human Services, Centers for Disease Control and Prevention, National Center for Health Statistics. (2005a). *Health, United States*. Retrieved April 26, 2007, from http://www.cdc.gov/nchs/data/hus/hus05.pdf

U.S. Department of Health and Human Services. (2005b). *National healthcare disparities report.* Rockville, MD: Agency for Healthcare Research and Quality. Retrieved October 31, 2006, from http://www.ahrq.gov/qual/nhdr05/nhdr05.htm

U.S. Department of Health and Human Services. (2006). *Healthy People 2010: Mid-course review.* Retrieved April 26, 2007, from http://www.healthypeople.gov/data/midcourse/default.htm#pubs

Williams, D. (2005). Patterns and causes of disparities in health. In D. Mechanic, L. B. Rogut, D. C. Colby, & J. R. Knickman (Eds.), *Policy challenges in modern health care.* Piscataway, NJ: Rutgers University Press.

World Health Organization. (2000). *The world health report 2000: Health systems: Improving performance.* Geneva, Switzerland: WHO. Retrieved April 26, 2007, from http://www.who.int/whr/2000/en/whr00_en.pdf

Grant-Writing for Community-Based Health Disparities Research and Services: The Role of Academic/Community Partnerships

13

In Language, clarity is everything.
Confucius

Brenda D. Hayes

Introduction

Excellent communication skills, experienced organizational ability, comprehensive planning, and subject matter expertise, coupled with an ability to demonstrate or deliver specific measurable outcomes, often characterize the attributes of successfully funded grant proposals. Those associated with an academic community-based health disparity initiative introduce additional requirements, such as evidence of historical partnership activities and a methodological approach that includes a conceptual framework for mutual collaboration aimed at the elimination of health disparities.

Writing proposals focused on health disparities in conjunction with community collaboration requires a variety of skills and resources. Proposal development activities developed within the parameters of community and population driven research activities must be collaborative and should be initiated this way, that is, with community partners included at the beginning of the process who contribute to the selection of high-priority health issues defined by the community. These community partners then work closely with academic representatives (investigators) in designing the proposal

The Morehouse School of Medicine's Center of Excellence on Health Disparities (NIH/NCMHD 5P20MD00272) partially supported this work.

and each of the proposal components, including the process for the dissemination of findings. With this kind of collaboration, the community's expertise is paired with academic resources in order to develop a successful project plan and proposal using community-based participatory research methodology.

> The primary purpose of building community coalitions is to empower communities to become self-reliant in addressing lifestyle-related diseases, deaths, unintentional injuries, violence and other health concerns. (Dr. Gerald L. Durley, Former Director, Health Promotion and Resource Center, Morehouse School of Medicine, as cited in Thompson-Reid, 1992)

The Morehouse School of Medicine (MSM) developed an approach to working in communities and implemented this community-based strategy more than 25 years ago. Based on this approach, a model was developed for health promotion and health planning. Braithwaite and colleagues described this as a model of "community organization and development for health promotion that borrowed from the empowerment education approach of Paolo Friere" (Braithwaite & Lythcott, 1989).

In the field of public health, the partnership between the community and academic institutions is the common vehicle for a community-based strategy. The Center of Excellence on Health Disparities (COEHD) at MSM received a project award funded by the National Institutes of Health/National Center on Minority Health and Health Disparities in 2002. The Center of Excellence continues to operationalize this MSM community-based approach through a variety of mechanisms including awarding community mini-grants (sub-awards) to community partners for health programs addressing six health areas with high disparities. The Center's areas of interest include programs addressing cardiovascular and related diseases, cancer, HIV/AIDS, mental health, diabetes and maternal and child health.

This chapter will provide background information intended to clarify common conceptual elements of community-based participatory research (CBPR) that influence the development of community-based projects and proposals. The primary focus is on an academic/community model for health disparity community-based initiatives, which often serves as the foundation for proposal and project development. The chapter includes recommended strategies for initiating and maintaining community partnerships for effective proposal development and program sustainability based on the historical and collective experience of Morehouse School of Medicine. This chapter argues the fundamental importance of community participation in all aspects of proposal development—from the definition of the problem or need to outcome evaluation.

What Is the "Community?"

Community has been defined in a variety of ways from a set of common attributes shared by one or more individuals (Evans, 2004, p. 32), as a "unit of identity" (Israel et al., 2003, p. 55) or as simply a description for those who reside in a common geographical area, or share personal and cultural attributes (e.g., ethnicity, social status, group affiliations, etc.) or some other mutually shared variable (e.g., religion, income, sexual orientation, etc.). These definitions can be loosely inclusive or selectively exclusive and confined to a few common attributes shared between individuals dependent on the focus and intent. In this discussion, "community" refers to populations that may be defined by geography; race; ethnicity; culture, gender; sexual orientation; disability, illness or other health condition; or to groups that have a common interest or cause, such as health or service agencies and organizations, health care or public health practitioners or providers, policy makers, or lay public groups with public health concerns. "Community-based organizations" refer to those non-profit, tax-exempt organizations founded to meet identified needs, which can include specific services, programs, or other activities. In this chapter, the community-based organizations most likely encountered and discussed provide medical, health or social services; interventions, or activity or research processes targeting those who reside in the area and/or belong to a group identified to receive the services (Syme, 2004).

Why Do We Partner With Communities?

In the past two decades, a large and still growing body of literature and research documents the efficacy of community-based approaches to personal health and public health issues. Substantial medical, behavioral, and policy research documents the reality of the inequitable distribution of morbidity and mortality in health status experienced by most African Americans and other minority groups as well as those who are socio-economically disadvantaged. Contemporary literary research documents the history of the unique African American health inequity disparity phenomenon as dating back to the introduction of slavery to the Americas, which Byrd and Clayton (2000, 2002) describe as "An American Health Dilemma." Therefore, it is not surprising to find that today any health program addressing a health issue in the African American, other minority or underserved community will most likely focus on a health disparity or health inequity spanning a variety of health issues from access to care to infant mortality, prostate cancer incidence, and HIV/AIDS, including the under representation of minority health professionals in the workforce. Collaborating with communities is an efficient and effective vehicle for public health interventions and for the development of strategies that address population-specific issues.

In this current context, we collaborate and partner with communities in order to eliminate health disparities. Part of the rationale for this approach is that in health settings, we have focused on individual change strategies and group interventions with some success but many obstacles and setbacks impede our progress. However, given all of the factors that initiate, support, and reinforce health behavior change, the community-based approach seems to offer the potential for better outcomes, given the commitment of groups, organizations, and other community forces. Most of the "partners" often include various kinds of community-based (and faith-based) organizations involved in some aspects of health promotion.

The term "community-based" has been used to (1) define the role of the community residents, (2) to depict the type of organization that will carry out the intervention, and (3) to identify the place of the intervention (Easterling, Gallagher & Lodwick, 2003). At times, these various usages of the term community-based occur simultaneously. Minkler and Wallerstein (2003) provide some insight into the number of descriptive phrases used to describe the community-based focus and distinguish the work that is done in this setting as more than just a *place for research*, such as a community "laboratory" or as a parallel to the biomedical research environment. These researchers cite Israel and colleagues (who have been at the forefront of community-based participatory research or CBPR), who characterize CBPR as having these fundamental characteristics: participatory; cooperative; a colearning process; includes system development and community capacity building; an empowering process; achieves a balance between research and action (Minkler & Wallerstein, p. 5).

This usage also points out the multi-dimensional quality of the community-based approach and to a model of community-anchored intervention. In fact, Blumenthal and DiClemente (2004) state that "the community is a *partner* in research (training, service, etc.) that is conducted for the mutual benefit of both the researcher and community."

Therefore, community-based research:

- Is population-centered;
- Utilizes a multi-disciplinary approach;
- Takes place in a natural environment with participants continuing their usual activities;
- Often has a prevention focus (primary, secondary or tertiary levels of prevention); and
- Occurs in partnership with the community (O'Fallon, 2000).

Numerous examples of successful community partnerships exist at Morehouse School of Medicine (MSM) in Atlanta, Georgia. MSM has focused on building community and academic partnerships in low-income, predominately African American sections within Atlanta's inner city and rural areas of Georgia since 1987. In 2002, MSM through its Center of Excellence on Health Disparities established a shared resource core (Community Partnerships Development) that focused on expanding a network of community partners inclusive of community-based organizations, faith-based organizations and academic centers. The conceptual framework for this network partially utilized an approach to community designed initially by faculty and staff at MSM in the late 1980s. The *Coalition Building Guide*, written by Patricia Thomson-Reid (1992) and published by the MSM Health Promotion Resource Center (HPRC), outlines this model approach to community empowerment. The philosophy of the model is that:

> [H]ealth promotion efforts are likely to be more successful in populations where the community at risk is empowered to identify its own health concerns, develop its own prevention and/or intervention strategies and form a decision-making coalition board to make policy decisions and identify resources for program implementation. (Thompson-Reid, 1992)

The community-based approach is a comprehensive conceptual model incorporating community empowerment, community strengths and needs, and a health belief model focused on individual and community health improvement. Designing programs to reach *populations*, not merely individuals, is at the heart of a public health orientation (Glanz, Lewis, & Rimer, 2000).

Community-based participatory research (CBPR) has also been defined as scientific inquiry conducted in communities and in partnership with researchers. The process of scientific inquiry is such that community members, persons affected by the health condition, disability or issue under study, or other key stakeholders in the community's health have the opportunity to be full participants in each phase of the work (from conception through design, conduct analysis, interpretation, conclusions and communication of results). One of the characteristics of CBPR is the substantial community input in the development of the grant application (http://www.niehs.nih.gov/translat/cbpr/cbpr.htm).

Community-partnered approaches to research promise to deepen our scientific base of knowledge in the areas of health promotion, disease prevention, and health disparities while addressing community priorities (Vishwanathan, 2004; Yancey, 2004). Community-partnered research processes offer the potential to generate better-informed hypotheses, encourage the development of more effective interventions, and enhance the translation of the research results into practice. Specifically, involving community and academic partners as research collaborators may improve the quality and impact of research by:

1) More effectively focusing the research questions on health issues of greatest relevance to the communities at highest risk;
2) Enhancing recruitment and retention efforts by increasing community buy-in and trust;
3) Enhancing the reliability and validity of measurement instruments (particularly survey) through in-depth and honest feedback during pre-testing;
4) Improving data collection through increased response rates and decreased social desirability response patterns;
5) Increasing relevance of intervention approaches and thus likelihood for success;
6) Targeting interventions to the identified needs of community members;
7) Developing intervention strategies that incorporate community norms and values into scientifically valid approaches;
8) Increasing accurate and culturally sensitive interpretation of findings;
9) Facilitating more effective dissemination of research findings to impact public health and policy; and
10) Increasing the potential for translation and adaptation of evidence-based research into sustainable community change approaches.

Tips for Partnerships

For the purposes of this discussion, we define a *partnership* as a mutually beneficial and well-defined relationship entered into by two or more organizations to achieve common goals.

There is a significant amount of literature written about partnerships and sustainability. The issue of the sustainability of academic partnerships and community organizations is critical and a source of concern by most communities. In fact, since 1996, *Community-Campus Partnerships for Health* (http://depts.washington.edu/ccph/), a nonprofit organization, has established guiding principles to support community-academic partnerships as the result of substantial research in this area. In addition, Community-Campus Partnerships for Health (CCPH) provide programs, funding opportunities and other resources that address viability and sustainability of these relationships (Allison et al., 2005).

What Does a Partnership Require?

A partnership requires the following:

- Shared responsibility;
- Defined common goals;
- Mutual accountability for success; and
- Shared resources and rewards (Blumenthal & Yancey, 2004).

Why Create These Collaborative Partnerships?

Collaborative partnerships are created, given the following:

- They give more "bang for the buck" (efficiency);
- These relationships make services more accessible, effective, and tailored to fit the specific community;
- The resulting synergy offers ways to overcome obstacles;
- The combination diversifies capability to accomplish tasks; and
- "Funders" like it (see http://www.epa.gov/seahome.grants.src/writing/open-write.htm).

Creating and Sustaining Community–Based Partnerships

There is substantial documentation about the efficacy of forging academic and community partnerships to address the elimination of health disparities and other inequities that affect underserved communities. Morehouse School of Medicine (MSM) has a long, rich history of community involvement including training, service, and other activities that have involved communities and community members in significant roles for more than two decades. Consequently, MSM and other academic institutions with a similar history have an advantage in developing programs that must involve community-based organizations, civic groups, faith-based programs and the business community. These well-established community relationships are based on mutual respect, shared strengths, and vision, and are vital to successfully implementing sustainable programs designed to ameliorate and eventually eliminate health disparities.

What Are Some of the Methods Used to Nurture These Collaboratives? Several methods are used to nurture these collaborations. These include the following:

- Breaking down institutional barriers;
- Working through cultural differences; and
- Facilitating strategic planning.

Rationale for Partnerships and Collaborations

A community-based approach to the elimination of health disparities requires the involvement of the community in significant and meaningful ways—including advisory groups composed of community participants, forming interconnected networks of community health providers, key community institutions (schools, churches, other organizations, etc.), private industry, and consumers (Alexander et al., 2003). The approach is a comprehensive conceptual model incorporating community empowerment, community strengths and needs, and a health belief model focused on individual and community health improvement.

> The process of empowerment through formation of coalitions for health promotion is a means of developing the problem-solving potential of communities so that they can become proactive instead of reactive on important health issues. It also enables historically-disenfranchised individuals or communities to obtain access to and gain control of valued resources. (Thompson-Reid, 1992)

In order to affect changes in the community's health profile effectively, change strategies often include health education and awareness, available and updated health information bureaus, health resources, leadership and accountability, monitoring and evaluation, policy changes, and other factors thought to be pivotal in changing a community's health indicators (Cottrell et al., 1996). The institutions' activities to ameliorate and eventually eliminate health status gaps can be furthered with the organized use and systematic approach to the creation of partnerships and collaborations.

General Objectives of Community Partnerships

The objectives of developing community partnerships are many. One objective involves formalizing the community partnerships through a Memoranda of Agreement (MOA) or a Memoranda of Understanding (MOU) between the institution and the program. Another objective involves the creation of consumer participant groups who are representatives from the community. It is important to develop culturally appropriate and culturally sensitive materials and interventions for health focused activities as a key objective.

Useful Strategies

There are also a number of useful strategies, as follows:

1) Identify the community, faith, and business organizations to involve in the partnership based on common mission, goals, vision, etc.;
2) Establish written, formal agreements with the identified groups;
3) Share resources;
4) Develop and implement a proposed scope of work for the partnership;
5) Conduct proposal development activities with the partners;
6) Implement a community grant program with funds (and other resources) from the lead organization to underwrite joint activities between the institution and the community partners;
7) Determine the evaluative activities and other ongoing technical assistance methods to provide to the partners; and

8) Create feedback loops that involve the partners and key institutional leaders in discussing the achievements of the partnership.

The establishment and maintenance of mutually beneficial community-based partnerships between academic centers and programs that promote health services and health care are vital to the eventual elimination of health disparities. These synergistic partnerships offer the possibilities of generating new resources to support programmatic operations, the development and proliferation of best practices and the enhancement of health promotion. The ramifications of positive, long-term sustained partnerships have tremendous implications for affecting positive health outcomes, disease prevention and treatment improving health behaviors and encouraging modifications where needed in lifestyle choices.

Beyond these tips for partnerships, there is the task of bringing the partnership or collaboration to bear on the problem of a health disparity of concern to the community. We may now explore what is meant by a health disparity.

What Is a Health Disparity?

In the National Institutes of Health "Strategic Research Plan to Reduce and Ultimately Eliminate Health Disparities" (HHS, 2006), health disparities were defined as differences in the incidence, prevalence, morbidity, mortality, and burden of diseases and other adverse health conditions that exist among specific population groups. These health disparities include shorter overall life expectancy, higher rates of cardiovascular disease, cancer, infant mortality, birth defects, asthma, diabetes, stroke, sexually transmitted diseases, oral diseases and disorders, and mental disorders, among others. Contributing factors include reduced access to health care, increased risk of diseases and disability due to occupation or exposure, and increased risk of illness due to underlying biological, socioeconomic, ethnic, or familial factors; cultural values, and education (see http://www.nih.gov/about/hd/strategicplan.pdf, p. 7). The specific population groups are African Americans, American Indians, Alaska Natives, Asian Americans, Hispanic Americans, Native Hawaiians, Pacific Islanders, subpopulations of all of the above and medically underserved populations (i.e., socio-economically disadvantaged individuals in rural and urban areas).

Other researchers have addressed the conceptual issues that surround the use of the term "health disparity," which is apparently unique to the United States. Internationally, other terms such as "health inequity" and "health inequality" are used. However, according to Carter-Pokras and Baquet (2002), health disparity "could be viewed as a chain of events signified by a difference in (1) environment, (2) access to, utilization of and quality of care, (3) health status, or (4) a particular health outcome that deserves scrutiny. The international connotations denote issues of injustice with implications of health equity and health as a right (Satcher & Rust, 2006). Today, public health and social scientists and others continue to examine and expand the definition of health disparity to apply not only to issues of incidence and prevalence but also to address these other issues as well (Smedley & Syme, 2000).

Successful Strategies for Partnering on Proposal Development Focused on Health Disparities

Successful proposal development in the area of health disparities implies active engagement/involvement with communities (this suggests a population-based approach); more than one organization or agency is going to be involved with the proposed activities, which also suggests collaborations and partnerships. A population or community-based approach is implicit in the work of ameliorating health disparities since the nature of these inequities includes a focus on community elements (access issues, environment, resources, organizations, etc.) and individual health status, lifestyles, and health behavior.

Once the principal investigators or lead researchers have addressed this major factor of involving (matching, selecting, recruiting, etc.) community partners and the group has agreed upon the community approach to address the identified health disparity, the process of systematically developing the proposal should proceed just as any other proposal.

The process of developing a collaborative proposal can proceed in any number of ways after the creation of the core writing team by the involved collaborators and the lead agency. However, it is critical to reach an early consensus about the development, the approach and the writing responsibilities for the major sections of the proposal and the establishment of a time line to complete the project. The writing team should be representative of the skills needed to write a competitive proposal and include a minimum of three people: the lead agency representative(s), the community organization(s) representative, and an evaluator. *Remember: An adequate time frame is necessary to develop a competitive proposal.* In the best of all possible worlds, a minimum of 4 to 6 months is often required for the development of a successful proposal. In the real world, this period can be a luxury practically; 6 weeks may be all the time available. Therefore, proactive planning is highly recommended, including storing sets of information, sections from previously written proposals or concept papers, bibliographies (annotated if possible), and an up-to-date literature review.

Competition to acquire extramural, internal, or external funding resources continues to increase among small and large organizations, between academic and biomedical research enterprises and is directed toward all levels of government and private funds. There exist a range of reactions experienced by many individuals, agencies, and organizations new to the competitive grant writing process when faced with the task of submitting a grant application. Generally, the majority of these initial reactions can be classified as less than enthusiastic with many other mixed emotions running rampant, including the competitive spirit, enthusiasm for the process, negativism or pessimism regarding the outcome, other anxiety-related concerns, fear and trepidation. Many of the individual reactions expressed by those involved in the competitive proposal development and grant-writing process come from individuals with a variety of educational backgrounds, professionals and nonprofessionals, teachers, academicians, volunteers, community board members, and others. However, one of the unifying factors shared by most of the members in this disparate group is that many have little prior experience and an absence of focused, formal training in what some have called the Art of Grantsmanship.

What Is the Art of Grantsmanship?

Grantsmanship is a term encountered often in the academic and biomedical research arenas and generalized to include other areas. One researcher explained this as the "art of acquiring peer-reviewed research funding" (Kraicer, 1997). Today, one finds an expanded meaning or a more general use of the term grantsmanship, which is used frequently to describe the overall presentation, the proposal contents, and the overall packaging of a competitive grant application or proposal for competitive funding. What are the pathways in acquiring this skill? How does one become proficient in this "art" if not through training? The simplest answer is through practice.

Why Do We Write Proposals?

There exist a myriad of reasons for proposal development, but the most common driving forces include:

- To acquire resources for projects, programs, their activities and services as well as personnel to conduct them;
- To develop and implement new research initiatives;
- To contribute to the generalizable pool of knowledge; and
- To establish an academic/scientific reputation for career and service development.

These and a host of other reasons fuel the competition for resources: to conduct a wide range of research activities; to conduct teaching and training programs; to provide an infrastructure for communities; and to support a host of services at all levels. In turn, all levels of public sources (federal, state, and local government) and a host of voluntary and private sources award many of their funds on a competitive basis.

Given a crowded field of competitors, a number of analyses exist that identify successful and unsuccessful applications from which we can develop guidance or a "lessons learned" strategy. These are summarized in Table 13.1.

Steps to a Successful Grant Writing Process

There are several essential factors and activities that contribute to a successful proposal, according to many successful proposal and grant writers. Successful proposal and grant writers consider these tenets as basic proposal building blocks. These are discussed in this section.

Table 13.1	Unsuccessful Applications vs. Successful Applications*	
	Unsuccessful Applications	**Successful Applications**
	<ul><li>Fail to follow directions</li><li>Lack of new or original ideas</li><li>Diffuse, superficial, or unfocused research; lack of clearly stated hypothesis and rationale</li><li>Lack of an overall research goal; uncertainty about future directions</li><li>Lack of knowledge of relevant literature</li><li>Demonstrate questionable reasoning in design</li><li>Lack of demonstrated experience in methodology (lacks details)</li><li>Portray format issues</li><li>Outline an over-ambitious plan</li></ul>	<ul><li>Are direct, concise, compelling, convincing, capable, and resourceful</li><li>Address a significant/important problem</li><li>Develop explicit goals, measurable objectives</li><li>Contain a comprehensive but succinct background review</li><li>Reflect a methodology that fits the problem</li><li>Use an appropriate funding mechanism</li></ul>

*Sources:
NIH pamphlet: National Institutes of Health, Division of Research Grants. *Helpful Hints: Preparing an NIH Research Grant Application* (1995), Bethesda, MD.
"Why Clinical Research Grant Applications Fare Poorly in Review and How to Recover," by Janet M. Cuca and William J. McLoughlin, 1987, *Cancer Investigation, 5*(1), pp. 55–58.
"Ingredients of a Successful Grant Application to the National Institutes of Health" by Stephen L. Gordon, 1989, *Journal of Orthopaedic Research, 7,* pp. 38–141.
"Obtaining Grant Funding for Clinical Research" by S. L. Gordon, 1988, in *Non-Cemented Total Hip Arthroplast*, R. Fitzgerald, Jr., ed., pp. 473–478.

Three Essential Laws of Successful Grant Writing

Three essential laws of successful grant writing include the following:

1) Do your homework
2) Follow instructions
3) Use common sense.

Essential Techniques of Grant Writing

In addition, there are a number of techniques to incorporate into the grant writing or proposal development process. Some of these fundamental considerations include:

- Begin with a good idea;
- Review the components of a successful grant;
- Evaluate and discuss the plan for the proposal with your collaborators;
- Conduct a thorough literature review;
- Maintain an updated analysis of current research/activity in the field; and
- Develop a proposal writing team (U.S. Environmental Protection Agency, n.d.).

Essential Skills for Grant Writing

Similarly, there is an array of varied skills needed to plan, write, and submit a successful proposal. The lead writer or investigator may have these skills or they may be present in other members of the writing team. These skills include (1) excellent oral presentation or speaking skills; (2) planning ability; (3) organizing ability; (4) ability to work in and with a group; (5) previous management experience; (6) mentoring ability or experience; (7) good to excellent writing ability; (8) an ability to plan and use work schedules/time lines; (9) ability to identify and work with collaborators; and (10) an ability to incorporate review criteria into the proposal. Many successful grant writers consider these as *the essential laws* of successful proposal development (Hall, 1998; Locke et al., 2000).

Four Preliminary Steps to the Actual Grant/Proposal Writing

There are four preliminary steps to the actual process of writing the grant. These may be detailed, as follows.

Step One: Setting the Framework. One of the crucial pitfalls in developing a successful application is the failure to "set the framework" for the proposal by beginning with a good idea. A number of new investigators "look for funding" or needlessly "worry about the budget" before they have thoroughly developed a "good idea." Therefore, setting the framework is a necessary first step in developing a successful proposal. The following suggestions are offered to make sure that the parameters of the task (the proposal) are outlined at the initiation of the writing process and lead to a successful proposal (Reif-Lehrer, 2005).

- Overall approach: Develop, discuss and sharpen your ideas.
- Conceptual framework: What is the rationale and approach?
- Funding sources: What does the potential funder expect you to do? How do you sustain the research, conduct your activities, and get more money to sustain the project? Are the funds adequate to conduct the project?
- Literature review: Is it thorough?
- Underpinnings-theory-application to methodology: Does it fit?
- Research design: What kind of project?
  - Human subjects: Have you addressed this issue?
  - Data collection: Have you described the methods?
  - Data analysis: Did you explain the plan?
- Role of evaluation: Develop a plan based on your objectives.
- Develop a Dissemination Strategy that includes your community organization.

Step Two: Develop Your Idea(s). In the second step, it is important to adequately develop the idea(s) behind the grant. Numerous strategies are recommended to develop the idea(s), as outlined in the following:

- Conduct or use a needs assessment approach
  - Show evidence of the problem
  - Use local, county, state and national data
- Capability assessment

- Organizational
- People
- Past and present history
- Resources (funds, expertise, etc.)

The assessment process considers the organizations that are planning to be involved in the project as well as an analysis of the potential funding source's priorities and grantee record.

Step Three: Considerations and Getting Started. Beginning the work of actually writing the proposal requires an adequate time line. Many unsuccessful proposals reflect an inadequate amount of development and review time. Often writers start the process too late, with insufficient lead time, little adequate literature review, or the writing team becomes a party of one. Some of the assessment questions that will help to start the process include the following:

- Do you have sufficient time and resources to write a compelling and convincing proposal?
- What do you wish to achieve?
- What specific activities/services can be planned and conducted?
- Have you the capability to conduct the activity?
- Have you analyzed your assets?
- Does your previous record support a new project?
- Have you identified your collaborators and partners?
- Are the goals and objectives focused, compatible and reasonable?
- Does the methodology fit the task?
- What is the organizational history of partnerships?
- Is there a supportive networking environment?
- Is this a results-oriented project?
- Can you provide any evidence of impact from other funded projects?
- Have you developed a realistic budget?
  - What is the amount of the needed funds to support the scope of required work or activity?
- Did you include an evaluation plan?

After completing this initial assessment satisfactorily, then it is useful to meet with the organizational representatives and the writing team to outline the findings from the assessment process and to establish time lines for the balance of the writing project.

Step Four: Proposal Development and Grant Seeking Overview. In broad terms, the team leader must:

- Identify potential funding sources for the identified project (see Table 13.2)
  - Assess, evaluate, and prioritize these sources

Table 13.2	**Identifying Potential Funders**

- Local networks
  - County and state government divisions
  - Local voluntary associations
  - Faith-based organizations
  - Partnerships (related programs, common mission, etc.)
  - Friends, associates, and colleagues
- Regional branches of national organizations:
  - National Association of Social Workers
  - American Public Health Association
  - American Cancer Society, and so on
- Voluntary/private foundations
- Federal agencies
  - NIH (National Institutes of Health)
  - CDC (Centers for Disease Control and Prevention)
  - EPA (Environmental Protection Agency)
  - DOE (Department of Energy)
  - NSF (National Science Foundation)
  - ACF (American Cancer Foundation)

- Contact potential funders for further information
- Plan proposal
  - Design an evaluation component
- Develop a project budget (include a justification)
- Write, review, critique, and revise the proposal
- Submit the proposal
- Follow up with the potential funding source

It is useful to consider all of the possibilities listed, as shown in Table 13.2, as potential sources for funding.

In preparing the proposal, the lead writer/researcher/investigator will need to engage in numerous critical tasks. First, review the purpose statement and capability of the agency/institution/organization in comparison with the funding opportunity and the mission of the proposed sponsor. Second, assure the inclusion of all of the necessary proposal components. Third, develop and include a comprehensive time line/time frame for the project.

The writing team will need to determine if there exists a match between the proposed project and the funding source. In other words, is there a "Goodness of Fit" between the expressed ideas, organizational or agency capability, and the funding solicitation or announcement?

In this process, it is important to analyze and compare the ideas suggested, the capability of the organization and lead individuals, the resources available and/or possible; any other opportunities; and the benefit of the proposed program. Or, how will the inclusion of the partners, population, strategies, and so on enhance the project?

Developing the Actual Proposal

After completing the preliminary steps outlined above, the writing team members should receive their key assignments determined by the key investigator and the other collaborators on the project. However, a general question asked by new investigators and new proposal writers (after answering the getting started question) is about the proposal's format. Generally, the solicitation or funding announcement provides the required format and any other pertinent instructions for preparing the proposal. However, it is useful to keep the following general outline in mind, as discussed in the sections below.

Basic Proposal Components

The following list contains the basic section headings often encountered in the suggested format used by a variety of funding sources. It is important to adhere to the guidelines offered in the funding application and not to deviate by adding unrequested sections or items. In writing the proposal, it is useful to keep these general guidelines in mind: take sufficient time to prepare a good letter of intent (LOI), a concept paper or an abstract; avoid using jargon and acronyms; be careful when/where you cut and paste; assure uniformity of font size and type, format coherence, and so on; whenever you include a budget, also plan to include a budget justification; and ALWAYS use a reader (plan on getting editorial assistance).

1. **The Proposal Summary.** This front section of the proposal is often described by different names, which may be dependent on the type of proposal that is being developed. This section can be called an executive summary or overview and is seen in many service or training focused applications (public or private sources) while the term "abstract" is often found in research focused proposals. Regardless of the terminology, this section is usually brief, one or two pages and offers a summary of the project or proposal. The same section headings seen in the body of the proposal can be used to summarize the scope of the project, which is described in more detail in the proposal (Miner & Miner, 2005, p. 16; Ward, 2006, pp. 21–22).

2. **The Introduction.** The introduction has many functions. The introduction provides specific descriptive and capability information about the grant applicant. Specifically, the introduction: states the purpose and/or goal of the project; describes the programs; describes the clients or target population and the focus; states the applicant's achievements; establishes the credibility of the applicant; and documents the credibility of the applicant with specific examples. It is important to keep the introduction brief and focused.

3. **Problem Statement (or Needs Assessment).** This section of the proposal establishes the background for the project by describing the current state of what is known about the problem or situation and outlines the justification for the project for which funding is being sought.

4. **Project Description.** This is the key narrative section of the proposal, which includes the vital components of your project activity. In this section, you will outline the basic

Table 13.3	**Goals and Objectives**

Goals are:

- A general statement phrased in abstract terms and denotes the "big picture"
- Focused on intent
- Related to the mission or purpose of the research study or service

Objectives are:

- Required
- Reasonable
- Measurable
- Stated as outcomes
- Reflective of a research focus and/or population focused
- Timed
- Not methods

Objectives can:

- Restate the intent of the project
- Indicate what the project will achieve
- Help to determine the parameters of your evaluation plan
- Be concise, specific, measurable and relate directly to need

purpose, objectives, methods, and expected outcomes for the project. This section should be comprehensive, compelling, convincing, and written clearly.

4. A. Goals and objectives. Many of the initial pieces written for the proposal are straightforward and set the organization framework and capability in conducting the project. However, the next challenge in the proposal development process, after addressing the needed preliminary work, is the conceptualization of program objectives. Although the abstract conceptualization of the long-term goal (and perhaps short–term milestones as well) may appear to be quite easy, it is more abstract, general and larger in scope than the objectives. The goals (or purpose) of the project can be viewed as part of the shared priorities for the potential funding source and the applicant organization or agency. Depending on the type of proposal, this section may need to include your hypothesis and the specific aims (objectives) for a research focused project. Objectives outline what the project intends to do or accomplish. See Table 13.3.

Project objectives (or specific aims) are often constructed as action statements with some implicit or explicit *performance measure.* The objectives tell what activities will be conducted as part of the project. The examples below suggest the inclusion of action or performance verbs in determining the primary action strategies that serve as the focus for the project. The examples below state some of the possible actions undertaken by the project: (1) Assess, analyze, answer; (2) Compare, conduct, compile; (3) Develop, determine, demonstrate; (4) Establish, evaluate, examine; 5) Identify, inform, increase; and (6) Modify, prepare, measure.

These examples stress the importance of identifying the scope of the project and should relate to specific strategies or action items that detail the strategies to attain the objectives. It is important to remember that objectives are **SMART**: that is, they are smart, measurable, action-oriented, realistic, and timely. In fact, the approach to the process, constructing the proposal and the overall assessment of the proposal should be Specific, Measurable, Action-oriented, Realistic, and Timely (**SMART**).

4. B. Project method and design. The project or research design framework and the specific activities employed define the methodology. The project's design is your approach to the work of the proposal—either research, activities, or service. This design could be a case study, a community needs analysis, or a quasi-experimental project. All of these approaches would be informed by community input (CBPR). This section includes the **HOW** of the project and includes details about specific activities. One or more methods may be identified for each objective. Specify for each objective: **Who** will do what? **When** will it be done? **How** will it be accomplished? How **long** will each take?

In this section, one should be prepared to write about the data collection process: what is collected, when data is collected, and the prescribed end points in the process are identified for the data analysis section.

Measurement. The discussion of measurement issues should be in terms of the data used to establish need (Ward, 2006, p. 6). The various types and sources of data are outlined below:

A. Use data to present an objective view of the situation or the problem
    1. References
    2. Preliminary studies
    3. Community voices
B. Types and sources
    1. Program data
        a. Evaluation results
        b. Client intake information
        c. Client or participant surveys
        d. Waiting lists
        e. Service records
    2. Journals, periodicals, newspapers, newsletters, books
    3. Reports and documents from governmental sources, advisory boards, offices, commissions, etc.
    4. Reports from foundations and community groups
    5. Interviews with experts
    6. Feasibility studies and assessments

An important point to remember is that the data you collect, as part of the project, will help inform the evaluation process!

Most of the time, you cannot measure what is not collected, and once the data collection process is over, you cannot return to collect any more information. If the data cannot be analyzed as planned, then there are dire implications (and consequences) for the evaluation process, if it is incomplete, or is missing vital elements necessary for the evaluation process. These deficits become fatal flaws for the integrity of the data analysis process.

It is also important to select outcome or performance objectives that can show that the project influenced the same measures. For example, if the focus is on improving reading ability, then the following need and objective would be specified:

Need. Problem of poor reading performance can be addressed by a strategy to increase reading performance (in a number of ways, through a number of methods).

Objective. Should specifically relate to some level or aspect of reading performance and not to other factors, such as program attendance.

4. C. Program/project/research activities. Each section of the proposal is important. However, this section provides the details about how the proposed project will implement the strategies to reach the objectives. After developing the SMART objectives, the next step is to outline the associated strategies to attain them. These strategies provide explanations about how the project will reach the stated objectives; focus upon what is necessary to the success of the project; undertake only those activities that will move the project toward realization of objectives; and, fully describe activities in the proposal.

This is another section where different terminology is used. It is useful to incorporate the headings identified in the proposal guidelines for this section. These headings might be the project description, the methods section of the research plan, methodology, or simply the project narrative. The potential funding source wants specific information about the details of what will be done, by whom, when, and so forth. This will cover the specific tasks, the personnel carrying out the tasks, the time frame, facilities, training needs, if any and other relevant information about the activities (Lauffer, 1997, pp. 258–293; Ward, 2006, pp. 7–11).

4. C.1 Project management. One often overlooked aspect of proposal and project development is one of management. This aspect is sometimes obliquely addressed in the personnel section (or the budget justification) of the proposal. However, proposals are strengthened by assuring the inclusion of the following information: Who will manage the activity? What management strategies will be employed? Is an advisory board required in the guidelines? What is the role of consultants, collaborators, and/or other institutions?

When the potential funder requests this section in the proposal's guidelines, it is customary to add an organizational chart that shows the relationships with the partnering organizations as well as specifying the project mechanisms that integrate this project with other organizational components. If there is an advisory board or a steering committee, include these in the organizational relationships as well. If this section is not requested explicitly, it is still appropriate to discuss: how the project will be managed, the reporting relationships, and the administrative monitoring of the project.

4. C.2 Time lines. Along with the administrative management of a project, it is useful to provide a graphic representation of the projected work flow or accomplishments of the project. Provide a visual (graphic) of expected milestones throughout the funding period. The visual can be a bar chart, a plain timetable, or a *Gantt chart* listing major activities and specific tasks and details. Many of these formats are available electronically and can enhance understanding about the manner in which the work will be accomplished. Visuals inform the sponsoring agency (funding source) of planned outcomes, deliverables, and so forth. Time lines can be a useful evaluative tool for internal monitoring.

4.C.3 Project evaluation. This section of the proposal should identify an evaluation plan, when and where required as provided by the proposal guidelines. Often these guidelines outline the parameters of assessment needs (informational or baseline measures) that become a part of the project focus in terms of outcomes or other types of impact. The identification of these assessment steps could be displayed in a logic model or other diagrammatical formats that capture quantifiable and qualitative date elements. Minimally, the evaluation should examine the attainment or assessment of the specific objectives initially identified as the scope of activity for the project. The inclusion of a diagram or logic model provides a visual for the reviewer and can act as a plan for the project staff. This diagram should contain what the funding source outlines or expects the project to accomplish (Ward, 2006, pp. 12–15).

Part of the challenge in writing the evaluation plan is the determination of the type of evaluation appropriate for the project. This early determination should be part of the initial project conceptualization and relates to developing the specific objectives or aims for the project. This may be part of the rationale for the involvement of an evaluator at the beginning of the project to help with the form of evaluation and connecting the objectives to the evaluation process. In addition, it is useful to involve the evaluation at an early stage of the proposal discussions in order to sort through some evaluation terminology for the proposal-writing team. Everyone is then consistent about the form for the evaluation. We can describe some of these evaluative forms as follows: *Formative or Process evaluation*: Was the project conducted in accordance with the stated plan? How effective were the various activities within the plan? *Summative or Product evaluation:* Can the results be attributed to the project, as well as the extent to which the project attained the stated objectives? and *Outcome Analysis and/or Impact evaluation*: What happened? What are the implications (or "So What")?

4. C.4 Evaluation and assessment. Your proposal should always include an evaluation plan that addresses the proposed program or project. This evaluation plan can simply reflect but is not limited to a brief discussion of the following elements: Structure; Process; Outcomes; Impact or Findings; and Conclusions or Next Steps.

Formative vs. summative evaluation. Some proposal developers define formative and summative evaluation approaches as two different perspectives in measuring program achievement. Formative evaluation examines the processes and steps taken to achieve the objective while the summative approach asks: What was the outcome of the steps or activities taken? (See the antonyms in the following paragraph.)

Process or product evaluations. These are antonyms for formative or summative evaluation. When proposal guidelines ask for information about the processes employed or the products (deliverables) generated by the project, this is often another way of asking for a formative or summative evaluation. In this instance, "formative" can be equated to "process," while summative could be seen as the product(s) delivered by a project or program.

Quantitative vs. qualitative. Other forms of outcome data can be used as part of the project evaluation, including quantitative data methods (e.g., surveys, questionnaires, etc.) or qualitative methods (e.g., key informant interview schedules, board development curriculum, etc.) that yield findings. One can generate new data collection materials and/different methods to collect information based on the information generated as part of project findings.

Specify analytic methods. It is important to define the process and specify the analytical methods used in the data analysis section of the proposal. This may be another point where a statistician is useful as a consultant for the proposal writing team, if there is a need for outside assistance to refine or clarify the statistical analysis.

Specifically it is important to reiterate what you intend to deliver based on the previously specified objectives.

There should be some measurement involved in the strategies or actions implemented by the project or program, such as a change in status, lifestyle or behavior, knowledge increase, identification of new risk reduction methods, number of participants served, new partnerships formed, brochures developed, contacts made, presentations given, and so on.

Limitations. A brief section of the proposal should address any limitations or procedures to modify the impact of any program or design limitations. The statistical consultant can assist with minimizing any research design or data collection obstacles, while an evaluation consultant can contribute to any possible limitations in the deliverables.

Planning for the next phase. This section of the proposal should address the next steps or replicability of the project. This section could also address some of the issues associated with future funding and project sustainability as well. It is acceptable to include an evaluator as part of the evaluation plan but that personnel decision does not substitute for the inclusion of an evaluation plan in your proposal.

5. Project Budget. Developing a project budget seems to strike fear in the hearts of the fearless and remains a substantial source of anxiety for most new (and some seasoned) investigators. It is simple to address this anxiety by seeking assistance as soon as some determination or sketch of the project exists. This is an area where assistance is usually available through the applicant agency or organizational resources. It is necessary to follow agency guidelines in developing the budget and this requirement allows one to seek assistance early in the developmental process. It is important to remember that developing the budget is another interrelated process where one must fit the scope of the project into a finite amount of available funding. It is also important to keep in mind the need to write a clear justification for each category of budgetary expense as the budget process develops (Ward, 2006, pp. 15–19).

Simplify the budgeting process. What is recommended is to simplify the budgeting process by following the agency's budgeting instructions; making the budget consistent with the narrative; providing an adequate justification for all expense categories; consulting with the internal budgeting units; using the appropriate facility rates; thoroughly checking all calculations; avoiding any inflation in the budget (*do not inflate the budget*); and recognizing the need for and seeking out assistance as often as needed (get help).

Future funding. If this is a multi-year project, be sure to project your budget accurately over the stated project period and include the appropriate justifications for each project budget year. The calculations should anticipate any cost-of-living adjustments permitted by the agency's guidelines and remain within the framework of the customary and usual budgetary plans of the institution or agency.

6. Appendices. This section of the proposal should contain additional items and pieces of information that support the proposal and often includes the following items: support letters; resumes or job descriptions; and survey items and/or questionnaires.

These miscellaneous items are important in showing the programmatic capability of the applicant organization. Remember that any information that is critical to understanding the proposal should be in the proposal, such as organizational charts, examples of previous work, et cetera. These items should not be in the appendix unless the guidelines provide instructions to place them there.

Conclusion

Developing and writing successful proposals to address the amelioration or elimination of health disparities can be enhanced by the inclusion of community partners and by using a community-based approach to develop the problem definition, the statement of need, and the creation of the interventions, processes, or products. Forming and sustaining partnerships require a substantial investment of time and hard work, mutual trust and vision, and a willingness to take risks. Community-based participatory research appears to offer an ideal theoretical and practical approach to utilize in developing collaborative proposals focused on the elimination of health disparities as well as other population focused initiatives. Academic and community-based partnerships in themselves confer an intrinsic value to these collaborative arrangements and reinforce the expectation that each unit brings its very best resources to the relationship. The development of successful proposals focused on health disparities in most instances requires the involvement and participation of a diverse and multidisciplinary group of academic and professional individuals, and community representatives from different kinds of organizations that all share a mission to eliminate health disparities. This form of collaboration in itself requires many of the same attributes required to develop a winning proposal: tenacity, commitment, and a willingness to leverage resources to combat pervasive and long-standing community health issues. Goethe said it best:

Knowing is not enough; we must apply.
Willing is not enough; we must do.

REFERENCES

Alexander, J. A., Weiner, B. J., Metzger, M. E., Shortell, S. M., Bazzoli, G. J., Hasnain-Wynia, R., et al. (2003). Sustainability of collaborative capacity in community health partnerships. *Medical Care Research and Review*, *60*(4) (Supplement), 130S–160S.

Allison, D., Kauper-Brown, J., & Seifer, S. D. (2005). *Community-engaged scholarship toolkit*. Seattle: Community–Campus Partnerships for Health. Retrieved from http://www.communityengaged scholarship.info

Blumenthal, D. S., & DiClemente, R. J. (Eds.). (2004). *Community-based health research*. New York: Springer Publishing.

Blumenthal, D. S., & Yancey, Y. (2004). *Community-based research: An introduction*. In D. S. Blumenthal & R. J. DiClemente (Eds.), *Community-based health research*. New York: Springer Publishing.

Braithwaite, R. L., & Lythcott, N. (1989). Community empowerment as a strategy for health promotion for black and other minority populations. *Journal of the American Medical Association*, *261*, 282–283.

Byrd, W. M., & Clayton, L. A. (2000). *An American health dilemma: A medical history of African Americans and the problem of race: Beginnings to 1900* (Vol. 1). New York: Routledge.

Byrd, W. M., & Clayton, L. A. (2002). *An American health dilemma: Race, medicine, and health care in the United States, 1900–2000* (Vol. 2). New York: Routledge.

Carter-Pokras, O., & Baquet, C. (2002). What is a "health disparity"? *Public Health Reports*, *17*, 426–434.

Cottrell, R., Davis, W., Schlaff, A., Liburd, L., Orenstein, D., & Presley-Cantrell, L. (1996). *Promoting healthy lifestyles in inner-city minority communities*. Atlanta, GA: Centers for Disease Control and Prevention.

Cuca, J. M., & McLoughlin, W. J. (1987). Why clinical research grant applications fare poorly in review and how to recover. *Cancer Investigation*, *5*(1), 55–58.

Easterling, D. V., Gallagher, K. M., & Lodwick, D. G. (2003). What do the case studies say about community-based health promotion? In D. Easterling, K. Gallagher, & D. Lodwick (Eds.), *Promoting health at the community level*. Thousand Oaks, CA: Sage.

Evans, C. (2004). Assessing and applying community-based research. In D. S. Blumenthal & R. J. DiClemente (Eds.), *Community-based health research*. New York: Springer Publishing.

Glanz, K., Lewis, F. M., & Rimer, B. K. (2000). *Health behavior and health education: Theory, research, and practice*. San Francisco: Jossey-Bass.

Gordon, S. L. (1988). Obtaining grant funding for clinical research. In R. Fitzgerald, Jr. (Ed.), *Noncemented total hip arthroplast*. New York: Raven Press.

Gordon, S. L. (1989). Ingredients of a successful grant application to the National Institutes of Health. *Journal of Orthopaedic Research, 7,* 138–141.

Hall, M. (1998). Developing the idea: A model for proposal development. In M. Hall, *Getting funded: A complete guide to proposal writing*. Portland, OR: Continuing Education Publications, Portland State University.

Israel, B. A., Schulz, A. J., Parker, E. A., Becker, A. B., Allen, A. J., & Guzman, J. R. (2003). Critical issues in developing and following community based participatory research principles. In M. Minkler & N. Wallerstein (Eds.), *Community-based participatory research for health*. San Francisco: Jossey-Bass.

Kraicer, J. (1997). *The art of grantsmanship*. Retrieved June 11, 2006, from http://www.hfsp.org/how/content.htm

Lauffer, A. (1997). *Grants, etc.* (2nd ed.). Thousand Oaks, CA: Sage.

Locke, L. L., Spirduso, W. W., & Silverman, S. J. (2000). *Proposals that work* (4th ed.). Thousand Oaks, CA: Sage.

Miner, J. T., & Miner, L. E. (2005). *Models of proposal planning & writing*. Westport, CT: Praeger.

Minkler, M., & Wallerstein, N. (Eds.). (2003). *Community based participatory research for health*. San Francisco: Jossey Bass.

National Institutes of Health (NIH), Division of Research Grants. (1995). *Helpful hints: Preparing an NIH research grant application*. Bethesda, MD: National Institutes of Health.

O'Fallon, L., Tyson, F., & Dearry, A. (Eds.). (2000). *Successful models of community based participatory research*. Research Triangle Park, NC: National Institute of Environmental Health Sciences.

Reif-Lehrer, L. (2005). *Grant application writer's handbook* (4th ed.). Sudbury, MA: Jones and Bartlett.

Satcher, D., & Rust, G. (2006). Achieving health equity in America. *Ethnicity & Disease, 16*(suppl 3), 8–13.

Smedley, B. D., & Syme, L. (Eds.). (2000). *Promoting health intervention strategies from social and behavioral research*. Washington, DC: Institute of Medicine, National Academies Press.

Syme, S. L. (2004). Social determinants of health: The community as an empowered partner. *Preventing Chronic Disease* [serial online]. Retrieved January 18, 2005, from http://www.cdc.gov/pcd/issues/2004/jan/03_0001.htm

Thompson-Reid, P. (1992). *Coalition building guide*. Atlanta, GA: Health Promotion Resource Center.

U.S. Department of Health and Human Services, National Institutes of Health. (2006). *Strategic research plan to reduce and ultimately eliminate health disparities. Fiscal years 2002–2006*. Retrieved from http://www.nih.gov/about/hd/strategicplan.pdf

U.S. Environmental Protection Agency. (n.d.). *Tips on writing a grant proposal*. Retrieved from http://www.epa.gov/ogd/recipient/tips.htm

Vishwanathan, M., Ammerman, A., Eng, E., Gartlehner, G., Lohr, K., Griggith, D., et al. (Eds.). (2004). *Community based participatory research: Assessing the evidence*. Rockville, MD: Agency for Healthcare Research and Quality.

Ward, D. (Ed.). (2006). *Writing grant proposals that win* (3rd. ed.). Sudbury, MA: Jones and Bartlett.

Yancey, A. K., Kumanyika, S. K., Ponce, N. A., McCarthy, W. J., Fielding, J. E., Leslie, J. P., et al. (2004). Population-based interventions engaging communities of color in healthy eating and active living: A review. *Preventing Chronic Disease*. Retrieved February 1, 2005, from http://www.cdc.gov/pcd/issues/2004/jan/yancey.htm

Addressing Cardiovascular Health Disparities of Chinese Immigrants in New York City: A Case Study of the Chinese-American Healthy Heart Coalition

Kenny Kwong,
Henrietta Ho-Asjoe,
Waiwah Chung,
and Sally Sukman Wong

Cardiovascular Health Disparities

The American Heart Association (AHA) defines cardiovascular disease (CVD) as a broad term for diseases of the heart and blood vessels, the most common forms of which are coronary heart disease (CHD) and stroke (AHA, 2005). In 2002 approximately seventy million Americans had one or more forms of CVD (AHA, 2005). Of these, about sixty-five million (93%) died from high blood pressure, thirteen million (18.5%) from CHD, and 5.4 million (7.7%) from stroke. CHD and stroke are the first and third leading causes of death among Asian Americans and Pacific Islanders (AAPIs) in the United States over the age of 65 (CDC, 2001). In New York State, CVD is the leading killer among both men and women and across all racial and ethnic groups. In 2002, more than 67,700 New Yorkers died of cardiovascular disease, accounting for 43% of all deaths. New York State ranks first in the Nation in deaths due to ischemic heart disease. However, New York State vital statistics did not designate AAPIs as a racial or ethnic group; thus prevalence data of heart disease in these populations is unknown.

Previous national surveys of hypertension conducted in the United States did not disaggregate AAPIs, a population already with limited CVD prevalence data, into subgroups such as Chinese Americans. Stroke is the only leading cause of death for which Asian American men experience higher mortality rates than White men (Louie, 2001). Although national data showed a declining trend of stroke mortality, the rate of decrease for AAPIs lagged behind those for Whites and Blacks

(Mensah, Mokdad, Ford, Greenlund, & Croft, 2005). In fact, AAPIs tended to have lower heart disease death rates in all age groups but higher stroke death rates, particularly at younger ages (Mensah et al., 2005). A cross-sectional study using data of 11,684 Asian Americans in Northern California from 1978 to 1985 found that 18.3% of the 5,951 Chinese Americans were hypertensive (Angel, Armstrong, & Klatsky, 1989; Klatsky & Armstrong, 1991). A more recent cross-sectional study of 708 Chinese Americans in San Francisco, CA, revealed that 489 (69%) participants had hypertension (Lau et al., 2005). Of these participants with hypertension, only 41% reported taking hypertensive medications and 64% reported following a low-salt diet regimen (Lau et al., 2005). A cross-sectional study in Boston, MA examined the prevalence of cardiovascular risk factors of 246 Chinese American elders and found that the characteristics of cardiovascular risk factors highly resembled those of urban settings in mainland China, where hemorrhagic stroke is the major cause of cardiovascular mortality (Choi et al., 1990).

A national cross-sectional study, the *Multi-Ethnic Study of Atherosclerosis* (MESA), recruited 6,814 men and women age 45 to 85 from 6 different U.S. communities and found that 39% of the 803 Chinese Americans were found to be hypertensive, compared to 38% in whites (Kramer et al., 2004). This study found that Chinese ethnicity was associated with a 42% higher odds of hypertension compared with whites and further indicated that the percentage of treated but uncontrolled hypertension among Chinese was 33%, compared to 24% among Whites, 32% among Hispanics, and 35% among African Americans (Kramer et al., 2004). These results suggested that Chinese Americans, along with Hispanics and African Americans, are subject to significant disparities in the control of hypertension in the United States.

Cardiovascular Disease Risk Factors

In 2005, the AHA determined age, gender, race, ethnicity, and heredity to be non-modifiable risk factors for CVD, and are useful in identifying high-risk groups. Modifiable risk factors include high blood cholesterol, high blood pressure, diabetes mellitus, obesity, poor dietary habits, physical inactivity, and cigarette smoking; these are factors that can be treated or controlled by lifestyle change or medications. These risk factors were established from research conducted in the West; therefore they may not be directly translatable to AAPIs. Kandula and Lauderdale (2005) found that the longer Asian Americans live in the United States, the higher their risk for CVD. However, little is known about the pathway through which modifiable risk factors such as diet and physical activity change after AAPIs immigrate to the United States.

Overweight and Obesity for Chinese Americans

A case-control study of individuals suffering from Acute Myocardial Infarction (AMI) in Hong Kong indicates that conventional CVD risk factors are important among the Chinese population (Donnan et al., 1994). Nevertheless, the thresholds established in the West may not be directly applicable to Chinese and Chinese-Americans. The following discussion on obesity demonstrates this point.

Overweight and obesity have been shown to play an important role in the clustering of cardiovascular disease risk factors in western populations (Hubert, Feinleib, McNamara, & Castelli, 1983). According to the World Health Organization, overweight is defined as BMI ≥ 25; and central adiposity defined as waist circumference ≥94 cm (37 in) for men and ≥ 80 cm (31.5 in) for women. However, body composition of Asians is different from other ethnic populations (Dhiman, Duseja, & Chawla, 2005). The average BMI values and the rates of overweight and obesity in the Chinese population are reportedly much lower than those in western populations when based on the western definition of overweight and obesity. In a prospective cohort study, Zhou and colleagues (2002) monitored 100,000 individuals in China from 1991 to 1995 to assess their incidence of stroke attacks, coronary heart disease, and all causes of death. The data revealed that the cohort had a relatively low mean body mass index (BMI), with an average of 19.7 to 23.6 for men and 19.5 to 24.3 for women at the baseline measurement. Yet, BMI was still found to be an independent risk factor for the incidence of both CHD and stroke, and not mediated by age, gender, blood pressure, serum total cholesterol, smoking, and alcohol drinking (Zhou et al., 2002). Furthermore, a cross-sectional study of 15,838 randomly selected individuals in China also found that BMI and waist circumference were independently associated with CVD risk factors in Chinese adults (Wildman et al., 2005). Similarly, although the mean serum cholesterol level among Chinese is low by western standards, low levels of serum cholesterol have still been shown to have a direct, continuous relationship to coronary heart disease mortality (Chen et al., 1991).

Several epidemiologic studies of Asian populations have shown that Asians have higher amount of body fat at lower BMIs and waist circumferences than do Western populations (Deurenberg, Yap, & van Staveren, 1998). Several studies have suggested a BMI cutoff of 22 to 24 for Asian men and women and a waist circumference cutoff near 75–80 cm for Asian women and 80–85 cm for Asian men (Ko, Chan, Cockram, & Woo, 1999; Zhou et al., 2002). Using a nationally representative sample in China, Wildman and colleagues (2005) found that of the 15,838 randomly selected individuals, a BMI value of 24 and a waist circumference value of 80 cm in both men and women were appropriate for use in the identification of high cardiovascular risk Chinese patients. In a cross-sectional study of 1,513 Chinese individuals living in Hong Kong, Ko and colleagues (1999) found that the risk of diabetes, hypertension, dyslipidemia, and albuminuria starts increasing at a BMI of about 23 (Ko et al., 1999). In addition, the same report suggested that the optimal BMI cutoff point to predict hypertension in Hong Kong Chinese is 23.8 among men and 24.1 for women; for dyslipidemia is 23.0 among men and 24.1 for women; and for type 2 diabetes among men is 24.3 and 23.2 for women (Ko et al., 1999). As a result, the Western Pacific regional office of the World Health Organization (WHO), the International Association for the Study of Obesity (IASO), and the International Obesity Task Force (IOTF) collaborated in establishing new definition and recommendations for BMI and waist circumference cutoffs among Asian populations (Wildman et al., 2005). Under these new recommendations, overweight is defined as a BMI ≥23, and the suggested waist circumference cutoffs are 90 cm (35.4 in) for men and 80 cm (31.5 in) for women (World Health Organization, 2000). These redefinitions are extremely important for health professionals working with Asian American communities in identifying those who may be at risk of developing cardiovascular disease and other chronic health conditions. In summary, all of the above studies indicated that uncontrolled hypertension and stroke are a major disease burden among Chinese Americans in the United States.

Chinese individuals with relatively low serum cholesterol levels are still at risk of developing coronary heart disease. Chinese with a lower BMI and waist circumference cutoffs can be overweight, thus attributing to a higher risk of developing cardiovascular disease and other health conditions.

Increased Risk Due to Acculturation and Dietary Changes

Dietary acculturation is defined as the process that occurs when members of a minority or immigrant group adopt the eating patterns/food choices of the host country (Chavez, Sha, Persky, Langenberg, & Pestano-Binghay, 1994; Satia-Abouta, Patterson, Neuhouser, & Elder, 2002). Chinese immigrants in the United States tend to adopt Western dietary patterns while maintaining traditional Chinese eating habits, rather than rejecting one of them (Nan & Cason, 2004). Changes toward a western-type diet or lifestyle have been found to increase the risk of many lifestyle chronic diseases, such as obesity, hypertension, diabetes mellitus, cardiovascular diseases, and cancers among immigrants (Satia-Abouta et al., 2002). Compared to Chinese living in Asia, those living in the United States have high rates of chronic disease attributable to poor diet and health (Campbell, Parpia, & Chen, 1998; LeMarchand, Wilkens, Kolonel, Hankin, & Lyu, 1997). The increased access to new food supplies resulting from acculturation has been associated with shifts from traditional diets of vegetables, meats, and whole grains to increased consumption of meat, fats, sweets, and highly processed foods by Chinese American immigrants (Nan & Cason, 2004; Satia-Abouta et al., 2002; Unger, Reynolds, Shakib, Spruijt-Metz, Sun, & Johnson, 2004). Some studies also cited that the number of meals and portion of meals greatly increase after immigration to the United States. For example, more than half (62%) of the 71 Asian American immigrant college students reported weight gain after immigrating to the United States, accompanied by a significant increases in the consumption of fats, sweets, and dairy products, and significant drop in the amount of vegetables consumed (Pan, Dixon, Himburg, & Huffman, 1999).

Barriers to Screening and Health Education Among Chinese Americans

Despite these health concerns, many Chinese Americans are underserved and face culturally specific barriers to health care access for early diagnosis and comprehensive treatments for CVD. One major barrier is the lack of financial resources among Chinese immigrants. According to the 2000 Census, AAPIs are more likely to live at or below 100% of the federal poverty level (22%) than the total population (20%). Since 1970, the Chinese population has increased by 300% according to the 2000 U.S. Census. Among AAPIs living in New York City, the Chinese population is the largest subgroup. It is estimated over 360,000; approximately 45% of AAPIs living in New York City are Chinese. Chinese immigrants are also more likely than other ethnic minority groups to experience language barriers. In the large Chinese immigrant enclaves of Manhattan, Brooklyn, and Queens, 50% of Chinese immigrants were found to have limited English proficiency compared to 22% overall in the same neighborhoods. Thirdly, AAPIs are considered to be at the highest risk for not receiving medical care (NYC DOHMH, 2003). Data show that 24% of AAPI New Yorkers lack health insurance coverage and only 11% are enrolled in public insurance programs and nearly 20% of AAPI New Yorkers reported that they could not obtain medical care when needed compared to 11% for whites (NYC DOHMH, 2003). Uninsured individuals are also less likely to have their own primary care physicians. As a result of these barriers to care, many Chinese immigrants have limited health literacy and self-management capability, and are unlikely to receive preventive health care such as routine checkups and screening. These consequences pose significant challenge to the management of chronic diseases such as CVD.

Promoting cardiovascular health education and improving access to screening services for early detection of hypertension and heart disease among Chinese Americans are becoming pressing clinical and public health issues. Bilingual health education and health care services, while helpful, do not do enough to close this gap. To close this gap, health care organizations must utilize a community-wide multipronged integrated approach to providing culturally competent and linguistically appropriate health education and health care services for medically underserved Chinese immigrants.

The purpose of this chapter is to present a case study of the Chinese-American Healthy Heart Coalition (Healthy Heart Coalition) and to discuss the innovative strategies used by the Healthy Heart Coalition in addressing cardiovascular diseases among Chinese Americans in New York City. In addition, discussion covers the process involved in capacity building, sustaining and managing a coalition, as well as lessons learned through this collaborative venture.

Addressing Health Disparity—Shifting Focus From Individuals to Community

While it is necessary to learn the behavioral, psychosocial, and economic pathways by which poverty may affect the health outcomes at the individual level, stress and material deprivation in poor families [and communities] originated from the inequality of income, wealth, and resources, and from the decline of social capital at the neighborhood level (Kaplan, Pamuk, Lynch, Cohen, & Balfour, 1996). Income inequality at a neighborhood or society level, indicating dispersion or distribution of income, wealth, or resources across individuals in a group, is conceptualized as a characteristic of a group or society (Kaplan et al., 1996), and has been found to be associated with community-level health outcomes (Kaplan et al., 1996; Kennedy, Kawachi, & Prothrow-Smith, 1996; Lynch et al., 1998).

The Framework: Social Capital and Asset-Based Approach

Social capital is defined by Putnam (2000) as features of the social structure, such as levels of interpersonal trust, norms of reciprocity, and mutual aid, which act as resources for individuals and facilitate collective action, mutual support, and community empowerment. Social cohesion and social capital are both collective (neighborhood or community-level) dimensions of a society, and should be distinguished from the concept of social networks and social support, which are characteristically measured at the level of the individual (Kawachi & Berkman, 2003). The use of asset-based community development intervention approach (Kretzmann & McKnight, 1993) alleviates health outcome disparities by increasing social capital and strengthening the scope of influence, resources, and assets of poor and medically underserved neighborhoods to address health disparity, ultimately altering social milieu or economic position at a community level. Such an approach is based on the assumption that a community cannot be rebuilt by focusing on the individual members' needs, problems, and deficiencies. Rather, community building starts with the process of locating the resources, assets, skills, and capacities of residents, citizens' associations, and local institutions.

Formation of the Chinese-American Healthy Heart Coalition

In response to the emerging needs for evidence-based, culturally appropriate interventions to decrease CVD disparities among the Chinese Americans, leaders from health care organizations, academic institutions, social service agencies, private business groups, and community health centers envisioned a community-based coalition using the asset-based community development approach to address these disparities in the community. In 2000, the Charles B. Wang Community Heath Center, the lead agency of the Coalition, received a grant from the New York State Department of Health Minority Health Community Partnerships to plan, coordinate, and implement all of the coalition's activities to promote heart health and address risk factors on both the individual and community levels. Other agencies that formed the initial core of Healthy Heart Coalition included New York Downtown Hospital Chinese Community Partnership of Health, Chinese American Planning Council, and a community cardiologist who also represents the Chinese American Medical Society and American Heart Association.

Although members of the Healthy Heart Coalition came from widely different sectors, they were unified by the common interest and desire to improve the cardiovascular health and quality of life of Chinese Americans residing in the New York City metropolitan area. In fact, the establishment of the Coalition enabled the health care organizations, health plans, social service organizations, businesses, mass media, other interest groups, and most importantly, the Chinatown community, to work together under one umbrella, integrating efforts and creating a synergy of purpose. As a result, the Coalition is able to ensure a full-range of capacity to accomplish its ambitious goals.

The primary goal of the Healthy Heart Coalition is to develop and implement a comprehensive, culturally, and linguistically appropriate community-based intervention to increase the awareness of CVD, and its risk factors and comorbidities. The Coalition also aims to promote hearth-healthy lifestyles and practices among low-income, medically underserved Chinese Americans in New York City. Several partnering organizations in the beginning phase of the Coalition received training on coalition development, the asset-based community development model, and program evaluation from the New York State Department of Health's Office of Minority Health. Coalition members agreed to embrace the following key concepts of the asset-based community development model (Kretzmann & McKnight, 1993): (1) *coalition-driven*: coalition members participated in defining and developing the coalition's mission, goals and objectives, roles and responsibilities, recruitment and communication strategies, and program planning and implementation; (2) *asset-based*: coalitions engaged local individuals, associations, and institutions in program planning, implementation, and communication strategies; and (3) *neighborhood-specific*: a variety of community sectors including local residents were involved in designing programs that were built on the strengths and resources of the community.

An Asset-Based Community Development Approach

In late 2000, the Chinese-American Healthy Heart Coalition conducted asset mapping, an innovative method to identify local resources rather than the needs of individuals and groups in the Chinese community, and developed an inventory of local and community assets. The asset-based approach enabled the Coalition to visualize its overall needs, and expanded its resources and scope of influence by leveraging various aspects of the Chinese-American community's social capital. Aspects of *social capital* can be categorized as individual, group, associational, and institutional capital (Putnam, 2000). In the case of the Healthy Heart Coalition, its individual capital includes professional health care staff and volunteers, materials, equipment, promotional items, facilities, and the member organizations' extensive personal networks with individuals of the Chinese community. Group capital includes the media, pharmaceutical and business groups, and faith-based groups and churches. Associational capital involves neighborhood and civic associations such as the Chinese Consolidated Benevolent Association. Institutional capital includes major hospitals and health programs, training institutes such as the Center of the Study of Asian American Health of NYU School of Medicine, Chinese American Medical Society, and national organizations such as the American Heart Association and the National Diabetes Education Program.

The essence of the asset-based approach is to rebuild social capital in poor Chinese neighborhoods by elevating the levels of interpersonal and organizational trust and establishing the norms of reciprocity and mutual support among these individuals and organizations. Since 2000, this approach has led to a rapid expansion of community resources and assets for individuals, groups, and community in addressing cardiovascular health disparity in the Chinese American community. As of 2006, the Healthy Heart Coalition has grown from 4 partner agencies at inception to a collaboration of more than 30 organization members from different sectors including health care, academic, social services, civic associations, neighborhood businesses, and ethnic-specific media.

Development of Multipronged Interventions at Individual, Group, and Community Levels

By utilizing different aspects of social capital, the Coalition designed and implemented a number of unique and innovative interventions and programs to address cardiovascular health issues in the community. The focus of these initiatives ranged from lifestyle habits, such as diet and physical activity, to specific diseases that especially affect the Chinese American community, including CVD. In addition, the Coalition tackled socio-economic and cultural barriers, including the community's lack of access to low-cost health services and culturally relevant education. In the 6 years since its inception, the Healthy Heart Coalition's initiatives have encompassed the following objectives: (1) to increase access to comprehensive health screenings for the detection of cardiovascular disease risk factors; (2) to increase knowledge and awareness of cardiovascular disease and risk factors through community education and ethnic-specific media campaigns; (3) to improve the Chinese

American community's awareness and ability to respond to cardiac emergencies through the "CPR for Family and Friend" program; and (4) to launch a healthy eating campaign to increase the ability of Chinese individuals to maintain healthy lifestyle habits.

Improving Access to Preventive Care: Community Health Screenings

Without access to culturally and linguistically competent clinical services and preventive health screening, educational efforts would be insufficient to bridge the gap between health knowledge and actual behavior change. Therefore, appropriate screenings and referrals are key components in the Healthy Heart Coalition programs. Since 2001, Coalition partners including New York Downtown Hospital, Bellevue Hospital Center, Charles B. Wang Community Health Center, and Pfizer, Inc., have pooled resources and provided free screening for blood cholesterol, blood pressure, blood glucose, and body mass index (BMI) to more than 500 community residents each year at health fairs and via a community outreach vehicle that particularly targeted the elderly and those at high-risk for CVD. Screenings took place at locations that had the most direct and extensive reach to the target population, and were accompanied by individual health education, clinical consultation, and referrals. Participants with abnormal screening results were followed up with phone calls to ensure that they seek proper health care and additional health services. These collaborative efforts through the Coalition not only successfully provided preventive services to a large number of Chinese Americans who otherwise might not have received them, but also was effective in conveying the importance of early detection and screening to the community as a whole.

Increasing Knowledge of CVD: Community Education and Media Campaigns

The Coalition launched education and media campaigns that were aimed to increase community residents' knowledge related to heart health, and to promote behaviors that would lower their risk for heart disease and cardiac-related morbidity and mortality. To maximize reach, these campaigns took place through various venues. Coalition partners conducted multisession educational workshops, community health forums at senior centers, social agencies, and business organizations, and distributed health education materials and resources at community health and street fairs to promote public awareness of heart-healthy lifestyles and habits. The printed education materials were bilingual in both Chinese and English, and were developed according to health literacy principles to ensure cultural relevance and linguistic appropriateness. Workshops, presentations, and seminars were conducted in Mandarin Chinese or Cantonese depending on the audience, and incorporated culturally suitable curricular and information. Discussions on diet and nutrition focused on Chinese foods and ingredients so that information was culturally relevant to the community. Between 2000 and 2005, more than 260 Chinese individuals who were at risk for cardiovascular disease and stroke attended these multisession workshops.

A half-day symposium on "Take Heart: Prevention, Education and Action," targeting health care professionals, academics, community leaders, media representatives, and other concerned individuals, was conducted in the spring of 2006. The objectives of the symposium were (1) to educate professionals on the modifiable risk factors related to CVD among Asian Americans, as well as culturally competent, model intervention programs; (2) to engage the target audience in the development of community level, multipronged strategies that address the underlying causes of CVD such as access to care, nutrition, physical activity, and community education; and (3) to expand community support for the Chinese-American Healthy Heart Coalition activities and recruit new members to the Coalition. The conference included presentations on innovative programs and research on effective interventions pertaining to CVD among Chinese and Asian Americans. Speakers were health care professionals and representatives from community, business, and media sectors.

In addition to the educational activities discussed above, one of the greatest accomplishments of the Coalition was to launch a culturally tailored media campaign employing a regular Chinese call-in radio program. This monthly radio program was hosted by experts in the health care field and addressed cardiovascular issues that were specific to the Chinese American community. Community members were encouraged to call in to the radio program and speak directly with the health care providers and specialists about their concerns. These interactive radio programs proved successful and well received in the Chinese American community. From 2000 to 2005, the Healthy Heart Coalition conducted 52 call-in or taped radio programs on several major Chinese radio stations. During the same period, the coalition also convened several press conferences and published over 50 news articles and stories on risk factors for heart diseases and diabetes, and the importance of adopting healthy lifestyles in preventing the onset of diabetes and heart disease.

Improving Response to Cardiac Emergencies: CPR for Family and Friends

According to the AHA, cardiovascular disease and sudden cardiac arrest claim the lives of 335,000 Americans each year before they have a chance to reach a hospital. About 80% of these cardiac arrests occur at home and are witnessed by a family member. Currently the survival rate of cardiac arrest victims is less than 5%. Cardiopulmonary resuscitation (CPR) can double a victim's chance of survival. Therefore, it is important for family members to learn CPR so that they are empowered and prepared to help their loved ones and neighbors during cardiac emergencies.

For the prevention of cardiovascular disease-related morbidity and mortality, the Coalition recognized the importance of training community residents on how to handle cardiac emergencies. Together with local partners such as the American Heart Association's Operation Heart Beat Committee and the Chinese Community Social Service and Health Council, several Coalition members developed a curriculum to educate and train the Chinese American community, health care professionals, and community leaders on the symptoms and early detection of stroke and heart attack, how to call 911, and how to conduct CPR and early defibrillation. Also, the Coalition sponsored a seminar titled the *American Heartsaver Day*: *What You Need to Know to be Heart Healthy* in 2002. Topics covered in the symposium included the prevention of heart disease, heart attack, and the importance of emergency care, and hundreds of community members and health professionals attended the event. Attendance was overwhelming, and these seminars and CPR trainings, conducted in Chinese (both Cantonese and Mandarin), were so well received by the community that demands for additional sessions continued for a long time.

This was a clear indication that the Chinese American community was keenly aware of the potential dangers of cardiac emergencies, and recognized the need for skill in the effectively handling of these emergency situations.

The "CPR for Family and Friends" program is geared toward laypersons who want to learn CPR but do not need the certification. This 2-hour course teaches the recognition and emergency resuscitation techniques used for heart attack, cardiac arrest, stroke, and choking in adults, and is available in both English and Spanish from AHA. With the generous support of AHA, the Healthy Heart Coalition translated and customized the program to meet the language and cultural needs, and offered the Chinese version of "CPR Family and Friends" program to the Chinese community. From 2000 to 2005, the program successfully trained over 180 community members, although not without obstacles. Recruitment and training of bilingual CPR instructors was difficult due to extensive time commitment. Translation of the original CPR course materials, both in printed and video formats, from English into Chinese proved more laborious and time-consuming than anticipated, and took more than a year to produce (longer than expected).

Improving Eating Habits: The Healthy Eating Campaign

The Healthy Eating Campaign began with a 1-year pilot project funded by the Bristol-Myers-Squibb Foundation in 2004 called "You Are What You Eat." The goal of the pilot project was to increase the availability of healthy food choices locally, and to promote hearth-healthy habits such as proper nutrition and physical activity. As part of this project, the Coalition organized a series of community forums and workshops for at-risk seniors to improve knowledge and self-efficacy related to heart health. In addition, the Coalition formed working partnerships with senior-serving organizations to provide supportive environments that enable healthy eating, physical activity, and active living. The Healthy Heart Coalition also collaborated with the Sweet-N-Tart Restaurant and the Golden Carriage Bakery in New York City during this pilot project to provide low-fat, low-cholesterol, low-sodium, and high-fiber food products for the community.

A registered dietitian (RD) from the Coalition worked with the restaurant and bakery to modify their menus and provide healthy alternatives to health-conscious customers or those with specific dietary requirements. Using information on ingredients and cooking instructions provided by these vendors, the RD determined the nutrition profiles, and presented the serving size, nutrient content per serving, and percent daily values of each food product in the standardized format used by the Food and Drug Administration. By making nutrition information readily available in pamphlets to consumers, community members were empowered to choose food that would meet their specific dietary needs.

In addition, an RD provided on-site nutrition education classes for restaurant and bakery employees on heart-healthy cooking methods, recipe modifications, and ways to promote healthy eating. Restaurants were encouraged to provide nutrition and food preparation information voluntarily and offer patrons the flexibility to customize food choices based on their needs and preferences. Follow-up evaluations conducted with participating restaurants and bakeries revealed that this pilot project greatly increased the availability of healthy food choices in the New York City Chinatown area. The success of this pilot intervention helped mobilize the community to increase demand for healthier food alternatives, resulting in the inclusion of heart-healthy food items in the menus of more local restaurants and bakeries.

The initial success of the pilot project led to the award of a 3-year grant from the Office of Minority Health of the U.S. Department of Health and Human Services in 2004. The Healthy Heart Coalition used the additional funds to expand the pilot and outreach to more restaurants and bakeries in the New York City region. As in the pilot phase, an RD and a health educator provided on-site basic nutrition education at eateries, constructed the Chinese Food Guide Pyramid, taught heart-healthy cooking tips, and offered technical support to all participating restaurant and bakery employees. Bilingual pamphlets with heart-healthy cooking tips were also developed and disseminated to food vendors and community members interested in heart-healthy cooking. Currently, 2 years into the grant period, the Campaign has 7 participating eateries (3 restaurants and 4 bakeries), and is expected to expand to more food vendors in the New York City region. This continuous partnership, by allowing the Coalition to create an enabling environment, proves to be a crucial factor in the success of the Healthy Eating Campaign.

Lessons Learned From Partnership Building and Coalition Development

Coalitions and partnerships are frequently used as a tool to promote community health issues and concerns (Wandersman, Goodman, & Butterfoss, 1999; Kass & Freudenberg, 1999). Coalition building emphasizes coordination and collaboration, and the elimination of competition and redundancy of community resources (Wandersman et al., 1999). Since its establishment, the Healthy Heart Coalition strived to develop and sustain strong partnerships by building upon community assets and utilizing the strengths of its community social network. It also endeavored to provide opportunities for individuals and/or organizations to get involved and stay connected, and to have a direct impact on their own community. All the cardiovascular health initiatives led by the Healthy Heart Coalition also aimed to improve engagement and increase contribution by all partners in the Coalition's planning and implementation. Each subsequent initiative also strengthened the Coalition's administrative processes, improved communication among partners, helped bolster community assets by providing training opportunities for professionals as well as residents, and gave a floor for social networking and support. The extensive collaboration illustrated by the Healthy Eating Campaign was an excellent example of the participation of its broad and diverse members who actively planned and worked with different eateries in the community.

A number of management challenges arose from the rapid growth and expansion of the Healthy Heart coalition over the past 6 years. The transition into a more diverse, inclusive, and participatory organizational structure changed the partnership dynamics, resulting in different points of view among partners on the definition, structure, and priority of the Coalition, as well as the roles and functions of the partners and of the lead agency. Several Coalition members demanded increased recognition and acknowledgement, more transparency in the decision-making process, and more direct involvement in Coalition management and future initiatives. To address these issues, key staff members from the lead agency met individually with core Coalition partners to define their level of involvement and to discuss ways to foster collaboration. The process was further formalized with the creation of a Steering Committee. The Steering Committee, consisting of core members, was convened to provide overall direction and management of the coalition; to develop strategic plans; to seek grant funding opportunities; and to oversee and recruit new partners. Efforts were made to clearly differentiate the roles of the lead agency and key partners to help manage tensions and competition among partners as they arose. The core partners were asked to rotate as the facilitator at both Coalition general membership and steering committee meetings, resulting in increased ownership and leadership shared among core partners. To strengthen communication, monthly updates of the Coalition activities were disseminated to all members. Several members also initiated to post the Coalition activities and campaign materials in their Web sites.

The problems arising from a coalition of diverse partners and possible solutions can be further illustrated by our experience in launching the Healthy Eating Campaign. Chinatown restaurants tend to be small businesses with limited resources and an eye on making a profit, not necessarily on what's healthy for the community. Recruiting eateries to join the campaign and modify their products and business processes was extremely challenging due to the intense competition among them. To make matters worse, since 9/11, many small businesses, including eateries and restaurants in Chinatown, have not fully recovered from the economic recession. The economic condition has also worsened for restaurants in recent years due to sharp increases in rents and utility costs. Under these economic strains, many Chinatown restaurants have closed down or relocated. When approached by the Healthy Heart Coalition, some eatery owners expressed concerns about staying in business and were reluctant to commit their time and resources to this project, which they considered risky, labor-intensive, time-consuming, and yielding little financial return. Other bakeries and eateries indicated that they were "too busy" or did not have enough resources to participate in the campaign.

The Coalition devoted much time, energy and resources working with partner eateries on improving the supply side of the Healthy Eating Campaign, but the results were less than optimal. Besides, the resources needed from the Coalition to ensure that the eateries maintain the quality of their signature healthy food options made this effort unsustainable. Consequently, project staff began to shift the focus from improving supplies to increasing demand for healthy food options. The Coalition recently stepped up efforts in launching educational workshops and social marketing campaign to promote smarter food choices and healthy eating. It is our hope that, once the community-wide demand for heart-healthy food options has reached a critical level, it would be in the business interest of the food vendors in Chinatown to supply these healthy choices.

The Coalition and its lead agency recognized several challenges in the team-building process. Expectations and outcomes from members could be varied, especially in their operational understanding of the Coalition objectives and decision making. Coalition management can be time consuming and requires commitment to share leadership, resources, responsibilities, and credits for accomplishments. In the attempt to overcome some of the challenges, the Coalition developed a leadership work plan through the Steering Committee and encouraged community building through its partners for better opportunities to share resources and requests for funding.

Guiding Principles. To continue to build and sustain a diverse Coalition, the following principles were used to guide the coalition development process:

- Articulating a clear mission and vision for the coalition.
- Defining ways to foster collaboration among participating organizations.

- Conducting strategic outreach to seek resources and funding and membership development.
- Creating leadership opportunities for everyone that promote ownership and sharing of resources, responsibility, and recognitions for the coalition accomplishment.
- Establishing a structure and operating procedures that reinforce open and adequate communication.
- Increasing transparency in decision making process, and equity in sharing responsibility and resources.
- Setting ground rules that maintain a safe and supportive environment.
- Designing and engaging in activities that are responsive to the diverse needs of the Coalition, members, and the community.

Even though the Coalition continued to face challenges in managing organizational change and growth and sustaining partner involvement, several key accomplishments over the past 6 years are worth mentioning. The Coalition as a collective was able to reach diverse community members by providing services that were more cost-effective and coordinated than would be possible if offered by partners individually. The broad-based public support for cardiovascular health promotion was evident throughout all the initiatives especially the Healthy Eating Campaign and CPR for Family and Friends program. As a result, these initiatives received high levels of media attention and public profile. Building on its popularity and accomplishments, the Coalition positioned itself to attract additional funding and business sponsorships to support future intervention activities.

The asset-based community development approach presented major challenges during its implementation. In our case, Coalition members had varied service philosophy, agendas, interests, and levels of commitment. We may also have the tendency to conceive social capital as an unqualified social good (Woolcock, 1998), and the common downside of social capital includes the interlocking network of obligations, the inhibitions of individual expression, and the intrusion of individual autonomy. Nevertheless when social capital is optimized as evidenced by using the asset-based community development approach, these interventions can significantly enhance social capital and increase community assets and resources for a particular neighborhood. Ultimately they can alter the social milieu and economic position at a community or neighborhood level.

Summary

Partnerships among diverse community-based organizations including health care institutions, social service agencies, business sectors, and individuals have great potential for growth and create new venues to improve community and public health concerns in a community. The case study presented in this chapter illustrates the substantial resources, time, and effort required in forming such partnerships, and discusses the strategies that the Healthy Heart Coalition used to counter some of the major challenges. In true coalition building, there is no final destination to be reached, as the cultivation of partnerships does not end; nevertheless, the tremendous benefits to the community are well worth the effort.

REFERENCES

American Heart Association. (2005). *What are healthy levels of cholesterol?* Retrieved from http://www.americanheart.org/presenter.jhtml?identifier=183

Angel, A., Armstrong, M. A., & Klatsky, A. L. (1989). Blood pressure among Asian Americans living in Northern America. *American Journal of Cardiology, 64,* 237–240.

Campbell, T., Parpia, B., & Chen, J. (1998). Diet, lifestyle, and the etiology of coronary artery disease: The Cornell China study. *American Journal of Cardiology, 82,* 18T–21T.

Centers for Disease Control and Prevention. (2001). *Deaths, percent of total deaths, and death rates for the 15 leading causes of death in selected age groups, by race and sex: United States, 2001.* Retrieved April 18, 2005, from http://www.cdc.gov/nchs/data/dvs/LCWK3_2001.pdf

Chavez, N., Sha, L., Persky, V., Langenberg, P., & Pestano-Binghay, E. (1994). Effect of length of U.S. residence on food group intake in Mexican and Puerto Rican women. *Journal of Nutrition Education, 26*(2), 79–86.

Chen, Z., Peto, R., Collins, R., MacMahon, S., Lu, J., & Li, W. (1991). Serum cholesterol concentration and coronary heart disease in population with low cholesterol concentrations. *British Medical Journal, 303,* 276–282.

Choi, E. S., McGandy, R. B., Dallal, G. E., Russell, R. M., Jacob, R. A., Schaefer, E. J., et al. (1990). The prevalence of cardiovascular risk factors among elderly Chinese Americans. *Archives of Internal Medicine, 150*(2), 413–418.

Deurenberg, P., Yap, M., & van Staveren, W. (1998). Body mass index and percent body fat: A meta-analysis among different ethnic groups. *International Journal of Obesity Related Metabolic Disorder, 22,* 1164–1171.

Dhiman, R., Duseja, A., & Chawla, Y. (2005). Asians need different criteria for defining overweight and obesity. *Archives of Internal Medicine, 165*(9), 1069–1070.

Donnan, S., Ho, S., Woo, J., Wong, S., Woo, K., Tse, C., et al. (1994). Risk factors for acute myocardial infarction in a southern Chinese population. *Annals of Epidemiology, 4*(1), 46–58.

Hubert, H., Feinleib, M., McNamara, P., & Castelli, W. (1983). Obesity as an independent risk factor for cardiovascular disease: A 26-year follow-up of participants in the Framingham heart study. *Circulation, 67*(5), 968–977.

Kandula, N., & Lauderdale, D. (2005). Leisure time, non-leisure time, and occupational physical activity in Asian Americans. *Annals of Epidemiology, 15,* 257–265.

Kaplan, G., Pamuk, E., Lynch, J., Cohen, R., & Balfour, J. (1996). Income inequality and mortality in the United States: Analysis of mortality and potential pathways. *British Medical Journal, 312,* 999–1003.

Kass, D., & Freudenberg, N. (1999). Coalition building to prevent childhood lead poisoning: A case study from New York City. In M. Minkler (Ed.), *Community organizing & community building for health.* New Brunswick, NJ: Rutgers University Press.

Kawachi, I., & Berkman, L. (Eds.). (2003). *Neighborhoods and health.* New York: Oxford University Press.

Kennedy, B., Kawachi, I., & Prothrow-Stith, D. (1996). Income distribution and mortality: Cross-sectional ecologic study of the Robin Hood index in the U.S. *British Medical Journal, 312,* 1004–1007.

Klatsky, A., & Armstrong, M. (1991). Cardiovascular risk factors among Asian Americans living in northern California. *American Journal of Pubic Health, 81,* 1423–1428.

Ko, G., Chan, J., Cockram, C., & Woo, J. (1999). Prediction of hypertension, diabetes, dyslipidemia or albuminuria using simple anthropometric indexes in Hong Kong Chinese. *International Journal of Obesity Related Metabolic Disorder, 23*(11), 1136–1142.

Kramer, H., Han, C., Post, W., Goff, D., Diez-Roux, A., Cooper, R., et al. (2004). Racial/ethnic differences in hypertension and hypertension treatment and control in the multi-ethnic study of atherosclerosis (MESA). *American Journal of Hypertension, 17*(10), 963–970.

Kretzmann, J. P., & McKnight, J. L. (1993). *Building communities from the inside out: A path toward finding and mobilizing a community's assets.* Evanston, IL: Institute for Policy Research.

Lau, D., Lee, G., Wong, C., Fung, G., Cooper, B., & Mason, D. (2005). Characterization of systematic hypertension in the San Francisco Chinese community. *American Journal of Cardiology*, *96*(4), 570–573.

LeMarchand, L., Wilkens, L. R., Kolonel, L. H., Hankin, J. H., & Lyu, L. C. (1997). Association of sedentary lifestyle, obesity, smoking, alcohol use, and diabetes with the risk of colorectal cancer. *Cancer Research*, *57*, 4787–4794.

Louie, K. (2001). White paper on the health status of Asian Americans and Pacific Islanders and recommendations for research. *Nursing Outlook*, *49*(4), 173–178.

Lynch, J., Kaplan, G., Pamuk, E., Cohen, R., Heck, K., Balfour, J., et al. (1998). Income inequality and mortality in metropolitan areas of the United States. *American Journal of Public Health*, *88*(7), 1074–1080.

Mensah, G., Mokdad, A., Ford, E., Greenlund, K., & Croft, J. (2005). State of disparities in cardiovascular health in the United States. *Circulation*, *111*(10), 1233–1241.

Nan, L. V., & Cason, K. L. (2004). Dietary pattern change and acculturation of Chinese Americans in Pennsylvania. *Journal of the American Dietetic Association*, *104*, 771–778.

New York City Department of Health and Mental Hygiene (NYC DOHMH). (2003). *Community Health Survey*. New York: New York City Department of Health and Mental Hygiene.

Pan, Y. L., Dixon, Z., Himburg, S., & Huffman, F. (1999). Asian students change their eating patterns after living in the United States. *Journal of the American Dietetic Association*, *99*, 54–57.

Putnam, R. D. (2000). *Bowling alone: The collapse and revival of American community*. New York: Simon & Schuster.

Satia-Abouta, J., Patterson, R., Neuhouser, M., & Elder, J. (2002). Dietary acculturation: Applications to nutrition research and dietetics. *Journal of American Dietetic Association*, *102*(8), 1105–1118.

Unger, J. B., Reynolds, K., Shakib, S., Spruijt-Metz, D., Sun, P., & Johnson, A. (2004). Acculturation, physical activity, and fast food consumption among Asian American and Hispanic adolescents. *Journal of Community Health*, *29*, 467–481.

U.S. Census Bureau. (2000). *Census 2000*. Atlanta, GA: U.S. Census Bureau.

Wandersman, A., Goodman, R. M., & Butterfoss, F. D. (1999). Understanding coalitions and how they operate: An "open systems" organizational framework. In M. Minkler (Ed.), *Community organizing & community building for health*. New Brunswick, NJ: Rutgers University Press.

Wildman, R., Gu, D., Reynolds, K., Duan, X., Wu, X., & He, J. (2005). Are waist circumference and body mass index independently associated with cardiovascular disease risk in Chinese adults? *American Journal of Clinical Nutrition*, *82*(6), 1195–1202.

Woolcock, M. (1998). Social capital and economic development: Toward a theoretical synthesis and policy framework. *Theory and Society*, *37*, 505–521.

World Health Organization. (2000). *The Asia-Pacific perspective: Redefining obesity and its treatment*. Melbourne, Australia: World Health Organization Collaborating Centre for the Epidemiology of Diabetes and Health Promotion for Noncommunicable Diseases.

Zhou, B., Wu, Y., Yang, J., Li, Y., Zhang, H., & Zhao, L. (2002). Overweight is an independent risk factor for cardiovascular disease in Chinese populations. *Obesity Review*, *3*(3), 147–156.

HIV/AIDS Risk Reduction With Couples: Implications for Reducing Health Disparities in HIV/AIDS Prevention

Nabila El-Bassel, Susan S. Witte, and Louisa Gilbert

Introduction

Twenty-five years into the epidemic, AIDS remains a significant public health issue that highlights the persistence of health disparities in the United States. HIV/AIDS continues to disproportionately affect communities of color, especially African American and Latino communities (Centers for Disease Control and Prevention [CDC], 2006a), and women. Women of color, particularly African American women, have been especially hardest hit and represent the majority of new HIV and AIDS cases among women, and the majority of women living with the disease (CDC, 2006a).

As of 2006, more than 1 million people in the United States are living with HIV (CDC, 2006a). During 2001–2004, based on data from 35 U.S. areas that have HIV reporting, 51% of all new HIV/AIDS diagnoses were among African Americans, who account for only approximately 13% of the U.S. population (CDC, 2006a). Of these, 54% (23,820) of HIV/AIDS diagnoses in women were in African American women infected through heterosexual contact. Today, women account for approximately one quarter of all new HIV/AIDS diagnoses, and heterosexual activity is the chief mode of transmission among women in the U.S., accounting for 71% of infection sources (CDC, 2006a). In 2005, the AIDS case rate for non-Hispanic black women was 49.9 per 100,000, a rate 24 times higher than that for non-Hispanic whites (2.1%), whereas the rate for Hispanic nonwhite women was 12.2 per 100,000, which was 6 times higher that for whites. In 2002, HIV infection was the leading cause of death for African American women aged 25–34 years (CDC, 2006a).

Although the vast majority of women are infected through heterosexual contacts, until recently, HIV prevention studies had not adequately focused on couples, nor addressed the relationship contexts (intimacy, closeness, trust, living together, dependencies) that have been found to be major HIV risk factors for women in long-term relationships. In light of this salient gap, this chapter is designed to (1) review current research on HIV prevention for couples and highlight the rationale for conducting couple-based intervention research; (2) describe the process of designing Project Connect, a cultural- and gender-specific HIV/STI prevention intervention; (3) present theories that guided the study; (4) describe the content of the intervention; and finally (5) discuss the implications of the efficacy of Project Connect for the design and dissemination of culturally-congruent interventions to address the AIDS epidemic among ethnically diverse women and their male partners.

Current Research and Rationale for Employing Couples-Based HIV Prevention

Almost two decades of accumulated research demonstrate that behavioral interventions can curb HIV sexual risk behavior in a variety of populations (Ehrhardt et al., 2002; Jemmott III & Jemmott, 2000; NIMH Multisite HIV Prevention Trial, 1998; O'Leary & Wingood, 2000). Studies have revealed significant increases in self-reported condom use (Belcher et al., 1998; DiClemente & Wingood, 1995; El-Bassel & Schilling, 1992; Jemmott III, Jemmott, & Fong, 1998; Kamb et al., 1998; Kelly et al., 1997; Kelly et al., 1994; Neumann et al., 2002; NIMH Multisite HIV Prevention Trial, 1998) and reductions in the self-reported frequency of unprotected sexual acts (Belcher et al., 1998; Jemmott III et al., 1998; Jemmott III, Jemmott, Fong, & McCaffree, 1999; Jemmott & Jemmott III, 1992; Kelly et al., 1997; Kelly et al., 1994; Neumann et al., 2002; St. Lawrence, Jefferson, Alleyne, & Brasfield, 1995) among people who received HIV risk-reduction interventions as compared with those in control groups. A number of randomized clinical trials (RCTs) have also found that HIV risk-reduction interventions reduced the incidence of biologically confirmed STIs (Jemmott III & Jemmott, 2000; Kamb et al., 1998; Neumann et al., 2002; NIMH Multisite HIV Prevention Trial, 1998; Shain et al., 1999). However, a recent meta analysis of HIV prevention intervention randomized control trials, which have addressed heterosexual risk reduction, noted that few intervention studies have focused on increasing condom use and negotiation skills among men or among steady couples. Moreover, traditional individual or group-based HIV prevention programs often fail to demonstrate increased condom use among women in long-term intimate relationships (Bryan, Aiken, & West, 1996; Ickovics & Yoshikawa, 1998; Schilling, El-Bassel, Hadden, & Gilbert, 1995). In addition, few interventions provided an alternative to the use of male condoms (Neumann et al., 2002).

To overcome these shortcomings, couple-oriented intervention models are being developed and evaluated to address condom use and HIV/sexually transmitted infections (STI) prevention (Allen et al., 1992; Deschamps, Pape, Haffner, Hyppolite, & Johnson, 1991; Ehrhardt & Exner, 2000; El-Bassel et al., 2001; Harvey, 2000; Higgins et al., 1991; Musaba, Morrison, Sunkutu, & Wong, 1998; Padian, O'Brien, Chang, Glass, & Francis, 1993; Voluntary HIV-1 Counseling and Testing Efficacy Study Group, 2000; Wingood & DiClemente, 2000). While there is evidence to suggest that couples counseling is effective in promoting condom use among couples with elevated HIV risk, (Allen et al.,

1992; Deschamps et al., 1991; Higgins et al., 1991; Padian et al., 1993), these approaches are limited by several methodological drawbacks, including small sample size, lack of a randomized control design, and lack of attentional control groups. In addition, none of the studies was designed to examine potential mediating factors that might clarify why the interventions succeeded. To date few studies have tested the efficacy of couple-based HIV risk-reduction interventions using an RCT design.

There are many potential advantages to bringing couples together to learn how to protect themselves from HIV and other sexually transmitted infections. Bringing the couple together may (1) increase trust, intimacy, and commitment in relationships; (2) reduce gender power imbalances associated with sexual coercion and inability to negotiate condom use; (3) increase couples' communication and negotiation skills about HIV risk reduction and sex in general; (4) allow partners to express their needs to take care of and protect each other by using condoms (Basen-Engquist, 1992; Ehrhardt, 1994; El-Bassel et al., 2001; Fisher & Fisher, 1992; Kelly, 1995; Nadler & Fisher, 1992; Tanner & Pollack, 1988); (5) allow information to be introduced by an objective, "knowledgeable" facilitator, who may normalize HIV/STI protection as a dimension of personal, interpersonal, and ethnic community protection, and not solely because of risky past or present behaviors (El-Bassel et al., 2001); and (6) provide a supportive environment that might enable those in intimate relationships to disclose more safely to their partners extra-dyadic sexual encounters, STI histories, injection drug use, or past experiences in abusive relationships (El-Bassel et al., 2001). Such disclosure may enable couples to gain a more realistic appraisal of their HIV risks.

Project Connect

Between 1997 and 2001, the Social Intervention Group (SIG) at the Columbia University School of Social Work (CUSSW) developed and tested a relationship-based, HIV/STI prevention intervention targeting heterosexual couples. The Project Connect trial was a randomized clinical trial (RCT) that tested the efficacy of Connect, a relationship-based intervention, in increasing condom use among 217 low-income, predominantly minority women and their regular sexual partners, who were at elevated risk for HIV/STIs. The objectives of this study were to examine (1) whether a six-session relationship-based intervention to prevent HIV/STIs would be efficacious in increasing the proportion of protected sexual acts and decreasing the number of unprotected sexual acts at 12-month follow up, compared to a control condition consisting of a single session of HIV/STI education, and (2) whether the intervention would be equally efficacious when the woman and her partner received the relationship-based intervention together or when the woman received the relationship-based intervention alone. "Connect" is also the name for the six-session relationship-based intervention itself, tested in the trial, and is described in more detail below.

Recruitment and Eligibility

Initiated in 1997, women were recruited to participate in the trial from hospital-based outpatient clinics in Bronx, New York. A women was eligible for the study if she (1) was between 18 and 55 years old; (2) had a regular, male sexual partner whom she identified as a boyfriend, spouse, or lover; (3) was in a long-term relationship, operationalized as involvement with this partner for the past 6 months and intent to stay with him for at least 1 year; (4) had at least one episode of unprotected vaginal or anal sex with this partner in the past 30 days; (5) did not report any severe physical or sexual abuse by this partner within the past 6 months, according to selected questions from the Revised Conflict Tactics Scale (Straus, Hamby, Boney-McCoy, & Sugarman, 1996); and (6) was a patient at one of the hospital's outpatient clinics. To be eligible, a woman also had to know or suspect that her partner met at least one of the following HIV/STI risk criteria: (1) he had sex with other women or men in the past 90 days; (2) he had been diagnosed with or exhibited symptoms of an STI in the past 90 days; (3) he had injected drugs in the past 90 days; and/or (4) he was HIV positive. At the end of the screening interview, female participants were asked to give written, informed consent. Prior to the baseline interview, the male partners were also informed about the purpose of the study and asked to give written, informed consent. Screening procedures were designed to identify a sample of heterosexual couples at high risk for sexual transmission of HIV and other STIs.

Study Procedures

At baseline, simultaneous but separate interviews with gender-matched interviewers took place with each partner. Couples were then randomly assigned to one of three study conditions (Figure 15.1): (1) the *couple condition* (C), six weekly relationship-based sessions, in which both a woman and her partner received the intervention; (2) the *woman-alone condition* (WA), in which only the woman received the same intervention; or (3) the *education control condition* (E), in which the woman alone received one HIV/STI information session. Each woman and her main male participated in a 3-month follow-up interview postintervention and the women also participated in a 12-month follow-up interview postintervention (see Figure 15.1).

Whether provided conjointly to both partners or one-on-one with the woman alone, the content of each intervention session was the same, incorporating concepts from the AIDS Risk Reduction Model (Catania, Kegeles, & Coates, 1990), the ecological perspective (Bronfenbrenner, 1979), previous related empirical research on HIV/STI prevention with couples (NIMH Multisite HIV Prevention Trial, 1998), and qualitative pilot data summarized from local community consultants interviewed during the developmental phase of the study (El-Bassel et al., 2001; Sormanti, Pereira, El-Bassel, Witte, & Gilbert, 2001).

The intervention (described in detail in the following pages) consisted of six sessions of a relationship-based HIV/STI prevention intervention (El-Bassel et al., 2001). Intervention sessions met once a week, lasted 2 hours, and began either the day of baseline or on a day scheduled within the following 2 weeks. Intervention sessions were generally completed within 7 weeks of enrollment. Couple sessions were rescheduled if one partner was absent.

Profile of Study Participants

Participants in the Connect trial were predominantly African American and Latina/o. Of the 217 couples randomized, 47.5% were African American couples, 29.5% were

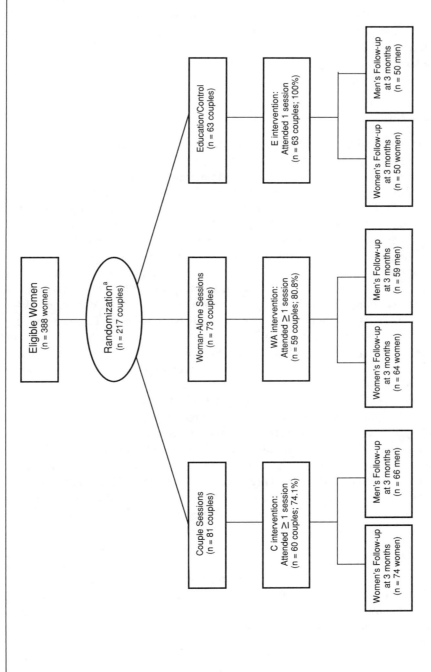

a. During a regular review of scientific integrity, it was determined that a few assignment envelopes had been omitted accidentally, resulting in an imbalance in the sizes of the groups assigned to each condition. Potential imbalance and resultant bias in our data analyses were explored as described in the text.

Overview of Project Connect

Latino couples, and 23% were mixed ethnic couples. The mean age of participants was 38 years; most (57%) were never married, and most (57%) had annual incomes of less than $5,000. Half of the participants had less than 12 years of education, while 14.5% of women and 34.9% of men were employed. The majority (67.9%) of couples were HIV negative; in 17% of the couples both partners were positive, while in 15% of the couples, one partner was positive, the other HIV negative.

Theoretical Framework

Two theoretical frameworks, the AIDS Risk Reduction Model (Catania et al., 1990) and the ecological perspective (Bronfenbrenner, 1979), guide the intervention. The ARRM was developed as a conceptual framework to organize behavior change information and skills directed at HIV risk reduction. This eclectic model integrates constructs from the theory of reasoned action (Ajzen & Fishbein, 1980; Fishbein & Middlestadt, 1989), social cognitive theory (Bandura, 1986, 1994), and health-belief approaches (Janz & Becker, 1984). The ARRM incorporates three stages: (1) recognizing and labeling one's sexual behaviors as high risk for contracting HIV, (2) making a commitment to reducing high risk sexual behaviors and increasing low risk activities, and (3) seeking and enacting strategies to attain these goals, such as communicating with one's sex partner about change, initiating condom use, and seeking help from one's network for changing risk behaviors. Although separated for conceptual purposes, these stages may occur concurrently (Catania et al., 1990). In our intervention, we modified the ARRM by adding an additional stage: the "maintenance" of behavioral change. While ARRM focuses on changing individual behavior, the emphasis on improving communication and negotiation skills for risk reduction may best occur with partners together in relationship-based sessions.

The AARM recognizes that knowledge of how to reduce risk and the motivation to act on such knowledge is not adequate without cognitive and behavioral preparedness and the ability to communicate with a sexual partner. Necessary self-regulatory skills include the ability to recognize situations likely to lead to unsafe sex, avoiding situations leading to risky behavior, controlling impulses that lead to risky sex, and anticipating sexual encounters so that one is prepared to use condoms. Also required are the abilities to assert a commitment to safer sex, to reduce the partner's opposition to these activities (i.e., problem solving, communication, and negotiation skills), and to develop and maintain relationships that are supportive of safer sex behavior (Kelly, St. Lawrence, Hood, & Brasfield, 1989). Structured, skill-based, experiential strategies enable individuals to anticipate problem or high-risk situations, and to develop specific behavioral competencies in solving problems, overcoming challenges, or avoiding risks. Skills training includes introduction and definition, modeling, and behavior rehearsal with coaching and feedback. Homework assignments promote generalization of skills. Positive reinforcement and social support facilitate "trying out" new behaviors and help maintain motivation over time.

The ecological perspective (Bronfenbrenner, 1979) provides a way to conceptualize a contextually- and relationship-specific approach to HIV risk reduction (Moss & Tarter, 1993). This perspective emphasizes the various levels of contextual factors that play a role in establishing and maintaining protective behaviors. These may include an individual's background, relationship context, immediate social context, and the broader cultural values and beliefs in which HIV risk behaviors occur. These four nested analytical levels of sexual risk and protective factors are (1) the *ontogenetic* level, which refers to the personal factors that are unique to an individual's developmental history, such as trauma (childhood sexual abuse, rape), psychological distress, self-efficacy, and communication skills; (2) the *micro system* level, which refers to the interactional and relationship factors that are part of the immediate context in which sexual activity takes place (i.e., power imbalances, intimacy, closeness, physical and sexual coercion); (3) the *exosystem level*, which refers to all risk factors both formal and informal that impinge upon the immediate setting by acting as external stressors or buffers on the likelihood of engaging in risky behavior, such as socio-economic and employment status, peer norms about safer sex, social networks and support, and access to HIV related services; and (4) the *macro-cultural level*, which includes the broad cultural values and belief systems that interact with all the other analytical levels and macro-level factors, such as social norms towards HIV and attitudes toward gender roles. Project Connect intervention components were designed to address predominantly micro and exosystem risk and protective factors, keeping ontogenetic and macro level factors in mind for cultural and community relevance.

While the ecological perspective is comprehensive, its application to HIV risk reduction poses a challenge in that risk and protective factors are analytically "nested" within each other (i.e., one factor operates within the limits set by other factors). Individual factors incorporated into the model have been empirically demonstrated to be associated with HIV risk or protective strategies (i.e., social support, condom use self-efficacy, etc.), although there is room for interpretation as to where any particular factor fits most appropriately into the multilevel framework (e.g., the lines between micro- and exo-level factors are not always clear). However, we believe that the significance of a nested ecological perspective resides not so much in the precise location of the factors but rather in their dynamic interplay.

The Connect Intervention

The intervention consists of an orientation session and five relationship-based sessions. It combines content related to safer sex practices and prevention of HIV and all other STIs as well as joint HIV testing and an emphasis on communication and negotiation skills. In addition to being guided by the two theoretical frameworks discussed above, we conducted focus groups with several couples recruited from the primary health care setting at the study site and incorporated their input and voice in the design of the intervention components in order to strengthen the cultural congruence and gender specificity of the intervention (for a more complete discussion see Sormanti et al., 2001).

The goal of the intervention's relationship-based approach is to reframe safer sex not as individual "protection," but rather as a way to preserve relationship and community, as an act of love, commitment, and intimacy. This approach emphasizes the importance of communication, negotiation, and problem-solving skills, and highlights how relationship dynamics may be affected by gender roles and expectations. The session content emphasizes the contribution each participant and their partner makes to enhancing the future health of their partnership, family, and community. Consistent with the U.S. National HIV Prevention Plan (CDC, 2001), the intervention also directed prevention messages to HIV-positive individuals and couples without changing its core elements, but with minor adjustments in the language used in some of the core elements. For example, the intervention emphasizes reducing risk for any new STIs, including HIV, with a secondary prevention emphasis for HIV-infected individuals, and highlights empirical data on the emergence of newer, drug-resistant strains of HIV, the particular susceptibility of HIV positive individuals to infection by other STIs, and the misperception of posing no transmission risk if one's viral load is undetectable.

The intervention also emphasizes responsibility for self, for each other as a couple, for community, and for family. The intervention focuses on a positive future orientation, for example, addressing change for preventive health as opposed to past risky behaviors. It also emphasizes the importance of individual contribution to enhancing the future health of ethnic communities hardest hit by AIDS, for example, by addressing the adverse effects of AIDS in the African-American and Latino communities and linking behavior change to commitment to one's community (Kelly, 1995; Schilling et al., 1995; DiClemente & Wingood, 1995; van der Straten, King, Grinstead, Serufilira, & Allen, 1995).

Orientation Session: "Preparing for the Journey." The purpose of the orientation session is to increase the couple's motivation to attend the remaining sessions together and to give each participant an opportunity to explore his or her concerns and questions about the intervention. Drawing from the ARRM model, the orientation session serves to heighten awareness of risk and to begin the cognitive preparedness required for risk reduction behavior change. Sessions are provided one-on-one to women and their partners separately by a same-sex facilitator. HIV prevention for couples is normalized through discussion of the relevance of the intervention for regular, intimate partners and presentation of current, local HIV and STI rates among long term partners. In this individual session, facilitators work with participants to reduce anxiety and clarify misperceptions about the intervention. Facilitators also highlight confidentiality procedures and reassure participants that they will not be compelled to share any information that they want to keep from their partners. Drawing from the ecological perspective, the session emphasizes how important the individual's relationship context and dynamics (microsystem) will be to the sessions. The facilitator emphasizes that the intervention will focus on the strengths of their relationship and will provide options and alternative ways of protecting themselves and their partners. In this individual session, participants are encouraged to weigh the pros and cons of participation and discuss attendance, thus strengthening their motivation to complete the intervention. At the end of this session, participants sign a contract of commitment to attend the sessions. This session is well-received by participants, and has been found to be useful as a cohesive mechanism to prepare the woman and her partner to work collaboratively with the facilitator.

Session 1: "Identifying Risks and Vulnerabilities in our Relationship." The objectives of this session are to (1) increase perceptions about vulnerability to STIs, including HIV, as a couple; (2) increase motivation for change by focusing on the couple's risk factors as well as their strengths; (3) set ground rules and confidentiality procedures; and (4) introduce a couple communication skills-building technique. These objectives draw from both the ARRM and ecological models as they integrate knowledge building, risk identification and awareness, and strengthening of communication skills.

Session 1 begins with a discussion of the pros and cons of session participation. Next, the facilitator helps the couple to clarify individual roles and expectations. Ground rules are discussed, with an emphasis on the importance of confidentiality, and the right to ask questions. Participants are discouraged from using drugs prior to the sessions and asked to withhold judgment and avoid "put downs." The couple is invited to share as much as they feel comfortable sharing, and are informed that the more they participate, the more they should benefit.

HIV/AIDS information is provided focusing on how the epidemic affects them (as a couple), their children, friends, and community. A myths and facts game format is used to initiate discussion of basic HIV/AIDS transmission information. Information about STIs other than HIV is provided in a video format, followed by a discussion of the couple's STI history and knowledge base. Facilitators emphasize that HIV is only one of many STIs from which couples must protect each other.

The couple is asked to identify any past individual risk factors for HIV (e.g., drug use, alcohol abuse, sex with risky partners). This exercise is critical to intervention success as it establishes the starting point of risk for each couple upon which they will build a repertoire of safer behaviors. As an introduction to communication skills, couples face each other and take turns speaking and listening, telling each other the qualities they value in each other and what they each hope to be doing 5 years in the future. Through coaching, feedback, and rehearsal, the couple is trained in the Speaker/Listener Technique (Markman, Stanley, & Blumberg, 1996), a communication skill designed to help them listen to and understand each other's differing perspectives better. This technique is first practiced with a relatively easy issue identified by the couple, then practiced with an issue specifically related to safer sex goals.

Session 2: "Protecting our Relationship." The objectives of this session are to (1) identify how relationship factors (closeness, love, respect, power imbalances) might be barriers to protected sex; (2) understand the importance of safer sex practices in the context of an intimate relationship; (3) learn the spectrum of behavioral options for safer sex; and (4) practice condom use negotiation. More cognitive preparation, education, and motivation from the ARRM is addressed, while the objectives expand to incorporate additional elements of the ecological perspective, specifically relationship context, power imbalance, patterns of sexual behavior, communication about sexual comfort and desire, and traditional gender/sex roles. These elements of the ecological perspective will be addressed through sessions 3, 4 and 5.

In Session 2, the myths and facts game format is again used, this time to normalize societal challenges to the maintenance of a long-term, monogamous relationship (i.e., if your partner loves you she will not have sex with someone else) and to normalize the risks facing women and men in long-term relationships (i.e., if you only have sex with your main, regular partner, you are not at risk for HIV). Through this exercise, the facilitator emphasizes that it takes both partners in the couple working together to establish one, solid, protective plan.

Moving to preparation for behavioral risk reduction, individual and couple strengths, as well as the ability to make behavioral change, is emphasized by asking the couple to share an experience where they (individually and together) have already taken control over their lives and made a positive change.

Later in this session the couple also explores issues related to "unspoken rules" in the relationship (e.g., relationship factors, gender differences, sexuality, fidelity in the relationship), and condom use between steady partners. The facilitator helps the couple to acknowledge that love for each other and a desire for intimacy may constitute barriers to condom use. The facilitator focuses on strengths by emphasizing the message that taking care of oneself and protecting each other as a couple is a sign of love and respect.

Under the topic "sexual decision-making," the facilitator leads an active discussion about how (stereotypically) men and women differ in terms of sexual decisions, condom use decisions, and sexuality (issues of comfort in talking about sex, requesting condom use, desire for pregnancy and condom use, etc.). The facilitator introduces a hierarchy or spectrum of sexual behaviors ranked from safer to least safe ways to prevent transmission of HIV: from abstinence to no protection at all. With the help of the facilitator, couples start exploring the complexity of safer sex and choose the best option for their situation. The hierarchy makes clear that the most protection is offered by abstinence or mutual or parallel masturbation. Options include using alternatives to intercourse for achieving orgasm, male or female condoms for vaginal or anal intercourse, dental dams and condoms for oral sex, or using HIV testing as a strategy to plan for mutual monogamy.

The couple is asked to indicate what behaviors they currently engage in on the hierarchy or spectrum of risk and to select safer behaviors that they would like to begin practicing together over the course of the intervention sessions. Because the couple's desire for a pregnancy may be a barrier to condom use, a discussion on how to conceive safely is initiated. The couple signs a contract of commitment to work together to achieve their goal of movement along the Safer Sex Scale. Through coaching and feedback, the couple again practices the Speaker/Listener technique, this time with respect to challenging gender differences or unspoken rules within their relationship that act as barriers to safer sex behaviors.

Session 3: "Making Choices That Strengthen our Relationship." The objectives of this session are to help the couple to (1) learn about male and female anatomy; (2) practice proper use of male and female condoms; (3) acquire information about the safest condom and lubricant types available; (4) increase couple safer sex options; and (5) discover how to make safe sex fun and enhance sexual communication skills. Skills and strategy building consistent with the ARRM are addressed, while the various contextual factors of the ecological model highlighted in Session 2 continue to be addressed.

The anatomy knowledge exercise names sexual and reproductive organs, encourages communication about anatomy, and aids in understanding how male and female condoms work to prevent STI infection and pregnancy. With coaching and feedback from the facilitator, anatomy and condom use knowledge and skills are reviewed and practiced by the couple together.

In this session the facilitator also encourages the couple to examine their sexual routines or everyday practices with regard to intimacy and communication around sexual issues: Do they ever explore barriers to communication? How might they be confined by social constructions to gender and culture? (In the language of the intervention, how often might their actions or choices be predetermined by what is the expected behavior of a man, or of woman?) The goal of this exercise is to encourage the couple to consider new sexual options, specifically, the adoption of safer sex practices.

To facilitate exploration of safer sex options and continue enhancement of sexual communication, couples are introduced to the "Connection Café Menu." This "menu" is a tool to help the couple identify ways to communicate intimate wishes in a non-threatening way. The menu offers several ways of having protected sex, including a number of "outercourse" (mutual and parallel masturbation) options, eroticizing female and male condom use, and a number of intimate behaviors not necessarily related to intercourse (reciting poetry, bathing together, walking in the moonlight). Participants apply the Speaker/Listener technique by taking turns "ordering" from the menu.

Session 4: "Working Together to Keep our Relationship, Family and Community Safe." The purpose of this session is to help couples to (1) identify triggers for unsafe sex, with an emphasis on relationship contexts (e.g., people, places, drug use, and mood and feelings such as love, trust, fear of rejection, loneliness, heightened or depressed sexual desires) and (2) introduce problem solving skills to avoid or negotiate high risk situations. Skills and strategy building consistent with the ARRM are addressed, while the various contextual factors of the ecological model highlighted in Sessions 2 and 3 are expanded to include the couple's impact on their broader community of family and friends.

The facilitator works with the couple to identify personal and couple risk triggers and helps them devise ways to prevent or address triggers through problem solving. Problem-solving involves a five step approach, including (1) identifying the problem; (2) identifying the trigger(s) leading to the problem; (3) brainstorming potential solutions to avoid the problem; (4) evaluating and choosing the best solution; and (5) developing an action plan to avoid the problem in the future. After presenting the model, the facilitator coaches the couple through their own risky behavior scenarios. The couple applies the Speaker/Listener technique to work through safer sex problem-solving scenarios. The safe sex hierarchy is reviewed and the couple discusses where they are on this hierarchy once more. Again, joint HIV testing is reinforced as an approach to prevention and an important way to determine current risk status. Finally, the couple is reminded of the importance of their role in supporting the health and welfare of their family, friends, and community by sharing their STI-related knowledge and skills. They are presented with personalized cards indicating that they are "prevention promoters" and encouraged to consider ways they can use what they have learned to impact prevention in the lives of family and friends.

Session 5: "Sustaining our Relationship Strength and Supports." The objectives of this final session are to assist the couple in (1) identifying social supports, both as individuals and as a couple, in order to assist each one in coping and maintaining safer sex behavior; (2) learning how to cope with challenges to maintaining safer sex practices over time in a long-term relationship; (3) enhancing social support from families and friends for initiating maintaining positive behavior changes in reducing sexual risk behavior; and (4) promoting HIV risk reduction in their community. The addition of the "maintenance" stage of the ARRM is addressed in this session, while the important role of the exosystem (specifically social supports) as conceptualized within the ecological perspective, is emphasized.

The facilitator highlights the progress that the couple has made since the first session. The couple is invited to talk about whether they have relapsed into unsafe sex. The skill of self-talk, telling oneself positive thoughts in an effort to maintain behavior change, is demonstrated and practiced. Three coping strategies—self talk, problem-solving, and the Speaker/Listener technique—are discussed as ways to avoid relapse triggers or ways to begin implementing risk reduction again should the couple relapse. They are asked to renew their commitment to protected sex as a couple and to review any new eroticizing skills they have employed as a result of the intervention. In order to promote maintenance of behavior change, the couple is encouraged to review issues related to their commitment to stay healthy. In addition, the couple identifies people in their network who will be supportive to healthy behaviors and safer sex practices. Again, the facilitator discusses how they can teach other people in their community to stay healthy. Couples are encouraged to promote safer sex messages to other couples, friends, family, children, and their community. Through discussion of these issues with their friends, relatives, and children, the participants are encouraged to sustain the changes that they have decided to make in their lives and also share and compare their successes and failures and renew their determination to do things differently in the future. Project Connect provides each couple with a certificate indicating completion of the intervention and suggests that their new knowledge and expertise about safer sex practices can be informatively shared with others in their community.

How Sessions Were Conducted. All sessions took place in a private office within the hospital outpatient setting where participants were recruited. Sessions lasted 2 hours and included didactic and experiential materials, and were conducted in English. In each session, one facilitator worked with one couple, providing feedback and coaching, and allowing the couple to practice the skills together. Most sessions included a modeling or educational video for variety in presentation media. Each session had several exercises and ended with goal setting, in which the couple was asked to select a goal for the next session that was related to the safer sex and communication skills content covered in the current session. Participants were provided with a selection of male and female condoms at the end of every session, and reminded of places in the community where they could access free condoms.

Facilitators employed a number of couple counseling skills. First, an attempt was made to provide equal attention to the two members of the couple throughout sessions. Second, facilitators maintained an "observer" stance to maximize productive interaction between the couple, but interceded as necessary and appropriate to clarify issues or concerns. Couples would sometimes disagree and digress into an argument. Disagreement between the couple was normalized and used to initiate and encourage compromise leading to behavior change. Third, facilitators created a "safe" context where the participants could express their thoughts and feelings, but not feel compelled to speak or participate. Facilitators capitalized on the couple's own dynamics to enhance communication and interaction between the dyad. One of the challenges that facilitators faced was balancing the need to adhere to the session content with the need to address specific issues and life concerns raised by each couple. To address extraneous concerns, facilitators were instructed to refer clients to treatment in the community. Such referrals were monitored and quantified for analysis.

Session Attendance. Most couples or women alone who attended at least one session completed all five sessions. Seventy-eight percent of participants randomized to either couples or woman alone treatment attended at least one session: 59% attended all five sessions, while the another 19% attended between 1 and 4 sessions. Twenty-two percent of participants randomized to treatment ($n = 33$) attended no treatment sessions.

Findings

Findings on the women's and their male study partners' reports from the 3 and 12 months follow-up are published elsewhere (El-Bassel et al., 2003), but are summarized briefly here. Findings suggest that the relationship-based intervention is efficacious in reducing HIV/STIs, particularly by reducing the number of unprotected acts at 12 months postintervention. Women assigned to an active intervention arm, irrespective of whether they received the sessions alone or with their partners, significantly decreased the number of unprotected sexual acts at 12 months and improved on the other two outcome measures (proportion of protected sexual acts and consistent condom usage). While the findings did not indicate that having a woman and her sexual partner together in the sessions necessarily yielded better risk reduction, findings did suggest that the Connect intervention is equally efficacious whether provided to a woman alone or together with her male sexual partner. These findings represent a new contribution to the HIV/STI prevention intervention literature and an important advancement in prevention strategies that would allow for the involvement of male partners in the risk reduction process.

In addition to primary outcomes assessment, we used qualitative methods to examine client satisfaction and intervention components perceived by clients as helpful, among men and women who participated in either of the two active treatment conditions. Participants completed this survey at the end of their last intervention session. Open-ended, qualitative evaluation questions explored levels of overall satisfaction, what participants liked best and least, what they learned, what they felt helped them in the intervention, and assessed reported frequency of male and female condom use pre- and postintervention. Data indicate that the intervention was very well received and highly regarded by participants. The most helpful components of the intervention identified were the couple's ability to communicate better with their main partner and the special strategies the facilitators used to engage the couple and to promote behavior change (e.g., the Speaker/Listener technique (Markman et al., 1996), problem solving and self talk). No negative components of the intervention were reported (see Schiff, Witte, & El-Bassel, 2003 for a compete discussion).

Cultural Congruence of the Connect Intervention

We employed several steps in order to make the Connect intervention culturally congruent and fit well with the needs and worldviews of the community in which the study was conducted. The community and consumers had considerable opportunities to make their voices heard during the grant preparation and conceptualization, research implementation and dissemination.

Step 1: Pre-Implementation. Before the submission of the grant application, the investigators met with a group comprised of: six community members who serve African-American/Latino HIV-affected populations, four staff from the primary health care clinics at the hospital were the study took place, and five potential couples (consumers). The group reviewed the study's aims and its benefits to the African American and Latino communities. Furthermore, a small pilot study was conducted with six couples to examine the feasibility of the proposed study. The feedback from the community, potential consumers, and the pilot informed the application of the grant.

Step 2: During the Implementation. During the intervention development phase of Project Connect, couples from the local community were engaged as consultants in a series of focus group discussions. Sixteen women and 13 male partners participated in a series of 18 focus groups of African American and Latino couples. Each individual participated in three focus groups of two single-sex sessions held over a 3-week time period and a third group that brought women and their male partners together. All couples met the same inclusion criteria that were required for the study participants. The format of the focus group discussions allowed us to explore cultural and gender-specific issues. The purpose of the focus group discussions were to explore couples' reactions and ideas about potential topics for the intervention, what they wanted to learn, what they thought that their main partner would like to learn and need to learn about HIV, what issues would be difficult to talk about, what would be gender and cultural obstacles. They also reviewed the language used in the content of the sessions and determined whether the content and message were culturally appropriate. Obstacles to attendance at sessions and follow-up were discussed. Couples raised concerns about issues of trust and infidelity that might arise during the implementation of the intervention. In addition, they provided feedback on the importance and utility of Project Connect to the African American and Latino communities. and on the sessions in terms of language (e.g., whether the content and messages are culturally appropriate, whether homework assignments are feasible).

In addition to the study intervention content, we worked during the early implementation stage of the Connect study with our consultants to develop a best practices model for the recruitment of African American and Latino couples (Witte, Campbell, & El-Bassel, 2004; Swanson & Ward, 1995). Until the inception of Project Connect, no studies had focused on the recruitment of African American and Latino couples into an HIV intervention trial. We were aware of existing disparities in the involvement of racial/ethnic minority participants in clinical research, and the growing emphasis by the National Institutes of Health on ensuring that racial/ethnic minorities, women, and other historically marginalized groups were represented in clinical research (National Institutes of Health, 2001; Varmus, 1994). Consultants provided feedback on recruitment and retention strategies and ways of introducing the study to the community and making sure that the community understood the overall benefits of the research. Following this protocol, we were able to successfully and safely recruit 217 predominantly African American and Latino heterosexual couples into the RCT. Details of the recruitment strategy development and implementation are provided elsewhere (see Witte, El-Bassel, et al., 2004 for details). This successful recruitment demonstrated the feasibility of engaging African American and Latino couples into RCTs, and highlighted the importance of (1) engaging community consultants into the protocol development process and (2) integrating lessons from empirical literature on best practices to address barriers to the engagement of historically marginalized groups of men and women into RCTs. (Harris, Gorelick, Samuels, & Bempong, 1996; Shavers, Lynch, & Burmeister, 2001)

Step 3: Main Phase of the Study Implementation. The consultants continued to be involved and provided feedback on issues related to recruitment and retention of couples. Their feedback remained critical and valuable throughout the life of the study.

Step 4: Preliminary Dissemination. After the completion of the research, the findings were shared with the consultants. The consultants were encouraged to present the findings at local, formal and informal conferences, and at meetings.

Connect Session for Facilitator Training and Supervision. All facilitators were female and possessed a Masters of Social Work (MSW) degree or were social work graduate students with clinical skills. A third of the facilitators ($n = 4$) were women of color (3 Latina, 1 Asian American). In order to control for facilitator gender while comparing an individual against a couple intervention in the research design, male facilitators were excluded. We believed that the nature of the intervention content (i.e., review and discussion of sexual risk and histories, male and female anatomy, etc.) precluded having a male facilitator work one-on-one with a female participant. Such a design might severely compromise feelings of safety on the part of women participating in the woman-alone sessions. To ensure the quality and consistency of the interventions, facilitators received a standard training course, used structured intervention protocols, met on a weekly basis with a clinical and task supervisor, and had routine monitoring (via audiotape) and feedback by an on site-supervisor (a random 10% of sessions were monitored). In the training, we paid attention to cultural competency by ensuring that the facilitators understood their own cultural biases understood different cultural worldviews, and felt comfortable discussing cultural differences and working with clients from a different cultural background. During supervision, we also paid attention to the facilitator's cultural competency and provided corrective feedback on ongoing basis, when needed.

A criterion of 80% compliance with intervention content and delivery process (timing of elements, etc.) was considered an acceptable standard. No facilitator failed to perform up to this standard. However, had it occurred, the facilitators whose performance deviated in quality or adherence would have been retrained or replaced. In addition, process evaluations assessing intervention content and client satisfaction were conducted by surveying participants in the final session (Schiff et al., 2003).

Discussion

Even though most women living with HIV/AIDS have been infected through heterosexual contact with regular partners, the science of couples-based HIV/STI prevention intervention in the United States is still in its early stages. The Project Connect study, targeting women at highest risk in the United States—African American and Latina heterosexual women—examined whether a relationship-based HIV/STI intervention could demonstrate sustained outcome effects at 3 and 12 month-follow-up, and whether the intervention participants demonstrated any more efficacious long-term effects when women received the intervention with their main partners versus women who received the intervention alone. To achieve cultural congruence and attend to gender-specific concerns, development of the study and intervention protocols was largely informed by community consultants representative of the Connect target population. Findings suggested that the relationship-based intervention is efficacious in reducing HIV/STIs, particularly by reducing the number of unprotected acts and increasing the proportion of protected sexual acts and consistent condom usage at 3 and 12 months post-intervention. The findings showed that that the women who completed either of the six session relationship-based conditions were more likely than their counterparts in the educational control condition to increase the proportion of protected sexual acts and decrease the number of unprotected acts. Thus, the intervention did not appear to be any more or less efficacious when a woman received the intervention with her partner compared to when she received it without him. Findings suggested that implementing the Connect intervention, which is relationship-based, to *either* an individual woman or to a woman with her male partner is an efficacious way to help reduce sexual risk behaviors to prevent STIs, including HIV.

We employed several steps in order to make the study culturally congruent and fit well with the needs and worldviews of the community for which the intervention was designed. The community and consumers were given voice during the grant preparation and conceptualization and research implementation.

Feedback from the "consultant" consumers and stakeholders was helpful in several ways: (1) it helped researchers to refine the intervention content (i.e., skills taught in the sessions and homework assignments); (2) it assisted researchers in ensuring the inclusion of cultural domains in the sessions, delivery style, and training of the researchers, as well as including gender-specific content; (3) it increased couples' attendance and participation in the research by apprising them that the study and the intervention were informed by couples like them and stakeholders from the community; and (4) it increased couples' recruitment and retention throughout the duration of the trial.

Implications for Culturally Congruent HIV/STI Prevention for Couples

The efficacy of the Project Connect intervention in reducing sexual risk among heterosexual couples is an important achievement in HIV prevention.

To date, ten peer-reviewed journal articles describing all aspects of the Project Connect trial, including the intervention development and content, implementation process, study design, fidelity and outcomes have been published or are near publication (El-Bassel et al., 2001, 2003, 2005; Schiff et al., 2003; Sormanti et al., 2001; Witte et al., 2004, 2006, in press; Wu, El-Bassel, Witte, Gilbert, & Chang, 2003; Wu et al., 2005). Most noteworthy is the impact and influence that the Project Connect intervention has evidenced in the HIV/STI prevention field. The Connect intervention has been the basis for several key adaptations currently under study in the United States and globally. Project Connect's core elements, each scripted for ease of use, have been adapted and built upon for use in Project Eban and Connect Two, clinical trials funded by the NIMH and NIDA, respectively, testing the efficacy of these Connect components with high-risk and underserved populations: African-American serodiscordant couples and drug-affected couples. Additional studies adapting and applying Project Connect have been completed in Colombia and in Trinidad, and a third international adaptation has demonstrated efficacy among couples in Kazakhstan.

The single largest impact to date that Project Connect may have on issues of health disparities in the United States is the contribution to Project Eban trial. Currently ongoing, Eban is an NIMH-funded study examining the efficacy of a couple-based HIV/STI intervention for African American couples with mixed HIV status. Eban is a multisite clinical trial, involving 4 U.S. sites, led by investigators with demonstrated leadership in culturally congruent HIV/STI prevention interventions. The authors of this paper are principal investigator and study investigator at one of the four sites. The intervention focuses on one ethnic group (African Americans), is guided by an Afro-centric paradigm (Karenga, 1994), and concentrates on the within-ethnic group strengths of African-descended people, as well as beliefs and practices that can shape an individual's understanding and worldview (Kambon, 1992). The structure of the intervention promotes the individualism essential to self-protection, as well as collectivism, which supports relationship building and peer support for behavior change (Karenga, 1988; Triandis, 1994). We selected the well-known paradigm of Nguzo Saba (Karenga, 1994) to guide our study design. The seven principles of Nguzo Saba—unity, self-determination, collective work and responsibility, cooperative economics, purpose, creativity, and faith—guide the Afro-centric worldview and belief systems of native groups of Africa (Karenga, 1988). In the context of this study, these seven principles guide the content of the intervention, the style of delivery, and the study design. The use of these principles sanctions the ethnic matching of facilitators and participants, which is essential to the peer support and modeling needed in a culturally congruent intervention. Nguzo Saba informs HIV prevention guidelines that bring couples, families, and communities together. The principles promote respect for traditions, and highlight the socio-political and racial realities that African-descended people affected by HIV continue to face. The intervention consists of eight weekly 2-hour sessions. The intervention includes four sessions with individual couples and four sessions with groups of 3–5 couples (paper under review). Positive outcomes of the Eban study will demonstrate the success of another culturally congruent adaptation of the original Connect intervention elements.

Implications for Widespread Dissemination

A significant limitation to the Project Connect findings and adaptations to date is that demonstrating efficacy of culturally-congruent HIV/STI prevention interventions is not enough to influence health disparities. Public benefit from the nation's investment in new scientific efforts will be realized only when we close the gap between research discovery and program adoption in service delivery settings (Lenihan, 1986). As noted at the beginning of this chapter, for over almost two decades, prevention scientists have demonstrated efficacy in HIV risk reduction approaches (NIMH Multisite HIV Prevention Trial, 1998; Exner, Seal, & Ehrhardt, 1997; Peterson & DiClemente, 2000; Prendergast, Urada, & Podus, 2001; Neumann et al., 2002; Semaan et al., 2002), while the science of program dissemination lags. There is a need for increased capacity, scale, and speed for HIV prevention intervention dissemination, and interactive multimedia technologies have the potential for achieving these goals (Strecher, Greenwood, Wang, & Dumont, 1999). Relatively little is known about how to best improve the availability and utilization of evidence-based HIV prevention approaches (Glasgow, Lichtenstein, & Marcus, 2003).

The existing body of literature on the transfer of HIV prevention interventions to community-based provider settings is largely based on the experiences of the CDC Replicating Effective Programs (REP) (Neumann & Sogolow, 2000; CDC, 2006b) and Diffusion of Effective Behavioral Interventions (DEBI) initiatives (CDC, 2006c). The Project Connect intervention was recently recognized by the CDC through the HIV/AIDS Prevention Research Synthesis (PRS) project (Sogolow et al., 2002; Des Jarlais & Semaan, 2002; Herbst et al., 2006)—the largest review of evidence-based HIV/STI prevention programming to date—as a best evidence intervention recommended for widespread dissemination. Simultaneously, the authors of this chapter were awarded funding as a CDC REP project to translate the Connect intervention and facilitator training into a package of materials for implementation in community-based settings, and to replicate the manualized version of Project Connect in two CBOs (PI: Witte). Project Connect is the first couple-based REP project; no DEBI projects are couple-based interventions.

In addition to the REP project funding, the Social Intervention Group (SIG) has engaged in a collaborative effort with the Columbia Center for New Media Teaching and Learning (CCNMTL) to develop the Connect intervention into an entirely multimedia-based and web-accessible intervention. The details of this process are defined more explicitly in the next chapter (see Moretti & Witte, chapter 16), and are the first step in a dissemination plan that includes a technology transfer study that will advance the science of HIV prevention dissemination research. This will be accomplished by testing whether employing multimedia and Internet-based technology for implementation of Project Connect improves adoption outcomes beyond existing technology transfer approaches, which use a combination of manuals, training, and technical assistance.

Real reductions in health disparities will take place at the point where cost-effective and easily disseminable applications of interventions, such as Project Connect, have demonstrated effectiveness in dissemination trials and are made available to all communities in need.

REFERENCES

Ajzen, I., & Fishbein, M. (1980). *Understanding attitudes and predicting social behavior.* Englewood Cliffs, NJ: Prentice-Hall.

Allen, S., Serufilira, A., Bogaerts, J., Van de Perre, P., Nsengumuremyi, F., Lindan, C., et al. (1992). Confidential HIV testing and condom promotion in Africa: Impact on HIV and gonorrhea rates. *Journal of the American Medical Association, 268*(23), 3338–3343.

Bandura, A. (1986). *Social foundations of thought and action: A social and cognitive theory.* Englewood Cliffs, NJ: Prentice-Hall.

Bandura, A. (1994). Social cognitive theory and exercise of control over HIV infection. In R. J. DiClemente (Ed.), *Preventing AIDS: Theories and methods of behavioral interventions.* New York: Plenum Press.

Basen-Engquist, K. (1992). Psychosocial predictors of "safer sex" behaviors in young adults. *AIDS Education and Prevention, 4*(2), 120–134.

Belcher, L., Kalichman, S., Topping, M., Smith, S., Emshoff, J., Norris, F., et al. (1998). A randomized trial of a brief HIV risk reduction counseling intervention for women. *Journal of Consulting and Clinical Psychology, 66*(5), 856–861.

Bronfenbrenner, U. (1979). The ecology of human development. *American Psychologist, 32,* 513–531.

Bryan, A. D., Aiken, L. S., & West, S. G. (1996). Increasing condom use: Evaluation of a theory-based intervention to prevent sexually transmitted diseases in young women. *Health Psychology*, *15*, 371–382.

Catania, J. A., Kegeles, S. M., & Coates, T. J. (1990). Towards an understanding of risk behavior: An AIDS risk reduction model (ARRM). *Health Education Quarterly*, *17*, 53–72.

Centers for Disease Control and Prevention (CDC). (2001). *HIV/AIDS surveillance supplemental report*. Atlanta, GA: U.S. Department of Health and Human Services.

Centers for Disease Control and Prevention (CDC). (2006a). Twenty-five years of HIV/AIDS—United States, 1981–2006. *Morbidity and Mortality Weekly Report*, *55*, 585–589.

Centers for Disease Control and Prevention (CDC). (2006b). *Replicating effective programs plus*. Retrieved August 6, 2007, from http://www.cdc.gov/hiv/projects/rep/

Centers for Disease Control and Prevention (CDC). (2006c). *Diffusion of effective behavioral interventions (DEBI)*. Retrieved August 6, 2007, from www.effectiveinterventions.org

Deschamps, M., Pape, J., Haffner, A., Hyppolite, R., & Johnson, W. (1991). *Heterosexual activity in at risk couples for HIV infection*. Paper presented at the VII International Conference on AIDS, Florence, Italy.

Des Jarlais, D. C., & Semaan, S. (2002). HIV prevention research: Cumulative knowledge or accumulating studies? *Journal of Acquired Immune Deficiency Syndromes*, *30*(Suppl. 1), S1–S7.

DiClemente, R. J., & Wingood, G. M. (1995). A randomized controlled trial of an HIV sexual risk-reduction intervention for young African-American women. *Journal of the American Medical Association*, *274*, 1271–1276.

Glasgow, R. E., Lichtenstein, E., & Marcus, A. C. (2003). Why don't we see more translation of health promotion research to practice? Rethinking the efficacy-to-effectivness transition. *American Journal of Public Health*, *93*(8), 1261–1267.

Ehrhardt, A., & Exner, T. (2000). Prevention of sexual risk behavior for HIV infection with women. *AIDS*, *14*(2), S53–58.

Ehrhardt, A. A. (1994). Narrow vs broad targeting of HIV/AIDS education: Response. *American Journal of Public Health*, *84*(3), 498–499.

Ehrhardt, A. A., Exner, T. M., Hoffman, S., Silberman, I., Leu, C.-S., Miller, S., et al. (2002). A gender-specific HIV/STD risk reduction intervention for women in a health care setting: Short- and long-term results of a randomized clinical trial. *AIDS Care*, *14*(2), 147–161.

El-Bassel, N., & Schilling, R. F. (1992). 15 month follow-up of women methadone patients taught to reduce heterosexual HIV transmission. *Public Health Reports*, *107*, 500–503.

El-Bassel, N., Witte, S., Gilbert, L., Sormanti, M., Moreno, C., Pereira, L., et al. (2001). HIV prevention for intimate couples: A relationship-based model. *Families, Systems, and Health*, *19*(4), 379–395.

El-Bassel, N., Witte, S. S., Gilbert, L., Wu, E., Chang, M., Hill, J., et al. (2003). The efficacy of a relationship-based HIV/STD prevention program for heterosexual couples. *American Journal of Public Health*, *93*(6), 963–969.

El-Bassel, N., Witte, S. S., Gilbert, L., Wu, E., Chang, M., Hill, J., et al. (2005). Long term effects of an HIV/STI sexual risk reduction intervention for heterosexual couples. *AIDS and Behavior*. *9*(1), 1–13.

Exner, T. M., Seal, D. W., & Ehrhardt, A. A. (1997). A review of HIV interventions for at-risk women. *AIDS and Behavior*, *1*(2), 93–124.

Fishbein, M., & Middlestadt, S. E. (1989). Using the theory of reasoned action as a framework for understanding and changing AIDS-related behaviors. In J. N. Wasserheit (Ed.), *Primary prevention of AIDS: Psychological approaches*. Newbury Park, NJ: Sage Publications.

Fisher, J. D., & Fisher, W. A. (1992). Changing AIDS-risk behavior. *Psychological Bulletin*, *111*(3), 455–474.

Harris, Y., Gorelick, P. B., Samuels, P., & Bempong, I. (1996). Why African Americans may not be participating in clinical trials. *Journal of the National Medical Association*, *88*, 630–634.

Harvey, S. (2000). New kinds of data, new options for HIV prevention among women: A public health challenge. *Health Education & Behavior*, *27*(5), 539–565.

Herbst, J. H., Collins, C. B., Kay, L. S., Crepaz, N., Lyles, C. M., & Team HAPRS. (2006). *Evidence-based HIV behavioral interventions in the United States identified through a systematic review, 2000–2004*. Atlanta, GA: Prevention Research Branch, Division of HIV/AIDS Prevention, CDC.

Higgins, D. L., Galavotti, C., O'Reilly, K. R., Schnell, D. J., Moore, M. M., Rugg, D. L., et al. (1991). Evidence for the effects of HIV antibody counseling and testing on risk behaviors. *Journal of the American Medical Association*, *266*, 2419–2429.

Ickovics, J. R., & Yoshikawa, H. (1998). Preventive interventions to reduce heterosexual HIV risk for women: Current perspectives, future directions. [Review]. *AIDS, 12*(Supplement A), S197–208.

Janz, N. K., & Becker, M. H. (1984). The Health Belief Model: A decade later. *Health Education Quarterly, 11*, 1–47.

Jemmott, J. B., III, & Jemmott, L. S. (2000). HIV behavioral interventions for adolescents in community settings. In J. Peterson & R. DiClemente (Eds.), *Handbook of HIV prevention. AIDS prevention and mental health.* New York: Kluwer Academic/Plenum Publishers.

Jemmott, J. B., III, Jemmott, L. S., & Fong, G. T. (1998). Abstinence and safer sex HIV risk-reduction interventions for African American adolescents: A randomized controlled trial. *Journal of the American Medical Association, 279*(19), 1529–1536.

Jemmott, J. B., III, Jemmott, L. S., Fong, G. T., & McCaffree, K. (1999). Reducing HIV risk-associated sexual behavior among African American adolescents: Testing the generality of intervention effects. *American Journal of Community Psychology, 27*, 161–187.

Jemmott, L. S., & Jemmott, J. B., III. (1992). Increasing condom-use intentions among sexually active inner-city black adolescent women: Effects of an AIDS prevention program. *Nursing Research, 41*, 273–279.

Kamb, M. L., Fishbein, M., Douglas, J. M. J., Rhodes, F., Rogers, J., Bolan, G., et al. (1998). Efficacy of risk-reduction counseling to prevent human immunodeficiency virus and sexually transmitted diseases: A randomized controlled trial. *Journal of the American Medical Association, 280*(13), 1161–1167.

Kambon, K. (1992). *The African personality in America: An African-centered framework.* Tallahassee, FL: NUBIAN Nation Publications.

Karenga, M. (1988). Black studies and the problematic paradigm. *Journal of Black Studies, 18*, 395–414.

Karenga, M. (1994). *Maat, the moral ideal in ancient Egypt: A study in classical African ethics.* Los Angeles: University of Southern California.

Kelly, J. A. (1995). Advances in HIV/AIDS education and prevention. *Family Relations, 44*, 345–352.

Kelly, J. A., Murphy, D. A., Sikkema, K. J., McAuliffe, T. L., Roffman, R. A., Soloman, L. J., et al. (1997). Randomised, controlled, community-level HIV prevention intervention for sexual-risk behavior among homosexual men in U.S. cities. *Lancet, 350*(9090), 1500–1505.

Kelly, J. A., Murphy, D. A., Washington, C. D., Wilson, T. S., Koob, J. J., Davis, D. R., et al. (1994). The effects of HIV/AIDS intervention groups for high-risk women in urban clinics. *American Journal of Public Health, 84*(12), 1918–1922.

Kelly, J. A., St. Lawrence, J. S., Hood, H. V., & Brasfield, T. L. (1989). Behavioral intervention to reduce AIDS risk activities. *Journal of Consulting and Clinical Psychology, 57*, 60–67.

Lenihan, G. O. (1986). Getting together, staying together: A workshop for couples. *Journal of College Student Personnel, 27*(4), 377–379.

Markman, H., Stanley, S., & Blumberg, S. L. (1996). Fighting marriage: Positive steps for preventing divorce and preserving love. *Contemporary Psychology, 41*(10), 988–990.

Moss, H. B., & Tarter, R. E. (1993). Substance abuse, aggression and violence: What are the connections? *American Journal on Addictions, 2*(2), 149–159.

Musaba, E., Morrison, C. S., Sunkutu, M. R., & Wong, E. L. (1998). Long-term use of the female condom among couples at high risk of human immunodeficiency virus infection in Zambia. *Sexually Transmitted Diseases, 25*(5), 260–264.

Nadler, A., & Fisher, J. D. (1992). Volitional personal change in an interpersonal perspective. In Y. Klar, J. D. Fisher, J. Chinsky & A. Nadler (Eds.), *Initiating self-change: Social psychological and clinical perspectives.* New York: Springer-Verlag.

National Institutes of Health. (2001). *NIH strategic research plan to reduce and ultimately eliminate health disparities.* Rockville, MD: National Institutes of Health.

Neumann, M. S., Johnson, W. D., Semaan, S., Flores, S. A., Peersman, G., Hedges, L. V., et al. (2002). Review and meta-analysis of HIV prevention intervention research for heterosexual adult populations in the United States. *Journal of Acquired Immune Deficiency Syndromes, 30*, S106–S117.

Neumann, M. S., & Sogolow, E. D. (2000). Replicating effective programs: HIV/AIDS prevention technology transfer. *AIDS Education and Prevention, 12*, 35–48.

NIMH Multisite HIV Prevention Trial. (1998). The NIMH Multisite HIV prevention Trial: Reducing HIV sexual risk behavior. *Science, 280*, 1889–1894.

O'Leary, A., & Wingood, G. M. (2000). Interventions for sexually active heterosexual women. In J. L. Peterson & R. J. DiClemente (Eds.), *Handbook of HIV prevention.* New York: Plenum.

Padian, N. S., O'Brien, T. R., Chang, Y. C., Glass, S., & Francis, D. (1993). Prevention of heterosexual transmission of human immunodeficiency virus through couple counseling. *Journal of Acquired Immune Deficiency Syndromes, 6*, 1043–1048.

Peterson, J. L., & DiClemente, R. J. (2000). *Handbook of HIV Prevention.* New York: Kluwer Academic.

Prendergast, M. L., Urada, D., & Podus, D. (2001). Meta-analysis of HIV risk reduction interventions within drug abuse treatment programs. *Journal of Consulting and Clinical Psychology, 69*(3), 389–405.

Schiff, M., Witte, S., & El-Bassel, N. (2003). Client satisfaction and perceived helping aspects of an HIV/AIDS preventative intervention for urban couples. *Research on Social Work Practice, 13*(4), 468–492.

Schilling, R. F., El-Bassel, N., Hadden, B., & Gilbert, L. (1995). Skills-training groups to reduce HIV transmission and drug use among methadone patients. *Social Work, 40*(1), 91–101.

Semaan, S., Des Jarlais, D. C., Sogolow, E., Johnson, W. D., Hedges, L. V., Ramirez, G., et al. (2002). A meta-analysis of the effect of the HIV prevention interventions on the sex behaviors of drug users in the United States. *Journal of Acquired Immune Deficiency Syndromes, 30*(Supplement 1), S73–S93.

Shain, R. N., Piper, J. M., Newton, E. R., Perdue, S. T., Ramos, R., Champion, J. D., et al. (1999). A randomized, controlled trial of a behavioral intervention to prevent sexually transmitted disease among minority women. *New England Journal of Medicine, 340*(2), 93–100.

Shavers, V. L., Lynch, C. F., & Burmeister, L. F. (2001). Factors that influence African-American willingness to participate in medical research studies. *Cancer, 91*(Supplement), 233–236.

Sogolow, E. D., Peersman, G., Semaan, S., Strouse, D., Lyles, C. M., & Team HAPRSP. (2002). The HIV/AIDS Prevention Research Synthesis Project: Scope, methods, and study classification results. *Journal of Acquired Immune Deficiency Syndromes, 30*(S1), S15–S29.

Sormanti, M., Pereira, L., El-Bassel, N., Witte, S., & Gilbert, L. (2001). The role of community consultants in designing an HIV prevention intervention. *AIDS Education and Prevention, 13*(4), 311–328.

St. Lawrence, J. S., Jefferson, K. W., Alleyne, E., & Brasfield, T. L. (1995). Comparison of education versus behavioral skills training interventions in lowering sexual HIV-risk behavior of substance-dependent adolescents. *Journal of Consulting and Clinical Psychology, 63*(1), 154–157.

Straus, M. A., Hamby, S. L., Boney-McCoy, S., & Sugarman, D. B. (1996). The revised Conflict Tactics Scales (CTS2): Development & preliminary psychometric data. *Journal of Family Issues, 17*, 283–316.

Strecher, V. J., Greenwood, T., Wang, C., & Dumont, D. (1999). Interactive multimedia and risk communication. *Journal of the National Cancer Institute Monographs, 25*, 134–139.

Swanson, M. G., & Ward, A. J. (1995). Recruiting minorities into clinical trials: Toward a participant-friendly system. *Journal of the National Cancer Institute, 87*(23), 1747–1759.

Tanner, W. M., & Pollack, R. H. (1988). The effect of condom use and erotic instructions on attitudes toward condoms. *Journal of Sex Research, 25*, 537–541.

Triandis, H. C. (1994). *Culture and social behavior.* New York: McGraw-Hill.

Van Der Straten, A., King, R., Grinstead, O., Serufilira, A., & Allen, S. (1995). Couple communication, sexual coercion and HIV risk reduction in Kigali, Rwanda. *AIDS, 9*, 935–944.

Varmus, H. (1994). NIH guidelines on the inclusion of women and minorities as subjects in clinical research. *Federal Register, 59*(59), 14508–14513.

Voluntary HIV-1 Counseling and Testing Efficacy Study Group. (2000). Efficacy of voluntary HIV-1 counselling and testing in individuals and couples in Kenya, Tanzania and Trinidad: A randomized trial. *The Lancet, 356*, 103–112.

Wingood, G. M., & DiClemente, R. J. (2000). Application of the theory of gender and power to examine HIV-related exposures, risk factors, and effective interventions for women. *Health Education & Behavior, 27*(5), 539–565.

Witte, S. S., Campbell, A., & El-Bassel, N. (2004). *Designing HIV prevention for drug-involved women exchanging street sex.* Oral presentation at the Annual Meeting of the Society for Social Work Research conference. New Orleans, LA.

Witte, S. S., El-Bassel, N., Gilbert, L., Chang, M., & Wu, E. (2006). Promoting female condom use to heterosexual couples: Findings from a randomized clinical trial. *Perspectives on Sexual and Reproductive Health, 38*(3), 148–154.

Witte, S. S., El-Bassel, N., Gilbert, L., Wu, E., Chang, M., & Steinglass, P. (2004). Recruitment of minority women and their main sexual partners in an HIV/STI prevention trial. *Journal of Women's Health, 13,* 1137–1147.

Witte, S. S., El-Bassel, N., Gilbert, L., Wu, E., & Chang, M. (in press). Predictors of discordant reports of sexual and HIV/sexually transmitted infection risk: Behaviors among heterosexual couples. *Sexually Transmitted Diseases.*

Wu, E., El-Bassel, N., Witte, S. S., Gilbert, L., & Chang, M. (2003). Associations between intimate partner violence and HIV risk among urban, low-income, minority women. *AIDS and Behavior, 7,* 291–301.

Wu, E., El-Bassel, N., Witte, S. S., Gilbert, L., Chang, M., & Morse, P. (2005). Enrollment of minority women and their main sexual partners in an HIV/STI prevention trial. *AIDS Education and Prevention, 17,* 41–52.

5

New Internet Technology—Achieving Wide Dissemination and Global Reach

Using New Media to Improve Learning: Multimedia Connect for HIV/AIDS Risk Reduction and the Triangle Initiative*

[We need] a new paradigm of scholarship, one that not only promotes the scholarship of discovering knowledge but also celebrates the scholarship of integrating knowledge, of COMMUNICATING knowledge, and of applying knowledge through professional service. [emphasis in the original]—Ernest Boyer, President, Carnegie Foundation (1994)

Introduction: The Digital Revolution and the State of our Educational Failure

Frank Moretti and Susan S. Witte

We live in a world that has been transformed by digital media. The changes have not been subtle, suggesting not a simple inflection, but a thoroughgoing transformation. Observe: the world of business and commerce, where corporations have developed the capacity to be everywhere and anywhere, transacting business globally by means of seamless, instantaneous interactions, liberating and destabilizing the balance between capital and labor hard-wrought through centuries of social dialectics; war, now pursued with smart weapons that find their targets effortlessly and produce their own press coverage at the same time, and soldiers who fight through interfaces that are extensions of their childhood Nintendo dreams; modes of entertainment that engage and enthrall so that people live in other worlds and create second lives; and, perhaps most fundamentally, science that has plumbed the secret of life and its forms, even healing illnesses and allowing us the opportunity to transform a world of HIV -infected victims into a healthy, self-sustaining citizenry.

---

*To view the images of Multimedia Connect referenced in this chapter, please visit http://ccnmtl.columbia.edu/connect/

Yet against the backdrop of these near-sci-fi scenarios that have become the warp and woof of daily life, we witness education, both narrowly and broadly defined, just as stymied as ever, with few demonstrable gains from the very same technologies. Digital media centers, research entities, educational corporations, and libraries chip at the edges of the traditional juggernaut but have thus far failed to mobilize digital media's potential to revitalize education as an enterprise or produce models of authentic education both within the academy and within the larger community of people.

In the past 10 years, two red herrings have produced misdirected energies in the field of technology and education. The first can be associated with the Clinton/Gore catchphrase, the "Information Superhighway," and the second is perhaps best captured by the notion of the "wisdom of crowds."[1] In the first, it was expected that simply sharing and making information accessible would somehow create educational equity and transformation. This was true at the school level, where the focus was on putting high-speed connections in every school, and at the university level, where the focus on digitization seemed to imply that digital technologies are best utilized as a bigger and better printing press. So go many of the educational aspirations of Web 1.0.

In the second, the expectation is that following the model of the open source software movement, education and culture will spontaneously be transformed through peer production. As goes Wikipedia, so goes the world. The most significant trait of this new idea is a naïve faith that technology, given its head, will lead us to a promised land through a kind of collective exertion. As Jarod Lanier (2006) asserts,

> What we are witnessing today is the alarming rise of the fallacy of the infallible collective. Numerous elite organizations have been swept off their feet by the idea. They are inspired by the rise of the Wikipedia, by the wealth of Google, and by the rush of entrepreneurs to be the most Meta. Government agencies, top corporate planning departments and major universities have all gotten the bug.—Digital Maoism

Although Lanier's critique of what he calls "Digital Maoism" is an attempt to save a place for the individual creator or intellect, more generally, he points out once again that technology inspires the desire for a shortcut, a bypass of the question of how individual collaborating minds achieve their depth and breadth before they enter the hive.

From this sweeping set of observations about the state of digital media and education, one can derive some basic inferences on how to proceed in the future. First and foremost, rather than looking to technology to provide economies or simply following commerce, pouncing on whatever emergent possibilities the next iTunes or iPods offer, the reinvention of education requires financial investment in appropriate forms of research and design. Secondly, the emphasis has to be on invention just as it has been in the worlds of business, science, and war (presented as separate with an awareness of

---

[1] The Information Superhighway refers to the Clinton/Gore effort to develop the Internet as a resource primarily for commerce, but also for education. In this essay, the expression "wisdom of crowds" is meant to stand for the present-day explosion of interest in peer production and social software. The expression itself is borrowed from the title of the book by James Surowiecki, *The Wisdom of Crowds: Why the Many are Smarter Than the Few and How Collective Wisdom Shapes Business, Economies, Societies and Nations*, 2005, Anchor. The book that has become the basic text for the movement is Yochai Benkler's *The Wealth of Networks: How Social Production Transforms Markets and Freedom*, 2006, New Haven: Yale University Press.

their connections). Third, the process of development and design must be deliberate, such that it draws on the wealth of past practice, and doesn't abjectly trust the future to a twenty-first century version of polytheism. Fourth, the powerful communications capacities of the Web should be allowed to topple artificial boundaries so that the academy and the community can share educational resources and opportunities more equitably.

This chapter describes the Columbia Center for New Media Teaching and Learning (CCNMTL: http://ccnmtl.columbia.edu), an organization constructed on the foundation of the principles described in the prior paragraph and devoted to providing service to University faculty, who aspire to use digital media as part of their educational efforts. We will also show how in conjunction with the Social Intervention Group (SIG) at the Columbia University School of Social Work (CUSSW), CCNMTL developed a multimedia version of Project Connect, SIG's already-successful prevention intervention (see El-Bassel, Witte, & Gilbert, chapter 15) which has been implemented in three distinct cultural settings: two in the United States and one in Central Asia, that may improve its efficacy, exponentially extend its dissemination, and also enhance classroom practice in related fields by repurposing Connect's assets for classroom use. Lastly, we will explain how CCNMTL's work with SIG led to the development of the Triangle Initiative, a new, more comprehensive strategic effort whereby through digital media, we are able to bring the three evergreen goals of the University—education, service to the community, and research—much more closely together in single projects.

The Columbia Center for New Media Teaching and Learning: Mission and Method

CCNMTL came into existence 8 years ago at the recommendation of a Columbia University faculty and administration committee charged to examine the state of digital technology on campus. Among the committee's recommendations, the first was the creation of an organization whose mission would be to provide service and support to the faculty in their use of digital technologies in the University's matriculated degree programs. In 1999, there was a significant awareness that the technology would not perform its own transformation any more than it did in the other domains of influence. In its short history, CCNMTL's original staff of three has grown to forty and has provided service to more than 3,000 faculty members with projects ranging from simple course management support to more than 150 larger projects, (see http://ccnmtl.columbia.edu/projects/). The Center, funded in large part through the University's operating budget, has received more than $5 million dollars in grants and $12 million in gifts.[2]

CCNMTL's mission is to provide service in the support of the purposeful use of digital media in education, and service is also the means of invention. Institutional arrangements and the language used to describe them are being challenged and reinvented

---

[2]CCNMTL was originally funded with a $10 million gift from a retiring member of the University Board of Trustees. After its first 5 years of operation, it was made part of the operating budget of the University with the expectation that it pursue grants and gifts to extend its efforts beyond the core subsidy. CCNMTL has received multiple grants from the National Science Foundation, the Department of Education, the Fund for the Improvement of Postsecondary Education, Ford Foundation, and others.

as digital technologies evolve and make new modalities of communication and engage-ment possible. This is particularly the case as one tries to define and manage organizations for which there are no historical antecedents. For instance, if one were to label CCNMTL a specialist support and service unit (as we do), it would not be absurd to assume that what it supports and serves is known in type and character, that it has a stable and universal identity. In fact, the process of "supporting and serving" in the digital age frequently includes a fundamental reconstruction of the enterprise of teaching and learning itself. This is as equally the case both in traditional institutional settings as it is with more customized and focused educational interventions, such as with Project Connect. If one is to call this work a service, therefore, then we must carefully define service as a proactive effort to attract faculty and other partners into simple and complex collaborations in the interest of inventing new possibilities for teaching and learning. One certain fact: we have barely begun to glimpse the landscape of education as it will be practiced in the future, no more than the pedagogues of the Early Renaissance could imagine how printing would shape the institutions of education.

Furthermore, just as these times require that new educational technology servicing organizations act as change agents within the broader pedagogical landscape, it is just as important that they play a similar role within the evolving landscape of organizational relationships. Being a good organizational team player has always carried the implication that it is important to know your place, especially in the necessarily conservative structures for memorializing knowledge and effecting its transmission. These structures have had a sacrosanct quality within the hermetic world of print. Within them one lived and worked. Now we know that we must reinvent them. Libraries are no longer "libraries" in the root sense of simply being places of the book. The computer support organizations of 20 years ago, which were specialized boutiques at the time, can only be viewed now as essential and can no longer exist in isolation; they are integral to the conduct of the business of education. The struggle for organizational clarity and effectiveness continues. We must be active and alive to possible opportunities for convergence and the reordering of these legacy enterprises, both in changing libraries with centuries of history, and digital organizations with only decades of habits, as well as research enterprises that in the print world would not have seen the links between the development of new pedagogical approaches and their efforts in the broader community.[3]

Digital service entities like CCNMTL provide motivation for bringing together traditionally separated activities of information provision, curriculum development, and tool construction. We must represent the new partnerships made possible by the fact that digital technologies are the common stuff of information in all media forms: of the tools of engagement—editing, analysis, authoring—as well as the scenarios that provide the context to make student work activity driven and purposeful. This is the new seamlessness of the pedagogical revolution. We need to recover from the Web-induced lapse into naive empiricism that dictated that simply providing the so-called "objects" to the learners

---

[3] See "Ménage a Trois: The Essential Computing, Library and Instructional Technology Partnership to Advance New Media Learning" by Frank Moretti, James Neal, and Patricia Renfro, all of Columbia University, at the Association of College and Research Libraries conference in April 2005. Session recording available from the ACRL. The PowerPoint presentation is available online at http://ccnmtl.columbia.edu/news/ACRLpresentation.ppt. Here, the argument is made that new forms of cooperation and new possibilities for the convergence of formerly separate elements of the information support structure of universities are now possible.

would magically occasion learning. We must recognize unique opportunities that the technologies provide to situate the learner in an active tool context connected to new emerging capacities to configure and present information. We must recognize similar opportunities to construct challenging and interesting use-scenarios. It must become as natural for libraries to suggest tools and context possibilities, as it must be for service entities to integrate information resources and digital libraries in their constructions. Lines between what had previously been discreet entities have become blurred, and it is necessary to grapple with the creation of their future connections and articulations. No one says this more eloquently than Dan Atkins, as quoted in the recently released report of the American Council of Learned Societies Commission on Cyberinfrastructure for the Humanities and Social Sciences.

The 2003 National Science Foundation report *Revolutionizing Science and Engineering Through Cyberinfrastructure* (hereafter referred to as the "Atkins report," after Dan Atkins, who chaired the committe that produced it) described *cyberinfrastructure* as a "layer of enabling hardware, algorithms, software, communications, institutions, and personnel" that lies between a layer of "base technologies . . . the integrated electro-optical components of computation, storage, and communication" and a layer of "software programs, services, instruments, data, information, knowledge, and social practices applicable to specific projects, disciplines, and communities of practice." In other words, for the Atkins report (and for this one), cyberinfrastructure is more than a tangible network and means of storage in digitized form, and it is not only discipline-specific software applications and project-specific data collections. It is also the more intangible layer of expertise and the best practices, standards, tools, collections and collaborative environments that can be broadly *shared* across communities of inquiry. "This layer," as the Atkins report notes, "should provide an effective and efficient platform for the empowerment of specific communities of researchers to innovate and eventually revolutionize what they do, how they do it, and who participates."[4]

Although these comments are directed to the research enterprise, the same exact characteristics and conditions are true for education. The issue is not information alone, but the "empowerment" of teachers and students through the provision of tools, best curricular practices, and the exploitation of the collaborative capacities of digital technologies.

Whether working with individual faculty members or larger groups, such as the Social Intervention Group, CCNMTL follows a methodology focused on beginning with the problem or opportunity and then proceeding to explore possible interventions. This process, which we call Design Research, is derived from the work of Ann Brown, Allan Collins, and Daniel Edelson, among others (Brown, 1992; Collins, 1999; Edelson, 2002). It is the common methodology shared by staff. Of course, no one person is expected to follow this in the exact order in which it is presented. This methodology acts as an anchor in a world of extreme motility that enables one, regardless of the different disciplines involved, to return to a common set of questions to be answered. (See http://ccnmtl.columbia.edu/dr/index.html for further information as well as Moretti & Pinto, 2005 and Moretti, 2005.)

---

[4]From *Our Cultural Commonwealth: The Report of the American Council of Learned Societies Commission on Cyberinfrastructure for the Humanities and Social Sciences*, American Council of Learned Societies, 2006. The full report is available online at http://www.acls.org/cyberinfrastructure/OurCulturalCommonwealth.pdf.

Here is their basic codification:

Step 1: **Understanding the curriculum and defining the challenge.** Each project requires that the faculty client and the Center representative(s) share a common understanding of the curriculum and its objectives. Just as many homeowners choose to buy tools before they have identified a need to use them, educational technologists are sometimes guilty of adopting technologies, quasi-technologies, and then looking for a place to apply them. Whether one is designing a simple course site or beginning to evolve the design of a larger solution, it is importan to locate all early discussions in the curricular context and its problems. With that understanding as a basis, it is then possible to identify the challenge, the area where significant improvement is possible.

Step 2: With the problem in mind, the next step in each case is to **hypothesize solutions** that include both inflections of the curricular context as well as changes in or developments of the technology.

Step 3: The **actual design and construction** of the environment, both curricular and technological, as outlined in Step 2.

Step 4: **Implementation** of the project in class. In each case the delivery of the project to the faculty member by the development team did not end the service involvement. Rather, the deployment and use of the project with students should be observed and supported as much as is feasible by the educational technologist.

Step 5: Based on criteria developed in Stage 3, the **intervention must be assessed** with the results used either to redevelop the project to increase its effectiveness or to corroborate the approach as an example of a best practice.

This cycle (understanding the curricular context and identifying the challenges, hypothesis, design, implementation, and assessment) is represented by the graphic in Figure 16.1.

Multimedia Connect and the Process of Its Development

Discovery

Working essentially within the design research structure, a CCNMTL team began working with senior researchers of the Social Intervention Group (SIG) at the Columbia University School of Social Work (http://www.columbia.edu/cu/ssw/sig/).

SIG is a multidisciplinary research center at the CUSSW that focuses on developing and testing effective prevention and intervention approaches and disseminates them to local, national, and international communities. The research addresses the co-occurring problems of HIV, substance abuse, intimate partner violence, and trauma, placing particular emphasis on the overlap and connections among these issues. A key aspect of SIG's mission is to move science-based medical, behavioral, and health service interventions from a research environment to community-based settings, making them more accessible to those who need them most.

Senior researchers and faculty at SIG, including Professors Nabila El-Bassel and Susan Witte, and Louisa Gilbert, had developed and tested Project Connect, the first couple-based, HIV/sexually transmitted infections (STI) prevention intervention that

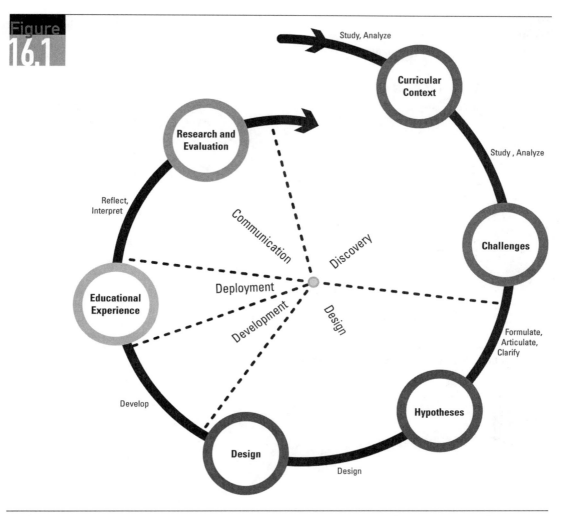

Illustrates how the Design Research methodology follows an iterative path of discovery, design, deployment, and communication.

was funded by the National Institute of Mental Health (NIMH) (for complete discussion see El-Bassel et al., chapter 15). SIG had proven the effectiveness of Project Connect in reducing sexual risk behaviors among heterosexual couples, but could not widely disseminate it because in its current form, implementation required the skills of an advanced clinician and a burdensome amount of peripheral material that was used during each session. (See articles by El-Bassel et al., 2001, 2003, 2005; Sormanti, Pereira, El-Bassel, Witte, & Gilbert, 2001.) During an extended discovery period, the CCNMTL/SIG team brainstormed many possibilities for the enhancement of Connect using digital media. This required, as a prerequisite, that CCNMTL become conversant with the content, process, and theoretical underpinnings of the intervention as well as all of the existing media SIG was accustomed to use, including videos, anatomical models, condoms and other prophylactics, and charts. SIG had to learn about the range of possibilities that

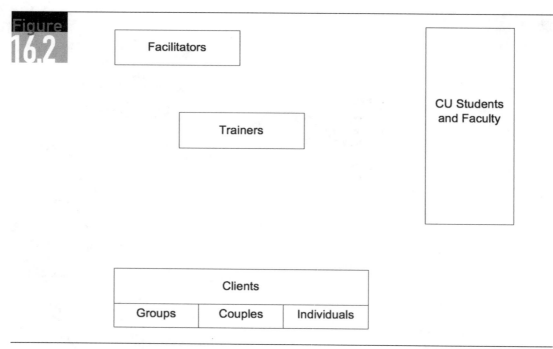

Potential beneficiaries of Multimedia Connect.

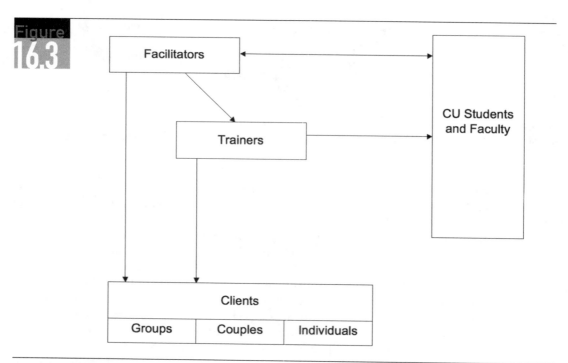

Plot of the different relationships among the identified groups.

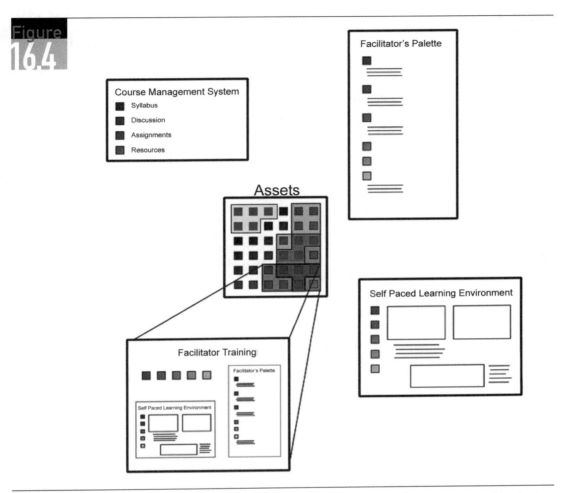

Figure 16.4

The diagrams in Figures 16.4 and 16.5 represent how a common set of assets, represented by the box in the middle, can serve all four projected audiences. In the original computer-based model, the lines connecting the assets to the audiences rotated.

digital media could support. Also from the very beginning, the team worked not only to imagine digital enhancements for Connect, but also to brainstorm how facilitator training might be improved and how what was developed might be repurposed for use in courses at the Columbia University School of Social Work. Here are the first series of visualizations developed during the discovery phase to describe the general landscape of audiences to be served and how the modularity of media allows for a common reservoir of assets to be deployed in different contexts to serve different groups (see Figures 16.2, 16.3, 16.4, and 16.5).

The discovery process continued using similar modeling techniques, from which the team derived basic strategies that were expressed in the form of a series of hypotheses. The following is a sample of these, along with the visuals developed to represent and communicate them.

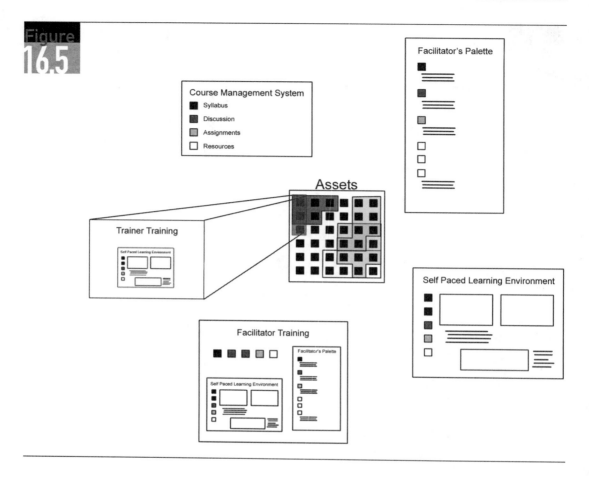

Hypotheses and Design

The effort begins by defining a problem that then leads to a hypothesis that directs development and that can ultimately be assessed in respect to its efficacy.

1. **Problem:** How can we help the participants better internalize (learn) what they need to institute healthier sex practices in their relationships?

Hypothesis: If we use multimedia to better communicate psycho–educational content, then, given the fact that most recipients of the intervention live in visual and significantly media-bound worlds, it would increase the probability of retention. The following example from the design research process demonstrates this approach to the myth/fact game, a part of the original intervention. Here, participants view the following myth/fact question shown in Figure 16.6.

They are then presented with an image of Magic Johnson along with the correct answer, explaining that a person does not necessarily display symptoms of illness even while they have HIV (see http://ccnmtl.columbia.edu/connect/mythfact.html).

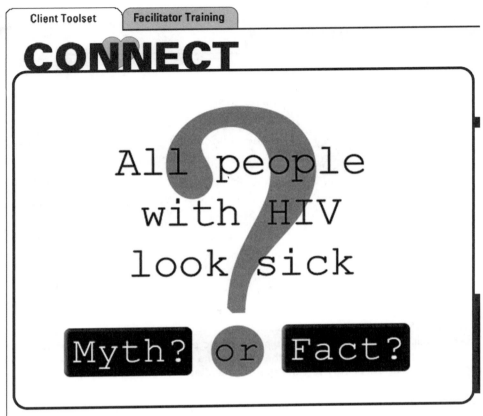

The question is posed.

2. Problem: Presently, it is more often the case than not that Connect is executed by highly trained clinicians. How can we broaden the base of facilitators so that a community-based health worker with some basic training could implement Connect?

Hypothesis: If Multimedia Connect could be organized so that its elements were represented in a computer environment as a roadmap used both to train facilitators and perform the intervention itself, then the training would be more consistently delivered to a broader base of community health workers who would use the same environment in their actual delivery of the intervention. Providing such a scaffold will relieve the facilitator from the anxieties related to managing the sequence of events in the intervention and, simultaneously, give both the facilitator and the participants a consistent and stable set of media objects and utilities that accompany them through the experience. See Figure 16.7.

3. Problem: Since the real world results of Connect depend on the capacity of the participants to maintain an open, frank, and collaborative way of making decisions, the

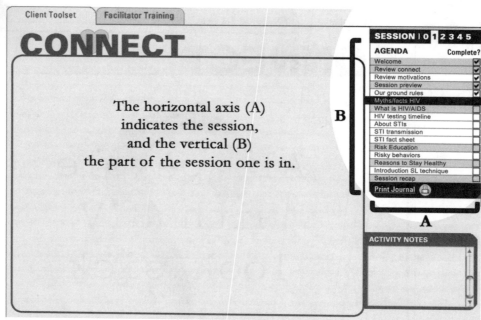

The roadmap is in the upper right-hand part of the screen. The horizontal axis indicates the session and the vertical axis indicates the part of the session one is in. As one moves through Connect, the menu highlights the current activity, and the appropriate related media is displayed on the screen.

importance of the part of the intervention that directly addresses and supports the development of these skills cannot be underestimated. How can Connect better support the communication and listening skills component that is part of the essential core in all six sessions?

Hypothesis: If we were to provide a video palette that would be present in every session with examples of people using speaker/listener skills addressing the specific topic of each session, these will improve client speaker/listener skills by providing the facilitator with a more flexible set of examples that can be used when deemed necessary.[5] (See speaker-listener process at http://ccnmtl.columbia.edu/connect/speakerlistener.html)

4. Problem: In Connect, participants often leave with things they have drawn or written in the process of the intervention on a session-by-session basis. Is there a way to extend this positive form of behavioral enforcement so that the materials participants leave with serve both as useful tools and more active memorials of their contract with one another as well as the successful completion of the intervention?

Hypothesis: If Multimedia Connect provides the capacity to print out all the specific information as well as general knowledge participants have learned and created

---

[5] *Speaker/Listener Technique* by H. Markman, S. Stanley, and S. Blumberg, 1996, Denver, Colorado: Educational Products, Inc.

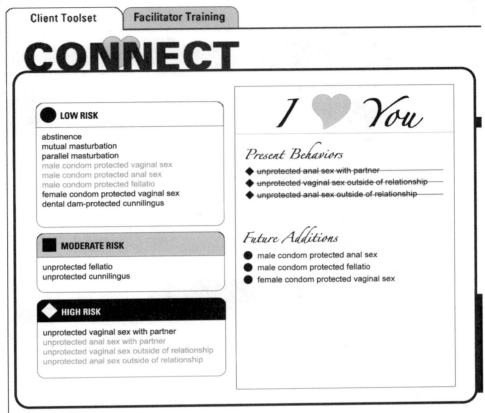

This visual comes from Session 2 and the Satisfying Safer Sex Scale. The participating couple makes selections from a random list provided by the facilitator, creating the ranking of the sex practices on the right. The middle list represents the couple's agreed upon goals. The activity note box has in it something the male member of the couple acknowledged and a new commitment he has made as part of the session. All of the information appearing on this screen is saved by the computer and becomes part of the customized manual that will be given to the couple upon the completion of Connect.

in the intervention (including the session-by-session notes participants create as they go through the intervention), then handing this material to the participants at the successful conclusion of the intervention will increase their sense of accomplishment and ownership of what they have agreed with each other, and may increase the length of Connect's positive effects (see Figure 16.8).

Development

Multimedia Connect is in the process of being developed across early months of the year 2007 as this is being written. Already completed are the Social Support Network Map (SSNM) and a prototype of Sessions 1 and 2 that were part of a pilot study produced in preparation for a National Institute of Mental Health research grant submission. Both

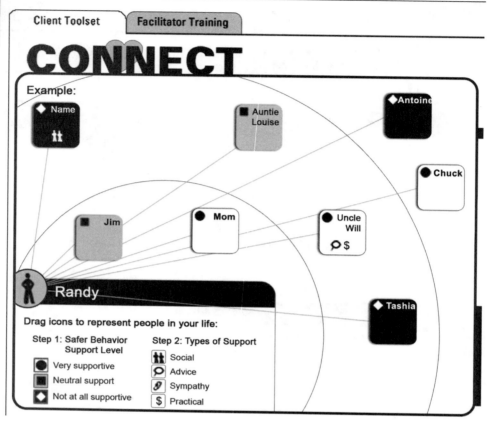

Figure 16.9

In the original design, the Social Support Network Map was called ECO Map and was the fourth element of the fifth session.

of these will be further described in the following section on the educational experience and evaluation.

Trial Run and Evaluation

Thus far, there have been two actual uses of already developed elements of Multimedia Connect. The SSNM has been used in classes at the Columbia University School of Social Work in clinical practice courses, and the pilot of Sessions 1 and 2 were used in an AIDS–related community-based services organization during the summer of 2006 with five couples. In developing the media-based version of the SSNM, which is a critical element of the intervention's fifth session, the design research process has produced the visual in Figure 16.9 as point of departure for the developers.

The working hypothesis was that if participants had a dynamic version of what was already a well–tested part of the Connect intervention, it would provide the facilitators and researchers the capacity to do quick modifications of the nomenclature with the goal of increasing the SSNM's effectiveness. In addition, by having a dynamic computer-based

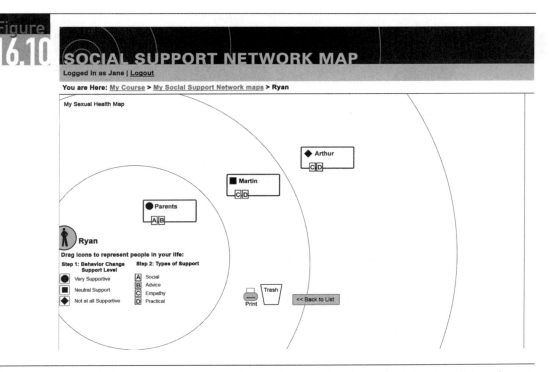

Figure 16.10

The dynamic characteristics of the map are obvious in the active language on the screen: click to change, save, discard, or drag icons. Less obvious is the fact that you can adjust the concentric circles to portray the proximity and distance of the influence of particular individuals.

(Web-based) version of the SSNM, it would be possible, as with many other elements of Multimedia Connect, to collect research data as it was being used, not only a significant economy and productive of an almost unfailing accuracy, but also capable of generating new information not possible without it, such as an account of the step by step use of the tool. The resulting actual SSNM appears in Figure 16.10.

The faculty member who used the Social Support Network Map in her course told us that

> Rather than stay in the abstract, we were able to actively engage the tool in the classroom, increasing each student's self-efficacy to use it and to implement it with clients in fieldwork settings. I feel more confident that these students would make use of the tool in settings where they have Internet access, compared to past years when I taught students to use a paper and pencil version. I am also aware of at least two students who have already used the tool with their clients in the course of their clinical work. A survey of students after the exercise revealed that 100% of students felt that the exercise better helped them understand the clinical technique of social support network mapping. [6]

---

[6] This comment is from an unpublished report of CCNMTL on the effectiveness of the Social Support Network Map in masters' level courses at the Columbia University School of Social Work.

The 2006 summer pilot test of a prototype of Sessions 1 and 2 produced very positive results, which are included in an NIMH research grant submission and are on the Multimedia Connect Web site. In summary, facilitators who participated in the pilot felt that the use of the computer greatly simplified the intervention delivery process, allowing them to focus more attention to the participants, making the content and skills-building more meaningful. They reported that the computer interaction did not compete with their ability to engage with participants, and that the multimedia was particularly engaging for participants with lower literacy, and younger participants who are more visually oriented. The staff reported no reluctance on the part of participants to engage the media. Further, staff felt that even the brief pilot appeared to be effective in imparting new knowledge and skills to the couples who attended.

In addition to learning much about the technical needs of the process, the pilot also showed that training the staff to implement the multimedia sessions was greatly enhanced by the multimedia facilitator-training curriculum. Compared with other onsite trainings for other large-scale National Institute of Health–funded prevention interventions, it was found that using multimedia reduces the amount of required peripherals and materials, as well as the preparation time and logistics that must go into traditional interventionist trainings.[7]

Unexpected Gifts of the Design Research Process

As the team proceeded with its design research, the significant long-term goals of Multimedia Connect began to emerge. The design research process had enhanced the team's vision of possibilities. The conversation moved from what was reasonably apparent at the beginning—that it would be possible to make Connect more effective through the use of multimedia and the incorporation of new technology-dependent forms of behavioral supports and that the training of facilitators would be largely enhanced and made more economical, to a far more embracive vision. One element of that vision came into focus when the team began to understand more fully the specific potentialities the modularity of digital media affords (Manovich, 2001).[8] The team began to see Multimedia Connect as a potentially global solution, ironically in part because the modularity of media allows for the localization process to take place more effortlessly. Multimedia Connect could be customized for language and cultural appropriateness without having to rebuild each version from scratch. In addition—and more obviously—the World Wide Web is exactly what it presents itself as, worldwide, and as such guarantees significant access to a majority of the earth's population. For those for whom the Web presents a problem because of either physical access or authorization, digital media make it possible to provide an optical disc (CD-ROM) or a smart disc for the network. As the team began to imagine these possibilities, some of its members began conversations with the 100 Dollar Laptop project people from MIT (See Negroponte, 2006.). The vision of a technology-powered

---

[7]These results are documented in an unpublished report, the substance of which has been included in a National Institute of Mental Health R01 research application, January 2007.

[8]See Lev Manovich's *The Language of New Media*, where he develops a description of the new palette of the digital media maker, the core concept of which is the flexibility, the modularity, of elements able to be reshaped and reconstituted both within and without the flow of time.

underclass making use of Multimedia Connect came one step closer to becoming a reality. At this point in the design research process, the team has elaborated three general goals: to improve outcomes within a social–cognitive framework through the use of digital media and new forms of behavioral support; to widen the range of facilitators through structure, standardization, and new approaches to facilitator training; and to make Multimedia Connect internationally deployable through the Web and other digital solutions as well as to gain the capacity to localize rapidly for culture and language.

A second unexpected result of the process was the creation of a completely new strategic endeavor for Columbia, the Triangle Initiative, the subject of the next section.

The Triangle Initiative: Digital Media and the Realization of the Three Evergreen Goals of the University

One of the unforeseen results of conceptualizing and designing Multimedia Connect was the realization that digital media provided a unique means to bring the often disparate goals of Columbia University in much closer harmony. In reflecting on what had been accomplished, it was apparent that the creation of Multimedia Connect had simultaneously contributed in direct and significant ways to advancing the research SIG had pioneered in by positioning them to study a large-scale dissemination of their proven intervention and to also explore the potential of new media in a more generic sense to provide unique support for community public health and human services efforts. Furthermore, both Multimedia Connect as a totality, as well as specific elements of it, such as the Social Support Network Map, will enrich the classrooms of social work and public health programs as well as others. And, most obviously, Multimedia Connect will have a direct and positive effect on the community, which is the target audience to begin with. In other words, a single media product maintaining its constructed identity without significant modification directly contributes to research, education and the welfare of the community.

This inspired the leadership of CCNMTL to look for other opportunities to accomplish the same triple play using Multimedia Connect as its heuristic. At present, we have three other Triangle Initiative projects, described below.

1. Collateral Consequences of Criminal Prosecution Knowledge Center

(http://www2.law.columbia.edu/fourcs/)
This resource compares the collateral consequences of criminal charges across of variety of doctrinal areas. CCKC will serve multiple communities in a variety of ways: faculty will build case studies around it, lawyers can use it to help them better counsel their clients, judges can use it to help assure appropriate sentencing, and public policy researchers can use it as a lens through which to examine the matrix of the New York State legal system.

Judge Kaye, Chief Justice of New York State, has supported the development of this tool, which she sees as a valuable social justice initiative. The project is in partnership with the Law School of Columbia University, specifically with Conrad Johnson, Clinical

Professor of Law and Director of the Lawyering in the Digital Age Clinic and member of the Collateral Consequences of Criminal Charges Working Group.

2. Women's Health Intervention: A Multimedia Approach

Working in collaboration with Dr. Denise Hien, Research Scientist, and Dr. Lisa Litt, Assistant Clinical Professor, both affiliated with the School of Social Work's Social Intervention Group, CCNMTL is developing a media-informed behavioral intervention for women with posttraumatic stress disorder and substance use disorder. The intervention, already proven successful in early iterations, will be developed to both enhance its efficacy and to improve and extend training possibilities for facilitators with the goal of extending it as a resource to a broader audience.

3. Multimedia Smart: Drug Adherence and Health

Working in conjunction with Dr. Robert Remien, Associate Professor of Clinical Psychology, Dr. Claude Ann Mellins, Associate Professor of Clinical Psychology, and Dr. Elaine Abrams, Associate Professor of Clinical Pediatrics and Clinical Epidemiology, at the HIV Center for Clinical and Behavioral Studies at the New York State Psychiatric Institute and Columbia University, and using as a point of departure Project SMART, already proved effective in research, CCNMTL will help construct a media rich version of the intervention with the goals of extending the target audience from couples/dyads to families, enhancing its efficacy and reaching a broader audience. In addition to research trials with the newly developed media interventions collaborating faculty will both deploy the resulting media assets in existing and new courses as well as recruit others to do the same in the Mailman School of Public Health, the School of Social Work, and the College of Physicians and Surgeons.

The Triangle Initiative has been well received by the Columbia community of faculty, researchers, and administrators. At present, it has received over one million dollars in support.

Conclusion and Future Possibilities

Anticipated Impact: Multimedia Connect and the Triangle Initiative

The Triangle Initiative will establish Columbia as a leader in extending its applied research in the human sciences into the classroom and community through the development of a new model of simultaneous classroom and community learning object development. The Triangle Initiative, through its specific projects, will seek to establish the efficacy of certain template approaches that will establish the "brand" of Columbia in the applied arena. This creates a unique new articulation of the University's often-disparate research, educational, and community objectives. Specific areas of interest include health and social welfare, law and justice, conflict resolution and, sustainable development.

The modularity of digital products enables Columbia researchers and field operatives to function in a global arena with the capacity to localize health and social welfare interventions for culture and language. It will be possible to substitute data within previously proven pedagogical formats in order to accommodate learning needs related to different ethnic and economic niches. For instance, SIG's Project Connect has been tested in three cultural settings, and with the extended capacity of Multimedia Connect, will reach a global audience. Additionally, the modularity of new media will allow for the substitution of different landscapes and settings as seen by field workers in various locations.

Columbia educators will build more profound bridges between the world of preparation and the world of practice because in the future, the tools of the teacher will be more often the tools of the practitioner. New fields of research will emerge as new forms of public and pedagogical intervention are realized. As an example, SIG researchers, by extending dissemination of their interventions with new media, will evolve new and deeper understandings of the significance of cultural difference in their work.

As always in human history, the battle continues between the forces of reform working towards the alleviation of human misery and the forces of mindless exploitation for profit and gain. Digital technologies have been enlisted on both sides and have exacerbated the differences among people, but also have shown the possibility and promise of reducing disparities and differences. As often has been the case in the past, there is a disproportionate investment in technology that anesthetizes and kills for the profit of the few. The challenge of the future is to leverage more in the interest of the many with little, and to create the conditions for a greater democratization of human possibilities that the explosive technology movements of our time makes possible, always remembering that the technology does not dictate its use, but we, its inventors.

REFERENCES

American Council of Learned Societies. (2006). *Our cultural commonwealth: The report of the American Council of Learned Societies Commission on Cyberinfrastructure for the Humanities and Social Sciences* (p. 13). New York: Author.

Benkler, Y. (2006). *The wealth of networks: How social production transforms networks and freedom.* New Haven, CT: Yale University Press.

Brown, A. L. (1992). Design experiments: Theoretical and methodological challenges in creating complex interventions. *Journal of the Learning Sciences, 2,* 141–178.

Collins, A. (1992). Toward a design science of education. In E. Scanlon & T. O'Shea (Eds.), *New directions in educational technology.* Berlin: Springer-Verlag.

Edelson, D. (2002). Design research: What we learn when we engage in design. *The Journal of the Learning Sciences, 11*(1).

El-Bassel, N., Witte, S. S., Gilbert, L., Sormanti, M., Moreno, C., Pereira, L., et al. (2001). HIV prevention for intimate couples: A relationship-based model. *Families, Systems, & Health, 19,* 379–395.

El-Bassel, N., Witte, S. S., Gilbert, L., Wu, E., Chang, M., Hill, J., et al. (2003). The efficacy of a relationship-based HIV/STD prevention program for heterosexual couples. *American Journal of Public Health, 93,* 963–969.

El-Bassel, N., Witte, S. S., Gilbert, L., Wu, E., Chang, M., Hill, J., et al. (2005). Long-term effects of an HIV/STI sexual risk reduction intervention for heterosexual couples. *AIDS and Behavior, 9*(1), 1–13.

Lanier, J. (2006, May 30). *Digital Maoism: The hazards of the new online collectivism.* Retrieved December 28, 2006, from http://www.edge.org/3rd_culture/lanier06/lanier06_index.html

Manovich, L. (2001). *The language of new media*. Cambridge, MA: MIT Press.

Moretti, F. (2005). Support in the use of new media. In M. Melling (Ed.), *Supporting E-learning: A guide for library and information managers*. London: Facet Publishing.

Moretti, F., & Pinto, L. (2005). What have we learned and how have we learned it? Examples of best practices of a new media services and development center in higher education. In B. Lehmann & E. Bloh (Ed.), *Online-Pädagogik* (Band 3). Baltmannsweiler, Germany: Schneider Verlag Hohengehren.

Negroponte, N. (2006, February). Retrieved December 28, 2006, from http://www.ted.com/tedtalks/tedtalksplayer.cfm?key=n_negroponte&gclid=CM_AnNPBl4kCFQQWUAods3FZSg

Sormanti, M., Pereira, L., El-Bassel, N., Witte, S. S., & Gilbert, L. (2001). The role of community consultants in designing an HIV prevention intervention. *AIDS Education and Prevention, 13*, 311–328.

A Role for Health Informatics and Information Technology (HIIT): Shaping a Global Research Agenda to Eliminate Health Disparities

Emerging Trends in Health Informatics Information Technology

Health professionals and consumers increasingly rely on various types of health-related data and information to support a broad range of functions ranging from public policy, research, service planning, and delivery through consumption. Informatics, the science of information management in health care, offers applications that can be used to support each of these functions and more. When used in conjunction with health information technology—computational systems that can perform a variety of information functions such as organizing, analyzing, and evaluating, compiling and coding information and/or statistics—then information can be managed, processed, and accessed more systematically by various users.

New advances in health informatics and information technology (HIIT) are constantly entering the marketplace. As one discovery is made another is on its heels waiting to enter the marketplace as an update or replacement. In the health care arena, providers and consumers are challenged to understand what technologies are available and how these tools with their multiple applications can be used to help improve services or manage various aspects of one's own health care.

Effective HIIT tools allow us to perform certain functions such as to receive, process, transmit, retrieve, protect and analyze a vast array of information. Each of these functions involves a high level of responsibility and a workforce that is knowledgeable and proficient in the use of appropriate tools to support these functions. Critical evaluations of the impact of emerging and new technologies alone have been significant (i.e., reducing medication errors and other adverse outcomes). Literature

Diane L. Adams
and Brenda A. Leath

reviews and information searches have shown that eliminating health disparities is a top strategic priority for most organizations globally. A demanding trend is to invest in research. This is essential if we are to use HIIT applications to address health disparities locally and globally.

Global Health Disparities, Health Informatics, and Information Technology

According to data in the World Factbook, as of July 2006, there were an estimated 6,525,170,264 people living in more than 268 nations around the globe. Approximately 27% of the population were 14 years of age or younger, over 65% were 15–64 years of age and about 7% were 65 years and older (Central Intelligence Agency [CIA], 2006). Indicators such as an infant mortality rate of 48.77 deaths/1,000 live births, a life expectancy of 64.77 years (CIA, 2006), and according to the World Health Organization (WHO), more than 39.5 million people living with HIV let us know about the health of our global community (WHO, 2006a). Almost 180 million people between the ages of 10 and 24 live with a disability. Most or about 150 million, live in the developing world and are routinely excluded from most educational, economic, social, and cultural opportunities (Groce, 2003). Our global society is also aging, which presents additional challenges for improving quality of care across the life span in order to support health and longevity. Yet, estimates indicate that less than 10% of the world's biomedical research funds are dedicated to addressing problems that are responsible for 90% of the world's burden of disease (Resnik, 2004). These statistics and trends, along with a host of other health indicators, provide insight into which population subgroups are overburdened with illness, disease and health disparities.

The National Institutes of Health (NIH) defines health disparities as "the differences in the incidence, prevalence, mortality, and burden of diseases and other adverse health conditions that exist among specific population groups in the United States." (NIH, 2000). This same definition is applicable to the global community. The manifestation of health disparities may surface in different subgroups based on various socioeconomic and cultural influences. In addition to these factors, Pfizer includes educational attainment level and geographic factors (Pfizer, 2004). In some instances excess disease burden is linked to gender, race, ethnicity, or disability. Despite how these disparities manifest, HIIT can be useful in many ways to address disease burden and disparities. For example, it can support surveillance of disease and health threats, manage services and resource allocations, track service utilization, document epidemiological and etiological relationships in disease processes, facilitate clinical decision making, and organize patient health information.

In our global society the health care needs of one community have implications for the larger worldwide community and vice versa. While industrialization of various nations has revolutionized life in countless ways, accompanying this growth has been an increasingly mobile society. People now travel distances for short-term visits to various countries or for long-term or permanent relocation to other geographic areas. In either case, each relies on information to support every aspect of daily living. At the same time, the combination of mobility and international growth and development has introduced increased opportunities for disease transmission from one region to another.

Diseases once regarded as problems of developing countries are increasingly being monitored to prevent their occurrence as threats to industrialized nations. One such example includes the reemergence of tuberculosis (TB). Researchers report that TB is a global epidemic with about one-third of the population infected and 9 million active cases. Knowledge of statistics is a result of a 10-year global project on Anti-Tuberculosis Drug Resistance Surveillance conducted by the World Health Organization and its partners (Aziz & Wright, 2005). Today's TB challenge relates to the prevalence of drug resistant strains (Multi Drug Resistant [MDR] and Extensive Drug Resistant [XDR]). Many international nations struggle to address the need for early detection and treatment of MDR-TB and XDR-TB and are working collaboratively to seek effective solutions. The convening of the 37th World Conference of the International Union Against Tuberculosis and Lung Disease in 2006 provided a venue for information exchange about community-based interventions and assessments of electronic record systems as a mechanism for maintaining comprehensive patient information and streamlining medical supply orders (Partners in Health, 2006).

Of relevance to this same issue is a recent survey conducted by the World Health Organization and the Centers for Disease Control and Prevention (CDC) on data from 2000–2004, which found that XDR-TB has been identified in all regions of the world but is most frequent in the countries of the former Soviet Union and in Asia. In the United States, 4% of MDR-TB cases met the criteria for XDR-TB. The World Health Organization also highlights separate data on a recent outbreak of XDR-TB in an HIV-positive population in Kwazulu-Natal in South Africa, which was characterized by alarmingly high mortality rates. In view of the underlying HIV epidemic, drug-resistant TB could have a severe impact on mortality in Africa (WHO, 2006b).

In these scenarios, the use of health informatics and information technology can prove to be useful tools in support of recommended disease surveillance and control measures. Relative to the TB cases described, Geographical Information Systems (GIS) also known as Geospatial Information Systems might be used as a tool to map TB outbreaks and/or HIV prevalence by location of communities affected. GIS could also be used to show patterns of the outbreaks over time as part of surveillance measures. GIS has many public health applications including disease and syndromic surveillance, supporting health research studies (i.e., health policy and epidemiological studies) and organizing clinical data geographically. Its use of computer hardware, software, and geographic data to capture, manage, analyze, and present geographically referenced data and information makes it an invaluable tool for various purposes. The Open Geospatial Consortium (OGC) is a key source working to provide interoperability solutions globally, adding capacity for global health research, policy, and services development. According to its mission, OGC is an international consortium that represents over 300 companies, government agencies, and universities. It serves as a global forum for the collaboration of developers and users of spatial data products and services, and to advance the development of international standards for geospatial interoperability (OGC Web site, n.d.).

Other examples of relevant HIIT applications to address the TB example might include public awareness communications focused on preventive precautions; use of clinical support tools that prompt provider diagnosis and treatment of drug resistant cases; and support of information management and collaboration between disease control programs. Communications between the HIV and TB control programs noted in the previous example would alert health officials of the special care needs of patients who are both HIV-positive and have contracted TB. Such communications would advance efforts to implement local and regional surveillance activities that support early detection and management of resistant cases.

Disease control measures must respond to a different threat today as a result of the evolution of different strains of agents that require new therapeutic interventions than those of yesterday. Surveillance systems are useful in monitoring and tracking the spread or decline of these diseases and help to support decision making about needed precautions or re-allocation of scarce resources.

Interconnections between the micro and macro level social networks within the global community are vast and require multidimensional approaches to the delivery of effective quality health care. Responsive global health strategies require attention to a variety of factors among which include population diversity, disparities, cultural and linguistic competence, workforce development and adoption and use of standards of care. Concurrently, it also requires development and adoption of a framework and infrastructure that support information and knowledge development, management, and use.

There are many perspectives on possible intersections between disparities and HIIT cited in the literature. One view includes that presented by Brennan (2003), who shares the following context for how informatics can address health disparities and the need for interdisciplinary collaboration. She describes how informatics professionals view the use of information to reach underserved populations, noting that disparities reflect:

- Differential access to health services
- Differential experiences of known health care problems
- Differential manifestation of health phenomena
- Differential response to health, illness, and disease challenges
- Differential approaches to management of health, illness, and development challenges

Addressing these challenges calls for collaboration between investigators with expertise in health disparities and informatics. A partnership between these two groups of professionals will help to leverage critical knowledge, skills, and tools that can be used to undergird integrative problem solving in support of efforts that foster health equity. Specifically, health disparities investigators offer language, stakeholders, a range of diversity, and vernacular, while informatics investigators offer representation schemes, terminology models, information models, and integration mechanisms (Brennan, 2003).

Gingrich and Dillione (2007) share a perspective based on growing evidence that health information technology can serve as a viable solution for reducing medication errors. They indicate that many of these errors are connected to more than 1.5 million injuries and deaths annually in the United States. Electronic prescribing, electronic health records, and clinical decision support systems are among the technologies that are increasingly being promoted as potential solutions.

In general, there seems to be some consensus among thought leaders that in order to integrate health disparities and information technology, there must be a coordinated effort among all of the entities involved. Therefore, integration of health informatics and information technology must involve all jurisdictions: state, local, federal, and international community in order for it to be effective.

Numerous research efforts are underway at various jurisdictional levels. At the federal level in the United States, the national health agenda includes a research component to address health disparities. For example, the Agency for Healthcare Research and Quality (AHRQ) has funded research to study overcoming health disparities (U.S. Department of Health and Human Services [HHS], 2006). Central to this effort must be collaboration among professionals in all disciplines of health care to improve functional and clinical outcomes as well as quality of care.

Another instance is documented in the Report Brief in March 2006, "In Examining the Health Disparities Research Plan of the National Institutes of Health (NIH): Unfinished Business," in which the Institute of Medicine (IOM) assesses NIH's response to the 2000 law, focusing on the development and implementation of the Strategic Plan across NIH Institutes and Centers. The report examines the Strategic Plan for fiscal years 2002–2006 and the as-yet unapproved Plan for 2004–2008. Congress passed a law to enhance the National Institutes of Health (NIH) work in the area: The Minority Health and Health Disparities Research and Education Act of 2000 (P.L.106-525). This legislation established the NIH National Center on Minority and Health Disparities (NCMHD) to administer special grant programs, coordinate minority health disparities research across NIH, and lead the development of an NIH-wide Strategic Plan on health disparities (IOM, 2006).

According to the IOM report, twenty-seven Institutes and Centers (ICs), along with two NIH Offices, developed individual plans as part of the 2002–2006 NIH-wide Strategic Plan. These units are conducting and planning valuable health disparities research. At the same time, the impact of this work is being mitigated by a lack of coordination and limited strategic planning. In short, when it comes to addressing health and fulfilling the promise of the 2000 law, NIH's business is unfinished (IOM, 2006). Health informatics should be explored as a mechanism to accelerate health disparities reduction/health equity efforts.

Lack of access to health care and barriers still exist for the poor and other vulnerable groups, where the cost of transportation, disabled individuals, geographic location (rural vs. urban community) and health literacy are major factors to consider. Implementation of effective interventions and policy changes are recommended to reduce these barriers. Funding research on access-related issues to ensure the quality of health information technology can help eliminate the digital divide, increase patient safety, and decrease medical errors. There must be a major transformation in the delivery of care to eliminate health disparities.

The National Bureau of Asian Research (NBR) (Mundie, 2007) points out that HIIT can be used to help transform global health by shifting the current focus on disease management to one of prevention and wellness. A shift of this type is likely to result in relief of significant health and economic burdens. The NBR (Mundie, 2007) specifically notes that

Technologies ranging from personal instrumentation and monitoring to nanotechnology and advanced robotics represent a huge opportunity to create an increasingly self-managed health care environment that facilities early health in a scalable way. [Further,] in the interconnected health care world of the future, general practitioners will have more expert system tools at their command; as a result of the ubiquity of information systems, those tools can be made available even in the most underserved areas.

On the international front, efforts are already underway to address the transformation of global health. In 2000, all United Nations members adopted the Millennium Development Goals (MDGs) as part of their commitment to reduce poverty and strengthen sustainable development (Singer et al., 2005). According to the Task Force on Science, Technology and Innovation (Task Force 10), one underlying factor of global health inequity is knowledge, particularly of science and technology (Singer et al., 2005). This observation suggests that health informatics and information technology can play a significant role in facilitating knowledge transfer. In view of various phases of knowledge transfer, concerted efforts should be made to link HIIT to relevant activities so that they occur across a continuum and are integrated throughout such phases as knowledge development (innovation or discovery), dissemination (sharing or exchange), and diffusion (assimilation or adoption).

The Genomic Working Group of Task Force 10 promotes the utility of genomics-related technologies in meeting some of the MDGs, namely those that promote gender equality and empower women, reduce child mortality, improve maternal health, combat HIV, malaria, and other diseases, and ensure environmental sustainability (Singer et al., 2005).

The Genomics and Global Health report encourages the creation of a Global Genomics Initiative (GGI), which could also lead to partnerships between industrialized countries and the developing world (Singer et al., 2005). Such partnerships could cultivate opportunities for the convergence of biotechnology, information technology, and cognitive technologies thereby offering enhanced potential to address global health disparities.

The World Health Organization asserts that the use of information and communications technologies (ICTs) provides a means to reach a series of desired outcomes, including:

- Health workers making better treatment decisions
- Hospitals providing higher quality and safer care
- People making informed choices about their own health
- Governments becoming more responsive to health needs
- National and local information systems supporting the development of effective, efficient and equitable health systems
- Policy makers and the public aware of health risks
- People having better access to the information and knowledge they need for better health

Chetley (2006) provides several descriptions of how ICT can and is being used in developing countries. These descriptions illuminate the potential impact various technologies or their combinations can have in under-resourced communities. Two such examples are summarized as follows. **The first case** involves a midwife with access to a personal digital assistant (PDA) and wireless router that stores surveillance data for a Ugandan district that uses the PDA to download health surveillance data. Two scenarios are highlighted about the potential uses of the data. One scenario involves access and use of data during the occurrence of a disease outbreak in a nearby community, which can serve as a warning to take preventive measures in the community that has not yet been exposed to the health threat.

Similarly, the transmission of data about a health problem that exists in the community where she is providing services can alert the Health District of the need to send medical support and assistance to aid in responding to a crisis. Large-scale use of PDAs could yield significant results. Developing viable mechanisms to systematically expand this capability to other groups of health workers in developing countries could lead to improvements in such areas as health equity, quality of life, productivity, and ultimately, enhance the economic solvency of communities adopting this and other similar strategies.

The second case involves health promotion activities in information dissemination centers in East and Southern Africa. Center coordinators gather existing research from institutions around the country on reproductive health and nutrition. Most centers collected research studies and produced annotated bibliographies. In some areas these were stored in searchable databases. Among the lessons learned was the need for appropriate formatting of information in order for it to be useful to various audiences. Use of multiple formats and channels are likely to result in greater use of the information.

In addition to these technology applications, the convergence of technologies in such areas as nanotechnology, biotechnology, information technology, and the cognitive sciences offer significant prospects aimed at cure, prevention and adaptation to assistive devices (Wolbring, 2004). As such, the convergence and/or combination of these technologies bring added capacity for improving health outcomes. Along these lines, telemedicine provides another option for providing services to vulnerable populations who are located in remote areas. Telemedicine has been extremely useful in improving the delivery of health care worldwide. There are many definitions of telemedicine. However, for the purpose of this chapter, we will use the definition that was included in the Office for the Advancement of Telehealth 2001 Report to Congress (HHS, 2002) as referenced in the article by Brantley, Laney-Cummings, and Spivack (2004), which states "the use of telecommunications and information technologies to provide health care services at a distance, to include diagnosis, treatment, public health, consumer health information, and health professions education." Brantley et al. indicate that, "this definition incorporates the concept of a comprehensive system for integrating various applications—clinical health care delivery, management of medical information, education, and administrative services—within a common infrastructure."

Other telemedicine services provided by health care professionals are mental health, radiology, psychiatry, and dermatology to underserved communities and individuals living in both urban and rural areas.

Certainly, building research capacity would be helpful in myriad ways. Effective data and information collection practices would enhance decision making among various audiences—policymakers, providers, and those who consume health services. Building the infrastructure to support such work has vast implications for health improvements not only in the directly affected communities but also in those to which they are connected.

In the age of the Internet, consumers are able to find just about anything they want to today because of information technology. Armed with more information, many consumers want to be active participants in decisions about their health care and are assuming greater responsibility in managing their health. Consumers are smarter than ever and are able to access patient and privacy information; clinical information; current research; quality of consumer health information; as well as health literacy materials. All of the aforementioned types of health information technologies have led to the coining of the term consumer health informatics.

According to Susannah Fox, eight million American adults look online for health information on a typical day. The typical search for health information online starts at a search engine, includes multiple sites, and is undertaken on behalf of someone other than the person doing the search. Most health seekers are pleased about what they find online, but some are frustrated or confused. Three-quarters of health seekers do not consistently check the source and date of health information they find online; and successful health information searches may bolster health seekers' confidence (Fox, 2006). Lastly, consumers are making better-informed choices and decisions through information and communications technology. The fact that consumers are more knowledgeable and have a proactive attitude about managing their own health should help to eliminate health disparities.

Advancing Service Delivery and Access Through Health Informatics Information Technology (HIIT)

Today, a patient goes to his health care provider and expects to see his medical record while the doctor is discussing his medical condition. However, what he sees is a computer with his *medical records* stored in the system electronically. C. Peter Waegemann (2003) spoke of four important reasons why the use of electronic health records (EHRs) were not implemented. They were (a) lack of a framework of standards; (b) lack of motivation; (c) lack of direct benefits for practitioners; and (d) confusion about the concept. He stated that the vision of EHR was a journey and listed the difference between EHR vs. CPR vs. EMR. The differences between these types of records include:

- EHR (electronic health record)—generic term for all electronic patient care systems
- CPR (computer-based patient record)—lifetime patient record that includes all information from all specialties (even dentist, psychiatrist) and requires full interoperability (potentially internationally); unlikely to be achieved in foreseeable future
- EMR (electronic medical record)—electronic record with full interoperability within an enterprise (hospital, clinic, practice)

The same year, The Institute of Medicine, listed "Key Capabilities of an Electronic Health Record System" (IOM, 2003) (see Table 17.1).

Waegemann also stated that, "although progress in implementing full EHRs has been slow, advancements are being made" (Waegemann, 2003). Approximately 3 years later, advancements in EHRs have been made and North Adams, Massachusetts, with a resident population of 14,000, will become the first city in the state of Massachusetts, in the United States to have electronic medical records that can be viewed in an instant by any physician and many nurses in the community, from their offices, the local hospital, or the visiting nurses association, according to Liz Kowalczyk (2007).

Table 17.1	The Eight Core Functions of an Electronic Health Record

- **Health Information and Data**
  Patients' diagnoses, allergies, and lab results
- **Results Management**
  New and past test results by all clinicians involved in treating a patient
- **Order Management**
  Computerized entry and storage of data on all medications, tests, and other services
- **Decision Support**
  Electronic alerts and reminders to improve compliance with best practices, ensure regular screenings and other preventive practices, identify possible drug interactions, and facilitate diagnoses and treatments
- **Patient Support**
  Tools offering patients access to their medical records, interactive education, and the ability to do home monitoring and testing
- **Administrative Processes**
  Tools, including scheduling systems, that improve administrative efficiencies and patient service
- **Reporting**
  Electronic data storage that uses uniform data standards to enable physician offices and healthcare organizations to comply with federal, state, and private reporting requirements in a timely manner
- **Electronic Communication and Connectivity**
  Secure and readily accessible communication among clinicians and patients

Note: Excerpt from *Key Capabilities of an Electronic Health Record System,* Institute of Medicine (IOM), July 2003.

Similar networks of shared patient information are scheduled to go live in other cities such as Brockton and Newburyport, MA in the summer of 2007, and doctors are working on a system for Boston as well as ways to link doctors and hospitals across the state. Patients typically are treated by multiple physicians, clinics, and hospitals, and a computerized records network allows doctors to find information quickly in an emergency, alerting them, for example, if a patient has a dangerous allergy to a medication, or if they are about to order an expensive test a patient has already had (Kowalczyk, 2007).

All of the news sounds good, however, according to a recent. Government Accountability Office (GAO) report, the increased use of information technology to exchange electronic health information introduces challenges to protecting individuals' personal health information. Key challenges include the following:

- Understanding and resolving data-sharing issues introduced by varying state privacy laws and organization-level practices
- Determining liability and enforcing sanctions in cases of breach of confidentiality
- Determining the minimum data necessary that can be disclosed in order for requesters to accomplish their intended purposes
- Obtaining individuals' authorization and consent for use and disclosure of personal health information (GAO, 2007)

A major recommendation of the GAO report was to address key challenges associated with legal and policy issues, disclosure of personal health information, individuals' rights to request access and amendments to health information, and security measures for protecting health information within a nationwide exchange of health information.

We must be able to protect and ensure the privacy of consumer's health information. Federal law protects a persons' health information. It can't be used or shared without written authorization. That is why in 1996, the U.S. Congress created the Health Insurance Portability Accountability Act (HIPAA). Through this Act, the U.S. Department of Health and Human Services issued regulations entitled *Standards for Privacy of Individually Identifiable Health Information*. (Office for Civil Rights, n.d.) For most covered entities, compliance with these regulations, known as the Privacy Rule, was required as of April 14, 2003. This Act provided a mechanism whereby implementation would prevent or reduce the misuse of personal information and restrict access to medical records by many (i.e., insurers, employers, clinical researchers, etc.).

According to the Healthcare Information and Management Systems Society (HIMSS), various national efforts are underway globally to fund health care information technology. In a 2007 report, HIMSS indicates that

> "the Canada Health Infoway, an independent not-for-profit corporation, leads the national effort with all 14 federal, provincial and territorial governments as shareholders. By 2003 the Canadian government had invested $1.2 billion in Infoway and by March 2007, Infoway will have committed more that $1 billion in co-investment within the jurisdictions. Australia's national approach combines both centralized and decentralized components to create an interoperable electronic health information infrastructure. England is the worldwide leader in the development of healthcare infrastructure and its funding has been through the government-funded National Health Service (NHS)."

In the United States on December 7, 2006, The Robert Wood Johnson Foundation (RWJF) kicked off a landmark program to design and test bold ideas for how consumers can use information technology to better manage their health and navigate the health care system. The program is called *Project HealthDesign: Rethinking the Power and Potential of Personal Health Records*. A $4.4 million initiative with nine multidisciplinary teams selected (see Table 17.2) will build new tools that advance the field of personal health record (PHR) systems.

According to RWJF, the teams were chosen from a pool of more than 165 applicants and each has been selected to receive an 18-month, $300,000 grant. Primary funding for the *Project HealthDesign* is provided by RWJF's Pioneer Portfolio, which supports innovative projects that may lead to breakthrough improvements in health and health care. RWJF collaborated with The California HealthCare Foundation, which contributed an additional $900,000 to the initiative.

In this two-phased initiative, design teams will first participate in a 6-month structured process to design user-centered personal health applications that address specific health challenges faced by individuals and caregivers. In the subsequent 12-month phase, prototypes of these personal health tools will be tested with target populations.

Table 17.2	Robert Wood Johnson Foundation HealthDesign: Rethinking the Power and Potential of Personal Health Records Project Teams	
Location	**Organization**	**Project Title**
San Francisco, CA	University of California, San Francisco Center for Excellence for Breast Cancer	A Customized Care Plan for Breast Cancer Patients— (Supported by The California HealthCare Foundation)
Rochester, NY	University of Rochester, Department of Computer Sciences	Personal Health Management Assistant
Boston, MA	Joslin Diabetes Center, Inc.	Personal Health Application for Diabetes Self-Management
Seattle, WA	University of Washington	Chronic Disease Medication Management Between Office Visits
Nashville, TN	Vanderbilt University Medical Center, Department of Biomedical Informatics	My-Med-Health: A Vision for a Child-focused Personal Medication Management System
Atlanta, GA	Research Triangle Institute	ActivHealth: A PHR System for At-Risk Sedentary Adults
Worchester, MA	University of Massachusetts Medical School, Department of Family Medicine and Community Health	Supporting Patient and Provider Management of Chronic Pain with PDA Applications Linked to Personal Health Records
Pasadena, CA	Art Center College of Design, Graduate Media Design Program	Living Profiles: Transmedia Personal Health Record Systems for Young Adults
Aurora, CO	University of Colorado at Denver and Health Sciences Center, Division of Internal Medicine	Assisting Older Adults with Transitions of Care

Grant teams will work collaboratively to design and test a suite of PHR applications that can be built upon a common platform to help people better meet their health care needs in an integrated fashion. Furthermore, RWJF states that PHR tools may remind a patient to take medications, provide tailored decision prompts to help people adhere to treatment regimens for diabetes or pain therapy, or transmit data to providers—such as blood pressure readings or exercise levels—that are collected from patient self-testing and biomonitoring devices in the home.

There have been many organizations over the years that have placed emphasis on using technology and communication to improve consumer's health through the use of electronic information systems. One such federal agency is the Centers for Disease Control and Prevention (CDC) who awarded approximately $5.2 million to fund two new Centers of Excellence in Health Marketing and Health Communication as well as two Centers of Excellence in Public Health Informatics in September 2005.

According to Dr. Julie Gerberding, Director of the CDC, "with these initial investments in four new Centers of Excellence, we hope to identify new tools, approaches, and strategies for managing health records, bringing together disease information from different places, understanding the questions and concerns of patients, and educating people about ways to improve their health. The more we learn about when and how to use health communication and electronic information systems, the better able we'll be to meet the needs of people in the community" (CDC, 2005).

The two new Centers of Excellence in Health Marketing and Health Communication are the University of Connecticut and the University of Georgia. Each Center is designed to examine better ways to improve the overall health and well-being of people who are at higher risk for disease and illness, especially those living in rural areas that have minimum access to medical care (CDC, 2005).

The CDC's two new Centers of Excellence in Public Health Informatics will improve the public's health through discovery, innovation, and research related to health information and information technology (e.g., better use of electronic or computerized information systems). The new Center at Harvard Medical School will be developing a computer-based system designed to rapidly identify disease outbreaks using patient and other medical records. The new Center at the University of Washington will work on two major research projects that focus on improving public health surveillance and epidemic detection methods and the development of an interactive digital knowledge management system including concept mapping services that will provide rapid access to answers from a variety of key resources (CDC, 2005).

Implementing Standards of Practice Via Public Policy and Governance

According to the HIMSS, ". . . all countries suffer from the same issues of lack of health-care IT standards and barriers to inter-system communication. France, Sweden and the Netherlands are trying to standardize EHRs, within their respective countries. A few countries such as Germany, the Netherlands and France are attempting to do this by using a variation of the Health Level Seven (HL7) standard to promote interoperability between countries" (HIMSS, 2007).

In the United States, e-health has garnered the interest of state and federal officials and policymakers. In 2004, President George W. Bush established the position of National Coordinator for Health Information Technology to serve as the chief advisor to the Secretary of the U.S. Department of Health and Human Services, Michael Leavitt. This position and responsibilities were created with the President's Executive Order 13335 on April 27, 2004 and responds to the President's call for the availability of secure, interoperable health information technology (HHS, 2007; GAO, 2007).

The next year in 2005, Secretary Leavitt announced the formation of a federal advisory committee comprised of public and private health care stakeholders to form the American Health Information Community, which was charged with the responsibility of making recommendations to the Secretary on strategies for accelerating the adoption of interoperable electronic health.

These two important steps paved the way for subsequent activities that support the continued development of a seamless technology platform to support electronic health records (EHRs). Underway are formal efforts to address such issues as the development of health IT standards, a certification process for health IT products, establishment of a National Health Information Network, advances in clinical decision support, as well as privacy and security policies and practices (HHS, 2007; GAO, 2007).

Secretary Leavitt's acceptance of 30 standards recommended by the Healthcare Information Technology Standards Panel in late January of 2007 marked another major milestone toward achieving broad-based adoption of electronic health records (ANSI, 2007). While many stakeholders may argue that such adoption will transform the U.S. health care system, as we currently know it, we should envision a seamless telecommunications system that supports interoperability rather than a single uniform system. Linking state efforts to the broader federal initiatives was embarked upon as state governors met for the first time on health IT (Pulley, 2007).

Of the numerous bills that included elements to address technology that were introduced during the 109th Congress, two were passed and became public laws. House of Representatives Bill 1812 was introduced by Representative Menendez of New Jersey in April of 2005 and became Public Law No.109-18, The Patient Navigator Outreach and Chronic Disease Prevention Act of 2005. This law amends the Public Health Service Act to authorize a demonstration grant program to provide patient navigator services to reduce barriers and improve health care outcomes, and for other purposes. Senate Bill 544 was introduced by Senator Jeffords of Vermont in March of 2005 and became Public Law No. 109-41, The Patient Safety and Quality Improvement Act of 2005. The law amends Title IX of the Public Health Service Act to provide for the improvement of patient safety and to reduce the incidence of events that adversely effect patient safety.

Workforce Development

As Kathleen Young (2000) highlights in her book, *Informatics for Healthcare Professionals*, health informatics is interdisciplinary in nature. Specifically, health informatics reflects a cross section of four science-based disciplines and draws from: (1) Health care science—the basic and clinical sciences overlaid with specialty knowledge that forms the basis of health care practice; (2) Information science—which focuses on messaging—the development, format, acquisition, transmission, processing, perception, and interpretation of information; (3) Cognitive science—focusing on the functions of the mind and the processes that involve thinking, understanding, remembering and acquisition of knowledge; and (4) Computer science—the development, configuration, and architecture of computer hard- and software. Since health informatics draws from each of these disciplines and is an emerging field, there are significant implications for knowledge development in today's health workforce.

Daniel R. Masys notes that information technologies have fueled another societal trend that will continue to have an impact on the health care workforce. The flag bearer of this trend is the Internet, which brings information access and interpersonal communication on an unprecedented scale to hundreds of millions of persons worldwide (Masys, 2002). What does this mean for informatics and health care?

It means we will need to develop a knowledgeable health informatics workforce that has both general and specific knowledge and skills needed to implement health informatics applications so that we are better able to inform health care providers, expand knowledge, and deliver efficient well-managed care or services.

In the United States, public policy and national workforce development efforts are underway in this regard. Two examples are referenced in press releases of Congressman David Wu (2006) and of the American Medical Informatics Association. Announcements focused on legislation, the "10,000 Trained by 2010 Act" introduced by Congressman David Wu, which supports the development of a workforce that is capable of innovating, implementing, and using communications and information technology. The American Medical Informatics Association (AMIA) and the American Health Information Management Association (AHIMA) creation of the 10x10 program reflects collaboration at the national level to help achieve the goals of the legislation (AMIA, 2006).

Developing competency-based curricula in health informatics is essential, if we are to improve the effectiveness of data assimilation, interpretation and representation. Similarly, William A. Yasnoff and colleagues (2000) have written,

> "that a cadre of public health informaticians with comprehensive training and experience in both public health and informatics is needed to serve in leadership, research and teaching roles, such as chief information officers for state public health agencies and informatics faculty at schools of public health. The competencies and knowledge needed by a public health informatician include an understanding of the respective roles and domains of information technology (IT) and public health team members; the ability to develop and use an IT architecture; a working knowledge of information system development, networking, and database design; familiarity with data standards; a clear understanding of privacy and confidentiality issues, as well as security technologies; and skills in IT planning and procurement, IT leadership, managing change, communication, and systems evaluations research. Curricula are needed for developing these competencies at a basic level for the entire public health workforce, an intermediate level for public health managers and leaders, and an advanced level for public health informatics specialists and researchers."

Efforts are currently underway to develop core competencies in public health informatics by the University of Washington (UW) School of Public Health and Community Medicine. In fact, the UW School of Public Health administered a survey during 2006 to solicit input from various stakeholders about the comprehensiveness of a proposed set of competency requirements for junior and senior professionals.

In a 2006 report by the Association of State and Territorial Health Officials (ASTHO), they indicated that there is a demand for a knowledgeable and skilled public health informatics workforce to support emerging data sharing and communications initiatives designed to improve public health programs, modernize health care, and increase the utility of public health data by linking disparate information systems. A few of the initiatives listed were: public health information network, health information exchange, biosurveillance, and vital statistics (ASTHO, 2006).

Various international communities are working toward gaining increased knowledge about the competencies needed by health professionals who will increasingly be faced with IT-related tasks as part of their work performance. A formal study to assess health professionals' perceptions of health informatics skills required in their roles was conducted using the Australian Health Informatics Skill Needs Survey (Garde, Harrison, Huque, & Hovenga, 2006). Limitations in knowledge and use of systematic approaches to process data and information have significant implications for effective decision making by health professionals. These factors have influenced heightened attention and focused efforts to consider global developments in health informatics and information technology educational curricula (Hovenga & Mantas, 2004). Additionally, authorities are linking new and emerging health information technologies with the need to develop a workforce that is educated and trained on their applications and uses.

According to Hovenga, "We are witnessing a paradigm shift in higher education as a result of technological advances, adoption of on-line learning and a greater participation in e-commerce by higher education providers. Given the dearth of academics with high-level expertise in health informatics in many countries, we need to explore how best to use our scarce resources to have the greatest possible impact regarding the preparation of health professionals such that they can make the best possible use of available informatics technologies to support health service delivery." Working toward this end of developing international standards for health informatics education and research, is the International Medical Informatics Association's (IMIA) education working group in collaboration with its academic members (Hovenga, 2004; Hovenga & Mantas, 2004).

Developing Infrastructure and Capacity: New and Adaptive Technology Applications

HIIT infrastructure development and capacity building must consider factors relating to accessibility and usability of technology and health information by diverse audiences. Diamond and Shreve (2007) indicate, "While advances in hardware and software design have been rapid, our understanding of user needs and how these needs can be translated into better system design has not advanced as rapidly." As a consequence, some population groups (i.e., persons with physical and/or cognitive disabilities) may experience access barriers to essential technology and pertinent health information. This could translate into restricted access and/or use as a result of the lack of appropriate technology, challenges experienced in manipulating hardware, complications in navigating sites hosting electronic health information, or difficulty understanding health information content. Diamond and Shreve (2004) posit the need for increased data collection about various population group needs along with the development and use of various interfaces, customized content, and adaptive techniques that may help to address some of these issues.

The work of researchers at the Georgia Institute of Technology along with physician scientists and medical staff at the Bascom Palmer Eye Institute (BPEI) in Miami, Florida is an example of a collaborative research effort focused on adaptive technologies for use among adults with visual impairments, specifically age-related macular degeneration (AMD). According to the Institute, "the study is to develop computer-based, low vision technologies that can automatically adapt, or morph themselves, to suit the visual capabilities of individual users" (Georgia Institute of Technology, 2003).

An emerging technology is robotics. Many scientists globally are testing equipment to make things better for consumers. In the United States, Scott Banks, an Assistant Professor of Aerospace and Mechanical Engineering at the University of Florida has designed a robot to shadow and shoot X-ray video of sufferers of orthopedic injuries as they walk, climb stairs, stand up from a seated position or pursue other normal activities – and maybe even athletic ones like swinging a bat (Science Daily, 2006a). On this project, he is working with Dr. Mike Moser, a University of Florida orthopedic surgeon. In the same Science Daily article, Banks states that,

> "He hopes his robot – actually, a system that uses two robots because one robot will be necessary to shoot the X-ray video and another to hold the image sensor—will lead to a radical improvement. He has one working robot currently. The robot, which has a one-meter mechanical arm, is a commercial product normally used in robotically assisted surgeries and silicon chip manufacturing that he and his graduate students have re-engineered. The robot can shadow a person's knee, shoulder or other joint with its hand as he or she moves.
>
> Improving the accuracy is one of several challenges that remain in the project. The University of Florida has applied for a patent on the new imaging technique, and it's possible that it could become standard equipment in hospitals. The biggest thing that this technology could offer in treating orthopedic injuries is that it has the ability to visualize joint motion dynamically, as it changes. He thinks this would be good for many different conditions of the shoulder, knee, elbow and ankle, and it could be extrapolated to pretty much any orthopedic injury or condition." Dr. Mike Moser said, "He thinks the robot system would be very useful to surgeons." (Science Daily, 2006a)

In a workshop description, Fran Berman of the San Diego Supercomputer Center and University of California-San Diego presents a cogent discussion on Cyberinfrastructure for the Social Sciences. She defines cyberinfrastructure, as "the coordinated aggregate of software, hardware, and other technologies along with human expertise, that is required to support current and future discoveries in science and engineering." While many are fascinated by its evolution, Berman cautions the need to be thoughtful about its design, development, and deployment to ensure its success in serving as a framework for contemporary science and engineering. Collaborative partnerships between and across such disciplines as the social sciences, computer sciences, technology and engineering will be a prerequisite for building a viable and successful cyberinfrastructure (Berman, n.d.).

An alternate definition of cyberinfrastructure from the computer science perspective is, "the comprehensive infrastructure needed to capitalize on dramatic advances in information technology" (Baru, 2005). Baru presents a conceptual model that highlights how cyberinfrastructure uses technologies to bring remote resources together through web-services-enabled science and engineering and its role in facilitating global connectivity. The National Science Foundation (NSF) is among key stakeholders and investors in cyberinfrastructure projects. As Baru also highlights, all of which require on-demand access to large computers for modeling, data analysis, visualization, and data assimilation. The NSF cyberinfrastructure projects include:

- Grid Physics Network (GriPhyN), which supports sharing of high-energy physics data from single, large data sources;
- National Virtual Observatory (NVO), which provides online access to digital sky surveys and the integration of heterogeneous sky surveys, also providing the context;
- Biomedical Informatics Research Network (BIRN), which supports sharing human and mouse structural and functional brain imaging data between independent remote research groups;
- Network for Earthquake Engineering Simulations (NEES), which shares experimental data and supports a central, persistent repository for data from shake-table and tsunami wave tank experiments;
- Geosciences Network (GEON), which integrates existing 4D multi-disciplinary data products and involves extreme heterogeneity in data (discipline, scale, resolution, accuracy); and
- Science Environment for Ecological Knowledge (SEEK), which provides the information technology structure support ecological modeling and access to distributed ecological data collections.

When addressing health problems, computer grid technology offers the capacity to use significant computing power and engage a broad range of expertise remotely located in a collaborative effort. Projects of this type create a milieu that is conducive to the generation of intellectual contributions in a virtual environment.

A description of an international computer grid project to address the Avian Flu was published in Science Daily (2006b). The project involved a large-scale collaboration among Asian and European laboratories in an international grid to analyze in this computer grid project, a large-scale collaboration among Asian and European laboratories participated in an international grid to analyze 300,000 possible drug components against Avian Flu Virus H5N1. The project used 2,000 computers during 4 weeks in April 2006. The computing power of this project reflected the equivalent of 100 years on a single computer, generating more than 60,000 output files with a volume of 600 Gigabytes. Subsequently, the focus of the project focused on identifying and ranking compounds against the avian flu. Similar to how the international community came together to address a critical health threat, a comparable process could be structured to address a large-scale health disparity problem. The combination of the computing power and intellectual capacity should enhance the production of viable solutions to health disparities reduction efforts, thereby, making health equity a real possibility.

Internationally, there are already a number of countries currently involved in HIIT-related activities. While the range of activities varies, Table 17.3 highlights selected countries engaged in such activities as Biomedical Cognitive Science; Imaging, Robotics, Virtual Reality; Bioinformatics; Computerized Clinical Guidelines; Nursing Informatics; Outcomes Assessment; Consumer Health Informatics; Public Health Informatics; Clinical Information Management; Standards, Social and Legal Issues; Decision Support Systems; Telemedicine; and Electronic Patient Records. As reflected in the chart,

Table 17.3

Selected International Community Health Informatics Activities

Country	BCS	BIO	CCG	CHI	CIM	DSS	EPR	IRV	NI	OA	PHI	SSL	TEL*
Argentina		▲							▲		▲		
Australia			▲	▲	▲	▲	▲	▲	▲				▲
Austria	▲	▲		▲	▲	▲	▲	▲	▲		▲	▲	▲
Belgium				▲				▲			▲		▲
Brazil	▲	▲	▲	▲	▲		▲	▲	▲	▲	▲	▲	▲
Canada	▲	▲	▲	▲	▲		▲		▲	▲	▲	▲	▲
China	▲												
Columbia								▲					
Croatia					▲				▲				
Cuba		▲		▲	▲	▲	▲		▲		▲		▲
Cypress (none)													
Czech Republic	▲	▲		▲		▲		▲			▲		▲
Denmark						▲	▲					▲	▲
Finland					▲	▲	▲					▲	▲
France					▲	▲	▲	▲			▲		▲
Georgia (none)													
Germany	▲	▲	▲	▲	▲		▲	▲	▲	▲	▲	▲	▲
Greece		▲		▲	▲		▲		▲	▲	▲	▲	▲
Hungary			▲								▲	▲	
India		▲		▲	▲	▲	▲	▲	▲	▲	▲	▲	▲
Indonesia (none)													
Ireland		▲				▲						▲	▲
Israel		▲	▲			▲	▲						
Italy	▲	▲	▲	▲	▲	▲	▲	▲		▲	▲	▲	▲
Japan					▲								▲
Korea (none)													
Lithuania					▲	▲	▲						▲
Luxembourg									▲				
Malaysia (none)													
Mali (none)													
Netherlands		▲	▲		▲	▲	▲	▲				▲	▲
New Zealand		▲	▲		▲	▲	▲		▲	▲	▲	▲	▲
Nigeria		▲		▲	▲	▲				▲	▲		▲
Norway			▲	▲		▲				▲			▲
Pakistan		▲	▲	▲				▲					▲
Peru						▲		▲					▲
Philippines					▲	▲	▲				▲		▲
Portugal												▲	
Romania	▲	▲						▲					▲
Russia (none)													

Table 17.3

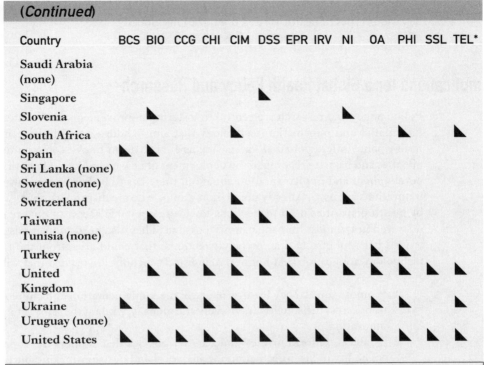

(Continued)													
Country	BCS	BIO	CCG	CHI	CIM	DSS	EPR	IRV	NI	OA	PHI	SSL	TEL*
Saudi Arabia (none)													
Singapore						▟							
Slovenia	▟								▟				
South Africa					▟						▟		▟
Spain	▟	▟											
Sri Lanka (none)													
Sweden (none)													
Switzerland					▟				▟				
Taiwan		▟			▟	▟	▟						
Tunisia (none)													
Turkey							▟	▟			▟	▟	
United Kingdom	▟	▟	▟	▟	▟	▟	▟	▟	▟	▟	▟	▟	▟
Ukraine	▟	▟	▟	▟	▟	▟	▟		▟	▟			▟
Uruguay (none)													
United States	▟	▟	▟	▟	▟	▟	▟	▟	▟	▟	▟	▟	▟

*Abbreviations Key	
BCS Biomedical Cognitive Science	**IRV** Imaging, Robotics, Virtual Reality
BIO Bioinformatics	**NI** Nursing Informatics
CCG Computerized Clinical Guidelines	**OA** Outcomes Assessment
CHI Consumer Health Informatics	**PHI** Public Health Informatics
CIM Clinical Information Management	**SSL** Standards, Social and Legal Issues
DSS Decision Support Systems	**TEL** Telemedicine
EPR Electronic Patient Records	

Source: Health Informatics World Wide, accessed February 8, 2007 at www.hiww.org

over 40 countries are involved, to some extent, in the HIIT activities previously mentioned. In instances where none appears by the country name, this indicates that this particular country is involved in other HIIT-related activities that are not mentioned. Having access to this type of information will be helpful in setting a global HIIT research agenda. Such information about areas of HIIT involvement by various nations provides insight into current gaps and capacity, infrastructure development needs, existing collaborative partnerships and opportunities for expansions or new partnerships, and opportunities for improving coordination efforts.

Increasingly leaders of national organizations are recognizing the importance of informatics and information technology in health. In the United States, the American Public Health Association (APHA) provides one such example through the formal establishment of the Special Primary Interest Group (SPIG) on Health Informatics Information Technology (HIIT) this year. The authors predict that emerging technologies and innovative HIIT applications will fuel growth trends over the next decade. As a result, we should expect to see increased prominence of HIIT within the infrastructures of various types of health-related organizations globally.

Implications for a Global Health Policy and Research

Public policy and research are central to fostering improvements in the effectiveness of informatics and information technology that aim to address health disparities. Global health policy offers potential for serving as a mechanism to overcome numerous complexities and barriers relating to the deployment of new technology. On both sides of the development and implementation equation, there has to be balance in how technology innovations are used. Already population groups who are disproportionately challenged by health disparities need protections to ensure equitable access to quality care that is delivered in the most humane manner possible. They also need protections from unintended harmful effects (i.e., privacy violations) that could arise from the use of novel technology applications. At minimum, political sanctions are needed that will:

1 Promote consistency in governance of the implementation of technology applications across jurisdictions nationally and globally, while at the same time supporting innovation.
2 Establish uniform privacy and security policies that support the appropriate accessibility of key information for analytical and decision-making purposes.
3 Standardize methods for developing, storing and managing data and information for retrieval and use by multiple users for various purposes.
4 Design secure system architectures that allow for system integration, coordination, and interoperability, enabling appropriate access to health information by various authorized users.
5 Address consumer mobility issues and the need for health information accessibility by various settings nationally and globally.
6 Support the development of human capital in the health care arena that reflect a knowledgeable workforce that is proficient in the various uses and applications of informatics and information technology concepts and tools.

Establishing an international research agenda is essential if our global community is to effectively address global health disparities. A comprehensive research agenda will require interdisciplinary collaboration across international communities to support knowledge transfer and capacity building activities that can address gaps where they may exist. In view of the plethora of disparities issues and the potential HIIT applications that are available to support various aspects of health care (i.e., assessment, treatment, surveillance, education, etc.), research capacity building must be a critical action step taken to develop a viable global research network and agenda.

In their article focused on strengthening a research agenda to achieve health equity, Sitthi-amorn and Somrongthong (2000) referenced four domains related to capacity building as identified by J. Simon during a WHO presentation. These domains include: (1) skills and competencies; (2) scientific activities; (3) outcomes; and (4) impacts on policies and programs. When these domains are linked to the four components of essential health research as identified by The Commission on Health Research for Development referenced in this same article, one can readily see how the domains and components can lead to the development of new information, knowledge, and improved outcomes. The Commission's components include:

- Analysis of the burden of illnesses and their determinants to identify and set priorities among health problems
- Research to guide and accelerate the implementation of research findings to tackle key health problems
- The development of new tools and methodologies to measure and promote equity
- Basic research to advance understanding of disease and disease mechanisms and to develop "orphan drugs and vaccines."

Linking the domains to the research components in an overarching disparity elimination/health equity research agenda would be central to a global health research design. Adding a component to the design that generates evidence about the impact and efficacy of infusing HIIT applications gives rise to a more comprehensive global research agenda. This expanded design would necessitate answers to a host of other questions that include the following:

1 To what extent has **political will** led to the development and growth of a biotechnology sector in the developing countries?
2 To what extent are **policies** focused on the translation of knowledge into products, practices, and services?
3 What **incentives** need to be put in place to build stable research enterprises?
4 Which strategies demonstrate the greatest promise for developing **workforce** capacity to manage the integration and convergence of cross-disciplinary technologies aimed at reducing health disparities?
5 What **metrics** need to be developed and/or employed to assess the impact of converging technologies on health disparities elimination?
6 What **benefits** are derived from combining certain technologies to address different health topics?
7 What **standards** are needed to advance interoperability when converging different technologies?
8 How has **health equity been advanced** as a result of research and public policy initiatives?

REFERENCES

American National Standards Institute (ANSI). (2007). *HHS Secretary Leavitt accepts recommendations from healthcare information technology standards panel (HITSP) data standards to support nationwide health information network*. Washington, DC. Retrieved February 4, 2007, from http://www.ansi.org/news_publications/print_article.aspx?articleid=1413

American Medical Informatics Association (AMIA)/American Health Information Management Association (AHIMA). (2006, June 9). *Support new workforce bill*. Retrieved February 11, 2007, from http://www.amia.org/inside/releases/2006/workforcebill_amia_ahima_june9.pdf

Association of State and Territorial Health Officials (ASTHO). (2006). *Issue report: The Public Health Informatics Workforce.* Retrieved August 9, 2007, from http://www.astho.org/pubs/mformatics WorkforceIssueReport.pdf

Aziz, M. A., & Wright, A. (2005). The World Health Organization/International Union Against Tuberculosis and Lung Disease global project on surveillance for anti-tuberculosis drug resistance: A model for other infectious diseases. *Clinical Infectious Diseases, 41*(Suppl 4), S258–S262.

Baru, C. (2005, September 29–October 1). *What is cyberinfrastructure? The computer science perspective.* A PowerPoint presentation during the SACNAS, Denver, CO.

Berman, F. (n.d.). SBE/CISE Workshop on Cyberinfrastructure for the Social Sciences, San Diego Supercomputer Center and University of California San Diego.

Brantley, D., Laney-Cummings, K., & Spivack, R. (Eds.). (2004). *Innovations, demand, and investment in telehealth.* Retrieved on February 16, 2007, from http://www.technology.gov/reports/TechPolicy/Telehealth/2004Report.pdf

Brennan, P. F. (2003). *Using the science of informatics to advance health disparities research.* University of Wisconsin-Madison, School of Nursing. Retrieved February 4, 2007, from http://www.son.washington.edu/centers/hdc/Brennan.asp

Centers for Disease Control and Prevention (CDC). (2005). *CDC working to improve ability to use technology and communication to improve health; First grants to establish centers of excellence are awarded.* Retrieved August 9, 2007, from http://www.cdc.gov/od/oc/media/pressrel/r050930.htm

Central Intelligence Agency (CIA). (2006). *World factbook.* Retrieved January 5, 2007, from https://www.cia.gov/cia/publications/factbook/print/xx.html

Chetley, A. (Ed.). (2006, May 31). *Improving health, connecting people: The role of ICTs in the health sector of developing countries—A framework paper.* Study commissioned by the InfoDev program Grant No. 1254.

Commission on Health Research for Development. (1990). *Health research: Essential link to equity in development.* Oxford: Oxford University Press.

Diamond, B. J., & Shreve, G. M. (2004). Informatics and society: The challenge of improving IT accessibility. *Journal of Systemics, Cybernetics and Informatics, 3*(6), 55–57.

Fox, S. (2006). Online health search. Washington, DC: *Pew Internet & American Life Project.* Retrieved August 9, 2007, from http://www.pewinternet.org/pdfs/PIP_Online_Health_2006.pdf

Garde, S., Harrison, D., Huque, M., & Hovenga, E. J. (2006). Building health informatics skills for health professionals: Results from the Australian Health Informatics Skill Needs Survey. *Australian Health Review, 30*(1), 34–45.

Georgia Institute of Technology. (2003). *An eye on adaptive computing.* Retrieved August 4, 2007, from http://www.gatech.edu/innovations/adaptive/index.php

Gingrich, N., & Dillione, J. (2007). Getting health-care field wired. *Philadelphia Inquirer.* Reprinted with title "Let's bring healthcare into the 21st century." Retrieved February 12, 2007, from http://www.healthtransformation.net/news/cht_in_the_news/5158.cfm

Groce, N. E. (2003). *Adolescents and youth with disability: Issues and challenges.* Retrieved February 15, 2007, from http://info.worldbank.org/etools/docs/library/81136/Nairobi2004/readings/hnp/youthdisability.pdf

Healthcare Information and Management Systems Society (HIMSS). (2007). *Electronic health records: A global perspective.* Retrieved August 21, 2007, from http://www.himss.org/content/files/DrArnold20011207EISPresentationWhitePaper.pdf

Hovenga, E. J. (2004). Globalisation of health and medical informatics education—What are the issues? *International Journal of Medical Informatics, 73*(2), 101–109.

Hovenga, E. J., & Mantas, J. (Eds.). (2004). Studies in health technology and informatics. Abstract. *Global Health Informatics Education, 1096.*

Institute of Medicine (IOM), Committee on Data Standards for Patient Safety, Board on Health Care Services. (2003). *Key capabilities of an electronic health record system: A letter report.* Washington, DC: National Academies Press.

Institute of Medicine (IOM). (2006). *Examining the health disparities research plan of the National Institutes of Health: Unfinished business.* Report brief. Retrieved from http://www.iom.edu/Object.File/Master/35/550/nih%20disparities.pdf

Kowalczyk, L. (2007). Hope challenges in computerizing medical records: North Adams blazes a trail. *Boston Globe.*

Masys, D. R. (2002). Effects of current and future information technologies on the health care workforce. *Health Affairs, 21*(5), 33–41.

Mundie, C. (2007). Information technology: Advancing global health. *NBR Analysis, 77*(2), 5–21.

National Institutes of Health. (2000). *Strategic plan to reduce and ultimately eliminate health disparities, fiscal years 2002–2006.* Retrieved February 4, 2007, from http://www.nih.gov/about/hd/strategicplan.pdf

Office for Civil Rights, U.S. Department of Health and Human Services. (n.d.). *Medical privacy—National standards to protect the privacy of personal health information.* Retrieved August 21, 2007, from http://www.hhs.gov/ocr/hipaa/

Open Geospatial Consortium (OGC). (n.d.). Web site. Retrieved February 1, 2007, from http://www.opengeospatial.org/ogc

Partners in Health. (PIH). (2006). *PIH fields strong presence at international tuberculosis meetings.* Retrieved February 20, 2007, from http://www.pih.org/inforresources/news/iuatld_2006.html

Pfizer, U.S. Public Policy Group. (2004, September). *Working to end health disparities.* Retrieved January 12, 2007, from http://www.pfizer.com/policy/public_disparities.pdf

Pulley, J. (2007). *Governors meet for first time on health IT, government health IT.* Retrieved February 3, 2007, from http://govhealthit.com/article97506-01-29-07-Web&RSS=yes

Resnik, D. B. (2004). The distribution of biomedical research resources and international justice. *Developing World Bioethics, 4*(1), 42–57.

Robert Wood Johnson Foundation (RWJF). (2006). *Expert teams to design new solutions for personal health records to help consumers manage their health.* (News release). Retrieved August 9, 2007, from http://www.rwjf.org/newsroom/newsreleasesdetail.jsp?id=10449

Science Daily. (2006a). *For orthopedic injuries: A robot that follows patients as they move.* Retrieved August 9, 2007, from http://www.sciencedaily.com/releases/2006/01/060123074657.htm

Science Daily. (2006b). *Computer grid helps fight avian flu.* Retrieved August 10, 2006, from http://www.sciencedaily.com/releases/2006/05/060504065526.htm

Singer, P. A., Bhatt, A., Frew, S., Greenwood, H., Persad, D. L., Salamanca-Buentello, F., et al. (2005). The critical role of genomics in global health. In S. Matlin (Ed.), *Global Forum Update on Research for Health, 2* (pp. 113–117). London: Pro-Brook Publishing.

Sitthi-amorn, C., & Somrongthong, R. (2000). Strengthening health research capacity in developing countries: A critical element for achieving health equity. *British Medical Journal, 321,* 813–817.

U.S. Department of Health and Human Services, Health Resources and Services Administration, Office for the Advancement of Telehealth. (2002, May). *2001 report to Congress on telemedicine.* Retrieved February 20, 2007, from ftp://ftp.hrsa.gov/telehealth/report2001.pdf

U.S. Department of Health and Human Services, Agency for Healthcare Research and Quality (AHRQ). (2006). *Fiscal year 2006 Agency for Healthcare Research and Quality performance budget submission for Congressional justification.* Retrieved December 29, 2007, from http://www.ahrq.gov/about/cj2006/cj2006.pdf

U.S. Department of Health and Human Services. (2007). *Health information technology initiative: Major accomplishments, 2004–2006.* Retrieved February 5, 2007, from http://www.hhs.gov/healthit/news/Accomplishments2006.pdf

U.S. Government Accountability Office (GAO). (2007). *Health information technology—Early efforts initiated but comprehensive privacy approach needed for national strategy.* GAO-07-238. Retrieved August 9, 2007, from http://www.gao.gov/new.items/d07238.pdf

Waegemann, C. P. (2003). EHR vs. CPR vs. EMR. *Healthcare Informatics Online.* Retrieved February 25, 2007, from http://www.providersedge.com/ehdocs/ehr_articles/EHR_vs_CPR_vs_EMR.pdf

Wolbring, G. (2004, November). *Disabled people science and technology and health research,* Global Forum for Health Research. Forum 8, Mexico City.

World Health Organization (WHO). (2006a.). *Global AIDS epidemic continues to grow.* Retrieved February 10, 2007, from http://www.who.int/hiv/mediacentre/news62/en/index.html

World Health Organization (WHO). (2006b). *Emergence of XDR-TB: WHO concern over extensive drug resistant TB strains that are virtually untreatable.* Retrieved February 4, 2007, from http://www.who.int/mediacentre/news/notes/2006/np23/en/index.html

Wu, D. (U.S. Congressman, House of Representative, D-OR). (2006, May 30). *Health informatics legislation press release.* Retrieved January 12, 2007, from http://www.house.gov/list/press/or01_wu/pr05302006healthcareIT.html

Yasnoff, W. A., O'Carroll, P. W., Koo, D., Linkins, R. W., & Kilbourne, E. W. (2000). Public health informatics: Improving and transforming public health in the information age. *Journal of Public Health Management and Practice, 6(6)*, 66–75.

Young, K. M. (2000). *Informatics for healthcare professionals*. Philadelphia: F. A. Davis.

RESOURCES

American Ethnic Geography: Provides links for maps containing statistics on ethnic groups, culture regions, language, religion, politics and socioeconomic factors in the United States: http://www. valpo.edu/geomet/geo/courses/geo200/HomePage.html

American Medical Association Cultural Competence Compendium: Minority Affairs Consortium: Comprehensive resource on the subject of cultural diversity and health care available online: http://www.ama-assn.org/ama1pub/upload/mm/20/policycompendium 2005 .pdf

American Medical Association Foundation Health Literacy: Contains information on patient education and links to resources on health literacy: http://www.amaassn.org/ama/pub/category/8115.html

American Public Health Association: http://www.apha.org provides link to the Health Informatics Information Technology (HIIT) Special Primary Interest Group (SPIG) at http://www. pubhiit.org

Center for Cross-Cultural Health: Contains an excellent set of approximately 50 cross-cultural links: http://www.crosshealth.com/

The Center for Linguistic and Cultural Competency in Health Care: A publication of the National Institutes of Health Office of Minority Health providing links to information on cultural competency in health care: http://www.ombrc.gov/cultural/

Cultural Diversity in Health Care: Provides information on caring for patients from different cultures: http://www.ggalanti.com/index.html

DiversityRX: Offers an information clearinghouse on cultural diversity: http://diversityrx.org/ HTML/DIVRX.htm

Harvard School of Public Health National Center for the Study of Adult Learning and Literacy: Offers information, tools, education and innovative materials, research reports, presentations and a comprehensive list for health literacy links: http://www.hsph.harvard.edu/healthliteracy/

Healthfinder: A service of the National Health Information Center that provides multilingual health information: http://www.healthfinder.gov/justforyou

Health Literacy: A Prescription to End Confusion: Free book online provided by the National Academies Press: http://www.nap.edu/catalog/10883.html

Language Access: A Resource for Helping Non-English Speakers Navigate Health and Human Services: Published by the National Conference of State Legislatures: http://www.ncsl.org/ programs/immig/languagesvcs.pdf

Medical Anthropology Web: Provides links to information on the cultural and biological study and understanding of health, illness, and health care: http://www.medanth.org

Minority Health & Health Disparities: Offers a link to national standards for culturally and linguistically appropriate health services: http://www.hrsa.gov/OMH/

National Institute for Literacy: Shares literacy information and resources, literacy research and funding opportunities: http://www.nifl.gov/

National Institute for Literacy Information and Communication System: Contains links to literacy research and statistics, multimedia curriculum, and national, regional, state and local networks: http://www.nifl.gov/lincs/t_index.html

National Institute for Literacy Special Collections: Provides health curricula for literacy ESOL classes, health resources in simple language, and other useful links: http://www.worlded.org/ us/health/lincs/

Pfizer Clear Health Communication Initiative: Provides health literacy resources and information on how to compute reading levels: http://www.pfizerhealthliteracy.com/improving.html

Qualitative Methods in Health Research: Opportunities and Consideration in Application and Review: A publication of the National Institutes of Health Office of Behavioral and Social Sciences Research: http://obssr.od.nih.gov/publications/Qualitative.PDF

The Center for Linguistic and Cultural Competency

in Health Care: A publication of the National Institutes of Health Office of Minority Health providing links to information on Cultural Competency in Health Care: http://www.ombrc.gov/cultural/

University of Maryland's Diversity Database: Contains general links and diversity resources: http://www.inform.umd.edu/EdRes/topic/Diversity/

World Education: Health and Literacy Compendium: An annotated bibliography of print and Web-based health materials for use with limited-literacy adults: http://www.worlded.org/us/health/docs/comp/

An Online Multimedia Peer Education Smoking Cessation Program for Korean Youth: A Film Script Contest for Stories on Quitting Smoking

Kyungmi Woo

Introduction

Within the global community, cigarette-related health inequities among Koreans stand out as most alarming. Gallup-Korea (1999) reported that the smoking rate among Korean adults was the highest in the world at 65.1%. The Korean Association of Smoking and Health (KASH) reported in 2006 that 20.7% of Korean adolescents currently smoke. This rate had gradually decreased from 33.4% in 1999; however, it still remains high compared to other developing countries, which show an average adolescent smoking rate of 15% (Grimshaw & Stanton, 2006). Newsis Communications (2006) reported that the age of initial smoking has declined each year, with the current age of initiation at 13.5 years of age—a decline of 1.6 years from 1998; most troublesome is how only 40.8% of youth reported exposure to anti-smoking education in school.

Given that most adult smokers start smoking in their youth (Park & June, 2006), adequate smoking prevention or cessation programs are essential to promote better health for Koreans—especially those targeting Korean youth. To date, almost all health education conducted in Korea has focused on simply delivering knowledge and has failed to capture the interest of and effectively engage adolescents (Park & June). Without passionate participation from the target group, no program can be successful.

The Internet emerges as a viable venue for health promotion with Korean youth, given the high rate of Internet usage. Approximately 62.8% of South Korea's 49 million people now use the Internet, according to government figures reported in 2004 (Korean Network Information

Center, 2004). Among them, more than 95% of those aged 6 to 29 periodically go online, compared with 86.4% and 58.3% of those in their thirties and forties, respectively.

The use of multimedia (i.e., the Internet, videos, music, etc.) has a viable role to play in delivering health promotion and disease prevention messages to Korean youth. Among the many published reports on smoking prevention or cessation with adolescents, some results were encouraging, indicating that complex approaches show promise (Grimshaw & Stanton, 2006). Other reports were discouraging, concluding that the evidence to date does not support the prevention of relapse (Lancaster, Hajek, Stead, West, & Jarvis, 2006). Group therapy was found to be better for helping people stop smoking than self-help or other less intensive interventions (Stead & Lancaster, 2006). A comparison of the effects of a face-to-face clinic-based brief intervention to Internet based therapy across 6 months to address adolescent smoking by Patten et al. (2006) found that the Internet approach was significantly more effective in reducing the average number of days smoked during the trial periods versus rates in the comparison group. Others also found that the Internet was useful in delivering treatment to address smoking, including recommendations for frequent e-mailing (Ota & Takahashi, 2005) and reinforcement using vouchers (Dallery, Glenn, & Raiff, 2006). Other studies evaluated the effects of media campaigns in various regions. For example, Biener et al. (2006) studied the impact of smoking cessation advertisements and mass media among recent quitters; they concluded that younger respondents and those who had remained abstinent for more than 6 months were most likely to report being helped by television advertisements; the most helpful advertisements were those that depicted illness due to smoking or provided inspirational tips on quitting. Moreover, Florida's "truth" campaign, a countermarketing anti-tobacco media campaign, resulted in a successful 19.4% decline in smoking among middle school students, and an 8.0% decline among high school students (Zucker et al., 2000).

The Anti-Tobacco Media Blitz (ATMB) was developed for middle and high school students in Virginia in the United States. In the program, students worked in teams to design, develop, and evaluate tobacco-free messages through posters, radio, television, and peer-led activities (Martino-McAllister & Wessel, 2005). A social marketing campaign was used to bring about social change with the goal of influencing behavioral action; they were successful in getting a number of students involved in the campaign, but the program showed limited success in helping the students accurately identify behavioral norms supportive of nonadoption of tobacco use behavior (Martino-McAllister & Wessel).

Peer education or training has proven its effectiveness in HIV/AIDS education (Ebreo, Feist-Price, Siewe, & Zimmerman, 2002; Kocken, Voorhan, Brandsma, & Swart, 2001; Morisky, Nguyen, Ang, & Tiglao, 2005), and is seen as "very much needed in contemporary times" (Wallace, 2005, p. 7). Research has found that the interpersonal influence of peer smoking has a huge impact on smoking behavior for adolescents in China (Grenard et al., 2006). Wallace (2005; see also chapter 19, this volume) has demonstrated how a model of peer education can be made culturally appropriate, allow peers freedom to create theatrical skits and songs, while remaining rooted in three evidence-based approaches—specifically, the concept of stages of change taken from the transtheoretical model (Prochaska & DiClemente, 1983), motivational interviewing (Miller & Rollnick, 2002), and relapse prevention (Marlatt & Donovan, 2005; Marlatt & Gordon, 1985).

As envisioned by Wallace (2005), the theatrical skits created by peer educators may result in theatrical productions that find wide dissemination. In this vein, the work of SenariosUSA is of note. SenariosUSA is a nongovernmental organization founded in 1999. SenariosUSA organizes a scriptwriting contest for anyone between the ages 13 and 18. The title of the contest is "Real Deal"; it encourages students to write stories about peer pressure, pregnancy scares, HIV testing, and so on. According to them, in the past 5 years 7,500 teens have participated in the contest and 12 films have been produced so far; and, 3 new films were launched in 2005. The possibility of one's story being made into a film can serve to further mobilize and galvanize the interest of youth.

Given this background, this chapter presents an innovative smoking prevention program—an online multimedia peer education intervention for Korean youth that provides a curriculum for training youth who become peer educators; includes a Web site for peer interaction and support; encourages the use of e-mail, chat room, and text-messaging communication among peers; and features a script writing contest for winning stories on quitting smoking that form the basis for the creation of films/videos. The program reflects contemporary social trends and interests among Korean youth, integrating an interactive Internet intervention, peer-led education, and the use of multimedia. The program model recently won a contest (2006) at Teachers College, Columbia University for the best most promising model for promoting global health for a problem behavior (i.e., adolescent smoking), while, specifically, integrating the use of three empirically derived models (stages of change, Prochaska & DiClemente, 1983; motivational interviewing, Miller & Rollnick, 2002; and relapse prevention, Marlatt & Donovan, 2005; Marlatt & Gordon, 1985).

Given cigarette-related health inequities among Korean adolescents, this chapter will introduce the online multimedia peer education smoking cessation program for Korean youth by: (1) beginning with a presentation of the three empirically derived models in which the program is rooted and from which the training curriculum arises; (2) presenting the training outline and program flow-chart/time-line for the overall online multimedia peer-education smoking cessation program; (3) providing a sample script of the kind deemed desirable for submission within the planned contest, illustrating the links between the curriculum content and what trained peer educators should produce in their scripts to achieve desired effectiveness; (4) an analysis of the script, highlighting how the script reflects the program's roots in the three evidence-based theories; and (5) conclude by offering key ingredients to success of the proposed program.

Three Evidence-Based Theories: Foundation of the Program

As the foundation for the innovative smoking cessation program tailored for contemporary Korean adolescents, three evidence-based theories hold the promise for going well beyond the primary use of health education strategies that seek to deliver knowledge—as Park and June (2006) noted. The three evidence-based theories will each be reviewed in this section, while also suggesting the basic information for use in the curriculum for training peer educators in the program—including key concepts, principles, and strategies for promoting and sustaining behavior change. The three evidence-based theories have also been described as core components of a viable manualized peer-education training program, while the basic framework can be adapted so it is culturally appropriate in various contexts (Wallace, 2005; and see chapter 19, this volume). Thus, the three evidence-based theories emerge as ideal for tailoring a smoking cessation program for contemporary Korean adolescents.

The Stages of Change

Taken from the Transtheoretical Model, the Stages of Change (SOC) (Prochaska & DiClemente, 1983) represents an integrative, stage-based model of behavioral change. The SOC are useful for tailoring interventions to a client's readiness to change (DiClemente & Velasquez, 2002). The largest number of studies related to the SOC has focused on smoking (Prochaska, Redding, & Evers, 2002). People in the *precontemplation stage* are either unaware of the problem behavior or are unwilling or discouraged when it comes to changing it. In the *contemplation stage*, a person acknowledges that he or she has a problem and begins to think seriously about solving it—even as they may feel a great deal of ambivalence. People in the *preparation stage* have made a determination to change; they may have tried and failed to change in the past, but have, once again, decided to pursue change. People in the *action stage* implement the plan for which they have been planning while in preparation—as a stage lasting up to 6 months. Finally, people in the *maintenance stage* aim to make the actions they have been taking enduring over time, as they seek to maintain change and prevent relapse—as a stage lasting from more than 6 months up to a lifetime (DiClemente & Velasquez, 2002, p. 212). There is a large body of support for SOC as an evidence-based intervention (Brogan, Prochaska, & Prochaska, 1999; Grimshaw & Stanton, 2006; see Prochaska, chapter 4, in this volume).

Motivational Interviewing

Motivational interviewing (MI; Miller & Rollnick, 2002) is also considered an evidence-based intervention. There is also a long tradition of integrating the stages of change and motivational interviewing (Miller & Rollnick, 1991). The most obvious connection between motivational interviewing and the stages of change discussed by DiClemente and Velasquez (2002) is that "motivational interviewing is an excellent counseling style to use with clients who are in the early stages" (p. 202). Motivational interviewing seeks to elicit the person's intrinsic motivation for change. One strategy in MI involves addressing ambivalence via a decisional balance, weighing the costs and benefits of change, or costs and benefits. Motivational interviewing has four general principles: *expressing empathy, developing discrepancy, rolling with resistance,* and *supporting self-efficacy.* Key methods involve *asking open-ended questions* that engage the client in conversation, *reflective listening,* and the use of periodic *summaries* of what the client has said, showing that one has been listening carefully—while serving as a stimulus for the client to elaborate further. Particularly important is the elicitation of *change talk.* Eliciting change talk in the client involves the client giving voice to reasons for change, or presenting arguments for change, as a form of self-motivating speech. Change talk typically covers the *disadvantages of the status quo,* potential *advantages of change,* covers *optimism for change,* or *intention to change.* It is very important that change talk is followed by the delivery of positive reinforcement, typically resulting in a further increase in the production of change talk. Miller and Rollnick (2002) elaborate further on the full dimensions of MI as either a prelude to another intervention, a stand-alone intervention, an intervention to be integrated with other approaches, or for use as a fall-back option when resistance to change is encountered. A body of evidence provides support for MI as an evidence-based intervention (Miller & Rollnick, 2002; Resnicow et al., 2002).

Relapse Prevention

Marlatt and Gordon (1985) advanced a model of relapse prevention (RP) that has been extended to a range of problem behaviors, including cigarette smoking. The innovation of relapse prevention constituted a major paradigmatic shift, emerging over the past two decades as an evidence-based approach. According to Marlatt and Witkiewitz (2005), the two specific aims of RP are preventing an initial lapse and maintaining abstinence or harm reduction treatment goals; and providing lapse management if a lapse occurs, in order to prevent further relapse. They also note that the ultimate goal of RP is to provide the skills to prevent a complete relapse, regardless of the situation or impending risk factors. Relapse has also been described as both an outcome and a process (Marlatt & Witkiewitz). Given this fact, one possible outcome of a relapse process is a return to the previous problematic behavior pattern (relapse). Another possible outcome is the individual getting "back on track" in the direction of positive change (prolapse). Most individuals who make an attempt to change their behavior in a certain direction (e.g., smoking cessation) will experience lapses that often lead to relapse (Marlatt & Witkiewitz).

Marlatt (1985) defines a high-risk situation as any situation that poses a threat to the individual's sense of control (self-efficacy) and increases the risk of potential relapse (p. 75). The probability of relapse in a given high-risk situation decreases considerably when the individual has a high level of self-efficacy for performing a coping response. If a coping response is successfully performed, the individual's self-efficacy will increase for coping in similar situations. In contrast, if an individual fails to cope with a high-risk situation, self-efficacy decreases, and the probability of relapse increases.

According to Marlatt and Witkiewitz (2005), if the individual lacks an effective coping response and/or confidence (self-efficacy) to deal with the situation, the person tends to give in to temptation. The decision to engage in or not engage in a problem behavior is also mediated by the individual's outcome expectancies for the initial effects of using the substance (Marlatt & Witkiewitz, 2005, p. 22).

The Abstinence Violation Effect (AVE) is defined as the self-blame, guilt, and loss of perceived control that individuals often experience after the violation of self-imposed rules (Marlatt & Gordon, 1985); the AVE can be extended to both abstinence and harm reduction goals. The AVE contains both an affective and a cognitive component. The affective component is related to feelings of guilt, shame, and hopelessness, often triggered by the discrepancy between one's prior identity as an abstainer and one's present behavior of a lapse. The cognitive component is dependent upon how a person views a lapse and the cognitive attributions in which they engage. If an individual attributes a lapse to factors that are internal, global, and uncontrollable, then relapse risk is heightened; this is undesirable. However, if the individual views the lapse as external and controllable, then the likelihood of a relapse is decreased; this is preferred and the goal of teaching clients about the AVE (Marlatt & Gordon, 1985). The RP approach values assessment of the potential high-risk situations and triggers for relapse an individual may face. Once potential relapse triggers and high-risk situations are identified, cognitive and behavioral skills training focuses on teaching effective coping strategies and enhancing self-efficacy for coping in specific high-risk situations. Emphasis is also placed on the value of social support, and declaring one's intention to stop smoking publicly. Educational components are especially central to RP, including teaching lapse management as an emergency procedure to be implemented in the event a lapse occurs (Marlatt & Gordon, 1985).

After providing education and intervention strategies, RP focuses on the implementation of global lifestyle self-management strategies (Marlatt & Gordon, 1985). The use of exercise, deep breathing, or meditation may be used by clients to foster the attainment of lifestyle balance, along with an analysis of the balance in their lives between things considered "shoulds" versus "wants" (Marlatt & Gordon, 1985). More recently, the use of mindfulness meditation is being systematically taught to clients, serving to further strengthen this part of the RP model, providing further evidence of efficacy of the overall model in evaluations done to date (Marlatt, 2007). Indeed, much evidence justifies viewing RP as an evidence-based intervention (Carroll, 1997; Marlatt & Witkiewitz, 2005).

Going Beyond Patient Health to Population Health

It is also important to go beyond considerations of individual patient or client or peer health, and to achieve maximum impact by considering population health (see Prochaska, chapter 4, in this volume). In this regard, Tucker, Donovan, and Marlatt (2001) seek to bridge clinical and public health strategies, recognizing how clinical approaches to individual level health (i.e., stages of change, motivational interviewing, and relapse prevention) need to be adapted so they impact entire populations and assist in improving public health. Tucker et al. (2001) compile perspectives that argue for making access to interventions low threshold (versus high threshold access to clinic-based interventions) so that members of the general public can be readily reached. Internet-based interventions, such as the kind Prochaska (chapter 4) describes as being readily accessible in people's homes via their home computers constitute what is desired. The prize winning model introduced in this chapter meets these criteria, being Internet/Web-based.

The Format of the Online Multimedia Peer Education Smoking Cessation Program and Script/Scenario Writing Contest

The premise of the approach taken in this chapter is that an online multimedia peer education smoking cessation program for Korean youth—rooted in the three evidence-based approaches described above—will capture their interest and effectively engage them. More specifically, the intervention will provide training to youth who become peer educators; include a Web site to support the training of peer educators and to foster peer interaction; encourage the use of e-mail, chat room, and text messaging communication among peers; and feature a script writing contest ("My Story of Quitting") for winning stories on quitting smoking that form the basis for the creation of films/videos.

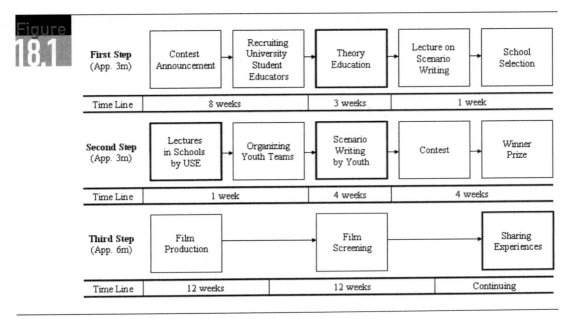

The three steps of the film script/scenario writing contest.

The First Step

As can be seen from Figure 18.1, the contest procedure consists of three steps. The first step will take approximately 3 months. This step involves promoting the contest and training university student educators (USE) in how to be peer educators. The use of university student educators (USE/peer educators) as youth team guides is adopted from The Anti-Tobacco Media Blitz (ATMB) developed for middle and high school students in Virginia in the United States (Martino-McAllister & Wessel, 2005). This type of model avoids the use of teachers who tend to be too busy to learn and teach new content to their students.

The USE/peer educators will be trained across 3 months by Korean health educators. The goal is to train the USE/peer educators to serve as mentors to the middle and high school students, who will primarily work on developing scripts for the script-writing contest; provide leadership to these teams of middle and high school students, as the teams work collaboratively in creating the scripts for submission to the script-writing contest; and convey the essence of the three evidence-based approaches in which the program is rooted, and which should be reflected in the scripts/scenarios. In this manner, a core part of the work by the USE/peer educators is to ensure that the scripts being developed by the younger students effectively implement key SOC, MI, and RP concepts. Hence, the expectation is that they will have to pass a test to become certified as USE/peer educators to ensure they possess adequate knowledge about these concepts. In addition, the USE/peer educators will also attend a lecture/training on screen-writing (led by a noted professional script writer) as further preparation for their work. Once so trained, the USE/peer educators will be linked to students in identified schools, while including opportunities for those who have dropped out of school, yet will be welcome to join school-based teams.

Vital to their training is the creation of an interactive multimedia Web site that will permit access to training materials and training videos. The Web site will also be created during this first step. The Web site will have the capacity to host videos created by the middle and high school students, as the project proceeds. The Web site will both store and serve to make accessible information about the key behavioral concepts to support smoking cessation (i.e., SOC, MI, and RP) as well as tips on effective script/scenario writing.

The Second Step

This second stage will take about 3 months. In this step, the USE/peer educators provide peer education in the schools with which they have been linked. They will recruit teams of students, organize their youth team, and begin to work on script/scenario writing. The goal is to have just one team per school and for teams to consist of smokers and nonsmokers.

Another goal is to have diverse student teams. There are several reasons for this. First, to avoid youth smokers feeling privileged (as might occur if only smokers could participate in this program), many diverse students are encouraged to get involved. Second, diversity in team membership allows nonsmokers an opportunity to learn about smoking risks by working with smokers, potentially helping them to avoid becoming future smokers. Lastly, due to cultural norms in Korea, Korean students prefer not to disclose their smoking status if they are smoking. Thus, providing a forum for youth to discuss and think about quitting without disclosing their status as smokers will permit reaching those who are actually smoking, potentially providing them with a good viable opportunity to stop smoking.

Given that some team members may be non-smokers, and those who are smokers may elect to not self-disclose, the youth will be encouraged to interview smokers outside of their teams. Using information accessible from the Web site, from their USE/peer educators, and from qualitative data they collect, the youth teams will proceed in creating original scripts/scenarios. The USE/peer educators ensure the scenarios incorporate SOC, MI, and RP theories. For example, students will be mentored in creating scripts/scenarios that accomplish the following: convey how people (i.e., the heroes of their story/script) may be in different stages of change; describe the process of people moving across stages of change as their intrinsic motivation to change increases; explain the manner in which people may experience lapses, relapses, and the importance of their learning how to effectively cope in high-risk situations so they avoid lapses/relapses; emphasize how to avoid the Abstinence Violation Effect (AVE); and, support increases in self-efficacy as effective coping prevails. In this regard, smokers on the teams or interviews conducted with smokers may contribute knowledge of high-risk situations for relapse, and successful ways of coping. In this manner, throughout this process, the youth will be experiencing an action-oriented curriculum that also results in them emerging as peer educators, themselves. The final products of the various teams will be submitted for evaluation to a volunteer team of screenplay writers, film directors, and professional health educators (well-versed in SOC, MI, and RP). They will select the winning scripts/scenarios.

Regarding the information available on the Web site, it will include quitting tips, health information on the hazards of smoking, and key summaries of the SOC, MI, and RP theories. Web site hosted interactive services include chat rooms, e-mail services so the youth can be closely mentored by their USE/peer educators, and a service where questions posed to health experts are answered. Over time, the Web site will host the movies that have been produced from the winning scripts/scenarios each year, accumulating a video library. Suggesting how population health may ultimately be impacted, members of the general public will be able to freely access the Web site to read scenarios, watch the winning films, and provide comments/feedback on the students' works/films.

The Third Step

The third step will take approximately 6 months. This final step involves the production of the film based on the winning scenario, ideally benefiting from the volunteer services of a professional film director, as well as professional actors; the goals are to benefit from their volunteer services, thereby generating great interest in the final movies. Ultimately, the winning films will be hosted on the project Web site, and can be freely viewed by all. In terms of the long-term vision, each year, annual winners will be featured.

A Sample Script/Scenario

A sample script/scenario may be provided to convey what is expected of the youth teams. The following sample may inspire them and give them an idea of what is expected.

Soo-Han and the Smoking Quitter's Chat Group

Soo-Han, an imaginary character, is a high school student who has been smoking for 2 years. He knows smoking is bad for adolescents because of TV campaigns, but does not have much knowledge about the impact on health. He has been thinking about quitting for months but has not attempted quitting and did not tell anybody about this issue—not knowing where to discuss it. His parents will be very angry if they find out about his smoking, but most of his close friends are smokers. He doubts the necessity of quitting, because he does not know what to do except smoke to reduce stress from studying. Even worse, Soo-Han worries that his friends would make fun of him if they knew his thoughts (**SOC: Contemplation for Soo-Han**).

One day, Soo-Han was surfing the Internet as usual and found a cyber chat room with the title "Smoking Quitters' Chat Group" in one of his favorite community sites. He hesitated for a while to enter the room but he was curious about what other smokers do to quit smoking. When he entered the virtual chat room and said hello to members in the room, the other members were discussing reasons why they wanted to stop smoking. One said that his new girlfriend does not like the odor of his breath from smoking, so he wanted to quit. Another said that her brother had recently been diagnosed with lung cancer due to smoking so she was scared of getting cancer if she kept smoking. While reading others' stories, Soo-Han also thought about reasons why he wanted to quit but no ideas came up. When other members asked him why he wanted to quit, he just answered that he did not know. One member with several trial experiences at quitting said that he was the same as Soo-Han, but found a good reason after thinking about his family and future. This member said he would listen carefully and could give Soo-Han good advice if he wanted (**MI: Reflective listening and expressing empathy**). Soo-Han was thankful to hear that. The conversation went smoothly, as members in the room were exchanging ideas about quitting and encouraging each other to quit. After many hours chatting, the five members promised to meet online regularly to support each other and exchange their quit attempt stories.

Soo-Han kept his promise and logged onto the cyber chat room where all original five members were waiting for him. Only 1 week had passed since the first meeting but some of the members had already started to quit and some had been successful so far. One said that he stopped smoking just after the first chat by throwing all of his cigarettes away; this was the one who had the girlfriend who complained about the odor on his breath. He told his girlfriend about his quitting and she was very happy with him, so they had a wonderful date last week. However, he said it felt hard to not smoke, especially in certain situations, like being surrounded by smoking friends or when alone late at night (**RP: Identifying high-risk situations**). He expressed wanting some help, and wondered if there was any place he could get it. When listening to his story another member who had tried to quit several times before strongly agreed with him and suggested they support each other by sending text messages to each other's cell phones. Everybody including Soo-Han agreed to this idea and shared their cell phone numbers so they could text message each other (**RP: Social support; SOC: Preparation for Soo-Han**).

Getting text messages frequently and chatting with his new friends, Soo-Han naturally started quitting. Whenever he feels like smoking, he sends a message to all the members and immediately receives messages reinforcing his behavior change from all the members (**SOC: Action for Soo-Han**). It was enough to keep him from smoking until 1 day he could not help smoking late at night. That day, Soo-Han had a test and he felt so miserable about it despite his hard efforts. He could not sleep until late so looked for some help. He sent messages to all the chatting friends but nobody answered him. It was too late to be woken up. Soo-Han finally smoked that night (**SOC: Relapse**).

Not only Soo-Han, but other members experienced some problems and challenges, so the chat group was inactive for a while. However, some members continuously sent messages trying to restore the chat group meeting. Finally all members gathered in the chat room and shared their stories of what had happened so far. Soo-Han felt miserable and helpless when he restarted smoking and had been angry with himself (**RP: Abstinence Violation Effect**). He told this story to other members and, to his surprise, all other relapsed members explained how they had the same feelings. The one who said she wanted to quit because of her brother's cancer had cheered others up by telling about her experience consulting with experts. Her mother arranged for her to meet a health expert who knew about her quit attempt and wanted to help her. According to the expert, almost all quitters lapse or relapse several times until finally becoming abstinent, so it is natural to lapse. The important thing is not to blame yourself for the lapse and to keep training yourself to cope with the identified high-risk situations by establishing one's own way of dealing with them (**RP: Lapse management**). Knowing this, Soo-Han felt relieved and encouraged to start again. He thought about situations when he felt the urge to smoke and asked for members' opinions, but all solutions seemed unrealistic to him. They decided that each member had to come up with at least one alternative activity as a coping skill, for example, running outside for a while (**RP: Coping skills training** and lifestyle modification). Soo–Han decided to drink a cup of water whenever he felt tempted to smoke—advice that he read from an anti-smoking Web site (**RP: Internet approaches; SOC: Preparation for a new behavior change**).

Soo–Han had been successfully coping with his urges to smoke by drinking water for a while (**SOC: Action**) when he met and fell in love with a girl from another school. He happened to see her on the way home from his school when he took the bus instead of the subway one day. Luckily, one of his friends knew her, so he had a chance to meet her. The girl seemed nice to Soo–Han, but she said that she wanted to focus on studying for entrance to a good university. Soo–Han felt heart broken and began smoking again (**SOC: Relapse**). Attending the cyber chat room meeting, he explained what happened to his cyber friends, receiving their understanding and encouragement, feeling better than before (**MI: Expressing empathy; RP: Social support**). This time, Soo–Han did not feel guilty for his lapse (**RP: No internal attributions or Abstinence Violation Effect**), but had not anticipated this kind of high-risk situation, nor planned how to cope with it, so he was not ready to cope with it. However, he said that he now knew what to do if he became disappointed in love in the future (**MI: Change talk; RP: Anticipating and planning how to cope in a newly identified high-risk situation**). Everyone was happy to hear his statement and felt he had changed and grown up after going through several relapse episodes and overcoming them (**MI: Positive reinforcement of change talk**).

Suddenly, one of the members suggested an off-line meeting of the group. Soo–Han was not sure whether he was ready for the meeting but eventually he agreed (**SOC: Preparation, having moved from the Relapse stage**). In the off-line meeting, Soo–Han made friends with a girl who's living near his house. She was the one who had a brother with lung cancer and had been successful in quitting thanks to support from her family, the chat group, and the expert she met with in person (**RP: Social support**). She was also the one who suggested the cyber chat group members meet from time to time outside of cyberspace to encourage each other to remain abstinent and to share successful stories. Soo–Han gratefully agreed with her, enjoying these meetings, and establishing his abstinence from smoking again (**SOC: Action**). As Soo–Han began meeting with this new girl and could claim being successful at quitting for more than 6 months (**SOC: Maintenance**), some of his smoking friends asked what happened to him. Many had not seen him in a while. He told them his story of joining the cyber chat group of quitters and what happened. Some of his smoking friends were genuinely interested in his story and said they were thinking about quitting, or were ready to try to quit also (**SOC: Contemplation and preparation, respectively**). Some of his other smoking friends just made jokes and teased him (**SOC: Precontemplation**). Soo–Han told his friends that quitting would be worth the try, inviting those ready to quit to join the cyber chat group.

Analysis of the Sample Script/Scenario

This sample script/scenario reveals how the hero, Soo–Han, moves across the SOC, while also demonstrating how MI and RP came into play. As the story unfolds, people can observe how Soo–Han, upon first joining the chat group, was in a stage of contemplation, doubting the necessity of quitting and balancing the pros and cons of not smoking. After chatting with some young smokers like himself, he entered a stage of preparation for quitting. Taking action to quit, but going through several relapse episodes, Soo–Han finally succeeded and moved to the maintenance stage by sustaining abstinence for more than 6 months.

While transferring from stage to stage, Soo–Han showed signs of change and received proper counseling and support from peers deploying interventions based in MI and RP. When he failed to find good reasons to motivate himself to quit smoking, other members of the chat group listened carefully. Notably, one of the members expressed empathy, which is one of the four general principles of MI. The use of MI, and especially the experience of genuine empathy, helped him to move to the next stage of change: action. In addition, after a second relapse, he engaged in "change talk" and also evidenced increased self-efficacy to deal with the same high-risk situation in the future. By motivating himself with "change talk," and receiving positive reinforcement from his peers for this change talk, he was able to return to the preparation stage from the relapse stage, then took action to re-establish abstinence from smoking, and was eventually successful in reaching the maintenance stage.

Strategies from the relapse prevention model helped Soo–Han with every challenge he encountered. Social support from the chat group members was the most important factor in this story. He was able to overcome all relapse crises as a result of peer support. When he first decided to quit smoking, when he was discouraged after failing an exam in school and started smoking again, and when he relapsed the second time due to a disappointment in love, support from other chat members enabled him to start again.

While social support, which is classified as a distal intervention (Shiffman, Kassel, Gwaltney, & McChargue, 2005), mainly led Soo–Han to stay abstinent, other proximal interventions, such as identifying high-risk situations and coping skills training, helped him to reach his goal. Specifically, he avoided being surrounded by his smoking friends as he had identified this as a high-risk situation. He also drank water whenever he felt the urge to smoke as a coping skill. Moreover, when the AVE occurred as a result of his first lapse, he managed the situation successfully by learning how to restructure his cognitions, changing his view so that he made external attributions, and not blaming himself.

What is also key is that the script/scenario takes place in cyber space, inside a chat room, while text messaging using cellular phones was also used. As such, the use of the Internet served to first connect the chat room members, which then led to off-line meetings that provided further social support and information on coping skills. Through the experiences of Soo–Han, the value of the Internet and contemporary technologies emerge as promising tools for use in health promotion and disease prevention for Korean youth. Ultimately, the overall Web site envisioned will permit a potential population-wide impact, going beyond the impact on health among a group of peers depicted via the script/scenario.

Conclusion

This chapter has introduced an online multimedia peer education smoking cessation program for Korean youth. There are several key ingredients to the success of this project, as follows:

Collaboration and Partnerships. The program requires collaboration on the part of universities (i.e., supporters of the USE/ peer educators), schools (i.e., supporters of the involvement of middle and high school youth, while also allowing use of their facilities for team meetings), health education experts, Internet/Web designers, and members of the film industry—movie/television script writers, producers, and actors. Also, students must collaborate and cooperate with each other on teams in order to create their scripts/scenarios—both learning from and educating each other. This model is rooted in the belief that students can learn most effectively when they collaborate with each other, think for themselves, communicate with their peers, and make things with their own hands. Other vital partners include government funders, while it is also important to build partnerships and coalitions with existing local Non-Governmental Organizations (NGOs). NGOs may assist with film production and have an interest in promoting and screening films with a health message—perhaps within fund-raisers for their organizations.

Linguistic and Cultural Appropriateness. Health education experts must ensure that the adaptation and use of the SOC, MI, and RP theories occurs in such a way (i.e., how they are taught to the USE/peer educators, youth, and conveyed on the Web site to the general public) that the result is linguistically and culturally appropriate for the Korean population. Given the critique of Western theories in chapter 1 of this volume, only Korean health education experts can determine if the integration of theory being used to underpin this project is properly adapted to the social context of Korean culture.

Creating an Engaging, Informative, and Interactive Multimodal Web site. Internet Web designers must ensure the creation of a Web site that can effectively engage youth and members of the general public. It must be a state-of-the art Web site that provides information (i.e., tips on quitting, information on the health impact of smoking, information on SOC, MI, and RP, etc.), has interactive components (i.e., chat room, question and answer service, e-mail service), and hosts/delivers videos/films that the Korean population, and especially adolescents, can freely access.

Although this prize-winning program has yet to be funded, implemented, and evaluated, I believe it will contribute to diminishing cigarette-related health inequities among Korean adolescents. In addition, this chapter offers a template for others to follow in designing online multimedia peer education training programs.

REFERENCES

Biener, L., Reimer, R. L., Wakefield, M., Szczypka, G., Rigotti, N. A., & Gonnolly, G. (2006). Impact of smoking cessation aids and mass media among recent quitters. [Electronic version]. *American Journal of Preventive Medicine, 30*(3), 217–224.

Brogan, M. M., Prochaska, J. O., & Prochaska, J. M. (1999). Predicting termination and continuation status in psychotherapy by using the transtheoretical model. *Psychotherapy, 36*, 105–113.

Carroll, K. M. (1997). Relapse prevention as a psychosocial treatment: A review of controlled clinical trials. In G. A. Marlatt & G. R. VandenBos (Eds.), *Addictive behaviors: Readings on etiology, prevention, and treatment.* Washington, DC: American Psychological Association.

Dallery, J., Glenn, I. M., & Raiff, B. R. (2006). An Internet-based abstinence reinforcement treatment for cigarette smoking. [Electronic version]. *Drug and Alcohol Dependence, 86*(2), 230–248.

DiClemente, C. C., & Velasquez, M. M. (2002). Motivational interviewing and the stages of change. In W. R. Miller & S. Rollnick (Eds.), *Motivational interviewing: Preparing people for change* (2nd ed.). New York: Guilford Press.

Ebreo, A., Feist-Price, S., Siewe, Y., & Zimmerman, R. S. (2002). Effects of peer education on the peer educators in a school-based HIV prevention program: Where should peer education research go from here? [Electronic version]. *Health Education and Behavior, 29*(4), 411–423.

GallupKorea. (1999). *Report about adult smoking in Korea.* Retrieved December 14, 2006, from http://www.lung.or.kr/statistics/smokingstat.html

Grenard, J. L., Guo, Q., Jasuja, G. K., Unger, J. B., Chou, C. P., Gallaher, P. E., et al. (2006). Influences affecting adolescent smoking behavior in China. [Electronic version]. *Nicotine and Tobacco Research, 8*(2), 245–255.

Grimshaw, G. M., & Stanton, A. (2006, August 15). Tobacco cessation interventions for young people. *The Cochrane Database of Systemic Reviews, 4.* Retrieved November 14, 2006, from http://www.cochrane.org/reviews/en/ab003289.html

Kocken, P., Voorhan, T., Brandsma, J., & Swart, W. (2001). Effects of peer-led AIDS education aimed at Turkish and Moroccan male immigrants in The Netherlands. A randomised controlled evaluation study. [Electronic version]. *European Journal of Public Health, 11*(2), 153–159.

Korean Network Information Center. (2004, August 11). *Ten years of Internet in Korea.* Retrieved December 12, 2006, from http://www.internetworldstats.com/asia/kr.htm

Lancaster, T., Hajek, P., Stead, L. F., West, R., & Jarvis, M. J. (2006). Prevention of relapse after quitting smoking: A systematic review of trials. [Electronic version]. *Achieves of Internal Medicine, 166*(8), 828–835.

Marlatt, G. A. (1985). Situational determinants of relapse and skill-training interventions. In G. A. Marlatt & J. R. Gordon (Eds.), *Relapse prevention: Maintenance strategies in the treatment of addictive behaviors.* New York: Guilford Press.

Marlatt, G. A. (2007, March 10). *The role of relapse prevention in closing the health disparities gap.* Plenary keynote at the Second Annual Health Disparities Conference, Teachers College, Columbia University, New York.

Marlatt, G. A., & Donovan, D. M. (Eds.). (2005). *Relapse prevention: Maintenance strategies in the treatment of addictive behaviors* (2nd ed.). New York: Guilford Press.

Marlatt G. A., & Gordon, J. R. (Eds.). (1985). *Relapse prevention: Maintenance strategies in the treatment of addictive behaviors.* New York: Guilford Press.

Marlatt, G. A., & Witkiewitz, K. (2005). Relapse prevention for alcohol and drug problems. In G. A. Marlatt & D. M. Donovan (Eds.), *Relapse prevention: Maintenance strategies in the treatment of addictive behaviors* (2nd ed.). New York: Guilford Press.

Martino–McAllister, J., & Wessel, M. T. (2005). An evaluation of a social norms marketing project for tobacco prevention with middle, high, and college students: Use of funds from the Tobacco Master Settlement (Virginia). [Electronic version]. *Journal of Drug Education, 35*(3), 185–200.

Miller, W. R., & Rollnick, S. (Eds.). (1991). *Motivational interviewing: Preparing people to change addictive behaviors* (1st ed.). New York: Guilford Press.

Miller, W. R., & Rollnick, S. (Eds.). (2002). *Motivational interviewing: Preparing people for change* (2nd ed.). New York: Guilford Press.

Morisky, D. E., Nguyen, C., Ang, A., & Tiglao, T. V. (2005). HIV/AIDS prevention among the male population: Results of a peer education program for taxicab and tricycle drivers in the Philippines. [Electronic version]. *Health Education and Behavior, 32*(1), 57–68.

Newsis Communications. (2006, October 13). *The age of initial smoking is now 13.5 years.* Retrieved December 14, 2006, from http://www.newsis.com/

Ota, A., & Takahashi, Y. (2005). Factors associated with successful smoking cessation among participants in a smoking cessation program involving use of the Internet, e-mails, and mailing list. [Electronic version]. *Japanese Journal of Public Health, 52*(11), 999–1005.

Park, S., & June, K. J. (2006) The importance of smoking definitions for the study of adolescent smoking behavior. *Taehan Kanho Hakhoe Chi, 36*(4), 612–620.

Patten, C. A., Croghan, I. T., Meis, T. M., Decker, P. A., Pingree, S., Colligan, R. C., et al. (2006). Randomized clinical trial of an Internet-based versus brief office intervention for adolescent smoking cessation. [Electronic version]. *Patient Education and Counseling, 64*(1), 249–258.

Prochaska, J. O., & DiClemente, C. C. (1983). Stages and processes of self-change of smoking: Toward an integrative model of change. *Journal of Consulting and Clinical Psychology, 51*, 390–395.

Prochaska, J. O., Redding, C. A., & Evers, K. (2002). The transtheoretical model and stages of change. In K. Glanz, B. K. Rimer, & F. M. Lewis (Eds.), *Health behavior and health education: Theory, research, and practice* (3rd ed., pp. 99–120). San Francisco: Jossey-Bass.

Resnicow, K., DiLorio, C., Soet, J. E., Borreli, B., Ernst, D., Hecht, J., et al. (2002). Motivational interviewing in medical and public health settings. In W. R. Miller & S. Rollnick (Eds.), *Motivational interviewing: Preparing people for change* (2nd ed.). New York: Guilford Press.

Shiffman, S., Kassel, J., Gwaltney, C., & McChargue, D. (2005). Relapse prevention for smoking. In G. A. Marlatt & D. M. Donovan (Eds.), *Relapse prevention: Maintenance strategies in the treatment of addictive behaviors* (2nd ed.). New York: Guilford Press.

Stead, L. F., & Lancaster, T. (2006, February 16). Group behaviour therapy programmes for smoking cessation. *The Cochrane Database of Systemic Reviews, 4*. Retrieved November 29, 2006, from http://www.cochrane.org/reviews/en/ab001007.html

Tucker, J. A., Donovan, D. M., & Marlatt, G. A. (Eds.). (2001). *Changing addictive behavior: Bridging clinical and public health strategies*. New York: Guilford Press.

Wallace, B. C. (2005). *HIV/AIDS peer education training manual: Combining African healing wisdom and evidence-based behavior change strategies*. Philadelphia: StarSpirit Press.

Zucker, D., Hopkins, R. S., Sly, D. F., Urich, J., Kershaw, J. M., & Solaris, S. (2000). Florida's "truth" campaign: A counter-marketing, anti-tobacco media campaign. [Electronic version]. *Journal of Public Health Management and Practice, 6*(3), 1–6.

6

Training Community Health Workers and Peer Educators

Training Community Health Workers and Peer Educators for HIV/AIDS Prevention in Africa: Integrating African Healing Wisdom and Evidence–Based Behavior Change Strategies

Barbara C. Wallace,
Ansumana Richard Konuwa,
and Nana Akomfohene
Korantema Ayeboafo

Introduction

Community health workers, or peer educators—by either name—have a vital role to play for the achievement of the goal of a global health transformation and equity in health for all. This chapter presents an approach to training community health workers and peer educators specifically created for contemporary Sierra Leone, Africa (Wallace, 2005a), successfully piloted there (Konuwa, 2006), and more recently used in Ghana, Africa (Ayeboafo, 2005). In so doing, the chapter also presents the results of the successful collaboration and partnership between the Research Group on Disparities in Health of Teachers College, Columbia University in New York City, and a Non-Governmental Organization (NGO) in consultative status with the economic and social council of the United Nations—StarSpirit International, Inc. (www.starspirit.com). This represents a model academic–NGO collaboration seeking to establish an international HIV/AIDS peer education certification program that will ultimately be Internet based, while this chapter reports on the results of the collaboration so far in creating and launching in Africa a culturally appropriate model for training peer educators and community health workers.

Seven Guiding Principles for Community Health Promotion

There are seven principles for community mental health promotion (adapted from Wallace, 1996) that may apply to both the training of community health workers and peer educators, while also specifying that in which they should engage once so trained.

1. *Training*: Provide training that is practical and easy to understand for professionals and paraprofessionals (in recovery, HIV +, Peer Educators). Training should give new tools, techniques, and terminology.
2. *Outreach*: Go to where the people in need are to be found in their very own communities and engage in community outreach—whether a school, worksite, church, prison, community, or country—and work alongside community members as respected equals.
3. *Acceptance*: Accept individuals in the condition, state of readiness to change, or stage of change (e.g., Prochaska & DiClemente, 1983) in which you find them, and always provide respect, empathy, hope, as you offer resources and foster enhanced motivation for whatever steps community members decide to take toward change and transformation.
4. *Self-Efficacy*: Facilitate practical and personal experiential learning (via work-books, role-plays, rehearsal, etc.) that increases the self-efficacy of all participants; and that facilitates the delivery of prevention, intervention, and treatment to others, in turn.
5. *Empowerment*: Support the empowerment of community health workers and community members to engage in the determination of their own community's health.
6. *Cultural Competence*: Provide culturally sensitive training that produces workers in the trenches who possess cultural competence and can engage in that which is culturally appropriate and linguistically appropriate.
7. *Determination*: Encourage self- and/or collective determination of a community's health and related standards and outcomes.

Wallace (1996) envisions training community health workers or peer educators who can, in turn, deliver the very same training they received, providing a manual for doing so, or training the trainers. More recently, following the same philosophy, a manualized workbook for training HIV/AIDS prevention peer educators has been developed (Wallace, 2005a).

The Context for Training: A New ERA With New Needs

The context for all such training manuals is what Elder (2001) describes as a new public health era—one where the emphasis is on health behavior and the environment in which it occurs, as well as on how societies and individuals have to take responsibility for health, rather than waiting for changes to be made for them. Thus, empowering community health workers and peer educators, and equipping them to be trainers of trainers, are a vital process consistent with this new era.

Elder (2001) explains how by emphasizing behavior change and the implications of changing behavior for health, in this new era, the responsibility and capacity for change can be seen as belonging to individuals and communities. This responsibility can also be seen as belonging not only to individuals and communities, but also to societies, in order to foster individual, family, and community health.

The model of training community health workers and peer educators being put forth in this chapter is consistent with what Elder (2001) envisions. Indeed, there is further support for this approach, given that there are also new emergent needs in this new era.

For example, LaVeist (2005) identifies keys to success in addressing health status and health care disparities that represent new emergent needs in this new era in which we find ourselves. For LaVeist, these three keys are (1) community-based participatory research; (2) the cultural tailoring of interventions in light of language and culture; and (3) the involvement of community health workers.

The training of community health workers emerges as an essential function, as is ensuring that the training they receive and the interventions they deliver are culturally tailored in light of language and culture. The training should, also, ideally, serve to prepare community health workers for valued roles in community-based participatory research (see Hayes, chapter 13, this volume).

The work in which community health workers and peer educators engage allows them to be on the front line and in the trenches, working alongside real people in real world contexts, perhaps in collaboration with Non-Governmental Organizations (NGOs). Together, they may also be able to act to ensure that health as a human right is attained in distant and rural settings around the globe, while also being able to witness and report violations of that right. Thus, another need in the new era is for those who can both work to ensure health is attained as a human right, and who can report violations—such as those NGOs in consultative status with the economic and social council of the United Nations.

Consider how the World Health Organization and its members asserted that health is a basic human right and essential for social and economic development, while prerequisites for health are peace, shelter, education, social security, empowerment of women, a stable ecosystem, sustainable resources use, social justice, and respect for human rights and equity, as articulated in the Jakarta Declaration of 1997 (Elder, 2001). With regard to the Jakarta Declaration, the following pertinent strategies to bring about health are highlighted by Elder (2001):

- Promote social responsibility for health (e.g., the public and private sectors should promote health via non-harmful policies and practices);
- Increase investments for health development (needs of women, children, older people, indigenous, poor, marginalized);
- Consolidate and expand partnerships for health (i.e., at all levels of government and society);
- Increase community capacity and empower the individual (e.g., health promotion is carried out by and with the people, not on to people; while there is a role for practical education, leadership training, and access to resources); and

- Secure an infrastructure for health promotion (e.g., new mechanisms of local, national, and global funding must be found).

The training of community health workers and peer educators represents an important means of increasing community capacity and empowering individuals to determine the health of their own communities. In this manner, community health workers and peer educators may assist in securing health as a human right, working to bring about equity in health for all as global health leaders.

Bambas and Casas (2003, p. 333) acknowledge how "the pursuit of equity is necessarily linked to issues of governance, which includes accountability, transparency, decision-making procedures, and the ability of the political sphere to allow for broad representation and the effective exercise of choice by all" in that society. Bambas and Casas conclude as follows: "Once a society embraces a political foundation of egalitarianism, whereby all citizens of a country are due equal regard under the law and have equal political voices, societies themselves become the ultimate arbitrators of equity in health or any other sphere" (p. 333).

However, even where larger societies and governments may or may not as yet be practicing egalitarianism, community health workers and peer educators can experience and work to create egalitarianism, especially via collaborations, coalitions, and partnerships with NGOs and academic professionals in community-based participatory research. Community health workers and peer educators can also provide a kind of broad representation of the health needs and experiences of their community members. Thus, another need in the new era is for those who can work to bring about egalitarianism and rebuild communities and social support networks.

With regard to the value of such egalitarianism, Kunitz (2007) notes the Roseto effect, arising from a detailed analysis of the Roseto town in Pennsylvania. This town was established in the late nineteenth century by immigrants from their town in southern Italy—in the United States. The town was known for an unusually low incidence of heart attacks, when compared to neighboring towns. The analysis of multiple sources of data led to the conclusion that this was due to "the egalitarianism and cohesiveness of the community and to the commitment of family members to one another" (p. 129). Also noteworthy is how over the first half of the twentieth century when the Roseto community was cohesive, this cohesiveness was also seen as "the result of hostility on the part of non-Italians in neighboring communities, as well as other hardships" (p. 130).

The training of community health workers and peer educators can represent an important mechanism for helping to bring about egalitarianism and community cohesiveness, while specifically addressing community hardships that are a threat to health. The HIV/AIDS pandemic in Africa brings with it the kind of hardships that may actually be harnessed as a cause for community mobilization toward cohesiveness so as to bring about health—within a movement ensuring the human right to health.

Kunitz (2007, p. 132) observes how social capital "is but the most recent manifestation of the quest for community." Thus, investing in the training of community health workers and peer educators may represent a vital investment in social capital, while also helping to build community cohesiveness. Bridglall and Gordon (chapter 27, this volume) discuss how human capital includes adults and peers who may serve as models of the behaviors others in a community can emulate, while social capital is represented in the networks of support, the connections to sources of information and resources, and the expectations of the group. Kwong, Ho-Asjoe, Chung, and Wong (chapter 14, this volume) note how when social capital is optimized through an asset-based community development approach, then the community assets and resources for a particular neighborhood are increased, holding the potential to enhance the social milieu and economic position on a community or neighborhood level.

Peter and Evans (2001) note how the new era also brings with it "the transnationalization of health risks . . . arising from environmental threats, communicable disease, social change, and so forth" (p. 32). Moreover, these health risks "make clear the importance of a global ethical framework for assessing inequalities in health"—suggesting a need for international institutions that can promote an inclusive discourse on health equity (p. 32).

Collaborations between academics and NGOs, especially when codified and made tangible via Internet Web sites, may begin to approach the kind of international institutions needed—of which Peter and Evans (2001) speak. Hence, a role for the academic–NGO partnership featured in this chapter, and for the training of community health workers and peer educators who constitute the "eyes and ears" centered in communities who can stand for the value of health and the human right to health, as global health leaders in their own right.

Indigenous Community–Based Arbiters and Gatekeepers Ensuring Cultural and Linguistic Appropriateness

Community health workers and peer educators are also the ultimate arbiters with regard to what is culturally appropriate in terms of interventions potentially deployed in their own communities. They are also the gatekeepers who can ensure that that which is done in their communities in the name of health promotion, health education, or disease prevention is consistent with their communities' own ethical standards, traditional values, spiritual orientation, worldview, and culture. They are also the ones who can ensure that all interventions delivered in their communities are both culturally appropriate, as well as linguistically appropriate. In fact, without community health workers and peer educators, no effective translation or meaningful health communication can occur, unless they are there, and able to search their internal data banks as the ones who know anywhere from two to five or more of the local languages, while reflecting on the lived experiences of their people, and discerning the very best words to convey a health concept. In this manner, without community health workers and peer educators, no academic–NGO partnership, or any other international agent seeking to work to bring about equity in health for all, can accomplish their work in the distant places around the globe where health needs are real and even urgent. Thus, only community health workers and peer educators who are indigenous to their own communities around the globe can ensure that all interventions are tailored to be culturally appropriate for their communities.

The Importance of the New Paradigm Guiding Collaborations

In order to benefit from the wealth of talents and resources community health workers and peer educators possess and bring to collaborations, they must be approached as equals, consistent with the new paradigm guiding this volume, where we can bring about equity in health only where $A = B$ (Wallace, 2003). While academics may know about evidence-based approaches and cutting edge approaches to bring about behavior change, a sense of empowerment, and equity in health, and while NGO representatives have links to indigenous communities around the globe, it is the indigenous community health workers and peer educators who know their own people the very best and what will "work" in that social context, and how to communicate in the local languages so what works can be effectively disseminated. To further underscore the value of this, it is noteworthy that in most parts of Africa, people speak two to five or more local languages, in addition to the language of their colonizers or some version of it. Thus, when one moves into the global realm and elects to work in Africa, indigenous community health workers and peer educators emerge as invaluable players on any viable team. Yet, the reciprocal and mutual training of all team members can still benefit from a focus on training community health workers and peer educators.

The Search for Relevant Theories for the Global Context: The Gates by Which We Enter

Given the importance of training community health workers and peer educators, the question arises as to which theories to draw upon in their training so they can work to bring about equity in health for their community members. Elder (2001) provides a telling critique, pointing out how epidemiology lacks theory development. In addition, health psychology and behavioral sciences judge interventions by the amount of individual behavior change achieved and extent to which broader generalizations can be made to other behavior-change efforts and phenomena. Many theories tend to be reductionistic, individualistic, and driven to some extent by biomedicine. Such theories also have limited applicability to developing-country populations and health issues, given how these are places where more traditional cultures and the subordination of individual to community identity prevail (Elder, 2001; see also Airhihenbuwa, 2007, chapter 1; and Airhihenbuwa & Okoror, chapter 3, this volume). Elder (2001) identified more practical general theories or models of behavior change for developing health promotion programs in developing countries (e.g., health communication and social marketing, operant psychology, social learning theory, media advocacy, community self-control).

Elder (2001) recommends an integration of epidemiology and behavioral sciences, referring to this as the emerging field of behavioral epidemiology. The new emergent field of behavioral epidemiology involves: the study of the distribution of health-related behaviors in populations; the association of these behaviors with health, morbidity, and mortality; and techniques for changing these behaviors on a population-wide basis. More-over, the results of the integration include how epidemiologists are discovering the behavioral connection with virtually all major threats to the health of humans—from chronic diseases and disabilities to infectious diseases and habitat destruction. To illustrate the value of this approach, Elder (2001) notes how small changes in an entire population will result in greater public health changes than large changes in a small group of high-risk individuals (see Prochaska, chapter 4, this volume). By way of an example, Elder (2001) points out how a 70% condom adoption rate in a patient population is a success; whereas a 10% effect in an entire community for condom adoption via a media campaign would be an extraordinary success. Meanwhile, Elder (2001) envisions potential applications to the goal of behavior change in several areas: vaccinations, breast feeding, nutrition, management of childhood diarrhea and acute respiratory infections, family planning, home hygiene, vector control (mosquitoes, fleas, etc.), and the prevention of the spread of HIV.

Of note, Airhihenbuwa (2007) offers the following caution, given how our guiding theories (closely tied up with identity) determine the gate by which the Western trained enter places such as Africa, and communities around the globe:

> It is necessary to identify the point of intervention entry with the understanding that there could be multiple entry points. The process removes the assumption that all interventions should focus on the individual, thus leading to the development of billboards and other media messages that may not address the context of behavior change. The three components of the domain of cultural identity are person, extended family, and neighborhood. (p. 187)

Hence, even as we are advised to embrace theories such as health communication, social marketing, and media advocacy advanced by Elder (2001), the work of Airhihenbuwa (2007) serves to point us back in the direction of needing to carefully consider how we enter the social context of Africa and other indigenous communities around the globe.

Again, a vital role emerges for those community health workers and peer educators who may provide assistance as those indigenous communities' gatekeepers to what is culturally appropriate—even as it may mean we draw upon their knowledge of the multiple languages and corresponding worldviews and traditions that will be the multiple entry points for delivering a health message in that social context. This emerges as a profound truth, regardless of our preferred theories and the paradigms they represent.

Toward Multiple Theories and Interventions to Choose From for the Global Health Context

Along these same lines, we may also need multiple theories that can be integrated or drawn upon—from a menu of evidence-based options or effective alternatives (Wallace, 2005b; see Nanín, Fontaine, & Wallace, chapter 22, this volume). Just as a menu of seven evidence-based approaches—all rooted in theory or theories—and seven state-of-the-art practices have been identified as available for use so that selections may be made by practitioners addressing disparities in addiction and substance abuse, as practitioners tailor treatment for multiproblem clients (Wallace, 2005b), the same may be a possibility for global health disparities in years to come. This is possible, given the goal also embedded in this edited volume to move the field of equity in health toward the identification of evidence-based strategies for bringing about a global health transformation. Ideally, within a decade there will be a range of evidence-based interventions from which to select, as they will constitute a menu, even as this volume begins to establish numerous approaches, models, interventions, and approaches as items all worthy of being on the menu of options for bringing about equity in health for all.

Communities may be like individual patients who may be in different states of readiness to change at different points in time, and may need different strategies depending upon various factors in the social context. Key factors include those reflective of indigenous cultures, traditions, and languages—perhaps with there being multiple cultures, traditions, and languages all in one community or region. In light of this possibility, if not reality, from among the seven evidence-based options on just one menu already described in the literature (Wallace, 2005b; see Nanín et al., chapter 22, this volume), three have been selected for application in creating a manualized model for training community health workers and peer educators for HIV/AIDS prevention in Africa.

The Three Evidence-Based Theories/Approaches for Training Community Health Workers and Peer Educators in Africa

While chapter 18 by Woo (this volume) presented the three evidence-based theories in detail, upon which the recommended model for training HIV/AIDS prevention peer educators or community health workers is based, this chapter will present the manner in which these theories can be adapted and summarized in brief; this allows the information to be readily accessible to those with low literacy, or are bilingual or multilingual in various international contexts. While Woo's chapter, which is the 2006 winner of a contest (2006) at Teachers College, Columbia University for the best most promising model for promoting global health for a problem behavior (e.g. adolescent smoking), illustrates the integration of the three evidence-based models (stages of change, Prochaska & DiClemente, 1983; motivational interviewing, Miller & Rollnick, 2002; and, relapse prevention, Marlatt & Donovan, 2005; Marlatt & Gordon, 1985), we present here a 2005 integration and application to the challenge of preventing HIV transmission in Sierra Leone (Konuwa, 2006). The resulting training manual (Wallace, 2005a) codifies and makes available for wide dissemination a recommended model for training community health workers and peer educators in Africa. The manual (Wallace, 2005a) also integrates the use of African Healing Wisdom (Ayeboafo, 2005), making it particularly well suited for use in Africa.

Manual Development

A focus group with people from Sierra Leone living in the United States was conducted to ensure that none of the finger positions or body gestures eventually incorporated in the manual to facilitate memorization among those with low literacy was culturally offensive (Konuwa, 2006). Five people from Sierra Leone living in the United States, who had traveled home within recent years, participated in the focus group. First they were presented with a meal prepared just for them and the principal investigator who was also from Sierra Leone (Ansumana Richard Konuwa)—the one planning to pilot the manual and peer education training program in Sierra Leone. Next, the participants were given 20–30 minutes to individually review an initial version of the training manual, with two men also discussing among themselves content on a few pages. Then the focus group began with all of the chapter authors present, with the first author taking the lead in asking the questions to stimulate dialogue.

Focus group discussion revealed that the participants were very pleased with the manual, found none of the hand or body gestures to be culturally offensive, but wanted much more knowledge information in the manual—effectively expanding the length of the manual by over 30 pages. Additional HIV/AIDS knowledge information was largely drawn from Kalichman (2003) and from Green (2003)—especially regarding prevention practices most appropriate for Africa. In addition, a nurse in the group, and the only female, very much wanted all the details of universal precautions to be included. Of great importance was information provided about HIV risk behaviors specific to Sierra Leone, including those common in the secret societies where rituals are performed with a knife that may be repeatedly used; and, the cultural belief that a syringe injection that hurts is the ideal medicine for literally any ill health condition, allowing charlatans to take one syringe to a village and inject countless people complaining about any malaise; one group member had a family member who dropped dead within 24 hours of receiving such an injection, while others had heard of similar stories. There was also consensus among group members that the visuals on how to use bleach to clean syringe injection equipment/needles would not be very helpful, as bleach was not readily available in most parts of Sierra Leone; hence, infection control guidelines were consulted. The nurse also put out a call for NGOs, foundations, and foreign governments to donate one-time use disposable scalpels for use in secret society rituals, as well as for one-time use disposable syringe injection equipment.

Pragmatics related to the implementation of the training model codified in the manual were also covered in the focus group. This included the manner in which 4 weeks was deemed sufficient to conduct the training across 4 weekdays, how lunch had to be served, and suggestions regarding what the appropriate stipend for participation would be upon completion and graduation as a certified HIV/AIDS prevention peer educator. Surprisingly, the focus group members felt very strongly that teachers, many of whom are unemployed, and other literate and educated people should be trained as peer educators—versus the initial plan to have good representation among many groups (e.g., youth, homeless, refugee camp participants, adults, elders, etc.). This recommendation was made so as to ensure maximum dissemination of the knowledge they would acquire, and the perception that those with more education and teachers might in the future (e.g., when teaching again) find more opportunities for sharing widely that which they learned.

Collectively, these suggestions were systematically incorporated into the manual, including information pertaining to infection control (Association for Professionals in Infection Control and Epidemiology, Inc., 1996), resulting in the final published manual (Wallace, 2005a) deemed culturally appropriate, given the application of findings from the focus group.

Interviews were also conducted with two physicians, one an internist and one a dentist—especially familiar with infection control procedures for use in sterilizing dental equipment. It became clear that in the absence of readily accessible bleach, and without the kind of dental sterilization equipment meeting optimum standards being available in rural parts of Sierra Leone, the best suggestion was for one-time use disposable scalpels and injection syringes being made available. The resulting application of their comments, in light of the focus group findings, resulted in a manual (Wallace, 2005a) also deemed scientifically appropriate—even if not totally realistic in recommendations that one-time use disposable scalpels and syringes be used in all cases; or, harm of contraction of other bacterial spores would continue to exist if equipment were only boiled—even as such boiling would destroy HIV.

Stages of Change as Stages of Safety

Consistent with values expressed some time ago, it is important to be able to effectively engage everyone within a training, regardless of their educational level, level of literacy, or primary spoken language (Wallace, 1996). Thus, techniques were sought that would allow for maximum dissemination of the training content. Toward this end, when simplifying the stages of change within the training of HIV/AIDS prevention peer educators, Wallace (2005a) introduced six stages of safety and six finger positions. The resulting HIV/AIDS prevention peer education training manual (Wallace, 2005a) introduces finger positions depicted in photographs. Another technique involves having peers make up a song to facilitate memorization of each stage and finger position. Further making the stages of change accessible and understandable, community health workers and peer educators are urged to accept how "our peers are in different stages of safety" (Wallace, 2005a, p. 60). The precontemplation stage is referred to as *not thinking about safety*, the contemplation stage as *thinking about safety*, the preparation stage as *decided to be safe*, the action stage as *taking safe action*, the maintenance stage as *staying safe*, and relapse as *unsafe/stopped taking safe action*.

Motivational Interviewing as Empowering Peers to Move Toward Safe Action

Wallace's model of training HIV/AIDS prevention peer educators (2005a, pp. 63–64) emphasizes the "six steps and six body positions for empowering our peers to move toward taking safe action," complementing the transformation of the stages of change into the stages of safety. Again, this is rooted in and extracted from motivational interviewing (MI) (Miller & Rollnick, 1991, 2002) as a simplification that serves to make this vast body of knowledge—summarized in detail by Woo (chapter 18, this volume)—readily accessible to anyone of any educational or literacy level seeking to promote health and behavior change literally anywhere (e.g., from a street corner where there is outreach to commercial sex workers, to someone doing outreach inside a bathhouse or brothel, to a hitchhiker riding with a truck driver, to an adolescent talking to a peacekeeper in a refugee camp).

The simplification of MI (Wallace, 2005a) emphasizes (1) avoiding argumentation or telling people what to do, (2) asking about concerns, (3) engaging in a decisional balance, (4) generating a menu of options, (5) exploring next steps, and (6) emphasizing a peer's free choice to decide what to do (Wallace, 2005a). More specifically, Wallace (2005) offers the following simplification:

1. *Rules/Hand*: The symbol is **a hand held up** to indicate stopping . . . or taking great care . . . a reminder to . . . not argue with your peers. Do not tell people what to do. Do not speak to people harshly. Talk to your peers with respect and in a calm manner. . . .

2. *Worries/Head*: The symbol is **a person holding their head with both hands**, as if they are concerned, worried, or thinking about problems.... [A]sk them, "What concerns do you have?" Or, "Do you have any worries, concerns, or problems?"

3. *Both Sides/Both Hands*: The symbol is a **person holding up each hand as if each hand represents the two sides of the argument, or two things being weighed in each hand**: Ask your peers about the two sides of the argument... in their mind.... Or... the pros (advantages) and cons (disadvantages) of changing.... You then summarize... and state: "On the one hand you say _____ (holding up one hand), and on the other hand you say _____ (holding up the other hand)...."

4. *List/Fingers*: The symbol is a person **using one hand to start to point to each finger on the other hand so each finger represents an item on a list**: ... Let's list all the things you can do, such as change, not change; and... all the options you have for changing. Let's make a menu of options.... The first smallest finger might represent not changing, the second finger changing.... Make the list with your peer, using your fingers....

5. *Next Steps/Feet*: The symbol is a person's **two feet with one foot in motion to suggest a next step is about to be taken on one of two roads—the safe road or dangerous road**: Ask your peer: "What's the next step?" "What do you feel ready to do now?" From the menu of options and all the things we listed, "What are you considering doing?"

6. *Choice/Pointer Finger*: The symbol is **a person's hand using the pointer finger to indicate two different directions, suggesting there is more than one direction to go in—the safe road or the dangerous road**: End by emphasizing with your peer: "The choice is up to you." (Wallace, 2005a, pp. 63–64)

Peer educators are also encouraged within each step to do the following: "Remember, if the person talks about already taking, wanting to take, or planning to take any actions to be safe, say 'good, good' " (Wallace, 2005a, pp. 63–64). In this manner, peer educators are trained to provide positive reinforcement for any "change talk"—consistent with MI.

Wallace (2005a) includes photographs of peer role models in each of the six body positions, and recommends that peer educators create original songs about the six body positions and corresponding techniques for empowering their peers to move toward taking safe action. The purpose of both the body positions and creation of songs is to facilitate memorization. The goal is for those with low literacy to also be able to access the information through songs and body gestures, while ensuring cultural appropriateness, since the peer educators determine content of the songs.

Relapse Prevention as Preparation to Pass Unexpected Tests and Avoid a Return to Being Unsafe

Wallace (2005a, p. 67) includes a segment in the curriculum on "empowering our peers to pass unexpected tests and avoid a return to being unsafe," using a metaphor of traveling along a road, while peer educators are likened to travel guides, giving advice to travelers. There are seven brief components, including teaching peers to anticipate in advance and plan how to cope with high risk situations for relapse; distinguishing between a lapse and a full-blown relapse; teaching avoidance of the abstinence violation effect (AVE) in the event of a lapse; and seeking to enhance self-efficacy through the creation and rehearsal of role plays for how to cope in high risk situations—even culminating in the creation of videos to educate others. The seven brief RP components (Wallace, 2005a) are shown below:

1. *Advice to Travelers*: "... *We all want to be safe and stay safe. But, there may be unexpected road conditions or dangerous situations along the road. So, we have to prepare by Learning* about all the dangerous situations; *Listing* all the dangerous situations [like a wet, oily, or slippery patch of road]; *Planning* a strategy for all dangerous situations; *Playing* out scenes for what to do in those situations; [and,] *Practicing* what to do in those situations. ..."

2. *Warn Travelers*: "... *You might slip or fall* ..." when ... there is a wet, oily, slippery spot. ... So, if a person has a slip or a fall ... we want to empower them to get up right away and to take action to be safe, again. ...

3. *Prepare Travelers*: "... *If you fall, don't give up and get up right away.* ..." After a person has a slip or fall, sometimes they feel bad, embarrassed, or ashamed. They may now doubt their ability. ... They may just give up and allow themselves to fall all the way. ... As a travel guide, warn travelers *before* they have a slip or a fall: "If you slip or fall, do not give up. Get right up after a slip or fall."

4. *Encourage Travelers*: "... *If you slip or fall, you will be a wiser traveler* ..." ... Instead of feeling bad, embarrassed, ashamed or doubting your ability to be safe, look at the slip or fall as a chance to learn. ... Because of the slip or fall, you now have new, important knowledge that will make you a better, wiser traveler in the future. ...

5. *Assist Travelers*: "... *A wiser traveler can plan what to do to avoid another slip or fall* ..." ... Remember, that the good thing about a slip or fall is that you learn about road conditions, and how to stay safe in travel by anticipating and *planning beforehand* how to deal with that road condition the next time you experience it in the future. ...

6. *Play Out What to Do*: "... *Let us play out what to do the next time we face the same dangerous situation.* ..." What can you do to avoid a slip or fall? ... What should you say and do next time? ... Let's pretend it is a scene in a play." Decide what seems to work best. ...

7. *Practice*: "... *Let us practice what to do over and over again, so we are prepared for the dangerous situation.* ..." Practice (play out) what to do again and again and again. ... You can also make a play (and video tape it). ... A play is one of the most powerful ways to teach and show others what to do to avoid a slip or fall. Practice! (Wallace, 2005a, pp. 66–68)

In this manner, all the key aspects of relapse prevention (Marlatt & Donovan, 2005; Marlatt & Gordon, 1985) are included in the training curriculum for community health workers and peer educators (Wallace, 2005a), as summarized by Woo (chapter 18, this volume). The manual even includes a focus on lifestyle modification (Marlatt & Gordon, 1985), which is also consistent with Marlatt's latest work (2007) integrating mindfulness meditation into relapse prevention—as explained next.

A Role for Deep Breathing

Given in-depth consideration of the potential stress and anxiety that might still be present among the displaced people of Sierra Leone, especially post-war (Konuwa, 2006), great value was placed upon incorporating an easy-to-learn and easy-to-teach method of stress reduction within the curriculum (Wallace, 2005a). The use of deep breathing is also consistent with the relapse prevention focus on lifestyle modification (Marlatt, 2007; Marlatt & Gordon, 1985). Thus, a breathing exercise (Hunter & Lewis-Coles, 2004) was incorporated into the training of peer educators very early on (Wallace, 2005a). According to Hunter and Lewis-Coles (2004), this breathing exercise is recommended for 5 minutes or at any moment when there is a need to self-calm, feel peace, think clearly, or strengthen your self for the next part of your journey. The recommended breathing technique comes from Ancient Egyptian culture and is also known as belly breathing, abdominal breathing, or proper breathing—as the natural breathing pattern when a person lies on his or her back. Wallace (2005a) includes photographs depicting the proper performance of this exercise, along with simple instructions. Peers are encouraged to start morning training sessions practicing deep breathing, as well as being instructed to teach others the technique (Wallace, 2005a).

A Role for Social Support

Also included in the training manual for peer educators are specific suggestions for seeking out social support, as well as optimistic and positive peers. Recommendations in this regard are taken from the work of Gaston and Porter (2001). Gaston and Porter acknowledge how when people are upset and angry, there are several possibilities for coping: (1) be passive and do nothing to get help from others; (2) be sneaky and try and get revenge against others without other people knowing; (3) be violent and strike out against others to get revenge so anyone and everyone can see and know about it—if they happen to be around or witness the event; and (4) make an assertive and positive response where you talk about what is bothering you to the person who made you upset or to others who are Supportive, Optimistic, and Positive Peers (SOPP). The training emphasizes the last option.

A context is provided for these possibilities, given the goal of providing training for HIV/AIDS prevention. Indeed, a story told in the focus group held with people from Sierra Leone was also incorporated into the training, emphasizing values other than seeking revenge. Wallace (2005a) offers the following, in this regard:

> There are some people who find out that they are HIV positive, become angry, and decide to be sneaky and get revenge against others without other people knowing it. For example. . . . a man gets HIV from a woman and decides to have sex with as many women as possible as a form of revenge against women. . . . It would be better for someone who is HIV positive to be assertive and positive and talk about what is bothering them to a buddy or a supportive, optimistic and positive peer. . . . This is why we want peer educators to be supportive, optimistic and positive peers who are available to people in the community. We need people trained so they can assist people in the community in accepting their HIV status . . . . getting tested and treated so they can stay healthy and live a long time—and not transmit HIV/AIDS to anyone else in the community.

No matter what we or our peers are going through, no matter what is bothering us, no matter why we are upset, the solution is to seek out Supportive, Optimistic, and Positive Peers (SOPP). By talking to SOPP, we are likely to end up with a more positive attitude that will help us to deal with the situation. (p. 22)

A Role for African Healing Wisdom

African Healing Wisdom (Ayeboafo, 2005) is also incorporated into the curriculum, actually being presented at the very beginning of the training, and being embodied in the daily affirmations or self-talk that peer educators are encouraged to practice as a group or with their buddy when they arrive to the training each morning. Their buddy is "a person of your same gender/sex who may live near you, or someone easy to contact on a regular basis" (Wallace, 2005a, p. 17). Furthermore, in "the West, this may be someone you talk with on the telephone," and "someone you may practice what you learn with, or with whom you will do your homework" (p. 17). This is yet another way in which social support is built into the training, while the relationship with the buddy is also pertinent to practicing values rooted in African Healing Wisdom.

The goal is for the African Healing Wisdom and cultural values brought forth by an African indigenous healer (Ayeboafo, 2005) to guide both the development of peers' relationships with their buddies, and the other peers in the training program, while also finding extension to their relationship with their community (Wallace, 2005a). The African Healing Wisdom and cultural values incorporated into the training of peer educators (Wallace, 2005a) follows:

> ... [Y]ou will practice **commitment** with your buddy (doing what you say will do all of the time, such as meeting your buddy at the correct time); and, if you fail to do what you say will do, you apologize and recommit; thus ... **apology** is very important. ... Suggesting how to **forgive** is also vital ... and ... to **pardon** another—deciding to withhold or not to deliver a punishment ... revenge.
>
> Also key ... is treating others with **equality and respect**. Another goal is to ... foster freedom of expression in others, so they feel able to open up and communicate with you. ...
>
> You will also practice **unity** with your buddy, learning to move and work as one unit, cooperating with each other, ... your entire training group, and ... your larger community. Also ... **harmony** ... focusing on what is the same ... instead of what is different, and cooperating ... to reach goals. ... You will also practice and experience **interdependence** .... focusing on how ... what affects "one" affects "all." (pp. 17–18)

Wallace (2005a, p. 18) explains how all "of these African cultural values are needed to alleviate the crisis and suffering in our communities, given the HIV/AIDS epidemic, as well as other community problems." They are further urged to "practice these cultural values and teach them to others," making them a part of one's individual, family, and community life (p. 18).

The rationale for incorporating African Healing Wisdom (Wallace, 2005a, p. 18) rests in one explanation offered by Dr. Erik Gbodossou, President of PROMETRA, The Association for the Promotion of Traditional Medicine in Senegal, as follows: *The West makes people who know how to make money. Africa makes human beings!* Moreover, in times of "crisis, community members around the world with people living with HIV/AIDS (PLWHA) need compassionate and caring human beings. Thus, there is great logic in embracing, learning, and practicing the African Healing Wisdom . . . and African cultural values" (p. 18).

Finally, to reinforce the learning of these cultural values, peer educators are urged to practice "the peer educators' daily affirmations, memorize them, and repeat them every day" (Wallace, 2005a). Peer educators are given the suggestion that these affirmations "will serve as a powerful guide in creating yourself anew as a compassionate and caring 'human being'" (p. 18). Of note, this is similar to Airhihenbuwa's (2007; and Airhihenbuwa & Okoror, chapter 3, this volume) discussion of what it means to be a real person in the Nigerian (*omwan*, or truly a person) and African worldview; this is a person with high standards within the community with regard to their ethics, principles, and values. Meanwhile, to create such compassionate and caring human beings, Wallace (2005a) recommends the following daily affirmations for peer educators, suggesting that peers also consider making up a short song to facilitate memorization of them:

> *COMMITMENT: "I am who I say I am. I do what I say I am going to do."*
> *APOLOGY: "If I ever fail to be who I say I am, or to do what I say I am going to do, I apologize and recommit."*
> *FORGIVENESS: "I ask others to forgive me, and forgive others."*
> *PARDON: "I ask others to pardon me, and pardon others."*
> *EQUALITY AND RESPECT: "I treat everyone with equality and respect."*
> *FREEDOM OF EXPRESSION: "I am trustworthy so others feel freedom of expression with me. I have an optimistic and positive attitude that helps people to feel free to express themselves with me."*
> *UNITY, HARMONY, AND INTERDEPENDENCE: "I am creating unity, harmony, and interdependence."*

Toward Songs, Theatrical Skits, Role-Plays, and a Graduation Play

The HIV/AIDS prevention training manual also challenges peer educators to increase their HIV/AIDS knowledge, requiring a pretraining and posttraining HIV/AIDS knowledge test, as well as the creation of songs and theatrical skits that convey how to prevent HIV transmission. For example, in Sierra Leone, the 32 peer educators and 4 trainers of peer educators broke up into 4 groups. Each group created its own play, conveying critical HIV prevention information. A special focus was specifically on how to move community members across stages of change so they might abandon high-risk cultural practices and related beliefs—taking action to be safe from HIV transmission, whether via knives and cutting instruments used in secret society rituals or the reuse of injection syringe equipment. Songs and skits emphasized harm reduction techniques of boiling such equipment after an instrument/syringe was used on any one person and before use on another person—being directed toward those unwilling to abandon or not yet ready to abandon such cultural practices. One play was directed toward village chiefs and their role in health promotion and disease prevention (Konuwa, 2006). All four plays created by each of the four groups were performed at a graduation ceremony, as the manual recommends (Wallace, 2005a). The plays were also performed in several languages.

A Note on Multiple Languages Used in Training. In Sierra Leone, Africa the training was actually conducted in five languages, reflecting the diverse ethnic backgrounds of the peer educators (Konuwa, 2006). This was essential to ensure that concepts were fully understood by all. The director of the training, Ansumana Richard Konuwa, both spoke and understood these five languages, and created a training atmosphere that comfortably moved back and forth from one language to another, while largely conducted in the Creole used in Sierra Leone.

The Impact in Sierra Leone

According to Dr. Konuwa, an assessment of the training manual was offered by the Team Leader for the National HIV/AIDS Secretariat and the Health Sector Response Group (ARG) of the Ministry of Health and Sanitation of Sierra Leone in Freetown; the Team Leader described the manual "an irresistible resource for HIV/AIDS prevention." The Manager of the Health Education Division in Sierra Leone who was profoundly impressed by the richness of the prevention messages in the manual referred to it as "an indispensable vaccine for HIV prevention in African countries, especially where the accessibility and affordability of antiretroviral medication is in the distant future." He extended his heartfelt thanks to Dr. Wallace, the producer of the manual, for work "well done." The peer educators similarly praised the manual and their training experience, having heartfelt gratitude.

A Second Training in Ghana, Africa and Role of the NGO, StarSpirit International, Inc.

StarSpirit International, Inc., as an NGO also played a role in sponsoring the Sierra Leone training. In this manner, it was StarSpirit, working in collaboration with its academic partner, the Research Group on Disparities in Health of Teachers College, Columbia University, that can claim having piloted the HIV/AIDS Prevention Peer Education Training manual that is the cornerstone of our approach to HIV/AIDS prevention. It was in Sierra Leone across 4 weeks in the summer of 2005 that 32 Peer Educators and 4 Trainers completed the training. Next, StarSpirit Press formally published the manual upon which the model of training is based—*The HIV/AIDS Peer Education Training Manual: Combining African Healing Wisdom and Evidence-Based Behavior Change Strategies* (Wallace, 2005a). This manual effectively codifies the model and allows for effective dissemination.

Under the leadership of the Founder and Head of StarSpirit International, Inc. (Ayeboafo), another cohort of 32 HIV/AIDS Prevention Peer Educators were trained across 4 weeks of intensive training in Larteh, Ghana, holding formal graduation ceremonies on February 3, 2006. At the graduation ceremony, the peer educators performed selected songs and skits from among the original 13 songs, 2 raps songs, 8 poems, and 7 theatrical skits they created to prevent HIV transmission. The group of 32 peer educators included 4 who graduated with the distinction of Trainers of Peer Educators. This was just the first cycle of 4 weeks of intensive training for peer educators to be held at what was also officially inaugurated as the StarSpirit International, Inc. Lighthouse HIV/AIDS Peer Education Training Center—located on the main street in Larteh-Kubease, Ghana.

The Impact in Ghana and Another Note on Language

The manual was embraced by the peer educators in Larteh, Ghana, using it as their guide, while also utilizing the Community Forum Model (Wallace, 2006) of free-flowing dialogue in response to key concepts in the book. In this manner, the peer educators who could readily read English, as well as those who spoke two or three languages but may have lacked adequate comprehension of the English language, collectively delved deeply into the material; by dialoguing amongst themselves, they ensured all acquired adequate understanding of the key concepts.

Other elements of the Larteh training program were also unique. For example, the training program was kicked off with a brass band and local rally. During the rally, community members of all ages paraded throughout the streets of Larteh, singing, dancing, and displaying some of the 50 placards and HIV/AIDS prevention slogans created to increase community awareness. In addition, a major FM radio station aired live a full 20 minutes of the songs and skits the peer educators created and performed within their formal graduation ceremonies. Over the 2 days following their graduation ceremony, this 20-minute segment was repeated on the radio. In this manner, the prevention program spurred widespread community awareness, while also gaining the support of both public health officials and heads of state—many of whom also attended the graduation ceremonies. The program also enjoyed the support of local Chiefs, as well as traditional healers, Shaman.

Effectiveness

A full discussion of the results of evaluating the HIV/AIDS prevention model in Sierra Leone and Ghana will be presented elsewhere later in 2007. What is noteworthy is that in Sierra Leone, data analysis showed that participation in the HIV/AIDS prevention peer education training model produced a significant increase in HIV/AIDS knowledge from preintervention to postintervention 4 weeks later (Konuwa, 2006). In addition, participants' self-ratings showed that they experienced significant increases in their HIV/AIDS knowledge, ability to move their peers across stages of safety, and ability to educate others about how to avoid a return to unsafe behavior, while also offering high ratings of the overall program (Konuwa, 2006).

Future Directions

The goal is to take the training all across Ghana, and eventually across all of Africa. We plan to do the same thing in America, focusing on Black enclaves and at-risk African American women in particular. The further expansion of these efforts with African Americans in the United States is much needed, given CDC (2006) data (and see

El-Bassel, Witte, & Gilbert, chapter 15, this volume). StarSpirit is pursuing this mission in collaboration with the Research Group on Disparities in Health of Teachers College, Columbia University. Indeed, the first such training in the United States was held across the Fall of 2006 in Philadelphia, while a training was also conducted in Albany, New York—both using African American churches as the base for training peer educators of African descent. In this manner, the academic–NGO collaboration expanded to include a faith-based organization, adapting a manual ideally suited for training peer educators and community health workers in Africa for use with African Americans. The presence of adolescents in the Philadelphia Fall 2006 training is also leading to a new adolescent version of the manual, containing multiple quizzes and further simplified HIV/AIDS knowledge for those with low health literacy. Plans include using this version in Haiti with adolescent schoolgirls in 2007.

It is our intent to establish an International HIV/AIDS Prevention Peer Education Training and Certification Program with the following objectives:

(1) To train volunteers in selected areas in America and communities in countries in Africa and the Caribbean to become certified HIV/AIDS Prevention Peer Educators and Trainers of other cohorts of Peer Educations. Next, Trainers, as new community leaders, will go on to conduct other training sessions; hence, the model is sustainable by local communities in America and the indigenous people abroad who emerge empowered to determine the health of their own communities, using their local talent, creativity, skills, and multiple indigenous languages.

(2) To support local and indigenous people in creating their own songs, prevention messages, and skits, while they also create traveling theatre troupes of peer educators, including specialized troupes that target youth, women as mothers/wives/girlfriends/commercial sex workers, and indigenous traditional healers/Shamans/herbalists (so they emerge trained to work together with medical personnel)—ideally, gaining exposure via radio and television.

(3) To procure technology for indigenous people to use in disseminating those culturally and linguistically appropriate HIV/AIDS prevention messages they create, using DVDs/videos and computers, as well as multimodal interactive Web sites launched by indigenous groups or NGOs working in collaboration with them.

(4) To adapt the HIV/AIDS peer education training model currently codified in a manual (Wallace, 2005a) so it is an Internet-based interactive multimedia training tool of the kind Moretti and Witte described (chapter 16), including the potential to adapt the basic template so it is culturally and linguistically appropriate, and can be delivered in one of a multiplicity of languages with a simple click onto a link. Such a tool could still be used during live face-to-face interactive trainings; it can be negotiated much like a PowerPoint presentation during live face-to-face trainings; research studies are planned using Web sites in such a manner. This can also standardize the training. Such a Web site would have been an asset in the Sierra Leone and Ghana trainings where trainers moved from one language to another during a single training session. Meanwhile, via the creation of such an Internet-based interactive multimedia training tool for peer educators and community health workers located around the globe, the curriculum can still reach and find dissemination within those areas of the global community plagued by war, daily acts of terrorism, or where conditions are extremely dangerous or unstable; such

areas could still receive access to trainings, given the vision articulated by Moretti and Witte and endorsed here.

(5) To create a central data bank containing information on the certification status of HIV/AIDS prevention peer educators and community health workers, including their status in updating their HIV/AIDS knowledge annually or bi-annually—allowing potential employers to receive information as needed, and creating a national and global resource pool; this builds both human and social capital and documents it. Members of this pool may also emerge as points of contact for future community-based participatory research projects, as well as consultants on future projects or interventions, or when any new health crises or epidemic emerges. They may also be important sources of information regarding human rights violations, also serving as global leaders in their communities ensuring continual movement toward equity in health for all.

It is also possible to adapt the basic model integrating African Healing Wisdom and the three evidence-based behavior change theories and replace the HIV/AIDS knowledge component with any knowledge base, adapting the curriculum to the training of peer educators and community health workers who might work on literally any health issue. This could lead to an adaptation of the model that permits training peer educators and community health workers to address health issues such as asthma, malaria, tuberculosis, water purification, community sanitation and waste disposal, or any other existing or newly emergent health issue. Global leaders trained within a vision where they are empowered to act autonomously could forge such adaptations of the basic curriculum summarized in this chapter (e.g., Wallace, 2005a), while, ideally, they find willing partners and collaborators who may help with such adaptations and their evaluation.

The model can also be integrated with other models. For example, a next step for the academic–NGO collaboration involves integrating the HIV/AIDS prevention peer education training model with a new Healing Drum Workshop piloted in February 2007 (Wallace & Ayeboafo, 2007) to rave reviews. The Healing Drum Workshop is well-suited for healing those with trauma, such as AIDS orphans or those displaced from their homes and living in refugee camps. The plan is to start with AIDS orphans and to combine the HIV/AIDS prevention peer education training model and the Healing Drum Workshop, along with computerized assessments of the AIDS orphans that can track their need for any additional psychological or psychiatric interventions—depending on their level of trauma and response to the workshop and training experiences. This model will depend on the kind of technological advances described by Adams and Leath in chapter 17 (this volume) that allow for the electronic storage of client health records—as one team of doctors or providers arrives at a site in Africa and is replaced by another team, allowing communication across time via electronic health records.

It is anticipated that the concept of being a peer educator, global health leader, or community health worker is something that AIDS orphans in Africa will embrace, giving them a new identity and purpose. In being given the certification and new identity, they will also be given a life purpose. Hence, there is a design and purpose in exposing them to both the Healing Drum Workshop and the HIV/AIDS prevention peer education training. This composite experience and training will give AIDS orphans a powerful and compelling purpose for living and new design for their lives. That purpose is to demonstrate through their lives and work (1) how they have gained something enduring by having the experience of a buddy with whom they trained as a peer educator, enjoying connection with a valuable partner in the learning process; (2) how their empowerment as peer educators and global health leaders who seek to determine their own health and that of other peers in their community is a tremendous victory—one that allows others to see how they, too, may excel, rising triumphant from their past traumas; (3) how they represent a new world and new way of seeing the world—powerfully demonstrating how one can move on, and carry the life of their parents/the deceased forward, while continuously showing others how they, too, can be healed and remain safe from HIV/AIDS; and (4) through the theatrical skits, songs, and raps they create, they will be able to powerfully demonstrate to others how to be free of HIV/AIDS.

In sum, this demonstrates how the HIV/AIDS prevention peer education training model presented in this chapter may serve as a stand-alone intervention, be adapted to an online interactive multimedia training format, or be integrated with other models that readers may have in mind, as well as adapted to other or new or emergent health problems. The intent is for others to embrace the model and adapt it to suit the needs of their communities.

However, ultimately what is needed is an evaluation and dissemination plan, especially when the model is adapted as an online interactive multimedia training format. This includes the kind of technology transfer studies discussed by El-Bassel et al. (chapter 15, this volume) "that will advance the science of HIV prevention dissemination research."

Thus, diverse communities around the globe may benefit from the model, stimulating fundamental behavior change in communities with the promise that the models may become sustainable over time—especially when promoted by peers as "each one teaches one to be and stay safe," avoiding HIV/AIDS transmission. All the technology in the world, such as that in resource rich countries, may not solve the problems presented by the HIV/AIDS epidemic if new norms about behavior change are not sustained over time by being actively promoted by community members—as "each one teaches one," as caring peers with a collective sense of community/identity and African cultural values might do. Thus, the goal is to create sustainable models of HIV/AIDS prevention that foster patterns of behavior change that endure over time (Wallace, 2005a, p. 8) by disseminating this innovative model for training peer educators and community health workers.

REFERENCES

Airhihenbuwa, C. O. (2007). *Healing our differences: The crisis of global health and the politics of identity.* Lanham, MD: Rowman & Littlefield.

Association for Professionals in Infection Control and Epidemiology, Inc. (1996). Guidelines for infection control practice (APIC guideline for selection and use of disinfectants). *American Journal of Infection Control, 24*(4), 313–342.

Ayeboafo, N. K. (2005). *Tigare speaks: Lessons for living in harmony.* Philadelphia: StarSpirit Press.

Bambas, A., & Casas, J. A. (2003). Accessing equity in health: Conceptual criteria. In R. Hofrichter (Ed.), *Health and social justice: Politics, ideology, and inequity in the distribution of disease.* San Francisco: Jossey-Bass.

Centers for Disease Control and Prevention (CDC). (2006). Racial/ethnic disparities in diagnoses of HIV/AIDS—33 States, 2001–2004. *Morbidity and Mortality Weekly Report, 55*(5), 121–124.

DiClemente, C. C., & Velasquez, M. M. (2002). Motivational interviewing and the stages of change. In W. R. Miller & S. Rollnick (Eds.), *Motivational interviewing: Preparing people for change* (2nd ed.). New York: Guilford Press.

Elder, J. P. (2001). *Behavior change and public health in the developing world.* Thousand Oaks, CA: Sage Publications.

Gaston, M. H., & Porter, G. K. (2001). *Prime time: The African American woman's complete guide to midlife health and wellness.* New York: Ballantine.

Green, E. C. (2003). *Rethinking AIDS prevention: Learning from successes in developing countries.* Westport, CT: Praeger.

Hunter, C. D., & Lewis-Coles, M. E. (2004). Coping with racism: A spirit-based psychological perspective. In J. L. Chin (Ed.), *The psychology of prejudice and discrimination* (Vol. 1), *Racism in America.* Westport, CT: Praeger.

Kalichman, S. C. (2003). *The inside story on AIDS: Experts answer your questions.* Washington, DC: American Psychological Association.

Konuwa, A. R. (2006, May). *The development, implementation, and evaluation of a peer education training program for HIV/AIDS prevention in post-war Sierra Leone, West Africa.* Dissertation. Teachers College, Columbia University, New York.

Kunitz, S. J. (2007). *The health of populations: General theories and particular realities.* New York: Oxford University Press.

LaVeist, T. A. (2005). *Minority populations and health: An introduction to health disparities in the United States.* San Francisco: Jossey-Bass.

Marlatt, G. A. (2007, March 10). *The role of relapse prevention in closing the health disparities gap.* A keynote address at the Second Annual Health Disparities Conference at Teachers College, Columbia University, New York.

Marlatt, G. A., & Donovan, D. M. (Eds.). (2005). *Relapse prevention: Maintenance strategies in the treatment of addictive behaviors* (2nd ed.). New York: Guilford Press.

Marlatt, G. A., & Gordon, J. R. (Eds.). (1985). *Relapse prevention: Maintenance strategies in the treatment of addictive behaviors.* New York: Guilford.

Miller, W. R., & Rollnick, S. (Eds.). (1991). *Motivational interviewing: Preparing people to change addictive behaviors* (1st ed.). New York: Guilford.

Miller, W. R., & Rollnick, S. (Eds.). (2002). *Motivational interviewing: Preparing people for change* (2nd ed.). New York: Guilford.

Miller, W. R., Wilbourne, P. L., & Hettema, J. E. (2003). What works? A summary of alcohol treatment outcome research. In R. K. Hester & W. R. Miller (Eds.), *Handbook of alcoholism treatment approaches: Effective alternatives* (3rd ed.). Boston: Allyn & Bacon.

Peter, F., & Evans, T. (2001). Health equity in a globalizing world. In T. Evans, M. Whitehead, F. Diderichsen, A. Bhuiya, & M. Wirth (Eds.), *Challenging inequities in health: From ethics to action.* New York: Oxford University Press.

Prochaska, J. O., & DiClemente, C. C. (1983). Stages and processes of self-change of smoking: Toward an integrative model of change. *Journal of Consulting and Clinical Psychology, 51,* 390–395.

Prochaska, J. O., DiClemente, C. C., & Norcross, J. C. (1992). In search of how people change. *American Psychologist, 47,* 1102–1114.

Wallace, B. C. (1996). *Adult children of dysfunctional families: Prevention, intervention and treatment for community mental health promotion.* Westport, CT: Praeger.

Wallace, B. C. (2003). A multicultural approach to violence: Toward a psychology of oppression, liberation, and identity development. In B. C. Wallace & R. T. Carter (Eds.), *Understanding and dealing with violence: A multicultural approach* (pp. 3–39). Thousand Oaks, CA: Sage Publications.

Wallace, B. C. (2005a). *HIV/AIDS peer education training manual: Combining African healing wisdom and evidence-based behavior change strategies.* Philadelphia: StarSpirit Press.

Wallace, B. C. (2005b). *Making mandated addiction treatment work.* Lanham, MD: Jason Aronson/Rowman & Littlefield.

Wallace, B. C. (2006). Healing collective wounds from racism: The community forum model. In M. G. Constantine & D. W. Sue (Eds.), *Addressing racism: Facilitating cultural competence in mental health and educational settings.* New York: Wiley.

Wallace, B. C., & Ayeboafo, N. K. (2007, February 17). *Call and response, drumming, dance, and communal celebration as indigenous African modalities: Implications as non-traditional approaches to diversity in race and culture for psychologists and educators.* A workshop presented at the 24th Annual Teachers College Winter Roundtable on Cultural Psychology and Education, Teachers College, Columbia University, New York.

The Social Education and Health Advocacy Training (SEHAT) Project: Training Peer Educators in Indian Prisons to Increase Health Awareness and Preventive Behavior for HIV

20

Amrita Bahl

Introduction

HIV is threatening the most affected nations with social and economic collapse while it continues its relentless spread to new regions. In the past year, 3 million people died of AIDS, more than ever before and more than from any other infectious disease. Meanwhile, about 5 million more became infected with HIV. More than 40 million people now carry the virus worldwide, almost 30 million of them in sub-Saharan Africa. This number includes more than 2 million children (UNAIDS, 2006). Despite local successes of prevention and treatment programs, national and international responses to the epidemic remain inadequate, and have barely made an impact on the course of the epidemic. It is estimated that at the end of 2005, only one in seven Asians and one in ten Africans who need antiretroviral therapy were receiving it; access to services for preventing transmission from mother to child is equally poor; and the most vulnerable group—young people—do not have enough information on protecting themselves from infection. Moreover, the distribution of treatment and prevention services remains profoundly inequitable (Wilson & Stabinski, 2004).

HIV/AIDS disproportionately affects those groups that are already vulnerable: children, women, and millions of people who do not have access to care and experience denial of basic human rights. There are four main population groups affected by this disease: homosexual men, heterosexual couples, intravenous drug users, and perinatal infection to children. In recent years, unequal rights of women, especially in developing countries, have made them increasingly vulnerable to HIV infection since most women do not have negotiation skills (rather, rights) for condom use in a sexual encounter.

Stigma and discrimination against people living with HIV or AIDS are pervasive; numerous studies have documented negative attitudes as well as active discrimination, ranging from social ostracism to employment discrimination to violence, in the developed as well as the developing world. Fear of infection (International Center for Research on Women, 2003; Monica, Tanga, & Nuwagaba, 2001) through casual contact and association with already stigmatized social groups or with behaviors considered immoral are potential sources of stigma. In particular, where the disease is strongly associated with prostitutes, intravenous drug users, or men who have sex with men, people with AIDS can inherit the strong burden of stigma often borne by these populations. It's a vicious cycle where association with AIDS can then in turn reinforce the despised status of these groups. Cultures where sexual behavior is weighed heavily with morality, HIV transmission through promiscuity or extramarital sex results in stigma, fueling the notion that people with AIDS "deserve" their fate, or that the disease is a punishment for sinful behavior. Sexual double standards common in many cultures mean that women suffer disproportionately from these assumptions, and are often blamed for the deaths of their partners from AIDS. Finally, AIDS, as an incurable, fatal disease, is a source of stigma that is exacerbated by the misconception that HIV infection inevitably progresses rapidly to AIDS and death. HIV/AIDS is not of course the first or only disease to be strongly stigmatized: people suffering from leprosy, tuberculosis (TB), and mental illness, among other conditions, have long been feared, shunned, and denied equal treatment. However, the taboos and gender inequalities surrounding sex add powerful new stigmatizing forces in the case of sexually transmitted diseases such as HIV/AIDS especially in developing countries.

Although the African continent has been hardest hit by the AIDS pandemic, countries of the former Soviet Union, China, and India, together home to a large share of the world's population, are currently the focus of increasing concern (U.S. Central Intelligence Agency, 2002). India is the land of one of the oldest civilizations in the world, a country where diversity is a norm, where people from the four corners of the country differ in language, food, culture and appearance—yet these people have a common thread binding them other than their citizenship . . . their vulnerability to HIV. It is estimated that by the year 2010, India along with Ethiopia, Nigeria, China, and Russia, with 40% of the world's population, will add 50 to 75 million infected people to the worldwide pool of HIV disease (Until There's A Cure, 2007).

India has had a sharp increase in the estimated number of HIV infections, from a few thousand in the early 1990s to a working estimate of between 3.8 and 4.6 million children and adults living with HIV/AIDS in 2002. In July 2007, this figure was officially revised to an estimated 2.5 million people living with the virus and HIV prevalence among adults to be around 0.36%. This revision was due to a new population-based survey, expanded sentinel surveillance and revised methodologies. Despite these revisions, with a population of over one billion, the HIV epidemic in India will have a major impact on the overall spread of HIV in Asia and the Pacific and indeed worldwide. One of the primary routes of transmission of the virus is through heterosexual contact in risky sexual behavior. As in Africa, one of the most affected populations is the commercial sex worker. In fact, the first case of HIV was diagnosed in a commercial sex worker; this has been a major reason for the stigma associated with disease. As 70% of the Indian population resides in rural areas, there is a significantly large migrant population that travels to its major cities. This flow of migrant workers as well as the long-distance truck driver population and their interaction with sex workers in roadside brothels along the highways is contributing to the increasing incidence of HIV in India. A second route of transmission is the use of illicit drugs especially in the North Eastern region of India.

Various programs are currently underway in India to educate commercial sex workers, truck drivers, and drug users about HIV prevention and the adoption of safer behavior in order to reduce the transmission of the infection to other segments of the population. However, little has been done to educate the incarcerated population in India. Of the three population groups mentioned, two engage in behavior that is prohibited in the country and is punishable by law. Truck drivers, too, are arrested for traffic and transport violations. Prisoners, therefore, are at higher risk for infection with HIV because of injection drug use, tattooing, consensual sex, and incidents of prisoner rape. Women prisoners who have engaged in prostitution and are also injection drug users may have come in contact with HIV-infected sex partners and therefore, are at additional risk for HIV infection. In fact, a study conducted in a Berlin prison by Stark et al. (1995) found that syringe sharing in prison was the most important independent determinant of HIV infection among injection drug users. Beyrer et al. (2003) found that incarceration was a known risk for HIV infection in Thai drug users. Their research indicated that through the 1990s, incarceration rates for drug-related offenses rose sharply, whereas HIV prevention and drug treatment in prisons remained limited. This being the case, the prison then, is a potential breeding ground where the transmission of infection can be prevented as the prisoners are easily available and they have fewer demands being made on their time. A literature search on PubMed and ProQuest for the keywords "HIV prevention education" generated more than a thousand studies. Refining the search to include "prisons" in the search criteria resulted only in a handful with most studies conducted in the United States.

The growth in the number of HIV infection cases and the resurgence of TB, including multiple drug resistant TB, are generating increased interest and concern among correctional and public health professionals. Both the diseases are found to a higher degree among the jail population than among the general population and more difficult to treat and manage in a jail setting because of crowded conditions and issues of confidentiality. Prior to incarceration, the lifestyle of many inmates includes activities such as risky sexual behavior, drug and alcohol abuse, poverty, homelessness, undereducation, and unemployment, all of which increase their risk of contracting HIV (Margolis et al., 2004). Nevertheless, research with ex-offenders supports the contention that high-risk behavior occurs inside prisons as well (Wohl, Johnson, & Jordan, 2000). A pilot study conducted by Singh, Prasad, and Mohanty (1999) in India indicated that sexually transmitted and blood-borne infections are highly prevalent in jail premises and pose a threat of rapid spread of these infections through intravenous drug use and homosexuality. Thus, a comprehensive program should address the increase in knowledge and awareness about HIV/AIDS in the context of postrelease high-risk behavior as well. In prisons, some inmates may be reevaluating the choices they made in their lives and may be open to receiving information that can help make appropriate health decisions. Access to medical and mental health services for little or no cost while in prison can also encourage and reinforce these positive changes.

Bearing these factors in mind, the author developed the Social Education and Health Advocacy Training (SEHAT) project, a peer-led client-centered participatory program that aims at increasing health awareness and preventive behaviors among the prisoners, with an emphasis on HIV prevention, during her Master's coursework. In Hindi, one of the official languages of India, the term "sehat" means health, which is why it was used to coin the name of this project. This chapter will discuss the value of peer-led prison-based interventions; the theoretical rationale for the SEHAT intervention; the process of designing SEHAT and developing strategic partnerships; the planning, funding, implementation, and time-lines for the SEHAT program; the accomplishments and evolution of SEHAT to date; and, finally, SEHAT's future directions and needs.

The Value of Peer-Led Prison-Based Interventions

Several research studies indicate that peer-led interventions are well received by their target population. For example, Grinstead, Zack, and Faigeles (2001) conducted an 8-week prerelease intervention in a California prison aimed at developing risk reduction strategies for HIV seropositive inmates. The researchers developed a peer-led intervention to prevent HIV among male prison inmates and their female partners. The results indicated that compared with men who signed up for the intervention but were unable to attend, men who received the intervention reported more use of community resources and less sexual- and drug-related risk behaviors in the months following release. Their findings also indicated that peer educators were an important resource as inmates preferred them and responded to them with increased attendance and attention.

In Russia, the results of a peer-led training program among drug dependent Siberian prisoners indicated that undergoing peer training proved beneficial for the participants. It led to an increased knowledge about HIV transmission, access to condoms, needle sterilization, as well as a decrease in the prevalence of tattooing while in prison (Dolan, Bijl, & White, 2004).

The Theoretical Rationale for the SEHAT Intervention

The SEHAT intervention drew upon various theories of health behavior change such as the Health Belief model, Transtheoretical Model (Stages of Change), Social Learning Theory, social support, as well as elements of relapse prevention in its skills training sessions. The objective of the SEHAT program is to initiate behavior change and empower prisoners to engage in positive health behaviors during incarceration and postrelease. To this end, the program required the involvement and participation of all the stakeholders, namely the staff, inmates, and the families of inmates during the different phases. In order to help prevent relapse, it was important to set up a postrelease network that will enable the released inmates to maintain the positive health behaviors.

Designing SEHAT and Developing Strategic Partnerships

Since there were no concrete data pertaining to the actual target population in New Delhi, international data was used as a guide for this program. Thus the initial project proposal included 12 modules for training the peer educators. Having written the proposal, the next step was to research opportunities to implement this project. A meeting with Dr. Kiran Bedi, the first and the highest ranking woman police officer in India, who was on deputation at the United Nations in the Department of Peacekeeping at the time, proved very inspirational and encouraging. Equally enthusiastic about the concept of peer education, she told the author that SEHAT would prove to be a pioneering addition to correctional reforms in India.

A vanguard of human rights, Dr. Kiran Bedi's name is synonymous with police and prison reforms that have won her international recognition. Known for her candor, she received a "punishment posting" to Tihar Prison as Inspector-General. Instead of being disheartened, she saw an opportunity to change the system and initiated several reforms and innovations. She arranged for every prisoner to attend school and had the prison schools declared government schools, staffed with regular teachers, and even provided vocational training recognized with certificates of completion. Additionally, she developed a "Panchayat" (council) system where prisoners who were respected for their age, education, or character represented other inmates and met every evening with senior officers to sort out problems—a major democratization that brought into play openness, transparency, accountability, and accessibility. She encouraged extracurricular activities for prisoners such as sports, yoga, prayer, Vipassana meditation, and the celebration of religious festivals. And most importantly, she declared the prison a no–smoking zone, a policy in effect even today. For her humane prison reforms, Dr. Kiran Bedi received the Ramon Magsaysay Award also known as the Asian Nobel Prize.

Planning, Funding, Implementation, and the SEHAT Time Line

The initial estimation of the time line for the entire SEHAT project was 1 year from the day the needs assessment was started to the day of the final data collection, an ambitious goal that at the time seemed achievable. A small grant from an Indian philanthropist helped initiate the needs assessment phase. The next step involved a partnership with the India Vision Foundation, a nonprofit started in 1994 by Dr. Kiran Bedi, after she received the Magsaysay Award. Over the years, the Foundation has worked with prisoners in Tihar teaching skills such as horticulture, bread making, embroidery, weaving, and so on, to starting a day care facility for children within the prison walls to mainstreaming these children into regular residential schools outside the prison walls. Seeking permission to work on sensitive subjects such as prisons and HIV can be a long drawn-out process in India, a process further complicated by bureaucratic red-tapism. Thankfully, the Foundation's goodwill came to the rescue, which helped speed up the procedure. While awaiting permission, a meeting with the United Nations Office on Drugs and Crime (UNODC) led to submitting a proposal for additional funds. It also led to the inclusion of another project site, Amritsar Central Prison, into the proposal. The logic for inclusion was that Amritsar, a border city in the state of Punjab, featured within the Golden Crescent of drug trafficking, could present us with comparisons and different challenges. So it was back to the drawing board, factoring in the cultural sensitivities of the particular region of the country as well.

Most prisons in India suffer from overcrowding (about 40% overcrowding exists countrywide). The Tihar Prison Complex in New Delhi, India is the largest maximum-security facility in South Asia and was initially built to house nearly 5,000 people. Today the actual population is over 13,000 inmates who endure in excess of 300% of the available capacity. Males consist of the majority of prisoners by far (96.2%) versus female inmates (3.8%). There are few, if any, public health prevention efforts toward the high-risk residents. In particular, sexually transmitted infections (STIs) and other communicable diseases, which tend to flourish in overcrowded situations, are largely left to chance. Some of the explanations for this include high prisoner turnover, where the prisoner is infected and then is released into the community and continues to spread disease. In addition to the aforementioned crowding issues, intravenous drug use and sharing nonhygienic needles also contribute to the STIs and other communicable disease spread.

Three Key Challenges: Stigma, Facilities, and Gender Modification

There were three major challenges that we needed to be sensitive to. The first was the stigma associated with HIV and some of the modes of transmission associated with the disease, for example, men who have sex with other men and intravenous drug users. Due to punitive actions associated with disclosure of these behaviors, there were very few statistics available. Next, there were no facilities for educating prisoners about the need for safer sex practices in the era of the HIV pandemic. Currently, there is no voluntary testing and counseling facilities for HIV at the two project sites, and drug use is common in the prison despite efforts to curtail it. Finally, the women in prisons would require a modified version of SEHAT. According to the Prison Statistics Report 2000, women inmates constitute 3.42% of the total inmate population in the country (and 3.8% in Tihar). In India social customs make women ex-offenders more vulnerable to suspicion and rejection versus their male counterparts. The stigma of having been in prison has more aftereffects that are adverse for women than for men.

The Needs Assessment

Nearly a month later, permission to conduct a needs assessment was received with access to only a select few jails within the prison complex. Although Tihar Prison is a fairly transparent system, any proposal for a research project had to be approved by the highest echelons in the system. Despite the suggestion of numerous scientists that correctional facilities offer an ideal opportunity for implementing HIV prevention interventions, as incarcerated individuals are logistically easier to reach with prevention and education programs, these have been slow to develop over the past two decades.

Braithwaite and Arriola (2003) found that the relatively slow development and implementation of HIV prevention programs in prison settings has occurred for several reasons. According to them, there is a duality and cultural divide between public health and corrections where correctional institutions focus on promoting the custody and security of inmates with some correctional officials being apathetic toward inmates' health and well-being. Additionally, the stigma associated with discussing HIV/AIDS, particularly in correctional settings where many HIV risk behaviors (e.g., injection drug use, unprotected anal intercourse) are not allowed, results in hesitation on the part of prison officers to accept HIV prevention messages. On their part, inmates fear that by expressing an open interest in learning about HIV prevention strategies or requesting testing, they may be perceived as admitting to engaging in homosexual or drug use behavior, which may have negative consequences for them. Moreover, difficulties in maintaining confidentiality can fuel an inmate's fear of being tested because of the stigma associated with having a positive test result, which might prompt him/her to choose to learn of his/her HIV serostatus only after release. Further, a lack of resources and interference with security procedures (e.g., lockdowns and the need for staff escorts) may be thwarting the implementation of these programs, even though many prison officials recognize the need for such programs. Despite these barriers, some prison officials recognize the value of delivering HIV education programs and have welcomed these services into their facilities. What is important is to develop programs that consider the logistical constraints of correctional settings.

To get a cross section of views and to evaluate specific issues that should be addressed within the context of the program, interviews were conducted with inmates as well as prison staff ranging from the Superintendent of the jail to the warders who came in daily contact with the inmates. The initial time line had a month slotted for the needs assessment, when actually it took nearly 3 months to complete all the interviews. The interviews took a long time, as rapport building was an important step in order to be able to discuss sexual behavior.

Results of the Needs Assessment: Revisions in the Curriculum

From the interviews, it emerged that the training modules needed to go beyond the initial topics decided upon; there was a need to incorporate more topics such as TB, scabies, and additional life skills components. The women inmates also expressed a desire to know more about reproductive health and child care issues. In order to truly succeed in their role as peer leaders, it was crucial for them to have basic knowledge about issues such as basic first aid, health, hygiene, nutrition, and so forth; and it was important to ensure that they were aware of cultural issues that they may encounter in their roles in the community.

Prison-based needle exchange programs, which have been found to be effective in Switzerland, Germany, and Spain (Dolan, Rutter, & Wodak, 2003), do not exist in India. Thus, harm reduction for intravenous drug users was also an important topic as

Table 20.1	The SEHAT Training Program Outline		
	Module 1: Introduction to peer health, education & human rights	**Module 2:** Principles of adult learning	**Module 3:** Cultural awareness & counseling skills
	Module 4: Health, hygiene and nutrition & basic first aid	**Module 5:** Introduction to immune system	**Module 6:** Common skin diseases
	Module 7: HIV/AIDS	**Module 8:** Sexually transmitted diseases	**Module 9:** Hepatitis
	Module 10: Tuberculosis	**Module 11:** Substance abuse & harm reduction	**Module 12:** Stress, coping & anger management
	Module 13: Communication & assertiveness skills	**Module 14:** Decision-making/negotiation skills	**Module 15:** Creative thinking/problem solving
	Module 16: Crisis intervention	**Module 17:** Presentation skills	Practice sessions, closure & graduation

research indicates that although most inmates who shared needle and syringes cleaned them, this was almost always only with water, which is likely to be inadequate to prevent HIV transmission (Millstein, 1993). Thus, to make the SEHAT program more comprehensive, 20 topics were decided on, which were grouped into 17 modules, as shown in Table 20.1.

Other Implementation Issues

Leadership changes at the Amritsar Central Prison prevented us from starting work there immediately, as the next Superintendent had to take charge, which meant starting rapport building all over again. Even then, chance interviews with a few inmates presented an opportunity to conduct an informal needs assessment in Amritsar. With the project now ready to operate at two sites, the task of hiring and training new team members also gained urgency.

In the interim period between the needs assessment and the module creation, funding from the UNODC for a pilot initiative at two sites was approved and released. Hence, we were ready to begin the process of implementation.

Inclusion Criteria for the 15 Peer Educators

It was decided that the pilot would be conducted with 15 peer educators at each site. There would be an additional 225 beneficiaries to be targeted by the peer leaders.

As with any proposal, there was a set of inclusion criteria namely, male and female inmates, between the ages of 18–50 years, former drug users and non–drug users convicted for long sentences, as well as those under trial for crimes such as murder, drug-trafficking, and the like. In addition, we required a minimum educational level of grade 8.

Prison Staff Sensitivity Training to Enhance Implementation

For any program to be successful, it was important that all stakeholders become actively involved. Logically, sensitivity training sessions with the prison staff were also factored in the program to encourage ownership and acceptance of the objectives.

Launching SEHAT as a Culturally Tailored Program

Finally, the program was launched at both the sites with a one-day site-specific training session for more than 200 inmates and prison staff where the inmates presented key messages about health, HIV prevention, and substance abuse through the medium of short skits/plays; poems written on the theme; speeches by inmates; folk songs and folk dances such as bolis/tappas and gidda dance (a form of folk dance) by the female inmates and bhangra dance (a form of folk dance) by the male inmates on the theme; kavishree (a form of folk music); shabad kirtan (religious hymns); religious discourses interpreting the teachings of Guru Granth Sahib which promote fidelity, monogamy, and no addictions of any kind; exhibition of their paintings on the themes; and participatory games based on the concept of "Who Wants To Be A Millionaire?"

Flexibility in Inclusion Criteria: A Role for Those With Low Literacy

When the time came for volunteers to sign up for the SEHAT pilot, the response was overwhelming. There were more volunteers than needed, including people who did not know how to read or write, some of who were influential in their respective barracks and could help disseminate information to other inmates who would ordinarily not listen to any outsider. And there were at least 8 of them at each site. A decision had to be made whether to include people with zero literacy levels in the program. Faced with a dilemma, a refusal would prove to be a damper on their spirit and desire to change their lives; it was decided to make them active participants while pairing them with more literate participants.

The Accomplishments and Evolution of SEHAT to Date

Since its inception there have been several achievements, albeit small steps that have helped strengthen the credibility of the project with the skeptics among the prison staff and the inmates. As the project had shifted into high gear with the receipt of funds, phases started overlapping. Consequently, module development and peer training happened on a real-time basis, which allowed field testing each module as it was developed and an opportunity to go back to the drawing board for revisions based on feedback provided by the participants. A modern version of Bloom's taxonomy, taken from Dr. Madhabi Chatterji's functional taxonomy (Chatterji, 2003) served as a guideline for the SEHAT benchmarks. Each module was developed keeping in mind the literacy levels of the inmates, while following the principles of adult learning. Thus, the modules included various participatory activities using role-plays, games, theater, and puppetry. Additionally, visual material such as charts and models was being developed to teach the more technical modules.

Hence, when the human immune system module was originally tested, it was found to contain technical terms. This module was revised to lower the jargon even further and to develop more activities and use visuals to explain the concepts. Yet another feedback was the ability of the modules to ease the flow of discussion for sensitive topics such as sexual orientation. In one incident, when the counselor was teaching a session on general health, one of the participants raised a question about sexual orientation. Since the group included a member who preferred people of the same sex, it was awkward for all the participants to open up and discuss initially. However, as the module progressed, this participant started talking about his/her own sexual orientation, and following this disclosure such discussions have not been an issue. In fact, we observed that there was an increase in team spirit, trust, and general bonding after this incident.

Moving from initially conducting a training session in any available space in the jail, the project has graduated to a dedicated "SEHAT room" at each site. The core group of peer leaders feels a great sense of ownership in decorating these rooms and keeping them clean, with a consensual agreement to rotate their duties underlying this pride. In the male ward in Tihar Central Prison a barrack has been allotted where our peer leaders live together to help and support each other and strengthen each other's resolve to be change agents. Some of the SEHAT peer educators have been released and prior to release they expressed a need to finish the course outside. Others have been delaying their bail, as they want to complete the course and get their certificate before they are released. The Amritsar Prison authorities have even provided an office space in the administrative section where continuation classes can be conducted and the postrelease network initiated.

One of the key successes is the development of a sense of identification of themselves first as SEHAT team members and then an inmate of the jail; this has been observed more strongly in the male ward in Amritsar Central Prison. Recently, the Deputy Inspector-General was on a routine inspection of the jail when the SEHAT male peer educators met with him. To the officer's query on grievances, they answered, "Sir, we are now reformed. Please ask the security man at the gate not to search us. We, the members of India Vision Foundation, associated with the SEHAT project want to start to reform the society from the jail itself."

The fact that SEHAT is actually succeeding in initiating change in attitudes and behavior can also be gauged from the following incident. Recently, one of the peer educators was hospitalized and when he saw the terrible conditions of the sick inmates and the corruption of the doctor present, he shared his observations with the Deputy Inspector-General, who, in turn, initiated an investigation and subsequently had the doctor removed from the hospital. The team has also started using the counseling skills they have learned amongst themselves and use these skills to avoid getting into fights and arguments. As they have started to lead by example, the adolescent team members have reported that their peers view them with more respect, which has helped increase their confidence and faith. In yet another incident, one of the SEHAT peer educators saved the life of an inmate using the CPR he was taught in the basic first aid module. Not only this, these peer leaders have also volunteered to get themselves tested for HIV first and then to motivate as many people as they can to volunteer for testing.

Today, the SEHAT project has a diverse team of peer educators, some of whom have not only started to learn to read and write, but also to actively voice their concerns to the authorities and to stand up for themselves and their team. One incident happened early in the project on the day after the session on Introduction to Peer Health Education Module. Payal, one of the peer leaders, who did not know how to read or write, sat the counselor down and asked if she knew what peer health education was. Needless to say, the counselor assumed that Payal wanted an explanation of the concept again, which she volunteered to do. Immediately, Payal said she knew and wanted to explain the concept to the counselor and went on to recite the definition of peer health education in simple terms. This episode was so encouraging because here was a person who did not know how to read and write and said she found it difficult to remember things, making an effort to learn the fundamental concept that forms the core of the project, thereby reinforcing the belief that nothing is impossible. This episode really strengthened the SEHAT team's resolve to involve more motivated people in the project no matter what their qualifications, as long as it promised to make a difference in their lives.

The past year has seen the prison staff observing a change in the inmates who are a part of the SEHAT team. They have realized the need for increased interaction and bringing about a change in their attitude toward the inmates who in turn have realized that the authorities are not the enemy. The wall created by the "us" and "them" attitude is slowly breaking down, with the most recent attempt being a joint presentation of a short drama where some of the actors were the Superintendent, the Deputy Superintendents, the Assistant Superintendents, and the Wardens enacting their roles themselves. This partnership between the prison authorities, the inmates, and the civil society is the first step toward a change in attitude, a change that will help fight the battle and defeat the growing AIDS epidemic in the country.

Prison–Based Condom Demonstrations and Voluntary Testing for HIV: Significant Milestones

The trust the authorities have in SEHAT is demonstrated by their willingness to permit a condom demonstration within the prison. India Vision Foundation was the first non-governmental organization (NGO) partner to successfully conduct a condom demonstration in both the male and female jails in Tihar Prison, perhaps the first NGO in the country to do so. The project has achieved another first. For the first time in the history of Indian Prisons, a voluntary HIV testing camp was conducted where more than 70 people, well above the expected number of initial volunteers, got themselves tested for serostatus.

These are huge achievements for the project and the NGO community as a whole, as any attempts to curb the AIDS epidemic involve adopting safer sex practices—the cornerstone for which is the use of condoms by sexual partners.

Among homosexual/heterosexual/bisexual prisoners there are reports of "survival sex" (i.e., trading sex for money, drugs, goods, or protection). In their study, Dolan, Bijl, and White (2004) found a small proportion of respondents reported engaging in sexual activity in prison, with some respondents trading sex for money or protection. Of those who reported sex in prison, less than a third reported using condoms. Despite the episodes of homosexual sex in prisons, the distribution of condoms to prisoners remains uncommon across the world. A primary obstacle to this is cultural attitudes toward homosexual behavior on the part of the prison authorities and officers. Studies have shown that condom provision (Dolan, Shearer, & Lowe, 2004) to inmates can be a simple and effective harm reduction strategy that can be implemented without harming either officers or other inmates. In India, sections of the Indian Penal Code also prove to be an impediment as they deem homosexuality as illegal and punishable by law. So a simple demonstration could be viewed as condoning sexual episodes punishable by law, a risk few officers are willing to take.

For all the sessions based on health topics, the Senior Medical Officer had been requested to be present to address any queries that the inmates had. Needless to say, her presence and initiation of the session for the condom demonstration proved to be an excellent ice-breaking exercise that helped pave the way for a truly interactive session where several questions were asked ranging from clarifications on use to the technicality of the product. The demonstration was conducted with an extended group of Indian as well as foreign inmates, which was a blessing as this section of inmates had been hitherto hard to reach as they had refused to be part of the project on numerous occasions. Consequently, these ladies signed up to be a part of the peer group of one of the peer leaders.

Dissemination of and Support for the Model

In August 2006, the SEHAT project was presented in a satellite meeting of the 16th International AIDS Conference held in Toronto, Canada. As more and more people are getting to know about the SEHAT project, they have started volunteering help. The President of the National Truckers Association and the owner of a trucking company committed his support to the project by agreeing to hire five peer educators on their release. Additionally, a local businessman in New Delhi volunteered to set up a gymnasium, the permission for which was denied due to security reasons. Not to be deterred, he and his staff have now volunteered time twice a week to conduct aerobic and cardio exercises, which started in the last week of October 2006.

The Need for Community-Based Supports Postincarceration

As a next logical step, the SEHAT team is working toward forming support groups for released inmates where they will meet twice a month and share their experiences and support other former inmates in rehabilitation. Margolis et al. (2004) found that even though substance abuse and sex occur during confinement, these rates do not appear sufficient to account for the high HIV/STD rates among inmates. Their findings suggest that HIV and STDs may often result from risk behaviors that occur in the community. So, while prevention efforts should address risks during incarceration, greater attention should be paid to develop inmates' ability, especially those at risk for HIV/AIDS, to adopt safer practices following release in order to break the vicious cycle of infection.

As one of the initiatives, the team has created a pocket directory listing the services available in New Delhi as well as Amritsar for services such as NA/AA meetings, HIV testing centers, TB clinics, and emergency services. These directories will be given to inmates prior to release. Additionally, theme based participatory games such snakes and ladders, flash cards for the HIV transmission game where the artwork has been done by the inmates have also been developed. Forging new partnerships with Rotary Clubs, as well as individual donors/partners who can help us in strengthening the postrelease network, is an on-going process. It is imperative to hand hold newly released inmates and try to prevent their return to a life of crime. As it happens, more often than not, when a female inmate arrested for immoral trafficking is released from the prison, it is her pimp who receives her at the gate and forces her back into the trade. By providing services at the postrelease level, a relapse may be averted. This also involves exploring avenues to provide employment to the released peer leaders in fields that match their skills so as to enable rehabilitation. In Amritsar, the details of hiring a released female peer educator as a member of the team are being charted out.

Meeting Challenges That Arise

This intervention has been a truly fulfilling experience for the SEHAT team as well. With each passing day, the team is evolving and learning something new every day from the peer educator team within the prison. Learning to be more patient with the obstacles that have presented—and there have been several—was the most valuable skill. The project has had to restart the peer leader batches on more than one occasion due to attrition or transfers, or people not taking too well to the task of discussing sexual behavior. It is so ironical that, in the land of Kamasutra, sex is a taboo topic for discussion even if it helps prevent an incurable illness. All this slows the team down, but then they bounce back, believing that at least some of them will spread the knowledge acquired during their time with the project. When one of the leaders says, "While we are attending the SEHAT sessions, we feel that we are not in the prison during those two hours"; when a young visitor writes to say "... the SEHAT program is by far the strongest in providing functional roles to inmates. I would like to see the program grow with more topics"; and when more and more inmates volunteer to be a part of the project, the team realizes a sense of accomplishment that nourishes the drive to perform harder.

What has worked for SEHAT has been the partnership with prison authorities. Rather than be critical and "anti" the system, the team has appreciated whatever the staff has been able to do in their resource-limited settings. If they said "no," to a request, reasoning and cajoling were the tools used with them to grant permission. If they did not prevail, the team just waited and bided time for the next opportune moment. The SEHAT team, on their part, has helped in trying to bridge the gap between the inmates and the authorities thereby gaining the trust of both parties.

Believing in India Vision Foundation's mission statement "to save the next victim," and not viewing them as criminals or the guilty party, inmates are given an opportunity to change their lives. Although there was an underlying respect for the team members, rapport building was a critical skill that the team invested in, as efforts that have led the peer leaders to confide very personal details, including accurate contact details for postrelease contact, something they would not ordinarily do in order to avoid the stigma of incarceration. The enormous support and freedom to innovate provided by the UN-ODC's Project RAS H71 team have allowed SEHAT team members to approach them for advice and has led to productive brainstorm sessions that have helped the intervention to evolve. And above all, the goodwill that Dr. Bedi and the Foundation enjoy in the field of reformative work in prisons paved the way for entry into an otherwise restricted zone.

Innovating and thinking on our feet has become an inherent part of the training techniques. Change has been the only constant in the lives of the SEHAT team. We have succeeded in meeting challenges to date.

Future Directions and Needs*

As the project moves forward, consolidation and documentation are taking place in order to ensure continuity. However, like any other project, there is a wish list of things that the team would like to accomplish in order to make the program more comprehensive and wholesome. To start with, setting up voluntary counseling and testing (VCT) facilities to service the clients who have volunteered and encouraging several more to come forward are pressing needs. With additional inputs to the curricula, if the SEHAT curricula can be approved and certified by a university, this can help provide employment for an emergent work force that can become either counselors in these VCT centers or community health workers in their respective communities—providing support at the grassroots level to the beleaguered public health system in the country. Establishment of a visitors' center on the lines of the House on the Hill in San Quentin, California, where family members of the incarcerated can be targeted with similar prevention messages and their help enlisted in making some changes in the environment that may help prevent relapse, is a new objective.

As the graduation ceremonies for the first batch of peer leaders approach, the project is going to go through the first litmus test. The Superintendent of the female jail at Tihar has scheduled an intensive training session for some of her staff members. She wants the SEHAT peer leaders to take some sessions. Of course, as usual the team has accepted the challenge head-on and the peer leaders are excited and apprehensive and feel honored that the Superintendent has faith in their abilities; this has invigorated them with that

---

* The author invites readers to contact her (amritabahl@gmail.com) for receipt of resource materials upon request (e.g., photographs, DVDs, posters, etc.).

extra dose of confidence. They have renewed their faith in the strength of the human spirit to endure and spring back; turning adversity to their advantage, believing it's always possible!

REFERENCES

Beyrer, C., Jittiwutikarn, J., Waranya, T., Razak, M. T., Suriyanon, V., Srirak, N., et al. (2003). Drug use, increasing incarceration rates, and prison-associated HIV risks in Thailand. *AIDS and Behavior*, *7*(2), 153–161.

Braithwaite, R. L., & Arriola, K. R. J. (2003). Male prisoners and HIV prevention: A call for action ignored. *American Journal of Public Health*, *93*(5), 759–763.

Chatterji, M. (2003). *Designing and using tools for educational assessment*. Boston: Allyn & Bacon.

Dolan, K., Rutter, S., & Wodak, A. (2003). Prison based syringe exchange programs: A review of the international research and development. *Addiction*, *98*, 153–158.

Dolan, K., Shearer, J., & Lowe, D. (2004). Evaluation of the condom distribution program in NSW prisons, Australia. *Journal of Law and Medical Ethics*, *31*(1), 124–128.

Dolan, K. A., Bijl, M., & White, B. (2004). HIV education in a Siberian prison colony for drug dependent males. *International Journal of Equity in Health*, *3*(7).

Grinstead, O., Zack, B., & Faigeles, B. (2001). Reducing post-release risk behavior among HIV seropositive prison inmates: The health promotion program. *AIDS Education and Prevention*, *13*(2), 109–119.

International Center for Research on Women. (2003). *Understanding HIV-related stigma and resulting discrimination in Sub-Saharan Africa: Emerging themes from early data collection in Ethiopia, Tanzania and Zambia*. Retrieved October 30, 2004, from http://www.icrw.org/projects/hivrelatedstigma/hivrelatedstigma.htm

Margolis, A. D., Wolitski, R. J., Seal, D. W., Belcher, L., Morrow, K., Sosman, J., et al. (2004). *Sexual behavior and substance use during incarceration*. Poster presented at the XV International AIDS Conference 2004, Bangkok, Thailand.

Millstein, R. (1993). *Community alert bulletin*. Rockville, MD: U.S. Department of Health and Human Services, Public Health Service, Alcohol, Drug Abuse, and Mental Health Administration.

Monica, S. M., Tanga, E. O., & Nuwagaba, A. (2001). *Uganda: HIV and AIDS-related discrimination, stigmatization and denial*. UNAIDS best practice collection. Retrieved October 30, 2004, from http://www.unaids.org/publications/documents/ human/law/HR_Uganda.pdf

Singh, S., Prasad, R., & Mohanty, A. (1999). High prevalence of sexually transmitted and blood-borne infections amongst the inmates of a district jail in Northern India. *International Journal of STD & AIDS*, *10*, 475–478.

Stark, K., Eller, R. M., Wirth, D., Bienzle, U., Pauli, G., & Guggenmoos-Holzmann, I. (1995). Determinants of HIV infection and recent risk behaviour among injecting drug users in Berlin by site of recruitment. *Addiction*, *90*(10), 1367–1376.

UNAIDS. (2006). *UNAIDS/WHO AIDS epidemic update: December 2006*. Retrieved February 15, 2007, from http://data.unaids.org/pub/EpiReport/2006/2006_EpiUpdate_en.pdf

Until There's A Cure. (2007). *The vital statistics section*. Retrieved February 15, 2007, from http://www.until.org/statistics.shtml

U.S. Central Intelligence Agency. (2002). *The next wave of HIV/AIDS: Nigeria, Ethiopia, Russia, India, and China*. Retrieved October 30, 2004, from http://www.cia.gov/nic/pubs/other_products/ICA%20HIVAIDS%20unclassified%20092302POSTGERBER.pdf

Wilson, P., & Stabinski, L. (2004). *Interim report of Task Force 5 Working Group on HIV/AIDS*. Retrieved October 30, 2004, from http://www.unmillenniumproject.org/documents/tf5hivinterim%20execsum.pdf

Wohl, A., Johnson, D., & Jordan, W. (2000). High-risk behaviors during incarceration in African-American men treated for HIV at three Los Angeles public medical centers. *Journal of Acquired Immune Deficiency Syndrome*, *24*, 386–392.

Training Peer Educators, Black MSM Leadership, and Partners for Ethnographic Community-Based Participatory Research

L. Philip Johnson and Barbara C. Wallace

Introduction

Where the challenge of delivering effective health education and promotion and disease prevention messages for the good of the public's health is concerned, there is no one size fits all remedy or solution that can effectively address all of the biopsychosocial risk factors, attitudes and beliefs, values, behaviors, and other issues associated with and stemming from a particular disease or condition. The challenge of delivering effective HIV/AIDS education is no exception. Due to the disproportional impact that the disease has had on the Black subpopulation in the United States, the Centers for Disease Control and Prevention (CDC) admit that "Continuing high rates of HIV infection among blacks underscore the need for effective, culturally tailored HIV-prevention strategies, including outreach testing strategies for identifying persons with undiagnosed HIV infection" (CDC, 2006, p. 123). Peer education and ethnography have a key role to play in these efforts.

To support this assertion, the authors draw upon their experiences training and working alongside paid peer educators in New York City, while also collecting ethnographic data with the peers, as well as designing culturally appropriate HIV/AIDS peer education training. Given this background, this chapter will discuss the challenge of reducing health disparities by training peer educators, and thereby effectively cultivating Black leadership and potential partners for participation in ethnographic community-based participatory research. Such community insiders may, also, ideally, be members of hard to reach subpopulations, such as Black men who have sex with men (MSM) and face intense cultural-based and societal-wide stigma and homophobia.

The Need for Partnerships That Include Peer Educators

In light of current trends in the HIV/AIDS epidemic (see more discussion by Nanín, Fontaine, & Wallace, chapter 22 in this volume), what has been recommended is a "comprehensive national program" that would "address the substantial racial disparities in HIV/AIDS diagnoses in the United States" (CDC, 2006, p. 125). As a part of this mission, the CDC suggests that "partnerships must be enhanced among a broad range of persons and groups, including governmental agencies, community organizations, faith-based institutions, educational institutions, community opinion leaders, and the public" (p. 125).

Partnerships may be enhanced through the training and employment of peer educators from the same communities hardest hit by the epidemic. Also, more health professionals are needed to train peer educators who are members of the communities being targeted for HIV prevention—such as MSM, HIV-positive, and undocumented immigrants. Peer educators and professionals can also join together to conduct community-based participatory research that uses ethnographic methods. There are many reasons to train and employ peer educators. Among these is the need to eliminate marginalization and reduce stigma. As Wallace suggested in her introduction (chapter 1, this volume), the investment of time and resources in training peer educators may result in their emerging as local community leaders, if not global leaders in the global transformation of health—toward the achievement of equity in health for all. The cultivation of such leadership is essential, particularly when drawing from among the ranks of those in the community who are MSM, HIV positive, undocumented immigrants, and unemployed. Cultivating this leadership through peer education training programs and involvement in community-based participatory research using ethnographic methods is highly recommended.

In a recent report commissioned by the National Minority AIDS Council (NMAC), Dr. Robert Fullilove (2006) outlined recommendations for confronting the HIV/AIDS epidemic in Black America. Dr. Fullilove lists as number three of five recommendations for confronting the epidemic in Black America, the following: "Eliminate the marginalization of, and reduce stigma and discrimination against, black gay and other men who have sex with men" (p. 8). Fullilove goes on to list several ideas for how to accomplish this task (Fullilove, 2006, pp. 22–23):

> There is only one randomly controlled HIV prevention program, "Many Men, Many Voices," specifically designed for black MSM. Investing in research to produce interventions that will work for a diverse population of black MSM is essential to a national prevention effort that will reverse the course of the epidemic in this population. The CDC and the National Institutes of Health must aggressively establish a robust research portfolio to achieve this goal.
>
> The empowerment of community leaders and organizations has been a critical element in our nation's effort to combat the HIV epidemic. More support must be leveraged to develop, promote, and sustain leadership among black MSM and in organizations serving them. Additionally, sustained investment must be made to build the capacity of organizations developed to serve black MSM in order to effectively change social networks, behavior and conditions contributing to HIV infections in this population.

Efforts should be supported to address homophobia evidenced through stigma, discrimination and violence that creates vulnerability to behaviors and conditions associated with risk for HIV infection among black MSM.

The NMAC (Fullilove, 2006) supports cultivating leadership among the ranks of those who are Black MSM, especially given how the HIV/AIDS epidemic is taking a tremendous toll on the health of urban minorities in America. These communities also increasingly include large numbers of undocumented immigrants and the unemployed, further compounding the challenge of homophobia by invoking other sources of stigma. Thus, now more than ever before, there is an urgent need for culturally appropriate and culturally tailored HIV-prevention strategies that can address the substantial racial disparities in HIV/AIDS diagnoses in the United States.

The report attempts to answer the question of how to frame and present the HIV prevention message to high-risk subgroup populations in a context that will result in intrinsically motivated health behavior change. An answer may be offered to this question through the use of peer education; and, more specifically peer education which utilizes evidence-based behavior change models rooted in a sound theoretical rationale, as we seek to train competent peer educators who can engage in outreach to their communities, emerge as valued leaders, and partner with professionals in not only HIV prevention to vulnerable stigmatized communities, but also in community-based participatory research that arises from and depends upon the ethnographic data such peers collect.

Rationale for Peer Education to Address HIV/AIDS

Green (2001) locates a rationale for the use of peer education in the work of Turner and Shepherd (1999). Turner and Shepherd offer ten key claims, as follows: peers are a credible source of information; peers are an acceptable source; peers tend to be more successful than professionals in conveying information; peers automatically serve to reinforce learning through ongoing contact; peers are positive role models; peer education is empowering for those involved; peer education is beneficial to those involved; peer education utilizes established channels of communication; peer education provides access to those who are hard to reach through conventional methods; and peer education is more cost effective (Green).

Other research confirms this rationale and demonstrates that there is definitely a role for peer education in national programs that address the HIV/AIDS epidemic. Peer education has been shown to be highly effective in filling gaps not covered by professionals (Burns-Lynch & Salzer, 2001), in accelerating health behavior change (Kelly et al., 1992), in developing social support systems (Sandstrom, 1996), and in engaging targeted clients in services (Wright, Gonzalez, Werner, Laughner, & Wallace, 1998).

Addressing Attitudes and Barriers Via Peer Education

Van Ryn and Fu (2003) discuss how public health personnel may contribute to racial and ethnic disparities in health. Potential personal and cultural barriers include factors related to an individual's knowledge, attitudes, and beliefs, as well as cultural barriers such as racism, language, sexism, and homophobia that can impact service delivery. Health care provider attitudes that impact peoples' ability to seek or use health care services are also considered to be cultural barriers (van Ryn & Fu, 2003). Peer educators may similarly have problematic attitudes that could be barriers in their delivery of education to peers.

Additional barriers to care that have been identified include lack of knowledge about HIV, stigma, language differences, concerns about confidentiality, immigration status, and cultural beliefs and practices. The moral association of HIV with "sin" and subsequent intolerance to those infected is a significant obstacle toward providing care (Wolf, Kemerer, Magaz, Romaguera, & Goldman, 2003). Hence, stigmatizing attitudes must be addressed for peer educators to be effective.

Community norms and cultural beliefs can impact negatively or positively on the attitudes and behaviors of persons living with HIV/AIDS. These findings are supported by the social science literature, which has found that the behaviors of individuals are affected by the social norms of their communities. Interventions that address social network and community-level phenomena have been shown to be effective in reducing HIV risk behaviors in diverse populations. These interventions have included enlisting peers who are trained to communicate, encourage, and reinforce health-protective messages (Kegeles, Hays, & Coates, 1996; Kegeles, Hays, Pollack, & Coates, 1999; Kelly et al., 1992).

Pertinent Theories to Support and Guide Peer Training

Turner and Shepherd (1999) assert that many peer education projects lack an explicit theoretical justification. They note that peer education does not derive from a single school of thought and, given its diversity, question the capacity of a single theory to offer universally applicable explanations of effectiveness. They explore the relevance of a number of theories deriving from different philosophical tradition, which, although not devised to explain peer education, are commonly cited in this context, or may be applicable.

They find evidence to support the application of some Social Learning Theory assertions (Bandura, 1997). Any training that seeks to increase self-efficacy and includes role-playing is likely to be effective. However, evidence for the contribution of modeling to the peer education process is found to be weak (Turner & Shepherd, 1999). They note the difficulty of measuring constructs such as self-efficacy and empowerment and suggest that, although the supporting evidence is limited, they are more relevant to the providers rather than the recipients of peer education (Turner & Shepherd).

The particular peer education training model being put forth here is most similar to that of Wallace (2005; see Wallace, Konuwa, & Ayeboafo, chapter 19, this volume), in being rooted in an integration of three evidence-based behavior change strategies: the stages of change (Prochaska & DiClemente, 1983, 1992; Prochaska, DiClemente, & Norcross, 1992); motivational interviewing (Miller & Rollnick, 1991, 2002); and relapse prevention (Carroll, 1997; Marlatt & Donovan, 2005; Marlatt & Gordon, 1985). Both motivational interviewing and relapse prevention focus heavily on increasing self-efficacy

(Marlatt & Donovan, 2005; Marlatt & Gordon, 1985; Miller & Rollnick, 1991, 2002). Bandura's (1997) self-efficacy theory is implicit in the recommended approach to peer education training. However, also worthy of note and embraced in training peer educators is a new paradigm embodied in a psychology of liberation (Wallace, 2003)—which is also seen as being supported by adult learning theory (Gallagher, 1996).

Addressing Stigma

Education alone does not change behavior (Zimmerman, Ramirez-Valles, Suarez, de la Rosa, & Castro, 1997). Attitudes guide behavior, and attitudes reflecting the internalization of homophobia and stigma may contribute to HIV transmission.

Most people in industrialized countries like the United States are educated about the disease, how it is spread, and how it can be prevented. Why then do the numbers of HIV/AIDS cases continue to rise? Some suggest that the belief that "it won't happen to me" and other inaccurate beliefs about HIV transmission are responsible for this phenomenon. Researchers like Herek, Widaman, and Capitanio (2005) suggest that stopping the spread of a communicable disease requires interrupting the process whereby it is transmitted from one person to another. They admit however, that the social construction of illness has a profound impact on the accomplishment of this task. The authors state that when the disease or some aspect of its transmission process is stigmatized, those affected are subjected to negative consequences such as personal rejection and social shunning, loss of employment and housing, deprivation of personal liberties, and even, in some extreme cases, violence and death.

Herek et al. (2005) further suggest that the stigma attached to a communicable disease (such as HIV) can also affect how the members of society understand its transmission, particularly when already-stigmatized groups are perceived to be disproportionately vulnerable to illness. It also requires confronting the public's personal anxieties about contracting AIDS, their negative attitudes toward sexual minorities, and the values that promote the equation of sex with disease. Herein lies the role that well-planned culturally appropriate evidence-based peer education can play, in the context of promoting the prevention of HIV transmission in hard-to-reach subpopulations.

Community health education and promotion programs, using peer educators from and directed at minority subpopulations—such as MSM, and men and women of African American and Caribbean American descent—as well as community-based ethnographic research involving these peer educators and subgroups, must be conducted in settings and spaces that are conducive to addressing issues of stigma. Therefore, correcting misconceptions about AIDS transmission requires more than simply disseminating accurate and detailed information about HIV (what is typically referred to as HIV 101) in these subgroups—as well-trained peer educators can readily do. It also requires confronting issues of stigmatization in a compassionate, safe, non-judgmental, non-threatening environment facilitated by meaningful others. Well-trained peer educators can play a vital role in addressing and facilitating dialogue around issues of stigma. Moreover, credible models for doing so exist (see Wallace, 2005, and Wallace, Konuwa, & Ayeboafo, chapter 19, this volume).

A Role for Ethnographic Research

Ethnography is a traditional method of sociology and cultural anthropology that involves the study of people performing activities and interacting in complex social settings in order to obtain a qualitative understanding of these interactions (Hawkins, 2003). Ethnographic research methodology can and does allow researchers to identify routine practices, problems, and possibilities for program development using adult peer educators. Ethnographic methods using individual and group interviews, as well as the collection of observational data, may readily benefit from the expertise of well-trained peer educators, especially in light of their membership in the communities being studied. Peer educators may also be ideal partners within collaborations involving multiple partners, especially within community-based participatory research.

Hayes (chapter 13, this volume) notes the manner in which community-based participatory research appears to offer an "ideal theoretical and a practical approach to utilize in developing collaborative proposals focused on the elimination of health disparities as well as other population focused initiatives." When peer educators are well-trained, they may meet Hayes's expectation that within academic and community-based partnerships "each unit brings their very best resources to the relationship." The resulting resources may be brought to bear to address and reduce stigma, in order to better reach populations at risk for HIV and prevent HIV transmission—reducing health disparities.

In this regard, Herdt (2001) also advocates the study of stigma as a means toward gaining a more complete understanding of HIV/AIDS and to enhance education and prevention efforts in cross-cultural research on AIDS. Herdt discusses how ethnography has traditionally been used for descriptive purposes, but how lately ethnographies of HIV/AIDS have become a useful tool for the study of resistance to stigma. It is also a powerful tool for studying the disruption of prejudice. And, it is an essential tool for studying changes within sexual cultures, as well as the production of new prevention practices or policy networks that effectively challenge stigma in real social contexts (Herdt). Herdt views the HIV/AIDS epidemic as a process that has occurred over time and space, and suggests that, if one begins looking at those areas and people hardest hit by the disease, then one may develop an understanding of how discrimination and stigma have played a significant role in affecting rates of HIV infection—whether by color, gender, sexual orientation, or socioeconomic status (SES). Herdt stated that people from vulnerable populations do not have the same power to protect themselves. In light of this view, it makes sense to benefit from the lens and viewpoint of those insiders most impacted by stigma, both via peer educators and the ethnographic data obtained through interaction with their own peers in their own communities.

Hence, there is support for a paradox. On the one hand, membership in specific subgroups carries with it a certain amount of stigma, and the more subgroup associations one has (i.e., experiencing multiple oppressions and sources of stigma), the less power individuals may have to advocate for themselves. Yet, on the other hand, members of such subgroups may emerge as empowered leaders who bring leadership to ethnographic community-based participatory research. Consider a portrait that conveys this paradox: imagine a case involving a Black, HIV positive, male, MSM, undocumented immigrant from the Caribbean, who is also uneducated and unemployed. Such a person may see himself as helpless and powerless to extricate himself from his circumstances, having very little choice but to remain hidden in obscurity—especially before receiving training as a peer educator. Yet, also consider what the first author has witnessed through training and employing such individuals across several years: the emergence of an empowered peer educator able to disclose his HIV positive and MSM status, enjoys paid employment as a peer educator, and provides leadership in peer support groups and on community-based participatory research teams collaborating with academics and effectively collecting ethnographic observations of what is happening among his peers in the community.

These kinds of outcomes can be achieved, as the first author has personally witnessed and participated in their creation across nearly a decade working with cohort after cohort of peer educators in New York City. Some researchers may find it extremely difficult to identify and recruit the participation of clients/patients for study projects or training as peer educators when they lack insight into the predisposing factors (e.g., values, beliefs, culture) associated with membership in these subgroups and a host of other enabling and reinforcing factors attributable to subgroup membership. Once potential peer educators and community-based participatory research partners are identified, care must be taken, and time must be taken to gain their trust. Next, our new partners must be seen as equals, as they bring vital resources to collaborative relationships with academic, community, and faith-based organizations. Then, our new partners deserve the receipt of skilled training, integration into our collaborative work and community spaces, and paid employment as peers educators and community-based participatory research partners. There is a central role for evidence-based behavior change models and peer education training models for those eventually employed and placed in paid service to their community.

Paying peer educators so trained is vital. For, according to Herdt (2001), social inequality is harmful to health in human society. Just as researchers and academics expect to be paid, peer educators need to be paid.

Peer educators must also be accepted for the stage of change they are in with regard to their sexual identity, for example, potentially being open about MSM behavior, or totally or partially closeted (Wallace, Carter, Nanín, Keller, & Alleyne, 2003).

In this regard, Herdt (2001) notes that, as diverse sexualities and sexual cultures confront stigma and discrimination, there are processes of resistance, marginalization, and social mobilization that also come into play. Herdt points out that it is important to recognize how, because of stigma and discrimination, individuals may seek to pass as normal to prevent having their identities spoiled from being stigmatized. All of these are issues best studied with ethnographic methods (Herdt), as well as issues that must be addressed in peer education training programs. Meanwhile, those training peer educators must respect and accept their choice, regarding when and if to disclose their MSM or HIV positive status.

Beyond Stigma: Training Supportive, Optimistic, Positive Peer Educators

In order for the role of peer educators to be effective, it is important that the training of peers be conducted in a manner consistent with full appreciation of factors operating in the larger socio-cultural context. This means exploring and addressing issues of stigma in the appropriate social context, including during the training of peer educators. For peer educators will undoubtedly encounter issues of stigma when working in the community on behalf of and reaching out to special populations—such as those including MSM, undocumented immigrants, and so forth. Moreover, whether they disclose it or not, they may have a history of personally experiencing stigma because of their own MSM behavior, for example, and the cultural mores common to the African, African American, or Caribbean populations that reject such behavior and those who engage in it—necessitating living in silence about MSM behavior. This complex cultural context must be understood and discussed in the training of peer educators, even if not a single peer educator elects to immediately or directly disclose his or her personal experiences; this kind of discussion is important so peer educators begin to move away from any internalized homophobia and/or tendencies to stigmatize others who engage in such controversial behavior. While one might assume that HIV peer education training needs to primarily cover biological, psychological, and social mechanisms that impact HIV transmission, time also needs to be spent in training covering these cultural issues.

Peer educators must also be trained to accept where various members of the community are with regard to issues of stigma. The stages of change can be adapted to facilitate understanding of where people are with regard to attitudes and behaviors that stigmatize others, or themselves (internalized homophobia), following the work of Prochaska and DiClemente (1983, 1992). For example, people may be in a pre-contemplation stage and not even thinking about how they contribute to the stigmatization of those who are MSM, or HIV positive; or they may be in a stage of contemplation, just having thought about such issues; or in a stage of preparation, having made a determination to begin to work on their stigmatizing attitudes and behaviors; or a stage of action, having taken action for more than 6 months in changing and working on their attitudes and beliefs; or in a maintenance stage, having done substantial work in this area for anywhere from 7 months to many years. Similarly, peer educators may themselves be in any of these stages, and in need of peer education training that guides them toward the acquisition of positive, optimistic, nonstigmatizing attitudes, freeing them from stigmatizing attitudes and any internalized homophobia. Wallace et al. (2003) have integrated the use of motivational interviewing (Miller & Rollnick, 2002) with stages of change (Prochaska & DiClemente, 1983, 1992) or identity statuses for stigmatized identities, such as those who are MSM; the result is a model holding promise, wherein motivational interviewing techniques are used to help facilitate movement for MSM across stages of change toward the possession of more progressive, differentiated identity statuses—such as one that embraces and celebrates an identity that includes MSM behavior. There is great utility in applying both stages of change theory (Prochaska & DiClemente) and motivational interviewing (Miller & Rollnick) when training peer educators.

In this regard, Wallace (2005; see also Wallace, Konuwa & Ayeboafo, chapter 19, this volume) has specifically integrated exposure to and training in the evidence-based motivational interviewing and stages of change—called stages of safety—into a model of training HIV/AIDS prevention peer educators. In addition, specifically seeking to assist peer educators in overcoming attitudes of stigma, the model includes the goal of peer educators' both being and learning to seek out Supportive, Optimistic Positive Peers (SOPP). In this way, carefully constructed peer education training models can move those being trained through stages of change toward taking action in adopting nonstigmatizing attitudes, replacing them with those that are supportive, optimistic, and positive when it comes to those who are MSM, undocumented immigrants, HIV positive, unemployed, or possessing any stigmatizing identity.

Furthermore, there is evidence to suggest that Wallace's model (2005, and Wallace, Konuwa & Ayeboafo, chapter 19, this volume) of training peer educators to engage in HIV prevention is effective. Data suggest that the model not only increases HIV knowledge from pre- to post-training across a 4-week training program, but also is embraced by peer educators, recommended by them, and enhances their skill set—based on their self-report.

Conclusion

This chapter has proposed reducing health disparities involving disproportionate rates of HIV infection by training peer educators. The goal is to cultivate Black MSM leadership and create viable culturally competent partners for ethnographic community-based participatory research.

While there is no one-size-fits-all approach to training peer educators or potential research partners among community members, there are available interventions that can be implemented that have been shown to be effective to motivate health related behavior change. Such interventions include training peer educators so they emerge as empowered leaders in their communities, capable of educating others, combating cultural-based stigma, and working alongside academic and other partners within community-based participatory research—including that which is ethnographic.

Health professionals and community health advocates and organizers can begin to address health concerns within communities by incorporating what has already been shown to be effective into community-based health education and promotion programs. More culturally appropriate health education and promotion programs that utilize evidence-based social behavioral change models (i.e., motivational interviewing, stages of change) are needed to provide as many varied options for consumers of health information in the community as possible. Additionally, more and better planned community-based ethnographic research needs to be done, including peer educators as partners, in order to investigate community norms and cultural beliefs that negatively and positively impact the attitudes and behaviors of persons affected by and living with HIV/AIDS.

This chapter has highlighted how the use of evidence-based and theory-based models can be useful in the design and implementation of effective peer education training programs that not only prepare peer educators to educate others, but also prepare peer educators to overcome any personal stigmatizing attitudes and behaviors, and empower them to address stigma when encountered in the community—all while assisting peer educators in developing personally and fostering in others the development of intrinsic motivation to pursue health behavior change.

By deploying culturally appropriate models for training peer educators, professionals may help to cultivate the Black MSM leadership being urgently called for to help stem the tide of the HIV/AIDS epidemic. In the process, we may also gain ideal partners for conducting community-based participatory research, such as that which uses ethnographic methods. The possibilities of such leaders taking models of HIV prevention and pertinent strategies beyond their physical communities, and even into prisons (see Bahl, chapter 20, this volume), or into Internet chat rooms are endless, but begin with the decision to train peer educators who are Black MSM.

REFERENCES

Bandura, A. (1997). *Self-efficacy: The exercise of control*. New York: W. H. Freeman.

Burns-Lynch, B., & Salzer, M. S. (2001). Adopting innovations—Lessons learned from a peer-based hospital diversion program. *Community Mental Health Journal, 37*(6), 511–521.

Carroll, K. M. (1997). Relapse prevention as a psychosocial treatment: A review of controlled clinical trials. In G. A. Marlatt & G. R. VandenBos (Eds.), *Addictive behaviors: Readings on etiology, prevention, and treatment*. Washington, DC: American Psychological Association.

Centers for Disease Control and Prevention (CDC). (2006). Racial/ethnic disparities in diagnoses of HIV/AIDS—33 States, 2001–2004. *Morbidity and Mortality Weekly Report, 55*(5), 121–124.

Fullilove, R. E. (2006, November). *African Americans, health disparities, and HIV/AIDS: Recommendations for confronting the epidemic in Black America*. New York: Columbia University, National Minority AIDS Council (NMAC).

Gallagher, D. M. (1996). HIV education: A challenge to adult learning theory and practice. *Journal of the Association of Nurses in AIDS Care, 7*(Suppl 1), 5–14.

Green, J. (2001). Peer education. *Promotion & Education, 8*(2), 65–68.

Hawkins, B. D. (2003). A predator in paradise. *Black Issues in Higher Education, 19*(25), 20–23.

Herdt, G. (2001). Stigma and the ethnographic study of HIV: Problems and prospects. *AIDS and Behavior, 5*(2), 141–149.

Herek, G. M., Widaman, K. F., & Capitanio, J. P. (2005). When sex equals AIDS: Symbolic stigma and heterosexual adults' inaccurate beliefs about sexual transmission of AIDS. *Social Problems, 52*(1), 15–37.

Kegeles, S. M., Hays, R. B., & Coates, T. J. (1996). The Mpowerment Project: A community-level HIV prevention intervention for young gay men. *American Journal of Public Health, 86*(8), 1129–1136.

Kegeles, S. M., Hays, R. B., Pollack, L. M., & Coates, T. J. (1999). Mobilizing young gay and bisexual men for HIV prevention: A two-community study. *AIDS, 13*, 1753–1762.

Kelly, J. A., St. Lawrence, J. S., Stevenson, Y., Hauth, A. C., Kalichman, S. C., Diaz, Y. E., et al. (1992). Community AIDS/HIV risk reduction: The effects of endorsements by popular people in three cities. *American Journal of Public Health, 82*(11), 1483–1489.

Marlatt, G. A., & Donovan, D. M. (Eds.). (2005). *Relapse prevention: Maintenance strategies in the treatment of addictive behaviors* (2nd ed.). New York: Guilford Press.

Marlatt, G. A., & Gordon, J. R. (1985). *Relapse prevention: Maintenance strategies in the treatment of addictive behaviors* (1st ed.). New York: Guilford Press.

Miller, W. R., & Rollnick, S. (Eds.). (1991). *Motivational interviewing: Preparing people to change addictive behaviors* (1st ed.). New York: Guilford Press.

Miller, W. R., & Rollnick, S. (Eds.). (2002). *Motivational interviewing: Preparing people for change* (2nd ed.). New York: Guilford Press.

Prochaska, J. O., & DiClemente, C. C. (1983). Stages and processes of self-change of smoking: Toward an integrative model of change. *Journal of Consulting and Clinical Psychology, 51*, 390–395.

Prochaska, J. O., & DiClemente, C. C. (1992). Stages of change in the modification of problem behaviors. *Progress in Behavior Modification, 28*, 183–218.

Prochaska, J. O., DiClemente, C. C., & Norcross, J. C. (1992). In search of how people change: Applications to addictive behaviors. *American Psychologist, 47*, 1102–1114.

Sandstrom, K. L. (1996). Searching for information, understanding, and self-value: The utilization of peer support groups by gay men with HIV/AIDS. *Social Work in Health Care, 23*(4), 51–74.

Turner, G., & Shepherd, J. (1999). A method in search of a theory: Peer education and health promotion. *Health Education Research, 114*(2), 235–247.

van Ryn, M., & Fu, S. S. (2003). Paved with good intentions: Do public health and human service providers contribute to racial/ethnic disparities in health? *American Journal of Public Health, 93*(2), 248–255.

Wallace, B. C. (2005). *HIV/AIDS peer education training manual: Combining African healing wisdom and evidence-based behavior change strategies*. Philadelphia: StarSpirit Press.

Wallace, B. C. (2003). A multicultural approach to violence: Toward a psychology of oppression, liberation, and identity development. In B. C. Wallace & R. T. Carter (Eds.), *Understanding and dealing with violence: A multicultural approach.* Thousand Oaks, CA: Sage.

Wallace, B. C., Carter, R. T., Nanín, J., Keller, R., & Alleyne, V. (2003). Identity development for 'diverse and different others': Integrating stages of change, motivational interviewing, and identity theories for race, people of color, sexual orientation, and disability. In B. C. Wallace & R. T. Carter (Eds.), *Understanding and dealing with violence: A multicultural approach.* Thousand Oaks, CA: Sage.

Wolf, R. C., Kemerer, V. F., Magaz, P., Romaguera, R., & Goldman, T. (2003, April). *Assessing the impact of Caribbean migration on HIV/AIDS care: Ryan White CARE Act consumer and provider focus groups and interviews.* Grant paper.

Wright, E. R., Gonzalez, C., Werner, J. N., Laughner, S. T., & Wallace, M. (1998). Indiana Youth Access Project. *Journal of Adolescent Health, 23*(S2), 83–95.

Zimmerman, M. A., Ramirez-Valles, J., Suarez, E., de la Rosa, G., & Castro, M. (1997). An HIV/AIDS prevention project for Mexican homosexual men: An empowerment approach. *Health Education & Behavior, 24*(2), 177–190.

Closing Gaps in Health for Special Populations

Recommendations for Researchers and Clinicians Working at the Intersection of the HIV/AIDS and Methamphetamine Epidemics With MSM

José Nanín,
Yves-Michel Fontaine,
and Barbara C. Wallace

Introduction

It is common knowledge in the health care field that health disparities exist among many populations in the Unites States. In a published commentary, Greenspan (2001) stated "[t]hat there are variations in the health status of different groups of Americans can come as no surprise to any health professional" (p. 417). Some of the most apparent disparities are among the poor and communities of color, as outlined in *Healthy People 2010* (HP 2010), the U.S. government's agenda for health promotion and disease prevention (U.S. Department of Health and Human Services [HHS], 2000). What is less apparent in discussions on health disparities is the fact that documented health disparities also exist among lesbian, gay, bisexual, and transgender (LGBT) individuals, especially men who have sex with men (MSM) (Gay and Lesbian Medical Association [GLMA], 2001). The MSM "community" is hard to define and difficult to reach because of stigma attached to complex identity, behavioral, cultural, and even geographical issues (see Johnson & Wallace, chapter 21, this volume). The term "gay community" is, at times, debated since in many cases there may not be a defined community to refer to. It has been argued that, especially among significant numbers of men of color, the term "gay" comes from a "racially insensitive white gay world" with which many MSM of color do not want to be associated (Boykin, 2005, p. 16). With this said, the term "MSM communities" will be used throughout this chapter to acknowledge the diversity that exists among MSM as well as the one factor that links these men together as a "community" regardless of identity, culture, or geography—they all have some level of attraction and sexual and intimate relationships with other men.

Knowing how to reach the multitude of sectors within this "community" can be helpful to health professionals in reducing disparities in disease prevention and health care services for the entire population of "behaviorally" gay/bisexual men, adapting a term used by Stokes, Damon, and McKirnan (1997). Because the original HP 2010 document did not address the issues of LGBT communities, the GLMA created an addendum to HP 2010 to fill this important information gap. This document, entitled *Healthy People 2010 Companion Document for Lesbian, Gay, Bisexual, and Transgender (LGBT) Health* (available for review and download at http://www.glma.org/_data/ n_0001/resources/live/HealthyCompanionDoc3.pdf) takes the original objectives outlined in HP 2010 and reframes them with the purpose of improving the health status of LGBT Americans and thus reducing related disparities (GLMA, 2001). An important consideration made by this document is that LGBT individuals, especially from ethnic minorities (referred to in the present chapter as *people of color*), are "hidden" client/patient populations within the health care world and that many do not feel empowered enough to disclose their sexual orientation or behaviors to their providers. An implication of this may be that, in order to conduct research about health disparities and provide services to reduce these disparities in LGBT populations, health professionals must be sensitive to LGBT-specific issues and offer what the communities say they need as opposed to what professionals *assume* they need.

Health Disparity Indicators for MSM

According to empirical evidence documented throughout the past decade, MSM experience as many negative health outcomes as other disenfranchised populations. Prevalence of HIV and other sexually transmitted infections (STIs) remains significantly high in many MSM communities around the Unites States (Buchacz, Greenberg, Onorato, & Janssen, 2005; Centers for Disease Control and Prevention [CDC], 2005, 2006; Klausner, Wolf, Fischer-Ponce, Zolt, & Katz, 2000; Purcell, Moss, Remien, Parsons, & Woods, 2005; Taylor et al., 2005). HIV/AIDS diagnoses increased 8% among MSM between 2003 and 2004; additionally, gonorrhea and syphilis cases increased more than two-fold between 1988 and 2003 (CDC, 2006).

Substance use continues to be a burgeoning issue, especially with recent reported increases in crystal methamphetamine and other drug use (CDC, 2006, 2007; Fontaine, 2007; Nanín & Parsons, 2006; Purcell et al. 2005; Purcell, Parsons, Halkitis, Mizuno, & Woods, 2001), as well as tobacco use (GLMA, 2001). Crystal methamphetamine (MA) use has been reportedly linked to unprotected sexual behavior among MSM; among those who are HIV-positive, there is a reported link to reduced HIV medication adherence (CDC, 2007). The Centers for Disease Control and Prevention regard these factors as challenges to HIV and STI prevention efforts (CDC, 2007). (The impact of crystal methamphetamine use on MSM health disparities and related clinical issues are discussed in more detail later in this chapter.)

This chapter acknowledges how, among MSM, those who are also using MA constitute a special subpopulation with special needs. Indeed, MSM who use MA are living at the intersections of the HIV/AIDS and methamphetamine epidemics, while also engaging in high-risk sexual behavior. For this reason, this chapter will discuss (1) the range of health disparities impacting MSM to place their lives in context; (2) research issues; and (3) clinical treatment issues.

The Range of Health Disparities Impacting MSM

Other health disparities abound. MSM are increasingly experiencing unwanted other-inflicted violence from prejudiced (homophobic) individuals as well as their own partners (Wallace, Carter, Nanín, Keller, & Alleyne, 2002). This, along with depression, childhood sexual abuse, and substance use, has been found to be related to risky sexual practices (CDC, 2006, 2007). In addition, published evidence shows how increased risk of cancer may be related to concealment of sexual identity among gay men (Cole, Kemeny, Taylor, & Visscher, 1996). Smoking has also been found to be higher in prevalence among LGB individuals than their heterosexual peers (Smith, Offen, & Malone, 2006). Smoking prevalence was higher in MSM samples (compared to heterosexual male samples) of two studies published within the past 3 years (Greenwood et al., 2005; Tang et al., 2004). Many of these disparities are further compounded by the fact that MSM still face much discrimination and stigma in health services (CDC, 2007).

Even though MSM seem to be receiving access to health care services they need, a major factor related to the receipt of substandard services is the increased likelihood among MSM to not disclose their sexual identity or details about their desires for and behaviors with other men (risky or otherwise) to their health care providers (GLMA, 2001). Health care access disparities are more emphasized among MSM of color who may have a more difficult time due to socioeconomic status, insurance status, as well as fear of stigma and disclosure by health care providers.

Health Disparities Among MSM of Color

The health status of men of color in general is dire. A recent study by the Kaiser Family Foundation (2006) reports that more black men suffer fatalities from prostate cancer than white men and other men of color because they do not receive early diagnoses and treatment or do not have access to appropriate and consistent health care. In addition, Black men reportedly have the shortest average life expectancy and highest mortality rate from heart disease and other cardiovascular conditions (Minino & Smith, 2001). On the HIV front, Latinos account for 20% of the total number of new AIDS cases, and the incidence rate is nearly four times that of non–Latino whites (CDC, 2004). A significant number of these cases are among Latino men.

For MSM of color, the disparities in HIV rates are astounding. In addition, the CDC (2004) report cited in the preceding paragraph highlights how a significant amount of the Latino HIV incidence rate is accounted for by Latino MSM. Recent reports show that, in a study of MSM across five U.S. cities, HIV-positive Black MSM report a staggering disproportionate rate of unrecognized HIV infection (64%) compared to Latino (18%), White (11%), and other races (6%) (CDC, 2005). The same report shows that HIV prevalence was highest among Black MSM (46%) compared to Whites (21%) and Latinos (17%).

Reaching out to and communicating with *all* communities in need of adequate health care as well as disease prevention services is an imperative part of all the work public health officials and other health service personnel conduct in order to reduce health disparities among MSM. Researchers are an integral part of the health field. Without researchers, much of the data we depend on for grant development and cited literature would not exist. In addition, researchers throughout the United States have created innovative methods to access "hard-to-reach" or "hidden" communities and to recruit individuals to participate in important research studies (Faugier & Sargeant, 1997; Muhib et al., 2001). Lessons can be learned from work conducted by researchers to recruit and maintain ethnically-diverse samples of MSM participants for their research studies.

Recruitment and Study Participation Issues With MSM Communities

Many efforts must be put forth in order to make participation in a research study attractive to a potential MSM participant, especially those with particular perceived health needs. When recruiting for studies, researchers need to gain and maintain trust with the MSM communities (Parsons, 2005). Many men may feel strange about disclosing personal or sensitive information to a perceived outsider. Even if the researcher is an MSM (gay-identified or not), he may still have to work hard at gaining and maintaining trust because of his affiliation with an institution that may be perceived as oppressive or not trustworthy (e.g., pharmaceutical company, college and university, the U.S. government).

MSM are also at different stages of readiness to change certain behaviors they may perceive as unhealthy (Parsons, 2005). For example, some men may be contemplating the adoption of safer sex practices while others have been practicing safer sex for years. A recent report has shown that, even in the face of crystal methamphetamine prevention campaign advertisements, some MSM may still feel tempted to use the drug (Nanín, Parsons, Bimbi, Grov, & Brown, 2006).

Acknowledging that *not* all MSM practice the same behaviors in the same way and that not all are in the same stage of behavior change is essential to reaching out to them (Parsons, 2005). In addition, it is important to acknowledge that all MSM do not participate in risk behaviors involving drug and alcohol use, unprotected sex, and other reported behaviors. When data from many studies on MSM risk behavior are reported, those who practice these behaviors are usually in the minority. What is usually not reported is how the majority of the men in these samples are *not* practicing these risky behaviors.

Many researchers who are sensitive to these phenomena can more effectively tailor their recruitment messages to certain factions of MSM communities, similar to how social marketers and health communication strategists conduct audience segmentation and tailor health promotion messages for individuals in certain stages of behavior change (Dearing et al., 1996). They realize that moralistic stereotyping of male-on-male sexual behavior (and anything related to it) is counterproductive to working with MSM communities as well as unethical for reducing health disparities among MSM and enhancing their sexual health (Robinson, Bockting, Rosser, Miner, & Coleman, 2002).

To ensure reaching out to a substantial diversity of men (with regards to race, ethnicity, and immigration status), researchers collaborate with community-based organizations, hospitals, and other entities that are experienced with providing services to communities of interest or catchment areas that are populated by diverse communities.

With MSM of color, this may entail reaching out to and offering to join efforts with AIDS service organizations, local and state health departments, and other social and health service agencies. The work may also involve visiting nontraditional venues (e.g., barber shops, parks, special events, social clubs, worksites, among others) and conducting work during nontraditional hours, as in late evenings and weekends, when access to MSM populations may be optimal. Efforts like these all involve using nontraditional methods in order to communicate with MSM from communities one is interested in accessing for research and service purposes (e.g., MSM of color who may *not* identify as gay) (see Millett, Malebranche, Mason, & Spikes, 2005).

An emerging issue in disease prevention, especially with HIV prevention, is the use of the Internet by MSM (CDC, 2003). Since significant numbers of MSM use the Internet to seek each other for friendships, romance, and sexual liaisons, among other reasons, it may behoove health professionals to increase use of the Internet as a venue to disseminate health promotion messages as well as to advertise health care services. The exposure to these messages and ads can increase the potential for more MSM to consider changing any perceived risk behaviors and/or to access health care services for determining their health status (e.g., prostate cancer screening, cardiovascular health screening, referrals to alcohol and drug use rehabilitation programs, as well as HIV testing services).

Reaching out to these communities in their own settings using nontraditional methods may be effective but one may also need to use communication strategies that appeal to these communities. Using humor can definitely make a health promotion message more appealing, especially when working with MSM who have been inundated with "fear-based" and moralistic messages about how their behaviors *need* to change (Nanín et al., 2006). Conway and Dube (2002) state how humor-based communication strategies can be used to persuade individuals to consider adoption of preventive health behaviors to diminish the threats of many diseases. Parsons and colleagues (2006) have been successful in using humor and entertainment to educate MSM about the "not-so-pretty" consequences of alcohol and party drug use. Approaches that use humor as well as entertainment may be effective with many MSM communities.

The work conducted by professionals in health care, health education, research, and similar fields is essential to enhancing the health status of all Americans, including MSM. Many professionals need to acknowledge that communities of MSM are very diverse when it comes to sexual identity development. Some MSM may have sex with men but do not feel ready or feel a compelling need to come out and proclaim themselves as *gay*. As mentioned earlier, some MSM may not want to adopt the term "gay" because of the stigmatizing link to white men (Boykin, 2005). It is necessary to provide support for MSM regardless of their position in the coming out process, whether they are completely out and proud of their sexual identity or if they are "in the closet" and having sex with other men. This support is critical in enhancing their psychological and physical well-being (Cole et al., 1996; Grov, Bimbi, Nanín, & Parsons, 2006; Kennamer, Honnold, Bradford, & Hendricks, 2000; Peacock, 2000; Ryan & Futterman, 1998). Improving psychological as well as physical well-being is an important determinant to reducing health disparities in many communities, especially MSM.

It is also important for providers to acknowledge that MSM are social beings. Many are parents or want to be parents (Weiser, Nanín, Parsons, & Bimbi, 2006). Many are employed in "traditional" types of employment but some may be involved in sex work and other types of "pleasure-based" employment (Bimbi et al., 2006). Nonjudgmental treatment of MSM regardless of their employment status, parental status, relationship status, or other social status is necessary for communicating with them and maintaining their trust.

Reaching out to and communicating with MSM communities require cultural sensitivity, cultural competence, and replacing any maladaptive responses (e.g., disdain disrespect, disregard, discrimination) with adaptive responses, such as acceptance, respect, and empathy—going well beyond tolerance. Recommended brief training is codified elsewhere (Wallace, 2005) and discussed later in this chapter. In addition, agencies benefit by diversifying their staff—ensuring the presence of MSM, along with culturally competent individuals of diverse racial/ethnic backgrounds. Staff members may need to participate in sensitivity training to understand the issues experienced by MSM as described in this chapter. Lastly, agencies may need to adapt their policies and procedures to incorporate nondiscrimination policies, ethical treatment of nonheterosexual individuals, and appropriate rules of conduct (including preventing sexual harassment and monitoring of inappropriate and biased language).

Without these efforts, many health professionals will find themselves in positions of not being able to qualify for governmental or privately funded grants focused on reducing health disparities in MSM communities. More importantly, without these efforts, many will find themselves trying to help individuals that they may be inadvertently offending or discouraging from accessing disease prevention and health care services. MSM communities deserve consistent, adequate, and sensitive prevention and health care services—just like everyone else in the United States.

Clinical Treatment Issues With MSM Using Methamphetamine (MA)

Clinicians find ample and increasing opportunities to work with men who fall into the categories of gay, bisexual, or men who have sex with men (MSM). Moreover, there is an intersection between the HIV/AIDS epidemic and the contemporary methamphetamine (MA) epidemic. MSM are the primary group living at the intersection of these two overlapping epidemics. In this manner, the experiences and needs of MSM who are using MA and engaging in high-risk sexual behavior for the transmission of HIV are unique, justifying a special focus on this subpopulation of MSM, in this section of the chapter. These contemporary MSM MA users may be active compulsive or infrequent users of crystal methamphetamine or other amphetamine type stimulants and in various stages of the recovery process.

When training other clinicians about crystal methamphetamine treatment, a popular exercise is to request that everyone step into the shoes of a methamphetamine user. They are asked to draw on anything that they have heard about methamphetamine either from their work in the public health sector, from personal experience, or from information they have picked up from the media. In this manner, the participants become the clients. They are then asked to share the reasons why they use methamphetamine. What tend to be mentioned as the most common reasons given include the following: to have the best sex of my life, to escape the reality of HIV, to feel more attractive, to have more energy, to have sex for extended periods of time, to be more social, to be more focused and productive, to lose inhibitions, and to lose weight. Next, they are asked, "With benefits like these, why would you want to stop using?" It is from this perspective of understanding the challenges of giving up a behavior with so many real and perceived benefits that the work begins. The perspective gained from this exercise powerfully connects practitioners with the experience of MSM using MA, facilitating understanding of the role MA use plays in their sexual and emotional lives, creating a starting point for approaching the task of assisting MSM MA users in changing their relationship to MA—ideally, relinquishing the drug.

So What Is Crystal Methamphetamine (MA)?

A next step for practitioners involves understanding the nature of the drug at issue as well as mechanisms of action via various routes (Schuckit, 2006). Methamphetamine is classified as a Schedule II drug, which are drugs or other substances that have been deemed to have a high potential for abuse. MA, also known by its many street names (e.g., "Meth," "Tina," "Crystal," "Ice," "Glass," "Crank," "Speed," and "Crack Methamphetamine"), is a synthetic stimulant that excites the brain and the central nervous system. MA triggers the release of large amounts of dopamine in the body—the chemical that sends pleasure messages to the brain, as well as the release of norepinephrine and serotonin. The high can last anywhere from 8 to 24 hours, depending on the duration of use, and takes roughly 12 hours before 50% of drug is removed from the body.

MA is a translucent crystal similar in appearance to rock candy or salt, and is sometimes made into capsules or pills. While MA can appear yellowish, brownish, or off-white in color, it is closer to a pure white powder when crushed, depending upon its purity and the integrity of the cooking process. In its rock/crystal form, MA can be inhaled by smoking. In powder form, MA can be snorted, injected, or taken orally or anally. Injecting methamphetamine is the riskiest way to use. A person is far more likely to become dependent if the user injects; users tend to build up tolerance for the drug more quickly. MA users are also at risk of other harms including vein damage, overdose, and exposure to infections such as hepatitis B/C and HIV (Schuckit, 2006). Because the culture of injection drug use is a social one, first-time injectors are usually shown the ropes by someone more experienced, so they are at the mercy of the injector.

Current Approaches to Methamphetamine Treatment

Unfortunately there is no magic bullet when it comes to treating MA addiction or dependence. However, some data support the view that MA users are responsive to treatment (Shoptaw et al., 2005), and various evidence-based approaches to addiction treatment with contemporary clients (Wallace, 2005) apply to MSM using MA. Some of the current treatment modalities being used are worthy of brief discussion.

Cognitive Behavioral Therapy (CBT) is a structured short-term therapy that looks at the relationship between thoughts, feelings, and behavior, to help the client explore the antecedents, behaviors, and consequences of their drug use. CBT can be delivered in either a group or individual setting and can be tailored to meet the individual needs of each client (Donovan & Marlatt, 2005; Wallace, 2005).

Motivational Interviewing is described by Miller and Rollnick (2002) as a client-centered, directive method for enhancing intrinsic motivation to change by exploring and resolving ambivalence. The emphasis is placed on eliciting self-motivational statements of desire for and commitment to change, and on a client's perceptions of his or her current drug-using behavior and the personal goals that he or she has for himself.

Relapse Prevention is described by Marlatt and Witkiewitz (2005) as tertiary prevention with two specific aims: (1) to prevent an initial lapse and maintain abstinence or harm reduction treatment goals, and (2) to provide lapse management if a laps occurs, to prevent further relapse. The ultimate goal is to provide the skills to prevent a complete relapse, regardless of the situation or impending risk factors.

Contingency Management is based on operant conditioning that provides stimulus for favorable responses. In the case of contingency management, clients are rewarded or given vouchers for producing clean urine samples indicating no recent drug use, which can in turn be used to purchase items that are in line with a drug-free lifestyle. Vouchers or rewards are withheld for producing dirty urines (Higgins & Silverman, 1999).

Crystal Methamphetamine Anonymous (CMA) has become an increasingly popular approach to recovery by many MA users. Some choose to go the CMA route without other forms of treatment, while others use CMA in addition to utilizing other forms of addiction therapy.

The Matrix Model is a manualized, 16-week, outpatient, evidence-based model that integrates the principles of relapse prevention, motivational interviewing, cognitive behavior therapy, contingency management, and 12-step participation (Rawson et al., 1995).

Pharmacological Treatment: There are currently no FDA approved medications for the treatment of MA dependence.

Methamphetamine Treatment Considerations

Although it can be difficult to do, it is important to screen all clients for preexisting and co-occurring psychiatric disorders when beginning treatment. One approach to a psychological assessment and psychiatric screening has been described in detail (Wallace, 2005). It is important to identify and diagnose clients, laying the foundation for matching clients to appropriate mental health and psychiatric interventions. Ideally, mental health/psychiatric treatment and substance use treatment are integrated and delivered in the same setting, as the preferred contemporary standard.

Treating the underlying psychiatric disorders can greatly improve treatment outcomes. Psychiatric treatment can also help ameliorate some of the MA withdrawal side effects—some of which can persist for several weeks (Kolodny, 2006).

Using Crystal for Reasons That Are Not So Apparent

While many MSM use MA for reasons similar to those named by the training participants described above, MSM also report using MA to manage the following: feelings of loneliness and boredom; sero-converting to being HIV-positive; wanting to connect with other men; wanting to feel part of something; having a negative self-image (e.g., body image, penis size, age, among others); lack of energy due to HIV-related fatigue; engaging in commercial sex work; medicating episodes of depression and other mental health issues; not wanting to deal with unemployment and homelessness; and experiencing loss of sex drive due to side effects from certain medications.

The Importance of Early and Meaningful Engagement in Treatment

Methamphetamine users tend to access care when they are most unstable (i.e., experiencing withdrawal). Ideally, MA users access treatment as early as possible in their addiction.

Having services that are flexible enough to meet clients where they are, in their particular state of readiness to change, serves to increase the chance for a meaningful engagement in treatment.

Critical to successful and meaningful engagement in treatment, especially in outpatient settings, is frequent contact between practitioners and MA-using clients. For example, Wallace (2005) suggests 4–5× per week, or at least 2–3× per week, depending on individual client needs and characteristics, such as their dose and frequency of MA use. Frequent visits should proceed until clients achieve stability. Engagement also occurs when treatment is low-threshold, or when programs offer easy access, having as few barriers as possible. In essence, this means that programs have multiple features that maximize client engagement, including the following: a combination of daily intensive programs, less intensive evening programs, drop-in hours, flexibility to meet with clients more often if needed, as well as flexibility in response to clients' (at times) sporadic attendance. All of these elements may support early and meaningful engagement in MA treatment with the goal of stabilizing the client as quickly as possible.

The Triage Model: What Needs Attention Now vs. Later

The Triage Model is most effective when working with MA users. The triage concepts help to identify and focus attention upon clients' most immediate needs, (i.e., sleep, food, shelter, containment), allowing clinicians to prioritize. Clients' immediate needs will dictate the immediate intervention and the goal. Consistent with a consideration of what is urgent and needs to be addressed now, versus later (Wallace, 2005), clinicians are urged to meet immediate needs, before attending to more complex issues (e.g., problem behaviors) later.

The Importance of Determining and Differentiating Nature of MA Use

Not all MA users share the same experience of their use. The mode of use can affect the user differently (e.g., taking orally vs. anally, by snorting, by smoking, or by injecting). Additionally, the frequency (i.e., daily, weekly, or weekend use vs. monthly, or yearly use), and quantity of use (i.e., how much MA is used during an episode, or the typical dose) are also important when assessing clients' use and which treatment intervention is appropriate. In addition to the mode and frequency and typical dose of MA use, the drug set and setting of use also play a significant part in the user's experience. The effects of drugs include drug pharmacologic effects, expectations about using, and the context in which drugs are used, which are factors clinicians need to consider.

The Importance of Properly Trained Staff

Because our first contact with a client may potentially be our only contact, the challenge is to be responsive to clients' immediate needs while giving clients accurate information about their use. It is important to have clinicians on staff who are knowledgeable about the biochemical and psychiatric effects of methamphetamine use (Levounis & Ruggiero, 2006). For instance, MA intoxication can range from feelings of euphoria and well-being to restlessness, insomnia, and loss of appetite. MA intoxication can also look like a number of psychiatric disorders, including mood, anxiety, and psychotic disorders

(Kolodny, 2006). People experiencing psychosis often present as confused, and can become agitated, irritable, and have excessive mood swings, which can sometimes leads to violence or paranoia. Staff will need to be able to recognize the signs of MA intoxication and how to respond accordingly (Schuckit, 2006) to MA use–induced states. Usually such states go away when the MA use has stopped and the drug has been metabolized from the body (usually a few days but may take longer with chronic use). Some people will require medical attention either during or after an episode of psychosis (Schuckit, 2006).

The Role of Stigma

For many MSM, stigma plays a large role in their sexual and emotional lives, and may be related to MA use. Whether it is stigma around identity as a gay or bisexual man, or a man who has sex with men (MSM), or stigma around sexual orientation or gender, or stigma around HIV status, or even stigma about being an MSM of color, there is a common task that arises: one of managing feelings or experiences of shame and stigma, given how this is something that most MSM face in their everyday lives. Feelings of shame and disappointment will oftentimes surface in sessions and should be handled with sensitivity. In working with MSM around themes related to shame or stigma, it is useful to help identify what the shame is around (e.g., sex in general, sex with men, drug use, being gay), in order to identify how these feelings might be related to triggers for using MA. Stigma around the use of MA and around sex can add to the difficulty clients have in wanting to share their stories with service providers, and engaging in a therapeutic interaction with clinicians.

Building Trust and Acquiring Adaptive Coping Responses as Clinicians

In any therapeutic relationship it is imperative that the health care provider create a safe therapeutic space. This is especially true when dealing with MSM around the treatment of MA. Having respect for the client, being sex positive (i.e., positive attitude about MSM sexual practices) and being nonjudgmental are important. An awareness of one's body language, while also maintaining eye contact, is important, as discomfort around clients' sexual, MSM, and MA use behavior can be communicated to the client nonverbally.

It is vital that clinicians follow what has been recommended (Wallace, 2005): specifically, acquiring adaptive coping responses to the diversity embodied in MSM MA users: acceptance, respect, and empathy. These adaptive affective coping responses are essential, and once established, reduce the chances of behavioral responses or bodily gestures and movements that suggest any maladaptive affective responses (e.g., affects of disdain, disregard, disgust); also, these reduce the chances that there are maladaptive behavioral responses in treatment (e.g., discrimination against MSM MA users, failure to adhere to recommended treatment protocols, ending sessions prematurely, or failing to give supportive or empathic responses) on the part of practitioners (Wallace).

Wallace (2005) describes the full range of adaptive affective, behavioral, and cognitive coping responses clinicians need acquire in order to be considered culturally competent in working with a diverse client population, such as that of MSM who use MA. Adaptive cognitive responses include having an optimistic, positive attitude and thoughts about

MSM who use MA, versus holding a negative prophecy or projecting negative and low expectations upon clients. This takes us into the realm of clinician negative counter-transference (i.e., any feelings or reactions on the part of clinicians in response to clients) reactions to clients. Meanwhile, Wallace is optimistic that clinicians can move across stages of change (Prochaska & DiClemente, 1983) or identity statuses themselves, acquiring more mature, differentiated, and progressive identities consistent with adaptive affective, behavioral, and cognitive responses to diversity—such as that presented by MSM who use MA. Practitioners can move from not thinking about their responses to client diversity and behavior (precontemplation), to thinking about them (contemplation), to determining to work on acquiring more adaptive responses (preparation), to actively working to acquire and refine adaptive responses to diversity (action stage, < 6 months), and to executing increasingly refined adaptive responses over time (maintenance stage, > 6 months). Thus, Wallace (2005) holds out the hope that practitioners can acquire cultural competence over time by systematically self-observing and self-monitoring their own affective, behavioral, and cognitive responses to diversity (e.g., to MSM who use MA), interrupting or stopping those that are maladaptive (e.g., negative, stereotypical, negative prophecies, cutting sessions short, not deploying evidence-based addiction treatment interventions, among others), and consciously deploying adaptive responses until they become increasingly refined and automatic.

Paying Attention to Counter-Transference Reactions

Clinicians working with MSM who are MA users can observe and utilize their counter-transference reactions, or any feelings that develop in them as information. Not all clinician counter-transference reactions mean that the clinician must change or do something more adaptive. In some cases, clinicians, being in the same room as the client, may begin to feel or sense the actual feelings of the client—even becoming filled up with the emotions of the client, as though they are a container for the client's emotions. Indeed, a variety of health care providers may end up having the experience of becoming a container for a client's ambivalent feelings about changing their use, feelings of loss around stopping their use, and feelings that sex will never be as good again—as common initially unspoken feelings. To the extent that clinicians begin to feel such feelings—even as they actually belong to the client—such a cue can be instrumental, leading to a clinician response of seeking to assist the client in moving forward, owning their own feelings (versus depositing them within the clinician, as some metaphoric container), and beginning to process and address their own inner feelings; the ability of clients to tolerate their own uncomfortable feelings can increase over time, along with their ability to communicate them during therapeutic interactions in an overt verbal manner.

A Role for Specific Motivational Interviewing Techniques

The exploration of ambivalent feelings also occurs within the context of the deployment of motivational interviewing techniques (Miller & Rollnick, 2002). Clients may also be asked about their concerns, or those things causing feelings of ambivalence; this may mean reviewing both the "con" side and the "pro" side of change. A *decisional balance* exercise can be utilized so clients clearly explore both the costs and benefits of using

MA and changing their use of MA, as well as any high-risk sexual behavior. This by necessity includes a discussion of how sexual practices, socialization patterns, and MA use are intricately intertwined with each other. As feelings are expressed and ambivalence fully explored, clients, ideally, begin to acquire the intrinsic motivation to begin to move toward change. Clients can also be assisted in generating a menu of options regarding how they might change (e.g., a harm reduction goal, reducing MA use, using condoms during sex when high on MA, or an abstinence goal of abandoning MA use, and/or continuing to engage in sexual practices or changing sexual practices—such as reducing sexual partners, and others). From among the menu of options that are generated, clients can be supported in exploring their next steps, or those options on the menu that they feel ready to take (Miller & Rollnick, 2002). In this manner, clients may also end up moving across stages of change (DiClemente & Velasquez, 2002; Prochaska & DiClemente, 1983), for example, as follows: from a stage of precontemplation where they were not thinking about changing MA use or related sexual practices, to a stages of contemplation where they begin to think about these issues, to a stage of preparation where they determine a need to make changes, to a stage of action where they begin to change some aspect of their behavior (<6 months), and, finally, to a stage of maintenance where clients are maintaining behavioral change over time so it is enduring (>6 months).

The Sex and MA Connection

What has emerged so far in this discussion is how the two behaviors—sexual behavior and MA drug use behavior—have become intricately intertwined in the lives of MSM who are MA users. Over time, MSM MA users tend to develop a "learned association" between MA use and sexual activity. Also tied up in such associations is client identity, to the extent that sexual activity may be directly linked to identity, especially in a society where that identity is not supported via a range of customs, such as gay marriage, for example. For whatever multitude of reasons, it seems as though gay, bisexual, and MSM identities can be so enmeshed with their sexual practices that the thought of stopping MA use may mean stopping or so fundamentally altering certain sexual practices that one's very identity is implicated as a focus of change—even if one does not seek to change one's identity; in other words, identity can feel threatened, because of the idea of having to change MA use may mean having to change some sexual behavior, which may implicate a shift in identity. Even as this takes us into the realm of speculation, what is observed clinically is how the thought of engaging in sex *without* MA drug use can trigger feelings of fear and anxiety. In addition, recovery from MA use is often also recovery from sexual activity that held a close association to MA use. The reality of such close interconnections has to be acknowledged and incorporated into any successful treatment intervention (Nanín & Parsons, 2006).

The Sex and MA Use and HIV-Positive Connection

Additionally, for HIV-positive MA users, the ongoing adjustment at the core of coming to terms with an HIV-positive diagnosis requires attention also being paid to the sex plus MA plus HIV-positive connection; this multiprong focus must also be incorporated into any successful treatment. This has implications when considering treatment interventions for MSM, as the intervention will most likely have to be multifaceted. Attention must be paid to multiple levels and to multiple interrelated behaviors. For example, attention must be paid to all sexual behaviors related to MA use; attention must be paid to those sexual behaviors and MA use behaviors that are related to being HIV-positive or the risk of HIV transmission; attention must also be paid to other HIV-positive related experiences and behaviors, such as medication adherence or side-effects of medication that may be linked to MA use, or identity issues around being HIV-positive and coping with one's status that may be linked to MA use and sexual behavior. Clients may be in different stages of change when it comes to working on (1) their MA use behaviors; (2) their MA related sexual behaviors (e.g., multiple partners or engagement in high-risk behaviors without condom use while high on MA across hours); (3) their HIV related behaviors (e.g., being medication adherent, having regular medical check ups, regular monitoring of viral loads, etc.); and (4) their sexual identity as a MSM (e.g., gay, bisexual, heterosexual, etc.). For each of these four elements, any given client could be in a different stage of change—following the stage-of-change scheme of Prochaska and DiClemente (1983).

For example, a client could be in an action stage for working on their MA use, via either a harm reduction or abstinence strategy (e.g., switching from a high-frequency and high-dose pattern of injection use to a low-frequency and low-dose pattern of intranasal use or oral use). They could also be in a contemplation stage for their related sexual behavior, only thinking about whether they should change, and feeling a great deal of ambivalence. For their HIV related behaviors, they may have once been in a maintenance stage for adherence to their HIV medication and viral load testing, but with escalating addiction to MA relapsed, stopped these behaviors, and are in a stage of precontemplation for resuming medication adherence, perhaps being depressed and grieving the loss of MA. In addition, with regard to their identity, the same client might be in a precontemplation stage, only acknowledging they enjoy MSM behavior, but lacking a gay or bisexual identity—not having thought through or processed what such an identity would mean; and, perhaps avoiding this task because of societal stigma.

Again, what is required is that health care practitioners respond adaptively to such clients and their multitude of characteristics, issues, and related stages of change—offering acceptance, respect, and empathy (Wallace, 2005). In addition, while acknowledging and accepting where a client is in the change process, or their stage of change, practitioners can also deploy motivational interviewing techniques to facilitate clients moving across stages of change (Wallace) as well as across corresponding identity statuses (Wallace et al., 2003) toward more mature, differentiated, and progressive identity statuses. Working on multiple levels either successively or simultaneously, practitioners can meet clients where they are with regard to multiple issues/behaviors.

Table 22.1 is adapted from Wallace (2005) in order to suggest the kinds of multiple issues MSM MA uses may present. The complexity of the challenge for practitioners emerges from this table.

Also, Wallace (2005) goes beyond a discussion of how to use motivational interviewing and the stages of change to tailor treatment to meet client's needs. Indeed, a total of seven evidence-based and seven state-of-the-art practices are recommended, as summarized in Table 22.2, including many mentioned earlier in this chapter.

Wallace (2005) recommends that practitioners learn to select from this menu of options in order to tailor treatment to the multiple needs of diverse contemporary clients, in light of their detailed and ongoing assessments of clients. Providing such training in

Table 22.1 Contemporary MSM Who Are MA Users: Characteristics/Needs

Diverse Demographics

- Representing all races, ethnicities, and religions
- Being of all sexual orientations—gay, bisexual, heterosexual MSM
- Representing all socioeconomic statuses

Varied Drug Use Patterns

- Methamphetamine (MA) use alone or with alcohol, other drugs (sometimes referred to as "trail mix" [see Nanín & Parsons, 2006])

Varied Multiple Addictive and Problem Behaviors

- Presence of more than one addictive behavior (alcohol, crack, marijuana)
- Presence of more than one problem behavior (violence, high-risk sex)
- Combinations of multiple addictive and problem behaviors

Clients With Challenging Comorbidity/Disability

- Combined/Multiple DSM IV-TR Axis I & Axis II Mental Disorders/Disability (i.e., depression)

Varied Health, Disability, and Medical Conditions

- HIV/AIDS and sexually transmitted diseases (STDs)
- Hepatitis B and C virus (HBV and HCV, respectively)
- Prostate problems/cancers
- Smoking-related disease (asthma, coronary heart disease, cancer)
- Chronic disease (diabetes, hypertension, etc.)
- Problems associated with aging: Visual and hearing impairments/disabilities
- Lifelong disabilities: Learning disabilities, speech impairments, etc.

Relationships Among Characteristics: The Mental, Behavioral and Physical Health Nexus

- Mental health compromises behavioral health
- Compromised behavioral health may lead to serious physical health problems

Being in Varied Stages of Change for Multiple Problems

- Stage of change for any one problem behavior varies from precontemplation, to contemplation, preparation, action, or maintenance
- A client may be in a different stage of change for each problem behavior

Histories of Abuse, Trauma, and Violence Across the Life Span

- Childhood neglect, abuse (emotional, physical, sexual), parental domestic violence
- Adolescent and adult rapes, battering/domestic violence, drug culture violence
- Varied patterns of both victimization from and perpetration of violence
- Varied experiences of stigma, homophobia, racism, bias/hate crimes

Source: Adapted from Wallace (2005) to reflect MSM issues.

Table 22.2

Practitioner's Menu of Options: Effective Alternatives

Category I: 7 Evidence Based Addiction Treatments

1. Special focus on building a strong Therapeutic Alliance/Social Support Network (TASS)
2. Motivational Interviewing (MI)/Motivational Enhancement Therapy (MET)/Brief interventions
3. Cognitive-Behavioral Therapy (CBT)/Relapse Prevention (RP)/Social Skills Training (SST)
4. Twelve-Step Facilitation (TSF)/Guidance using Alcoholics and/or Narcotics Anonymous
5. Individual Drug Counseling (IDC) and/or Supportive-Expressive Psychotherapy (SEP)
6. Community Reinforcement Approach (CRA)/Vouchers: Contingency Management (CM)
7. The MATRIX Model—Or, a day treatment approach or "IEC" outpatient model that is "I" or Intensive (4–5 days per week), "E" or Extensive (6–12 months), and "C" or Comprehensive (TASS, CBT/RP, IDC, Group Drug Counseling (GDC), drug testing, etc.).

Category II: 7 Recommended State-of-the-Art Practices

1. Integration of motivational interviewing and stages of change
2. Integration of stages of change and phases of treatment and recovery
3. Integration of harm reduction, moderation approaches, and abstinence models
4. Integration of psychoanalytic and cognitive-behavioral theory and technique
5. Acquisition of affective, behavioral, and cognitive coping skills—learning new "A,B,Cs"
6. Integration of motivational interviewing, stages of change, and identity development theory for a diverse identity involving race, sexual orientation, and/or disability
7. Incorporating contemporary trends in psychology: multiculturalism, positive psychology, the strengths-based approach, and optimistic thinking/learned optimism

Source: Wallace (2005).

an easy-to-follow guide (see Wallace), while using extensive case examples, what emerges is an optimistic view that the most challenging clients with multiple needs—including those that are urgent and must be addressed now (e.g., food, etc.) and those that can be addressed in time (e.g., a decision to practice harm reduction or abstinence for MA use)—can be assisted in cultivating the intrinsic motivation to change.

Moreover, clinicians can assist clients in skills training. Through skills training clients can learn to adaptively affectively, behaviorally, and cognitively cope in response to the challenges they face, while receiving therapeutic services in an atmosphere of acceptance, respect, and empathy. Perhaps most importantly, this process is most successful when clinicians are free of stigmatizing, rejecting, homophobic affective, behavioral, and cognitive responses, and assist clients in also being free of such responses (Wallace, 2005). This also begins to suggest the underlying mechanisms by which the population of MSM who are using MA may begin to experience equity in health care delivery, and experience reductions in disparities in health. A holistic approach that addresses their multiple needs across many closely related domains, while drawing upon evidence-based approaches is recommended, and tailoring interventions for clients, emerges as important, given what appears in Table 22.2. In this manner, what is desired is an approach that is both holistic and integrating evidence-based approaches, while meeting individual client's multiple and varied needs, yet acknowledging their varied stages of change for and willingness to change specific behaviors.

How We Measure Change Matters

Oftentimes treatment providers miss what has changed about clients MA drug use because the focus is on what has not changed. As discussed in this chapter, MA treatment with MSM usually involves addressing multiple issues related to addiction, sexuality, identity, and HIV; and, unlike some other substances, MA treatment tends be a protracted one, with change coming in small increments—often via the introduction of harm reduction as a first step in the change process. Hence, it is vital that practitioners recognize and appreciate all the cumulative steps that constitute progress.

Because there can be multiple issues to address when working with MSM and delivering individually tailored MA treatment, how we measure change matters. How clients see, understand, and feel about their MA use are all important things to consider when assessing behavior change and treatment outcome. Such standards may go above and beyond what practitioners are trained to consider when measuring treatment outcome.

As another important indicator of whether treatment is "working," retention plays a big part in the treatment of MA; and, to the extent that the health care provider is able to keep clients engaged in the treatment process, the greater the likelihood that the underlying issues driving MA use will be able to be addressed; again, adaptive affective responses of acceptance, respect, and empathy are key throughout this process. The goal is to ensure that both practitioners and their treatment programs reflect at their very core an essential feature of cultural competence, effectively managing not only clients' MSM issues, but also issues related to sexual identity, sexual shame, stigma, and all that goes along with being HIV-positive, or a part of a community impacted by the HIV/AIDS epidemic.

Also, given the common characteristics of clients shown in Table 22.1, a discussion of many of which was beyond the scope of this chapter, treatment and program staff not only must be knowledgeable about MA, but also must work collaboratively to create programs that effectively integrate the delivery of mental health and addiction treatment services. The goal is to be able to address the treatment of co-occurring psychiatric disorders, (Levounis & Ruggiero, 2006), as also suggested by Table 22.1.

Conclusion

Among the special populations experiencing disparities in health, MSM who use MA emerge as not only living at the intersection of two epidemics—the HIV/AIDS and methamphetamine epidemics—but also among the most stigmatized groups. This more than justifies researchers learning how to engage the MSM community in studies, as well as clinicians pursing training to ensure that they possess knowledge of evidence-based approaches to treatment, as well as cultural competence. Herein lies the justification for discussing these issues in this chapter, in order to provide training to researchers and clinicians seeking to work toward reducing health disparities involving MSM.

REFERENCES

Bimbi, D. S., Inan, E., Parsons, J. T., Nanín, J. E., Metler, J., & Smith, M. (2006, November). *Entry and motivation for becoming sex workers among gay/bisexual Internet escorts.* Paper presented at the National Conference of the Society for the Scientific Study of Sexuality, Las Vegas, NV.

Boykin, K. (2005). *Beyond the down low: Sex, lies, and denial in Black America.* New York: Carroll & Graf/Avalon.

Buchacz, K., Greenberg, A., Onorato, I., & Janssen, R. (2005). Syphilis epidemics and human immunodeficiency virus (HIV) incidence among men who have sex with men in the United States: Implications for HIV prevention. *Sexually Transmitted Diseases, 32*(10), S73–S79.

Centers for Disease Control and Prevention (CDC). (2003). Internet use and early syphilis infection among men who have sex with men—San Francisco, California, 1999–2003. *Morbidity and Mortality Weekly Report, 52,* 1229–1232.

Centers for Disease Control and Prevention (CDC). (2004). *HIV/AIDS among Hispanics fact sheet.* Retrieved May 20, 2006, from http://www.thebody.com/cdc/pdfs/hispanic2.pdf

Centers for Disease Control and Prevention (CDC). (2005). HIV prevalence, unrecognized infection, and HIV testing among men who have sex with men—Five U.S. cities, June 2004–April 2005. *Morbidity and Mortality Weekly Report, 54,* 597–601.

Centers for Disease Control and Prevention (CDC). (2006). *CDC HIV/AIDS fact sheet: HIV/AIDS among men who have sex with men.* Retrieved January 31, 2007, from http://www.cdc.gov/hiv/topics/msm/resources/factsheets/pdf/msm.pdf

Centers for Disease Control and Prevention (CDC). (2007). *Prevention challenges for prevention partners.* Retrieved July 20, 2007, from http://www.cdc.gov/hiv/topics/msm/challenges_partner.htm

Cole, S. W., Kemeny, M. E., Taylor, S. E., & Visscher, B. R. (1996). Elevated physical health risk among gay men who conceal their homosexual identity. *Health Psychology, 15,* 243–251.

Conway, M., & Dube, L. (2002). Humor in persuasion on threatening topics: Effectiveness is a function of audience sex role orientation. *Personality and Social Psychology Bulletin, 28*(7), 863–873.

Dearing, J. W., Rogers, E. M., Meyer, G., Casey, M. K., Rao, N., Campo, S., et al. (1996). Social marketing and diffusion-based strategies for communicating with unique populations: HIV prevention in San Francisco. *Journal of Health Communication, 1,* 343–363.

DiClemente, C., & Velasquez, M. M. (2002). Motivational interviewing and the stages of change. In W. R. Miller & S. Rollnick (Eds.), *Motivational interviewing: Preparing people for change* (2nd ed.). New York: Guilford Press.

Donovan, D. M., & Marlatt, G. A. (Eds.). (2005). *Assessment of addictive behaviors* (2nd ed.). New York: Guilford Press.

Faugier, J., & Sargeant, M. (1997). Sampling hard to reach populations. *Journal of Advanced Nursing, 26*(4), 790–797.

Fontaine, Y. (2007, March). *Crystal methamphetamine use and HIV risk and prevention among African American men who have sex with both men and women (MSMW).* Paper presented at the 2nd Annual Health Disparities Conference at Teachers College, Columbia University, New York.

Gay and Lesbian Medical Association (GLMA). (2001). *Healthy People 2010 companion document for lesbian, gay, bisexual, and transgender (LGBT) health.* San Francisco: Gay and Lesbian Medical Association.

Greenspan, B. (2001). Health disparities and the U.S. health care system. *Public Health Reports, 116,* 417–418.

Greenwood, G. L., Paul, J. P., Pollack, L. M., Binson, D., Catania, J. A., Chang, J., et al. (2005). Tobacco use and cessation among a household-based sample of US urban men who have sex with men. *American Journal of Public Health, 95*(1), 145–151.

Grov, C., Bimbi, D. S., Nanín, J. E., & Parsons, J. T. (2006). Race, ethnicity, gender, and generational factors associated with the coming out process among gay, lesbian, and bisexual individuals. *Journal of Sex Research, 43*(2), 115–121.

Higgins, S. T., & Silverman, K. (1999). *Motivating behavior change among illicit-drug abusers: Research on contingency management interventions*. Washington, DC: American Psychological Association.

Kaiser Family Foundation. (2006, December 19). *Health disparities report: A weekly look at race, ethnicity and health*. Washington, DC: Kaiser Family Foundation.

Kennamer, J. D., Honnold, J., Bradford, J., & Hendricks, M. (2000). Differences in disclosure of sexuality among African American and White gay/bisexual men: Implication for HIV/AIDS prevention. *AIDS Education and Prevention, 12*, 519–531.

Klausner, J. D., Wolf, W., Fischer-Ponce, L., Zolt, I., & Katz, M. H. (2000). Tracing a syphilis outbreak through cyberspace. *The Journal of the American Medical Association, 284*, 447–449.

Kolodny, A. (2006). Psychiatric consequences of methamphetamine use. *Journal of Gay & Lesbian Psychotherapy, 10*(3/4), 67–72.

Levounis, P., & Ruggiero, J. S. (2006). Outpatient management of crystal methamphetamine dependence among gay and bisexual men: How can it be done? *Primary Psychiatry, 13*(2), 40–45.

Marlatt, G. A., & Witkiewitz, K. (2005). Relapse prevention for alcohol and drug problems. In G. A. Marlatt & D. M. Donovan (Eds.), *Relapse prevention: Maintenance strategies in the treatment of addictive behaviors*. New York: Guilford Press.

Miller, W. R., & Rollnick, S. (2002). Ambivalence: The dilemma of change. In W. R. Miller & S. Rollnick (Eds.), *Motivational interviewing: Preparing people for change* (2nd ed.). New York: Guilford Press.

Millett, G., Malebranche, D., Mason, B., & Spikes, P. (2005). Focusing 'down low': Bisexual black men, HIV risk and heterosexual transmission. *Journal of the National Medical Association, 97*(Suppl 7), 52S–59S.

Minino, A. M., & Smith, B. L. (2001). Preliminary data for 2000 National Center for Health Statistics. *National Vital Statistics Reports, 49*(12), 2–5.

Muhib, F. B., Lin, L. S., Stueve, A., Miller, R. L., Ford, W. L., Johnson, W. D., et al. (2001). A venue-based method for sampling hard-to-reach populations. *Public Health Reports, 116*, 216–222.

Nanín, J., & Parsons, J. (2006). Club drug use and risky sex among gay and bisexual men in New York City. *Journal of Gay and Lesbian Psychotherapy, 10*(3/4), 111–122. (Simultaneously published in *Crystal meth and men who have sex with men: What mental health care professionals need to know*, Milton L. Wainberg, Andrew Kolodny, & Jack Drescher, Eds.)

Nanín, J., Parsons, J., Bimbi, D., Grov, C., & Brown, J. (2006). Community reactions to campaigns addressing crystal methamphetamine use among gay and bisexual men in New York City. *Journal of Drug Education, 36*(4), 285–303.

Parsons, J. T. (2005, April). *How to reach out and touch gay men: Approaches to sexual health research*. Presentation at the 2005 Fall Sexual Health Seminar of the Indiana University Sexual Health Research Working Group.

Parsons, J. T., Bimbi, D. S., Nanín, J. E., & Moran, J. (2006, November). *An educational video targeting club drug use among gay and bisexual men: The biggest mess*. Paper presented at the annual meeting of the American Public Health Association, Boston, MA.

Peacock, J. R. (2000). Gay male adult development: Some stage issues of an older cohort. *Journal of Homosexuality, 40*, 13–19.

Prochaska, J. O., & DiClemente, C. C. (1983). Stages and processes of self-change of cigarette smoking: Toward in integrative model of change. *Journal of Consulting and Clinical Psychology, 51*, 390–395.

Purcell, D. W., Moss, S., Remien, R. H., Parsons, J. T., & Woods, W. J. (2005). Illicit substance use as a predictor of sexual risk taking behavior among HIV-seropositive gay and bisexual men. *AIDS, 19*(S1), S37–S47.

Purcell, D. W., Parsons, J. T., Halkitis, P. N., Mizuno, Y., & Woods, W. (2001). Relationship of substance use by HIV-seropositive men who have sex with men and unprotected anal intercourse with HIV-negative and unknown serostatus partners. *Journal of Substance Abuse, 13*(1–2), 185–200.

Rawson, R. A., Shoptaw, S. J., Obert, J. L., McCann, M. J., Hasson, A. L., Marinelli-Casey, P. J., et al. (1995). An intensive outpatient approach for cocaine abuse treatment: The matrix model. *Journal of Substance Abuse Treatment, 12*(2), 117–127.

Robinson, B., Bockting, W., Rosser, B. R., Miner, M., & Coleman, E. (2002). The Sexual Health Model: Application of a sexological approach to HIV prevention. *Health Education Research, 17*(1), 43–57.

Ryan, C., & Futterman, D. (1998). *Lesbian and gay youth care and counseling: The first comprehensive guide to health and mental health care*. New York: Columbia University Press.

Schuckit, M. A. (2006). *Drug and alcohol abuse: A clinical guide to diagnosis and treatment* (6th ed.). New York: Springer.

Shoptaw, S., Reback, C. J., Peck, J. A., Yang, X., Rotheram-Fuller, E., Larkins, S., et al. (2005). Behavioral treatment approaches for methamphetamine dependence and HIV-related sexual risk behaviors among urban gay and bisexual men. *Drug and Alcohol Dependence, 78*, 125–134.

Smith, E. A., Offen, N., & Malone, R. E. (2006). Pictures worth a thousand words: Non-commercial tobacco content in the lesbian, gay and bisexual press. *Journal of Health Communication, 11*(7), 635–649.

Stokes, J. P., Damon, W., & McKirnan, D. J. (1997). Predictors of movement toward homosexuality: A longitudinal study of bisexual men. *Journal of Sex Research, 34*(3), 304–312.

Tang, H., Greenwood, G. L., Cowling, D. W., Lloyd, J. C., Roeseler, A. G., & Bal, D. G. (2004). Cigarette smoking among lesbians, gays, and bisexuals: How serious a problem? (United States). *Cancer Causes and Control, 15*(8), 797–803.

Taylor, M., Montoya, J. A., Cantrell, R., Mitchell, S. J., Williams, M., Jordahl, L., et al. (2005). Interventions in the commercial sex industry during the rise in syphilis rates among men who have sex with men. *Sexually Transmitted Diseases, 32*(10), S53–S59.

U.S. Department of Health and Human Services (HHS). (2000). *Healthy People 2010: Understanding and improving health* (2nd ed.). Washington, DC: U.S. Government Printing Office.

Wallace, B. C. (2005). *Making mandated addiction treatment work.* Lanham, MD: Jason Aronson/Rowman & Littlefield.

Wallace, B., Carter, R., Nanín, J., Keller, R., & Alleyne, V. (2002). Identity development for "diverse and different others": Integrating stages of change, motivational interviewing, and identity theories for race, people of color, sexual orientation, and disability. In B. Wallace & R. Carter (Eds.), *Understanding and dealing with violence: A multicultural approach.* Thousand Oaks, CA: Sage.

Weiser, J., Nanín, J. E., Parsons, J. T., & Bimbi, D. S. (2006, November). *Attitudes toward parenting among childless members of the LGB community.* Paper presented at the National Conference of the Society for the Scientific Study of Sexuality, Las Vegas, NV.

Lesbian and Bisexual Women of Color, Racism, Heterosexism, Homophobia, and Health: A Recommended Intervention and Research Agenda

23

Introduction

Beverly Greene,
Marie L. Miville,
and Angela D. Ferguson

The delivery of health care services in the new millennium challenges providers in many ways rarely addressed in practice or training as a matter of routine. Similarly, the AIDS epidemic continues to challenge health care researchers and practitioners to examine their methods for the most effective ways of getting needed information to consumers about protecting themselves, seeking treatment when applicable, and getting them to actually use that information. Consider the following: approximately 143.4 million people (50.9%) in the United States are women; approximately 42.1 million people (29.3%) are of racial–ethnic minority groups; and, many women of color experience the same health problems as White women (Office on Women's Health, 2003).

However, as a group, women of color are relatively in poorer health, use fewer health services, and suffer disproportionately from premature death, disease, and disabilities. According to the Office on Women's Health (2003), the leading causes of death among women of color include: heart disease; cancer; cerebrovascular disease, including stroke; diabetes; unintentional injuries; and HIV/AIDS, as a major concern.

Regarding the health status of lesbian and bisexual (LB) women, the following is also known: they are represented in all racial–ethnic groups, socioeconomic strata, and all age groups; no single type of family, community, culture, or demographic category is characteristic of LB women; and, the differences in health risks among LB women can be attributed to these women's health behaviors, stress, and the nature of their experiences with the health care system (Office on Women's Health, 2000).

According to the Gay and Lesbian Medical Association (GLMA, n.d.), common health concerns for LB women include breast cancer, gynecological cancers, depression, physical fitness, domestic violence, and heart health. It has also been reported (Office on Women's Health, 2000) that LB women share the four primary health risk behaviors characteristic of many people living in the United States: tobacco use; alcohol and drug use; poor nutrition and diet; and physical inactivity.

However, we suggest that the underlying stressors for engaging in these health risk behaviors among LB women are likely different from the mainstream population. To better understand health disparities both in the development of illness and health risk behaviors, as well as the resultant differential treatment and outcomes, we believe it is essential that health care providers better understand the significant social, economic, and cultural barriers to achieving optimal health that LB women of color must negotiate. In this chapter, we describe the impact of intersecting identities that affect LB women of color, communication and legal concerns that may lead to complex and difficult diagnostic and treatment considerations and problems of access to health care, and offer recommendations for health care researchers and practitioners.

Multiple Identities

Health and mental health interventions often require behavior change. Any attempt to understand, influence, or change behavior requires an analysis of both the historical and contemporary context of that behavior. One important element of that context can be considered culture, in its broadest sense. We often think of culture as a single identity, such as a persons' ethnicity. However, culture applies far more broadly and encompasses other identities as well, particularly when culture and other identities have a reciprocal effect on one another. Every individuals' personal, social, familial, and intrapsychic history and current life circumstances are embedded in the context of the sociopolitical realities of their lives and the history of those realities. It is also embedded in the sociopolitical history of the group or groups that they belong to or identify with in some way. These realities include, among other things, where people's identities place them on the social hierarchy of privilege and disadvantage with respect to those identities and how each of those positions moderates the other (race/ethnicity, gender, sexual orientation, physical or emotional disability, socioeconomic class, etc.), as well as the prevailing reality of social inequalities and their effects on those peoples' opportunities to develop their abilities, their understanding of who they are, what they may or may not do and what they are entitled to. These sociocultural and sociopolitical matrices have shaped their development and shaped their response to health, challenges to health, as well as other stressors; hence it will shape the degree to which they are likely or unlikely to present themselves for or comply with treatment. Therefore these factors must be understood by those of us who attempt to provide members of this population with care.

It is also important to understand the ways that no one locus of identity totally defines an individual. Each aspect of that person or identity is conflated by others requiring that we view our clients and patients from a perspective that understands that they have multiple, overlapping, kaleidoscopic, rather than static, monolithic, compartmentalized, or fixed identities. Lesbian and bisexual women of color represent a group with a complex matrix of identities in which one identity may be valued or highlighted in one setting and devalued in another. The level of psychosocial stressors that are inherent in the lives of most of these women may put them at higher risk for developing certain health and mental health problems; however, it also places them at higher risk for getting no or inferior care from service providers for a variety of reasons as well as less attention in the research arena. We will briefly discuss some of the perhaps less than obvious factors that contribute to this problem and include a few that are more familiar.

An important factor contributing to the access and quality of health care rendered to lesbian and bisexual women of color patients is the provider's beliefs about the client; however, it is perhaps the least examined aspect of care. Just as patients and clients are shaped by their sociocultural histories, so are providers (Greene, 1996, 1998a). The attitudes, feelings, and beliefs that providers harbor about their patients may have profound effects on the services they render to them; however, training rarely teaches providers the importance of understanding their role in this way. Providers as well as patients are socialized in a broader, dominant culture that gives us all kinds of information about people and groups whom we may have never met. Racial and ethnic differences, lesbian sexual orientations, gender differences, disability, the impoverished, the wealthy and the social tensions that surround them are issues that most people have feelings about, some of them, intense feelings. Providers are no exception.

In March 1999, *The New England Journal of Medicine* published an article whose findings suggest that the race and sex of the patient independently influenced how physicians in the study managed the same complaints of chest pain. Racist, sexist, heterosexist, and other biases have had a profound impact on the health and mental health literature in theoretical paradigms, as well as practice. Generally, it is important that providers be culturally literate, that is that they have some broad familiarity with the general characteristics of their patient's culture as well as the special health or mental health needs, pressures, or vulnerabilities that are a function of group membership, but more. Mental health practitioners are ethically required to scrutinize their own personal attitudes, feelings, and responses to clients who are members of many social groups, and to be aware of the negative stereotypes and beliefs about those clients and their impact on diagnostic and treatment decisions. We assume that when unexamined these factors predispose clinicians to make a range of unwarranted and inaccurate assumptions about their patients and their patients experiences, and hence, less than helpful interventions.

Women of Color: African American, Asian, Latina, and Native American

It is important to understand the ubiquitous reality of racism and sexism for women of color and the coping mechanisms that they must utilize to negotiate this reality; the way that racism colors the gender discrimination that most women face; and the role of racism, heterosexism, and social class in contributing to barriers to access of health and mental health care. Women of color have endured a history of discrimination and bias that does not exclude the medical and mental health professionals. Many members of this large and diverse population do not trust doctors, western medicine, or the medical establishment. For some, their distrust is based on a history of negative or harmful experiences (directly experienced or told to them) encountered when seeking professional assistance. Others base their distrust on disgraceful historical episodes in which members of minority groups were used in medical research in ways that were harmful to them. The sexual objectification of African Americans during slavery and other women of color during various periods in our history has been reinforced by images propagated of them, fueling a range of negative stereotypes and myths about their aberrant sexual desire and practices (Greene, 1996, 1998a). These myths are relevant to the development of the images that women of color have of themselves, particularly their sexuality.

For women of color who have internalized the negative stereotypes of their sexuality, sexual behavior outside of dominant societal norms can be experienced as a negative reflection on all members of their groups (Greene, 1996). Lipsky (1987) suggests that narrow, limited views of any given culture, of what authentic cultural behavior is, and anger about anything that differs too much from the mythical ideal of the middle class of the majority culture exemplifies internalized racism.

Lesbians

There has been significant movement in both the mental health and medical professions toward viewing lesbian sexual orientations as normal variations in developmental outcomes. Despite the growth and prominence of research in both areas, bias in health and mental health practice still persists. A majority of professional training programs do not routinely address the special considerations in the treatment of such patients, nor do they address the effects of a history of biased research on practitioner attitudes toward lesbian patients.

A physician's ability to properly diagnose and treat health care problems, particularly those that have a psychosocial component, is facilitated by having accurate information about the lifestyle of the patient. Many health and mental health practitioners presume the heterosexuality of patients, rather than taking a more neutral stance to the potential for the patient to fit anywhere on the spectrum of sexual orientation, even if they are presently in a heterosexual marriage. The answer to the question about whether or not someone is married does not necessarily tell us about all of his or her sexual partners, nor does it tell us about the gender of all partners. There are many women who have sex with women who do not label themselves lesbian nor do they construct an identity around whom they have sex with; many women who are formally married to men have sex with other women; and many women who label themselves lesbian have or have had sex with men. The assumption that the patient could be heterosexual, lesbian, or bisexual or that any range of sexual behavior is possible, leaves the practitioner free to ask a range of questions about their behavior and particularly sexual behaviors that are not typically explored when only one assumption is made. This is particularly important in the treatment of lesbian patients in general because they may be accustomed to withholding information about their sexual orientation and lesbians of color may do so to a greater extent than white lesbians. This level of caution may represent the culmination of experiences where disclosing it was used against the patient.

For example, Stevens (1995) interviewed a racially and socioeconomically diverse group of 45 lesbians and asked them to describe their access to and experience with health care. Findings suggest that heterosexist structuring of health care services delivery was designed and distributed with the assumption that heterosexual sexual orientation was universal, superior, natural, and/or required for women. The women interviewed observed that clinical, health education practices and policies were organized around the assumption that all female clients were heterosexual. Bias was apparent in written forms, brochures, posters, comments by office or hospital auxiliary and clerical staff, in advertisements for clientele, reading materials in the waiting room and pictures on the walls. For example, forms routinely required women to identify themselves as married, divorced, single, or widowed and went on to ask about the spouse's income, occupation, health insurance, and where *he* can be reached. The only opportunities to give information about a partner were through questions about a husband's activities.

Many women complained that messages about health and prevention were geared toward heterosexual women and that they had to translate or read between the lines to figure out what applied to them—some come away thinking that certain risk factors don't apply to them (although some women who consider themselves lesbian do have sex with men). Others reported concerns about the lack of legal recognition of their relationships that becomes particularly problematic when one is ill. For example, in the absence of the ability to legally marry, next-of-kin rules prevented them from seeing partners in ICUs (e.g., one woman reported that when her partner was hospitalized and she would ask questions, staff would look at her as if to ask: who are you?) Other clients of mine have responded to the dilemma by saying they are the patient's sister, and so on. The woman's partner may not be seen as the important source of intimate information about the patient that she is such that valuable information about the patient may be lost. Nor is the partner seen as the person who will be the primary caregiver (who in turn needs information from health care staff to do that properly); they may not be allowed to accompany them in ambulances.

Overall, findings suggest that lesbian patients have a wide range of health concerns and needs, and that they perceive medical practitioners as having little background information for understanding their concerns and an atmosphere in which it was not safe to pursue their questions.

This speaks to the issue of safety in disclosure. Cochran and Mays' survey in 1988 suggests that lesbians were reluctant to disclose their sexual orientation to their doctors to the extent that roughly only a third had done so. Patterns such as this complicate the ability to determine patterns of gynecologic and other forms of health risk. White and Dull (1997) observe that many lesbians in their study report feeling that their doctors are not sensitive to or knowledgeable about the specific health risks or needs of lesbians. Many of those who sought health care were uncomfortable with the relationship with their provider and as a result fail to disclose information that may be pertinent to their health. Sixty-one percent of the lesbians in this study reported that they felt unable to disclose their sexual orientation to their doctors and some 20% (almost half of those who did disclose) reported negative reactions from their provider after doing so. These experiences confirmed their feeling that they should not have done so. Issues of disclosure or nondisclosure can have important implications. Gomez (1995) observes that while lesbians who do not inject drugs and who have sex exclusively with women may fall on the low end of the risk for HIV continuum, they can never be presumed to have no risk at all. In her research, the potential for infection may not differ but the perception of one's risk does.

The failure to disclose sexual orientation may also represent a way of having to make conscious decisions about when, and whom to tell, rather than simply having it known. Such a patient may enter such encounters with a heightened level of suspicion of the medical establishment, white practitioners, and heterosexual practitioners as well. Because of the history of misinformation about lesbians and gay men and about people of color, even when sexual orientation is known, practitioners may make a range of assumptions about what it means that are disparaging and untrue. Heterosexual therapists who are uncomfortable with these issues may be even more likely to harbor such questionable beliefs. For example, they may assume that lesbian patients are preoccupied with sexual matters and that women or color are similarly preoccupied, that a lesbian is more like or wants to be a man, are more sexually active or engage in a wide range of unsafe sexual practices than do heterosexual women. They may also assume that a lesbian sexual orientation is synonymous with being promiscuous. Similarly, such assumptions may be made about women of color for whom historically racist stereotypes foster a view of, for example, African Americans as sexually promiscuous or preoccupied (Greene, 1996).

It may not be unusual for the lesbian client to express reluctance or refusal to discuss sexual practices with their health or mental health practitioners. Such reluctance is understandable as many lesbian clients have accurately experienced such inquiries as voyeuristic on the part of homophobic doctors who then attribute the patient's problems to their sexual orientation. It is important to be sensitive to the client's feelings about making such disclosures; however, that does not mean that inquiries should remain unexplored if the information needed is important to the patient's effective treatment. It is, however, the practitioner's responsibility in this realm to earn patients' trust and to help them understand how the information is of importance to their care. Heterosexual practitioners who respond to the patient's reluctance by avoiding asking any other questions in this realm may view this as respecting the patient's feelings. It can also serve as an avoidance on the practitioner's part that is designed to circumvent his or her own discomfort. The culturally sensitive treatment of lesbians of color occurs amidst a history of misinformation about them and brings those provocative issues together in a profound way. This can raise a range of challenges to even the most experienced practitioner (Greene, 1996, 1998a).

Initially, we must be culturally literate in our familiarity with the broader characteristics of the client's culture as well as the special needs and vulnerabilities of lesbian of color clients. As many training programs do not routinely provide assistance with such challenges, practitioners must be willing to augment their training elsewhere.

White, heterosexual therapists may have difficulty understanding and believing the reality of the barriers and stressors imposed by racism and homophobia in the patient's life. They may respond by becoming frustrated with the patient's presumed noncompliance without recognizing the obstacles the patient may encounter in attempting to comply with the doctor's treatment plan. They may also bend over backwards in ways that infantilize the patient. Striking an appropriate balance is a challenge (Greene, 1998a). Earlier in this chapter we referred to the concept of multiple identities or the notion that most patients have more than one important locus of identity and that they may include more than one identity that is disadvantaged. This is particularly relevant for lesbian and bisexual women of color.

Lesbian and Bisexual Women of Color

Lesbian and bisexual women of color are members of two groups whose needs are underrepresented in both the health and mental health scholarly literature and practice and as such face the potential of being poorly understood. The predominance of research on lesbians is based on groups of white lesbians. Similarly, the research on men and women of color rarely makes distinctions between the sexual orientation of participants and by inference presumes the heterosexuality of group members. In this realm, we are left with a paucity of information about the complexity of ethnic identity development and its interaction with sexual orientation identity development, and an ensuing gap in our knowledge base about a significant group of patients. Practitioners who are not sensitive to many of the unique stressors that impinge on lesbians of color may fail to ask questions relevant to their life circumstances in ways that are detrimental to their appropriate treatment.

Heterosexist and ethnic biases may lead practitioners to make a range of assumptions about lesbians, and about people of color that are erroneous. A commonly accepted belief is that lesbians wish to be men and are therefore confused about their appropriate gender role. In such a framework women are expected to be sexually attracted only to men. Being sexually attracted to the other gender culminating in reproductive sexuality has been traditionally deemed intrinsic to being a normal man or woman, as that which is psychologically normal and morally correct. Historical support for this premise from traditional psychological and medical perspectives facilitated the acceptance of viewing lesbians as defective women. It remains a persistent belief among some practitioners despite a recent burgeoning research literature to the contrary. Hence, an understanding of the meaning of being a lesbian of color requires a careful exploration of the importance of cultural gender roles, and both the nature and relative fluidity or rigidity of the culture's traditional gender stereotypes. For members of some oppressed groups, specifically African and Native Americans, reproductive sexuality is viewed as the means of continuing the groups' presence in the world. Hence, birth control or sexuality that is not reproductive may be viewed even by one's own group members as instruments of genocide. As sexuality is contextual, what it means to be a lesbian will be related to the meaning assigned to sexuality in the culture. An understanding of the role of ethnic stereotypes in the creation of sexual mythologies about people of color is another important component. The overarching task is that of understanding the ubiquitous reality of heterosexism for all lesbians; the ways that racism complicates the experience of heterosexism for lesbians of color; the range of negative stereotypes of lesbians; and the presumption of the heterosexuality of clients and their effects (Greene, 2000a, 2000b).

Social Class and Poor Women

Rarely do we pose questions regarding the effect of socioeconomic class on the development of identity. We know that class status and income affects variables like physical health, life span, quality of primary education, access to higher education, likelihood of arrest or imprisonment, and the general quality of life of all persons. We all know that money has a concrete and tangible effect on the kind of health care people receive, if at all; and, at what stage of mental or medical illness they seek care and what they get. It determines whether or not patients can fill a prescription, and whether or not they can keep appointments if transportation to offices, clinics or hospitals costs money—also depending on how far away they live from those services. All of those factors affect compliance. While we may not always be able to affect the kinds of financial resources patients have access to, we can address the issue of the clinician's attitude toward poor patients and not displace our frustration with the paucity of their resources or negative stereotypes about poor lesbian and bisexual women of color onto them (Greene, 2000b).

Women of Color, Lesbians, and Women With Disabilities

It is crucial that we understand the impact of the invisibility of women with disabilities in our society that makes the visibility of lesbians of color even more stark. Overall we are socialized to view women with disabilities as if they were asexual. Other factors influencing their care are the realistic physical barriers that such clients must negotiate when seeking care, and the cost and the ways that the effects of their disability is conflated by racism, sexism, classism, and homophobia.

Another invisible minority of women are those who are physically challenged. Research on heterosexual women, lesbians, and on women of color who have physical challenges are conspicuously absent from the literature. This omission can suggest that sexual orientation or ethnicity is the master identity, that heterosexism or racism is the primary locus of oppression, that there are no lesbians or gay men who have physical challenges, which we know is not so, or that the presence of a physical challenge does not have a salient impact on the identity or life of heterosexual women, lesbians, or women of color, or that the impact on one of these groups is the same on all of them (Greene, 2000b).

Fine and Asch (1988) observe that in research on disability, sexual orientation, gender, race, and class seem to be regarded as similarly irrelevant, suggesting that having a disability overshadows all other dimensions of social experience. They suggest that disability (as opposed to the mere presence of physical challenges), like gender, sexual orientation, ethnicity, and so forth, is a social construct. Solomon (1993) writes that it is the interaction between the presence of physical challenges or biological impairments and social, environmental, and cultural factors and social prejudice that determines whether or not the physical impairment becomes a disability. In their reviews of the literature on disabled women, Fine and Asch (1988) found

> no data on the numbers of lesbians with disabilities or on their acceptance by nondisabled lesbians as partners, but comments made by many disabled lesbians indicate that within the community of lesbians the disabled woman is still in search of love (p. 3).

Lesbians are the victims of the stereotype of being less attractive and less feminine than heterosexual women just as women with disabilities are regarded. Yet, we have virtually no information about the ways that these identities triply stigmatize lesbians of color with disabilities. Generally, research on most disabled women makes it clear that they are not seen as sexual beings (Greene, 2000b). The paucity of data on lesbians with disability challenges is such that making any generalizations would be questionable at best. Often, we are left with more questions than answers. What is it like for women in these communities who as a function of their physical challenges are not even seen as sexual beings and what effects do these perceptions have on the health care they receive?

Despite reports from men and women with disabilities that social factors influence their sexual experiences more profoundly that physiological factors, social factors are rarely discussed in the psychological literature (Greene, 2000b; Linton, 1998).

Communication and Legal Issues

Communication and legal issues may be illustrated via two brief cases.

Gloria is a 38-year-old African American woman. When completing the intake information form, she indicates that she is married, has used contraceptives, and that she is currently sexually active. This is her first office visit to a gynecologist in several years.

Carmen is a 24-year-old Latina. On her form, she indicates that she is single, sexually active, and does not use contraceptives. She reports that she is experiencing vaginal itching and irritation. This is her first visit to the gynecologist.

The two cases described above demonstrate a number of communication issues that often arise in the acquisition of important medical information from LB women of color. Most practitioners in private settings and hospitals presume the heterosexuality of their patients, and thus their intake forms, doctor–patient consultations, and other means of collecting important medical data (as well as the ensuing treatment regimens) often reflect this inaccurate presumption. Moreover, there are many patients who (a) may not label themselves lesbian or bisexual nor do they construct an identity around whom they have sex with; (b) may be married or who label themselves as heterosexual yet have sex with other women; or (c) label themselves lesbian who have or have had sex with men.

For example, many intake forms often identify relationship status markers as including single, married, widowed, or divorced, without allotting any space for patients to clearly identify their same-sex partners as spouses. This is particularly the case for medical practices whose primary patient base is made up of women (e.g., obstetrician, gynecologist). Moreover, given the extreme legal and social consequences that many LB women of color face for being "out" regarding their sexual orientation, they may be reluctant to describe same-sex behaviors or partners on these forms, given concerns for the confidentiality of this information and how this might be used against them. Indeed, it is not unusual for LB patients of color to express reluctance or refusal to discuss sexual practices with their health care practitioners. Such reluctance is understandable as many LB patients of color have accurately experienced such inquiries as voyeuristic on the part of racist or homophobic doctors who then attribute their patients' problems to their race-ethnicity or sexual orientation or both. It is important for health care practitioners to be sensitive to patient feelings about making such disclosures; however we do not suggest that such inquiries remain unexplored if the information is needed for effective treatment. Heterosexual practitioners who respond to patient reluctance by avoiding asking any other questions in this realm may view this as respecting their patients' feelings. However, we caution that avoidance can be a means of masking practitioners' own discomfort.

We also suggest that the answer to a question about whether or not someone is married, does not necessarily provide sufficient information about all of their patients' sexual partners, nor does it indicate the gender of all partners. This is particularly important in the treatment of lesbian patients in general because they may be used to withholding information about their sexual orientation. This level of caution may represent the culmination of experiences where self-disclosure was used against the patient.

In Gloria's case, it is possible that the information she has provided about being "married" refers to a long-standing same-sex relationship or a man, but health care providers would likely be unaware of the former situation. Moreover, Gloria indicates that she has used contraceptives, leading to a potentially erroneous conclusion that she is engaged in exclusively heterosexual behaviors. In contrast, Carmen's non-use of contraceptives may reflect a lack of information on her part, but it also may indicate a lesbian orientation and perhaps a need for information regarding safe sex practices (e.g., dental dams) for sexual behaviors with other women (this at least should be assessed by the health care worker).

Another common area of misinterpretation is the provision of contact information of another person should there be a medical emergency. Some LB women of color may indicate a "friend" as this contact who in reality is a spouse. More broadly, the lack of inclusive or accurate requests for information on forms or in doctor–patient consultations indicates to LB patients of color the lack of awareness and perhaps acceptance of their sexual orientation or same-sex sexual behaviors, reinforcing the assumption of heteronormativity. This may lead many LB women of color either not to come back, leading to further delay in obtaining prevention or treatment of their illnesses and conditions, or to distort important personal information due to their concerns about receiving caring and well-informed treatment. At a psychological level, these heterosexist experiences with health care services may reinforce internalized homophobia, perhaps leading to increased stress levels and risky health behaviors. We suggest that both premature termination as well as limited or inaccurate provision of important personal information thus may be a cause of some of the early deaths of LB women of color.

The lack of knowledge and understanding concerning racial–ethnic and sexual orientation identities also may lead practitioners to engage in neglectful, prejudicial, and even abusive behaviors with some of their patients. A majority of professional training programs do not routinely address these considerations in the treatment of their patients, nor do they address the effects of a history of biased research on practitioner attitudes toward LB patients. Because of the history of misinformation about lesbians and gay men and about people of color, even when sexual orientation is known, practitioners may make a range of assumptions that are disparaging and untrue (Greene, 1996, 1998a). Heterosexual health care workers who are uncomfortable with sexual orientation issues may be even more likely to harbor questionable beliefs. For example, they may assume that LB patients are preoccupied with sexual matters, are more like men, or are more sexually active or engage more in a wide range of unsafe sexual practices than do heterosexual women. They also may assume that an LB is synonymous with being promiscuous. Similarly, such assumptions may be made about people of color for whom historically racist stereotypes foster a view of, for example, African Americans as sexually promiscuous or preoccupied, or of Asian Americans as nonsexual or ascetic. White, heterosexual health care workers in particular may have difficulty understanding and believing the reality of the barriers and stressors imposed by both racism and homophobia/heterosexism in their patients' lives. They may respond by becoming frustrated with their patients' presumed noncompliance without recognizing the obstacles their patients may encounter in attempting to comply with their doctors' treatment plan. Physicians also may bend over backwards in ways that infantilize the patient. Unfortunately, many physicians are simply unaware that their abilities to properly diagnose and treat health care problems, particularly those that have a psychosocial component, is facilitated by having accurate information about the lifestyle of their patients (Greene, 1998a; Schulman et al., 1999).

Research conducted by Stevens (1995) provides support for several of these concerns. Many women complained that messages about health and prevention were geared toward heterosexual women and that they had to translate or read between the lines to figure out what applied to them. Some even came away thinking that certain risk factors may not apply to them. In sum, Stevens' findings suggest that lesbian patients have a wide range of health concerns and needs, and that they perceive medical practitioners as having little background information for understanding their concerns and an atmosphere in which it was not safe to pursue their questions (Cochran & Mays, 1988; Stevens, 1995).

Legal issues may lead to further complexities regarding accurate diagnoses and effective medical treatment, since in most states same-sex relationships have no legally recognized status. Indeed, many states have passed anti-gay legislation regarding marriage, which may preclude the inclusion of same-sex spouses in the notification and consultation about serious medical concerns. Stevens (1998) found that lesbian patients reported concerns about the lack of legal recognition of their relationships becomes particularly problematic when one is ill.

Access to Health Care

The overriding health care concern for LB women of color is *access* to health care. Due to concerns we already have described, many LB women of color delay health-seeking behaviors until they are symptomatic or the symptoms are at their worst (White & Dull, 1997). Still others may find health care procedures traumatizing. For example, some anecdotal evidence suggests that "butch" or male identified LB women may find visits to the gynecologist difficult or impossible to endure (Mautner Project, n.d.). A major dilemma for these women involves their self-perception as always being in control and minimizing their feminine selves, including their physical anatomy. Placing their feet in stirrups or undergoing a mammogram may lead to deeply felt experiences of anxiety, perhaps even depression. At the same time, like all women, these patients are most effectively treated with annual exams. Acknowledging their difficult feelings will go a long way toward more effective and consistent treatment. Traumatic experiences with previous practitioners who were insensitive, uninformed, even abusive, also may keep many LB women of color from pursuing health care that would save their lives or receiving accurate diagnoses and treatment. Further, estrangement from families and fears of power struggles in emergency situations may keep LB women of color from seeking needed services until too late. Finally, given the heterosexist nature of most medical practice, unique medical needs of LB women of color are rarely identified, let alone treated (Greene, 1998b).

At more systemic levels, several important barriers have been identified for treating women of color. For example, Dennis (2004) notes that major treatment procedures varies by race and gender with women of color having significantly lower rates of common medical procedures than White women. She further notes that health insurance rates vary by race and gender with women of color typically having lower occurrences of coverage. Economic barriers also play a major role, given the lower incomes and educational levels and higher poverty rates of many women of color (Office on Women's Health, 2003). Social and cultural barriers are important as well, particularly language and religious differences, as well as differing cultural beliefs about health and health care.

The Office on Women's Health (2003) has identified barriers within the health care system itself that have traditionally ignored the needs of women of color. With regard to *Medical Practice*, these include: an inadequate numbers of practitioners; practitioners not located where many patients live; and communication barriers, such as language differences. In terms of *Medical Education* pertinent barriers include little training in cultural competence and, little training in community practice. Under the category of *Medical Research* barriers involve: how people of color and women are not included in many studies; there is misreporting of demographic information; and data are collected in small subgroups that may inaccurately represent the population of interest. With regard to *Medical Leadership*, barriers include: too few practitioners are women of color; there is inadequate communication between practitioners and patients; and medical services are insensitive to cultural attitudes and health needs.

Thus, it is apparent that multiple and interlocking barriers exist that prevent even knowledgeable and motivated LB women of color from seeking and obtaining effective health care services. We turn now to recommendations for health care workers in their work with patients who are LB women of color.

Summary and Recommendations

There is the potential for negative effects on the physical health and psychological well-being of many of the women who belong to the groups we have discussed. It is important for all health practitioners to be aware of the unique combinations of stressors and psychological demands impinging on LB women of color, particularly the potential for barriers and maltreatment in encounters with service providers.

Overall, it is the practitioner's responsibility to make the treatment setting one that is safe for the client to disclose important information and be regarded with respect. A proactive understanding of the potential for barriers in that realm with these patients may serve to facilitate negotiating those barriers should they arise (Greene, 1996, 1998a).

Sexism and heterosexism affect women of color and White women differently. Racism affects African American heterosexual, lesbian, and bisexual women differently. Being a person of color shapes the construction and understanding of that person's sexuality, just as their sexuality shapes the construction of their ethnic identification. It also shapes the construction and manifestations of heterosexism and internalized homophobia as well. Gender, race, and sexual orientation oppression interact with one another in particular ways, and all shape and interact with the personality dynamics of each individual. Any analysis which fails to take this complex interaction of experiences and their effects into account can neither sensitively nor appropriately address the treatment of lesbian and bisexual women of color. Cultural literacy includes understanding the plight of women from the groups we have discussed in the context of the following factors:

1. The prevailing reality of the convergence of race, gender, and sexual orientation and other forms of bias (age, disability, etc.) and the interpersonal and institutional barriers which result in a patient's life experience. This includes a familiarity with the dominant culture's view of women's roles in general, and the roles or the place if you will of the women of that group; and their histories as distinct from its view of White women's roles and histories. It also requires an explicit understanding of the ethnosexual mythologies about women of color, as well as the sexual myths about poor women, women with disabilities, and lesbians.

2. A willingness on the part of the practitioner to validate the patient's accurate perceptions of discrimination and bias and their impact on the patient's life.

3. The wide range of similarities and diversities that exist within all women as a group, the subgroups we have discussed herein and the heterogeneity within those subgroups.

4. The individual client's intrapsychic and familial endowments and personal history as they are embedded in the aforementioned context.

5. An acknowledgment of the practitioner's own feelings and attitudes about the patient and their potential impact on our ability to maintain an empathic relationship with the client. This includes the practitioner's personal scrutiny about his or her feelings and motivations for working with clients who are members of the groups discussed, and how our practice and thinking is organized around considering their particular needs, whether or not the structure of our facilities even consider those needs.

Ultimately we are charged with the task of developing paradigms that assist us in better understanding the ongoing, dynamic, and interactive nature of constituents of human identity, in a context in which any single aspect of identity colors, transforms, and informs the meaning of others in reciprocal ways. Incorporating diverse perspectives and concerns in our paradigms should facilitate a more authentic understanding of all human beings. Omitting these diverse perspectives leaves us with a narrow and distorted view of women's worlds and realities. In this inclusive paradigm we will no longer need to see people as the same in order to treat them with fairness. We can make the important leap from equal treatment, which presumes sameness, to fair and sensitive treatment, one that acknowledges and even celebrates the richness of human differences (Greene, 1996; 1998a).

REFERENCES

Cochran, S. D., & Mays, V. M. (1988). Disclosure of sexual preference to physicians by Black lesbian and bisexual women. *Western Journal of Medicine*, *149*, 616–619.

Dennis, S. W. (2004). *Breaking down barriers to health care for women with disabilities*. Retrieved February 24, 2007, from www.hhs.gov/od/summit/dennis.ppt

Fine, M., & Asch, A. (Eds.). (1988). *Women with disabilities: Essays in psychology, culture, and politics.* Philadelphia: Temple University Press.

Gay and Lesbian Medical Association (GLMA). (n.d.). *Guidelines for care of lesbian, gay, bisexual, and transgender patients.* Retrieved February 24, 2007, from http://ce54.citysoft.com/_data/n_0001/resources/live/GLMA%20guidelines%202006%20FINAL.pdf

Gomez, C. A. (1995). Lesbians at risk for HIV: The unresolved debate. In G. Herek & B. Greene (Eds.), *AIDS, identity & community: The HIV epidemic and lesbians and gay men.* Thousand Oaks, CA: Sage.

Greene, B. (1996). African American women: Considering diverse identities and societal barriers in psychotherapy. In J. A. Sechzer, S. M. Pfafflin, F. L. Denmark, A. Griffin, & S. J. Blumenthal (Eds.), *Annals of the NY Academy of Science: Women and mental health, 789,* 191–209.

Greene, B. (1998a). Stereotypes and erroneous presumptions: Barriers to effective practice with lesbian and gay patients of color. *Medical Encounter, 14*(2), 15–17.

Greene, B. (1998b). Family, ethnic identity and sexual orientation among African American lesbians and gay men. In C. Patterson & A. D'Augelli (Eds.), *Lesbian, gay and bisexual identity: Psychological research & social policy* (pp. 40–52). New York: Oxford University Press.

Greene, B. (2000a). Homophobia. In A. E. Kazdin (Ed.), *Encyclopedia of psychology.* Washington, DC: American Psychological Association and Oxford University Press.

Greene, B. (2000b). Beyond heterosexism and across the cultural divide: Developing an inclusive lesbian, gay and bisexual psychology. In B. Greene & G. L. Croom (Eds.), *Education, research and practice in LGBT psychology: A resource manual* (pp. 1–45). Thousand Oaks, CA: Sage.

Linton, S. K. (1998). *Claiming disability: Knowledge and identity.* New York: New York University Press.

Lipsky, S. (1987). *Internalized racism.* Seattle, WA: Rational Island Publishers.

Mautner Project. (n.d.). *Lesbian health risks: Factors facing a medically underserved population.* Retrieved February 24, 2007, from http://www.mautnerproject.org/health%5Finformation/Provider%5FResources/

Office on Women's Health. (2000). *Lesbian health fact sheet.* Retrieved February 24, 2007, from http://www.4woman.gov/owh/pub/factsheets/lesbian1.pdf

Office on Women's Health. (2003). *The health of minority women.* Retrieved February 24, 2007, from http://www.4woman.gov/owh/pub/minority/minority.pdf

Schulman, K. A., Berlin, J. A., Harless, W., Kerner, J. F., Sistrunk, S., Gersh, B. J., et al. (1999). The effect of race and sex on physicians' recommendations for cardiac catheterization. *New England Journal of Medicine, 340*(14), 618–626.

Solomon, S. (1993). Women and physical distinction: A review of the literature and suggestions for intervention. *Women & Therapy, 14*(3/4), 91–103.

Stevens, P. E. (1995). Structural and interpersonal impact of heterosexual assumptions on lesbian health care clients. *Nursing Research, 44*(1), 25–30.

Stevens, P. E. (1998). The experiences of lesbians of color in health care encounters: Narrative insights for improving access and quality. *Journal of Lesbian Studies, 2*(1), 77–94.

White, J. C., & Dull, V. T. (1997). Health risk factors and health seeking behavior in lesbians. *Journal of Women's Health, 6*(1), 103–112.

Ethnic/Racial Disparities in Gay-Related Stress and Health Among Lesbian, Gay, and Bisexual Youths: Examining a Prevalent Hypothesis

24

Margaret Rosario, Eric W. Schrimshaw, and Joyce Hunter

Introduction

Lesbian, gay, and bisexual (LGB) individuals are more likely than their heterosexual peers to experience a variety of mental health and health-related problem behaviors, including emotional distress, suicidality, substance use, and sexual risk behaviors. However, demonstrably less research has examined health disparities *within* the LGB community—particularly the potential for ethnic/racial disparities in LGB health. Indeed, there has been much discussion proposing that Black and Latino LGB individuals experience more gay-related stress than White LGB individuals due to various cultural pressures against homosexuality that exist within the Black and Latino communities. These higher levels of stress—both gay-related and non–gay-related—are expected to lead to ethnic/racial disparities in health and health-related behaviors among LGB individuals. In this report, we investigate potential ethnic/racial differences in gay-related and non–gay-related stress among a sample of Black, Latino, and White LGB youths in New York City. We further examine whether ethnic/racial disparities exist in various mental health and health-related behaviors of LGB youths. We then examine whether gay-related stress may account for (i.e., mediate) the potential ethnic/racial disparities among LGB youths. We begin this report by reviewing the research on sexual orientation disparities in health among LGB youths, followed by a review of what is currently known about potential ethnic/racial disparities in stress and health among LGB youths.

Health Risks of LGB Youths

A growing literature—much of it with large representative samples—has documented that LGB youths (and adults) are more likely than heterosexuals to experience poorer health, more health-related risk behaviors (including greater emotional distress), and a higher prevalence of suicidality, substance use and abuse, and sexual risk behaviors. These disparities have been found regardless of the definitions used to assess sexual orientation (i.e., LGB self-identification, same-sex behavior, same-sex attractions, or some combination thereof).

Studies have found that LGB youths report poorer mental health than heterosexual youths (Safren & Heimberg, 1999; Williams, Connolly, Pepler, & Craig, 2005), such that they are 1.6–4.0 times more likely to report depression and anxiety than heterosexual youths (Fergusson, Horwood, & Beautrais, 1999; Udry & Chantala, 2002). In addition, LGB youths are 1.5–2.6 times more likely to have suicidal thoughts and 2.0–7.1 times more likely to have attempted suicide than heterosexual youths (e.g., Bontempo & D'Augelli, 2002; Faulkner & Cranston, 1998; Garofalo, Wolf, Wissow, Woods, & Goodman, 1999; Remafedi, French, Story, Resnick, & Blum, 1998; Russell & Joyner, 2001; Udry & Chantala, 2002).

Sexual orientation disparities also have been noted in substance use and abuse. LGB youths have been found to be 1.5–10 times more likely than heterosexual youths to smoke cigarettes, drink alcohol, smoke marijuana, and/or use other drugs, such as cocaine (e.g., Austin et al., 2004; Bontempo & D'Augelli, 2002; Faulkner & Cranston, 1998; Russell, Driscoll, & Truong, 2002; Udry & Chantala, 2002). Further, more LGB youths than heterosexual youths have been found to have problems with substance use, such as binge drinking (Faulkner & Cranston, 1998; Robin et al., 2002) and substance abuse (Fergusson et al., 1999; Russell et al., 2002).

Sexual orientation disparities extend to sexual risk behaviors. Both male and female LGB youths are more likely than heterosexual youths to report sexual intercourse, more sexual partners, sexual debut at a younger age, unprotected sexual activity, and exchanging sex for money or drugs (Blake et al., 2001; Bontempo & D'Augelli, 2002; Udry & Chantala, 2002). Male and female LGB youths also are more likely than heterosexual peers to have had sex while using alcohol or drugs (Blake et al., 2001).

Gay-Related Stress and Health

Theory and research have focused on the critical role of gay-related stress as the most likely explanation for the poorer mental health and greater risk behaviors found among LGB individuals (e.g., Meyer, 2003; Savin-Williams, 1994). Gay-related stress refers to the experience of stigmatization for being LGB in a society in which homosexuality is negatively sanctioned (Rosario, Schrimshaw, Hunter, & Gwadz, 2002). Gay-related stress is multidimensional, including both external and internal dimensions. External gay-related stress includes experiences of victimization, rejection, and other stressful events perpetrated against LGB individuals (Rosario et al., 2002). Internalized gay-related stress includes the LGB individual's internalization of society's negative attitudes toward homosexuality, which is frequently termed "internalized homophobia" (e.g., Meyer, 1995; Nungesser, 1983), as well as discomfort with other individuals knowing about the individual's LGB sexual orientation (Rosario et al., 2002).

The literature has documented that LGB individuals are more likely than heterosexual peers to be the victims of threats, violence, and ridicule. Large representative samples have found that many more LGB youths are threatened and physically victimized than heterosexual youths (Blake et al., 2001; Bontempo & D'Augelli, 2002, Faulkner & Cranston, 1998; Russell, Franz, & Driscoll, 2001; Williams et al., 2005). In addition, LGB youths frequently experience more subtle forms of stress, including arguments with parents and peers, experiences of rejection, the loss of friends, and being called names or insulted (Rosario, Rotheram-Borus, & Reid, 1996; Rosario et al., 2002).

External gay-related stress and health. A growing literature has suggested that experiences of gay-related stressful events are associated with poorer mental health and greater risk behaviors among LGB individuals. Among LGB youths, experiences of victimization have been found to be associated with poorer mental health (Hershberger & D'Augelli, 1995; Huebner, Rebchook, & Kegeles, 2004; Rosario et al., 1996; Williams et al., 2005), a greater likelihood of attempting suicide (Bontempo & D'Augelli, 2002; Garofalo et al., 1999; Russell & Joyner, 2001), greater likelihood of smoking, drinking, and using other drugs (Bontempo & D'Augelli, 2002; Rotheram-Borus, Rosario, Van Rossem, Reid, & Gillis, 1995), and a higher prevalence of sexual risk behaviors (Bontempo & D'Augelli, 2002; Rotheram-Borus et al., 1995). Further, when controls were imposed for gay-related stress, health disparities between LGB youths and heterosexual peers were no longer significant (Bontempo & D'Augelli, 2002; Garofalo et al., 1999; Russell & Joyner, 2001; Safren & Heimberg, 1999; Williams et al., 2005). These findings provide evidence that it is victimization, rather than sexual orientation itself, that may be the putative cause of the health disparities between LGB and heterosexual individuals. Nevertheless, external gay-related stress has not been universally associated with negative health outcomes (Rosario et al., 2002; Rosario, Schrimshaw, & Hunter, 2004b; Rotheram-Borus et al., 1995).

Internal gay-related stress and health. In addition to experiences of gay-related stressful events, LGB individuals who experience internal forms of gay-related stress (e.g., negative attitudes toward homosexuality) are more likely to experience poorer mental health and greater risk behaviors (see Williamson, 2000, for review). Although internal gay-related stress has been associated with poorer mental health (Herek, Cogan, Gillis, & Glunt, 1997; Meyer, 1995) and more sexual risk behaviors (Meyer & Dean, 1995; Stokes & Peterson, 1998), these studies have primarily examined LGB adults. However, at least some research has documented that internal gay-related stress is associated with poorer mental health (Rosario, Hunter, Maguen, Gwadz, & Smith, 2001) and greater sexual risk behaviors (Rosario, Schrimshaw, & Hunter, 2006; Waldo, McFarland, Katz, MacKellar, & Valleroy, 2000) among LGB youths as well.

Non–gay-related stress and health. LGB youths also experience a number of stressors that are unrelated to their sexual orientation (e.g., parental divorce, poor grades, and relationship break-ups). Indeed, LGB youths may also report more non–gay-related stress than heterosexual youths for two possible reasons. First, non–gay-related stress may be the result of spillover effects from gay-related stress (e.g., being ridiculed at school for being gay leads to poor grades, which then becomes an additional stressor). Second, some LGB youths may be unaware or unwilling to attribute some stressors to their sexual orientation (e.g., attributing teasing to lack of athleticism rather than sexual orientation). Thus, non–gay-related stress may be important in understanding the mental health and risk behaviors of LGB youths. Rotheram-Borus and colleagues (1995) found that academic and other non–gay-related stressors were correlated with various mental health, substance use, and sexual risk behavior outcomes among gay and bisexual male youths.

Ethnic/Racial Disparities in Gay-Related Stress

Despite the well-documented prevalence of health disparities between LGB and heterosexual youths, far less research has examined health disparities *within* the LGB community. In particular, there has been little research examining potential ethnic/racial disparities in the mental health and risk behaviors of LGB individuals. However, there is significant reason to believe that ethnic/racial minority LGB individuals may experience higher levels of stress—both gay-related and otherwise—than White LGB individuals. Such differences in stress should result in ethnic/racial disparities in mental health and risk behaviors.

Extensive writings have offered several cultural factors that could lead Black and Latino LGB individuals to experience greater gay-related stress (e.g., Diaz, 1998; Greene, 1998; Loiacano, 1989; Martinez & Sullivan, 1998; Rosario, Schrimshaw, & Hunter, 2004a; Savin-Williams, 1996). Specifically, it has been argued that, as compared with White peers, ethnic/racial minority LGB individuals are more likely to possess cultural values regarding the importance of family, traditional gender roles, and conservative religious beliefs that may lead them to hold more negative attitudes toward homosexuality. Further, their families and communities are more likely to share these same cultural values and hold more negative attitudes toward homosexuality, which in turn may cause Latino and Black LGB individuals to experience greater interpersonal conflict and greater gay-related victimization than White LGB individuals. In addition, ethnic/racial minority LGB individuals may confront racism within the predominantly White LGB community (e.g., Icard, 1986; Loiacano, 1989; Martinez & Sullivan, 1998; Savin-Williams, 1996), resulting in an additional source of (non–gay-related) stress that may contribute to health disparities.

Ethnic/racial differences in external gay-related stress. Despite the hypothesis that Black and Latino LGB individuals experience more gay-related stress than White peers, little empirical examination of potential ethnic/racial differences in gay-related stress is available because most studies have included too few ethnic/racial minorities for adequate statistical comparisons. Nevertheless, the available studies do not support the hypothesis. One study found that more White LGB youths than ethnic/racial minority youths were ever victimized or experienced three or more acts of victimization (Pilkington & D'Augelli, 1995). In addition, ethnic/racial minority LGB youths were no more likely to experience negative reactions from their families than were White LGB youths (Pilkington & D'Augelli). Similarly, in a large study of young gay and bisexual men (Huebner et al., 2004), Latinos were no more likely to report gay-related physical violence, discrimination, or harassment than young White gay and bisexual men. In addition, studies of LGB adults have found that Black LGB individuals experience more stress than White or Latino peers, with no significant difference between Latinos and Whites. Specifically, Black gay men reported more discrimination, verbal harassment, and negative interactions with homophobic people than White or Latino gay men (Siegel & Epstein, 1996). These findings that Black LGB individuals differed from Latino and White peers contradict the hypothesis that Black and Latino LGB individuals experience more gay-related stress than White peers.

Ethnic/racial differences in internal gay-related stress. The failure to support the hypothesis that both Black and Latino LGB individuals experience more gay-related stress extends to internalized stress. Black and Latino gay and bisexual male youths have not reported more negative attitudes toward homosexuality than White peers (Dubé & Savin-Williams, 1999). Although Black gay and bisexual men experienced more stress regarding being open about their sexuality with others than their White peers, the Black men experienced more stress than the Latino men, and the Latinos and Whites did not differ (Siegel & Epstein, 1996). Similarly, Black gay and bisexual male adults have been found to have more negative attitudes toward homosexuality than their White peers (Stokes, Vanable, & McKirnan, 1996), but Latinos were not included in the study.

Ethnic/racial differences in non–gay-related stress. Just as potential ethnic/racial disparities exist in gay-related stress, there also may be ethnic/racial disparities in non–gay-related stressors. Indeed, ethnic/racial minority youths (predominantly heterosexual) have been found to experience greater non–gay-related violence and victimization, as well as witnessing such violence, than White peers (e.g., Crouch, Hanson, Saunders, Kilpatrick, & Resnick, 2000; Singh & Yu, 1996). Such ethnic/racial disparities in non–gay-related stress may also account for potential ethnic/racial disparities in health and risk behaviors among LGB youths.

Ethnic/Racial Differences in Mental Health and Risk Behaviors

The literature reviewed to this point indicates that gay-related stress may explain the health disparities between LGB and heterosexual youths. It also suggests that some ethnic/racial minority LGB youths may experience higher levels of gay-related stress than White LGB youths. Therefore, it is reasonable to suggest that ethnic/racial differences in gay-related stress should lead to ethnic/racial disparities in the mental health and risk behaviors of LGB youths. However, despite the widespread discussion of ethnic/racial differences in gay-related stress, the corresponding ethnic/racial disparities in health have been little examined.

The available literature on LGB youths does not support the hypothesis. Although no data were identified that address ethnic differences in the emotional distress or suicidality of LGB youths, Thiede et al. (2003) found that young White men who have sex with men (MSM) consistently reported more (rather than less) drug use, polydrug use, and frequent drug use than young Black, Latino, or Asian young MSM. Similarly, young White and Hispanic MSM have been found to report more use of cocaine, stimulants, inhalants, and injection drug use than young Black MSM (Harawa et al., 2004). Concerning sexual risk behaviors, two large representative samples of young MSM found, as expected, that Black and Latino MSM reported more sex partners than White peers (Goodenow, Netherland, & Szalacha, 2002; Harawa et al., 2004). However, young Black MSM reported less unprotected anal sex than young White MSM (Goodenow et al., 2002; Harawa et al., 2004). This last finding is inconsistent with the higher rates of HIV infection found among young Black and Latino MSM relative to White peers (Valleroy et al., 2000).

The research on potential ethnic/racial disparities among LGB adults is also limited and inconsistent. With respect to mental health, Black, Hispanic, Asian, and Native-American gay and bisexual men do report more depressive symptoms than White peers (Mills et al., 2004) and Native-American gay and bisexual men are more likely to have attempted suicide than men of other ethnic/racial backgrounds (Paul et al., 2002). With respect to substance use, adult Hispanic MSM report more alcohol-related problems than White MSM (Stall et al., 2001). However, no differences have been found among adult gay/bisexual men's cigarette use (Greenwood et al., 2005); few differences have been found among adult MSM on illicit drug use (Irwin & Morgenstern, 2005; Stall et al., 2001); and adult Black MSM have been found to consume more alcohol than Latino and White MSM (Irwin & Morgenstern, 2005). Lastly, as compared with the research on LGB youths, no ethnic/racial differences in number of sexual partners or unprotected anal sex have been found among adult MSM (Xia et al., 2006).

Insufficient information exists on potential ethnic/racial disparities in the mental health, substance use, and sexual risk behaviors of LGB youths. Such information may be necessary to target intervention efforts most efficiently. Even the research that examines potential ethnic/racial disparities is limited in that it has focused exclusively on gay and bisexual males, with no studies identified that address ethnic/racial disparities in the health of lesbian and bisexual female youths. Our own earlier reports from this study also were limited because ethnic/racial disparities in health were never the central focus; rather, ethnicity/race was examined as a potential covariate of various health outcomes (e.g., Rosario et al., 2002, 2004b).

The current report examines potential ethnic/racial differences in the mental health, substance use, and sexual behaviors of LGB youths. It also examines ethnic/racial differences in the potential explanatory factors of gay-related stress and non–gay-related stress. If ethnic/racial differences are found in health and stress, we also will examine whether potential ethnic/racial differences in gay-related stress and other life stressors account for the health disparities. In keeping with the theoretical literature, we hypothesize that Black and Latino youths, relative to White peers, experience more gay-related stress and non–gay-related stress, as well as poorer health and health-related behaviors.

METHOD

Participants

Youths between the ages of 14 and 21 years were recruited from organizations serving LGB youths in New York City. These included three LGB-focused community-based organizations (CBOs; 85% of youths) and two LGB student organizations at public colleges (15% of youths). Attempts were made to recruit every youth at each organization, and approximately 80% agreed to participate. Of the 164 youths interviewed at baseline, 8 did not meet eligibility requirements (i.e., too old or heterosexual) or they provided invalid or duplicate data.

Of the resulting sample of 156 youths, 51% were male and 49% were female. The mean age was 18.3 years ($SD = 1.65$). The youths self-identified at baseline as gay or lesbian (66%), bisexual (31%), or other (3%). Youths were of diverse ethnic/racial backgrounds: Latino (37%), Black (35%), White (22%), Asian (5%), and other ethnic backgrounds (2%).[1] Because of the small number of youths from Asian and other ethnic backgrounds ($n = 11$), they were excluded from the present report. A third of youths (34%) reported having a parent who received welfare, food stamps, or Medicaid. Although 15% were recruited from colleges, 31% of the sample reported currently attending college.

Procedure

All youths provided signed informed consent. Parental consent for youths under age 18 was waived by the Commissioner of Mental Health for New York State. An adult at each CBO served *in loco parentis* to safeguard the rights of each minor-aged participant. The study was approved by the university Institutional Review Board and it received a Federal Certificate of Confidentiality.

Youths participated in a structured interview of 2–3 hours conducted at baseline, with follow-up assessments 6 months and 12 months later. Baseline interviews were conducted in 1993–1994, with follow-up interviews conducted through 1995. Interviews were conducted in a private room at the recruitment sites or in a private location convenient for the youths. Interviews were conducted by college-educated individuals of the same sex as the youth; no attempt was made to match the interviewer and the youth on ethnicity/race. Every interviewer was trained on all facets of the questionnaire battery, including conducting interviews on sexually sensitive topics. The interviewers conducted practice interviews and received ongoing supervision. Their audio-taped interviews were monitored throughout the study to ensure quality and consistency.

Youths were recontacted by telephone either directly or through members of their social network to schedule follow-up interviews. Retention was 92% ($n = 143$) for the 6-month interview and 90% ($n = 140$) for the 12-month interview. Overall, 85% ($n = 133$) completed all three assessments; only 5 youths were lost to both follow-up assessments.

Measures

Stress. Four aspects of stress were assessed at all three times: gay-related stressful life events, non–gay related stressful life events, negative attitudes toward homosexuality, and discomfort with other individuals knowing about the youths' sexuality. Gay-related

---

[1]We categorized the self-identified ethnic/racial background of youths into four mutually exclusive groups. The "Black" category included African Americans, Africans, and Caribbean Islanders of Black-non-Latino background. The "Latino" group was composed of youths from Latino ethnic backgrounds (e.g., Cuban, Dominican, Puerto Rican), regardless of racial background. The "White" group consisted of White-non-Latino ethnic groups (e.g., Italian Americans, Irish Americans). A similar classification identified the "Asian" group.

stressful events were assessed with a 12-item checklist (e.g., "Losing a close friend because of your [homosexuality/bisexuality]"; Rosario et al., 2002). The number of events experienced in the past 3 months (at baseline) or since the last interview (at Times 2 and 3) was computed as the indicator of gay-related stressful life events. Because the responses were skewed, we recoded the scale to indicate whether the youth experienced zero, one, or two or more stressful events. Because not all stress experienced by LGB youths is gay-related, the 32–item Life Events Checklist for adolescents (Johnson & Mc-Cutcheon, 1980) was used to assess the number of non–gay-related stressors experienced in the past 3 months or since the last interview. The number of such experienced events was computed as the indicator of non–gay-related stressful life events.

Aspects of internalized gay-related stress were assessed using a modified version of the 33–item Nungesser Homosexual Attitudes Inventory (Nungesser, 1983; see Rosario et al., 2002 for description of the modifications), using a 4-point response scale ranging from "disagree strongly" (1) to "agree strongly" (4). Factor analysis of the items identified two factors. The first factor included 11 items (e.g., "My [homosexuality/bisexuality] does not make me unhappy") that assessed attitudes toward homosexuality. The mean of these 11 items was computed (Cronbach's alpha = .83–.85 across all assessments). Because youths reported few negative attitudes (i.e., the data were skewed), a median split was used to identify youths who were above (1) or below (0) the median on negative attitudes; this dichotomy was used in subsequent analyses. A second factor was composed of 12 items (e.g., "If my straight friends knew of my [homosexuality/bisexuality], I would feel uncomfortable") that assessed discomfort with others knowing about the youths' homosexuality. The mean of these 12 items was computed, with a higher score indicating greater discomfort (Cronbach's alpha = .89–.91 across all assessments).

Emotional distress. Six aspects of emotional distress and well-being were assessed: depression, anxiety, conduct problems, self-esteem, suicidal ideation, and suicide attempts. Depressive and anxious symptoms during the past week were assessed using the Brief Symptom Inventory (BSI; Derogatis, 1993) at all three time periods. Items were completed using a 5-point response scale from "not at all" (0) to "extremely" (4) distressing. The mean of the 6 items of the depression subscale (Cronbach's alpha = .80–.82 across all assessments) and the mean of the 6 items of the anxiety subscale (Cronbach's alpha = .81–.83 across all assessments) were computed such that higher scores indicated greater depression or greater anxiety. Conduct problems during the past 6 months were assessed at all three time periods using a 13–item index constructed from the conduct problems identified in the DSM-III-R (American Psychiatric Association, 1987), such as skipping school, vandalism, stealing, and fighting. A count of the number of problems endorsed was computed. Self-esteem was assessed at all three times using Rosenberg's (1965) 10-item scale and its 4-point response scale ranging from "strongly agree" (1) to "strongly disagree" (4). The mean of these items was computed with higher scores indicating greater self-esteem (Cronbach's alpha = .83–.86 across all assessments). The prevalence of lifetime suicide attempts and suicidal ideation was assessed only at baseline using two items developed by Shaffer and Gould (1986). Youths were asked "Have you ever seriously thought about killing yourself? By seriously, I mean every day for a week or more." This was followed by asking, "Have you ever hurt yourself or tried to kill yourself at any time in your life?"

Substance use and abuse. Four aspects of substance use and abuse were assessed at all three assessment times: quantity of both cigarettes and alcohol used, frequency of marijuana use, and symptoms of substance abuse. Substance use and abuse in the past 3 months (or since the last assessment at Times 2 and 3) was measured using the Alcohol and Drug Schedule (ADS; Rosario, Hunter, & Gwadz, 1997), an instrument that has demonstrated acceptable test–retest reliability (Rosario et al., 1997). The average quantity of cigarette use per day was assessed using a 7-point scale ranging from "Did not smoke cigarettes in the past [three/six] months" (0) to "About 2 packs or more a day (over 35 cigarettes)" (6). The quantity of alcohol was assessed by asking youths how many drinks they typically have in a day when they drink. Because the quantity of alcohol use was positively skewed, the quantity of alcohol was recomputed to reflect whether youths reported zero, one, two, or three or more drinks. The frequency of marijuana use was assessed by asking the number of times they had used marijuana in the past 3/6 months. Finally, symptoms associated with alcohol or illicit drug abuse were assessed using 11 items (e.g., "Felt you needed or were dependent on alcohol and/or drugs") taken from the Diagnostic Interview Schedule for Children (National Institute of Mental Health, 1992). Items use a 5-point response scale from "not at all" (1) to "very often" (5). The mean of the items was computed as the index of substance abuse (Cronbach's alpha = .81–.90 across all assessments).

Sexual behaviors. Various sexual behaviors were assessed using the Sexual Risk Behavior Assessment Schedule for Youths (SERBAS-Y; Meyer-Bahlburg, Ehrhardt, Exner, & Gruen, 1994), an instrument that has demonstrated strong test–retest reliability among both male and female LGB youths in this sample (Schrimshaw, Rosario, Meyer-Bahlburg, & Scharf-Matlick, 2006). To assess lifetime number of sexual partners at baseline, youths were asked to "count up" all the same-sex partners with whom they had "any kind of sex within their whole lifetime," and similarly for other-sex partners. Similar questions were asked to assess the lifetime number of sexual encounters with same-sex and other-sex partners. The prevalence of recent same-sex and other-sex sexual behavior in the past 3 months (or since the last interview at Times 2 and 3) was assessed. Youths also were asked about the lifetime prevalence of having potentially risky sexual partners, meaning partners who injected drugs, had a sexually transmitted disease (STD), or had tested HIV positive. The lifetime prevalence of prostitution was assessed by asking youths if they had ever received money, drugs, or a place to stay in exchange for having sex with either a same-sex or other-sex partner; both same-sex and other-sex prostitution were combined into a single indicator of lifetime prevalence of prostitution.

At both the 6-month and 12-month assessments, male youths were asked about the number of episodes of receptive anal sex and insertive anal sex, as well as the number of such episodes in which condoms were used. The total number of unprotected receptive and insertive anal episodes across partners was computed by subtracting the total number of protected episodes from the total number of episodes. These data were dichotomized to assess whether youths reported (1) or did not report (0) having unprotected receptive and insertive anal sex across the 6- and 12-month assessments. Finally, the lifetime prevalence of having an STD was assessed by asking youths if they had ever had each of seven different STDs (i.e., gonorrhea, syphilis, genital herpes, venereal warts, chancroid, chlamydia, and any others); youths who reported any one of the seven STDs were categorized as having had an STD.

Data Analysis

Bivariate comparisons of Latino, Black, and White youths were made using analysis of variance (ANOVA) for continuous variables (e.g., gay-related stress, depressive symptoms) and chi-square (χ^2) for categorical variables (e.g., prevalence of suicide attempts, same-sex behavior). Effect sizes (i.e., the percent of variance explained) for each comparison were made using eta-square (η^2) for continuous variables and Goodman-Kruskal's tau (τ) for categorical variables. Further, significant findings were followed by the protected t-test for ANOVA or χ^2 to conduct all possible pairwise comparisons of means or frequencies. In order to rule out potential confounds of socio-demographic characteristics and social desirability, multivariate comparisons of Latino, Black, and White youths were made using a series of hierarchical linear regression models for continuous variables and hierarchical logistic regression models for categorical variables. Specifically, potential confounds were entered in the first step of the regression equation, with ethnicity/race entered in the second step of the regression equation to determine if ethnicity/race was still associated with each outcome variable after controlling for the potential confounds. Effect sizes are reported, specifically the standardized regression coefficient, beta (β), for multiple regression and the comparable odds ratio (OR) for logistic regression.

RESULTS

Ethnic/Racial Differences in Sociodemographic Characteristics and Social Desirability

We examined the associations between ethnicity/race and other sociodemographic factors and social desirability. No significant differences ($p < .10$) among Black, Latino, or White youths were found on sex, age, and socioeconomic status. A marginally significant difference on social desirability was found, $F(2, 142) = 2.51$, $p < .10$. Pairwise comparisons, using Fisher's Protected t-test, indicated that Black youths significantly ($p < .05$) provided more socially desirable responses than White youths. Ethnic differences also were found for recruitment site, $\chi^2(N = 145, df = 6) = 24.08$, $p < .001$. A more focused analysis examining ethnic/racial differences by whether the youths were recruited from the colleges as compared with the CBOs found a significant difference, $\chi^2(N = 145, df = 2) = 10.70$, $p < .005$. These data indicated that fewer numbers of Black (7%) and Latino (12%) youths were recruited from the colleges than were White youths (32%).

Bivariate Analyses of Ethnic/Racial Differences in Stress and Health

Ethnic/racial differences in stress and its potential outcomes—emotional distress, substance use, and sexual risk behaviors—were examined. Table 24.1 contains the findings for stress. Although nonsignificant differences predominated, ethnic/racial differences were consistently found in discomfort with others knowing about their homosexuality. Specifically, Black youths were more uncomfortable with others knowing about their homosexuality than were Latino or White youths.

Table 24.1	Ethnic/Racial Differences in Stress				
	Black M (SD)	Latino M (SD)	White M (SD)	F	η^2
Gay-Related Stressful Life Events					
Time 1	0.74 (0.94)	0.63 (0.86)	0.74 (0.86)	0.25	.00
Time 2	0.79 (0.85)	0.55 (0.79)	0.70 (0.84)	1.18	.02
Time 3	0.60 (0.73)	0.51 (0.70)	0.34 (0.61)	1.24	.02
Non-Gay-Related Stressful Life Events					
Time 1	7.22 (4.16)	9.0 (4.35)	6.68 (3.39)	4.38**	.06
Time 2	5.92 (2.85)	6.75 (4.23)	5.90 (4.11)	0.80	.01
Time 3	5.60 (4.12)	6.51 (4.96)	5.14 (2.71)	1.12	.02
Discomfort With Others Knowing Their Sexuality					
Time 1	2.41 (0.76)	2.12 (0.62)	1.91 (0.67)	5.81**	.08
Time 2	2.29 (0.75)	2.05 (0.53)	1.81 (0.63)	5.30**	.08
Time 3	2.20 (0.78)	1.93 (0.56)	1.80 (0.63)	3.78*	.06
	n (%)	n (%)	n (%)	χ^2	τ
Negative Attitudes Toward Homosexuality					
Time 1	33 (61%)	30 (54%)	15 (44%)	2.44	.02
Time 2	25 (52%)	27 (49%)	13 (45%)	0.38	.00
Time 3	22 (45%)	30 (59%)	17 (59%)	2.34	.02

Note: Means with differing superscripts are significantly different at $p < .05$.
* $p < .05$. ** $p < .01$

Significant ethnic/racial differences for emotional distress were fewer in number than nonsignificant findings (Table 24.2). However, differences at baseline (Time 1) indicated that Black youths reported more depressive symptoms and lower self-esteem than Latino youths. Black youths reported fewer conduct problems than Latino youths at baseline.

No ethnic/racial disparities were significant for substance use and abuse (Table 24.3) and nonsignificant ethnic/racial differences predominated for sexual risk behaviors (Table 24.4). The youths differed only on lifetime number of other-sex partners, with Black youths reporting more such partners than Latino youths.

Multivariate Analyses of Ethnic/Racial Differences in Stress and Health

Potential ethnic/racial differences where re-examined by controlling for social desirability and recruitment from colleges in multivariate analyses. We also controlled for sex as male or female because such differences have been found among (predominantly

Table
24.2

Ethnic/Racial Differences in Emotional Distress

	Black M (SD)	Latino M (SD)	White M (SD)	F	η^2
Depressive Symptoms					
Time 1	1.30 (0.97)	0.88 (0.84)	1.00 (0.62)	3.49*	.05
Time 2	0.93 (0.89)	0.85 (0.77)	0.94 (0.77)	0.17	.00
Time 3	0.82 (0.91)	0.68 (0.66)	0.78 (0.67)	0.46	.01
Anxious Symptoms					
Time 1	1.09 (0.89)	1.26 (0.99)	1.34 (0.80)	0.94	.01
Time 2	0.88 (0.90)	0.94 (0.83)	1.06 (0.88)	0.39	.01
Time 3	0.63 (0.79)	0.88 (0.84)	0.76 (0.49)	1.34	.02
Conduct Problems					
Time 1	1.52 (1.21)	2.21 (1.76)	2.12 (1.75)	2.99*	.04
Time 2	1.35 (1.45)	1.51 (1.36)	1.37 (1.47)	0.18	.00
Time 3	1.20 (1.43)	1.43 (1.36)	1.38 (1.08)	0.41	.01
Self–Esteem					
Time 1	3.19 (0.60)	3.45 (0.45)	3.37 (0.40)	3.75*	.05
Time 2	3.36 (0.48)	3.44 (0.45)	3.45 (0.48)	0.46	.01
Time 3	3.45 (0.47)	3.52 (0.43)	3.49 (0.46)	0.24	.00
	n (%)	n (%)	n (%)	χ^2	τ
Ever Suicidal Ideation					
Time 1	29 (54%)	27 (47%)	17 (50%)	0.45	.00
Ever Suicide Attempt					
Time 1	24 (44%)	19 (33%)	10 (29%)	2.45	.02

Note: Means with differing superscripts are significantly different at $p < .05$.
* $p < .05$

Table
24.3

Ethnic/Racial Differences in Substance Use and Abuse

	Black M (SD)	Latino M (SD)	White M (SD)	F^*	η^2
Quantity of Cigarettes					
Time 1	1.00 (1.39)	1.35 (1.53)	1.50 (1.91)	1.22	.02
Time 2	1.23 (1.48)	1.29 (1.47)	1.30 (1.70)	0.28	.00
Time 3	1.21 (1.32)	1.39 (1.51)	1.59 (1.74)	0.50	.01
Quantity of Alcohol					
Time 1	1.26 (1.17)	1.47 (1.24)	1.38 (1.23)	0.44	.01
Time 2	1.27 (1.05)	1.67 (1.31)	1.57 (1.19)	1.51	.02
Time 3	1.86 (0.91)	1.89 (1.17)	1.89 (1.15)	0.01	.00
Frequency of Marijuana					
Time 1	0.54 (0.75)	0.44 (0.68)	0.56 (0.66)	0.89	.01
Time 2	0.92 (0.87)	0.69 (0.88)	0.70 (0.84)	1.01	.02
Time 3	0.94 (0.91)	0.76 (0.86)	0.62 (0.73)	1.35	.02
Substance Abuse Symptoms					
Time 1	1.35 (0.71)	1.45 (0.73)	1.57 (0.77)	0.96	.01
Time 2	1.31 (0.42)	1.39 (0.59)	1.29 (0.48)	0.40	.01
Time 3	1.42 (0.58)	1.54 (0.73)	1.58 (0.84)	0.53	.01

Note: *All F tests were nonsignificant at $p > .05$.

Table 24.4 Ethnic/Racial Differences in Sexual Behaviors

	Black M (SD)	Latino M (SD)	White M (SD)	F	η^2
Lifetime Number of Same-Sex Sexual Partners	1.21 (1.08)	1.53 (1.28)	1.32 (1.21)	1.07	.02
Lifetime Number of Same-Sex Sexual Encounters	3.35 (2.29)	3.36 (2.09)	3.01 (2.11)	0.92	.01
Lifetime Number of Other-Sex Sexual Partners	1.00 (1.21)[a]	0.44 (1.07)[b]	0.81 (1.38)	3.14*	.04
Lifetime Number of Other-Sex Sexual Encounters	2.13 (2.06)	1.70 (2.21)	2.13 (2.56)	0.65	.01
	n (%)	n (%)	n (%)	χ^2	τ
Ever Same-Sex Sex					
Time 1	49 (91%)	53 (93%)	32 (92%)	0.38	.00
Ever Other-Sex Sex					
Time 1	42 (78%)	37 (65%)	22 (65%)	2.69	.02
Recent Same-Sex Sex					
Time 1	35 (65%)	39 (68%)	24 (71%)	0.35	.00
Time 2	42 (88%)	44 (82%)	22 (73%)	2.50	.02
Time 3	39 (78%)	42 (82%)	24 (83%)	0.40	.00
Recent Other-Sex Sex					
Time 1	8 (15%)	8 (14%)	8 (24%)	1.58	.01
Time 2	9 (19%)	7 (13%)	7 (23%)	1.53	.01
Time 3	15 (30%)	9 (18%)	7 (24%)	2.12	.02
Recent Risky Same-Sex Partner					
Time 1	12 (22%)	9 (16%)	6 (18%)	0.79	.01
Time 2	6 (13%)	8 (15%)	4 (13%)	0.12	.00
Time 3	6 (12%)	5 (10%)	4 (14%)	0.30	.00
Unprotected Anal Sex in the past year (males only)	11 (48%)	12 (50%)	6 (33%)	1.31	.02
Unprotected Receptive Anal Sex in the past year (males only)	7 (30%)	9 (38%)	4 (22%)	1.13	.02
Unprotected Insertive Anal Sex in the past year (males only)	9 (39%)	11 (46%)	6 (33%)	0.68	.01
Ever Engaged in Prostitution	6 (11%)	7 (12%)	7 (21%)	1.95	.01
Ever had an STD	3 (6%)	4 (7%)	3 (9%)	0.35	.00

Note: Means with differing superscripts are significantly different at $p < .05$.
* $p < .05$.

heterosexual) youths in mental health, substance use, and sexual risks (e.g., Kilpatrick et al., 2003; Rosario & Schrimshaw, 2006). After imposing these controls, we regressed each health factor on a set of dummy coded ethnic/racial variables comparing Latino (1) with Black (0) youths and White (1) with Black (0) youths because the bivariate findings indicated that differences predominated between Black youths and their Latino and White peers.

Table 24.5	Multivariate Associations Between Ethnicity/Race and Health Outcomes			
	Latino (1) vs. Black (0)		White (1) vs. Black (0)	
	β (SE)	OR (95% CI)	β (SE)	OR (95% CI)
Discomfort With Others Knowing Their Sexuality				
Time 1	−.21 (.09)*		−.32 (.10)***	
Time 2	−.19 (.10)*		−.34 (.10)***	
Time 3	−.22 (.10)*		−.30 (.10)**	
% Negative Attitudes Toward Homosexuality				
Time 1		ns		0.32 (.12, .88)*
Non-Gay-Related Stressful Life Events				
Time 1	.21 (.09)*		ns	
Depressive Symptoms				
Time 1	−.26 (.09)**		−.21 (.09)*	
Conduct Problems				
Time 1	.19 (.09)*		ns	
Self-Esteem				
Time 1	.27 (.09)**		.19 (.09)*	
Lifetime Number of Other-Sex Sexual Partners				
Time 1	−.25 (.09)**		ns	
% Recent Same-Sex Sex				
Time 2		ns		0.25 (.07, .90)*

Note: Multivariate analyses examined the association of ethnicity/race and health outcomes after controlling for sex, recruitment site (colleges vs. CBOs), and social desirability. Only significant ethnic/racial differences are presented; thus, variables and assessment time periods not presented did not differ significantly by ethnicity/race. Beta (β), the standardized regression coefficient, theoretically varies between negative one and one, with zero supporting the null hypothesis of no difference between the groups on the outcome variable. The odds ratio (OR) of logistic regression theoretically ranges between zero and positive infinity, with a value of one supporting the null hypothesis of no difference between the groups on the outcome variable. SE = Standard Error and CI = Confidence Interval. * $p < .05$, ** $p < .01$, *** $p < .001$, ns = not significant.

The multivariate findings for stress (Table 24.5) generally replicated the bivariate findings presented in Table 24.1. The significant multivariate findings indicated that Black youths were more uncomfortable with others knowing about their homosexuality than were Latino or White youths across all three assessments. Black youths also were more likely to report negative attitudes toward homosexuality than White youths at baseline. However, Black youths experienced less non–gay-related stress than Latino youths at baseline.

The majority of significant and nonsignificant bivariate findings pertaining to emotional distress (Table 24.2) were replicated (Table 24.5). The significant multivariate findings indicated that at baseline Black youths reported more depressive symptoms than both Latino and White youths, as well as lower self-esteem than both Latino and White youths. Black youths reported fewer conduct problems than Latino youths at baseline.

As with the bivariate findings for substance use (Table 24.3), multivariate analyses found no ethnic/racial disparities in substance use or abuse.

The multivariate findings for sexual behaviors (Table 24.5) generally replicated the bivariate findings (Table 24.4). One significant multivariate finding confirmed that Black youths reported more lifetime numbers of other-sex partners than Latino youths. A new finding indicated that more Black than White youths had at least one recent same-sex partner at Time 2.

DISCUSSION

We examined ethnic/racial differences in stress and health-related outcomes among LGB youths because LGB individuals of racial or ethnic minority backgrounds are hypothesized to experience more gay-related stress in their ethnic/racial communities than do their White peers and they are hypothesized to experience ethnic/racial stress in the predominantly White LGB community. If the hypotheses are correct, Black and Latino LGB individuals, as compared with White peers, should report more gay-related stress and poorer health-related outcomes, such as more emotional distress, substance use/abuse, and sexual risk behaviors. Despite the importance of these hypotheses, few investigations are available because most LGB samples are composed predominantly of White individuals; thus, precluding racial/ethic comparisons. Therefore, we examined the hypotheses among LGB youths of Black, Latino, and White backgrounds.

The Findings and Their Implications

With respect to gay-related stress, we found no ethnic/racial differences in external gay-related stress, but differences were found in internalized gay-related stress (i.e., comfort with others knowing, negative attitudes). Specifically, Black youths were consistently more uncomfortable with other individuals knowing about their homosexuality than were Latino or White youths across all assessment periods. These findings held even after controlling for potential rival explanations, such as social desirability. Furthermore, Black youths were more likely to report negative attitudes toward homosexuality than White youths at baseline in multivariate analyses. In sum, internalized gay-related stress was elevated among Black youths in 4 of 6 possible tests. Such findings would lead one to expect differences in health-related outcomes; specifically, Black youths should report poorer health than Latino or White youths.[2]

Examination of ethnic/racial differences in health-related outcomes was characterized by a pattern of nonsignificant findings for substance use (12 of 12 tests) and sexual

---

[2]This new hypothesis, which is empirically derived, is at odds with the theoretical hypothesis advanced at the beginning of this chapter (i.e., Black and Latino youths experience more gay-related stress and poorer health than White peers). However, the new hypothesis is consistent with some past empirical research that has failed to identify differences between Latino and White youths (e.g., Huebner et al., 2004). The implications of the findings for the theoretical hypothesis will be discussed later.

risk behaviors (19 of 20 tests). Nevertheless, of 14 tests involving emotional distress and well-being, 3 significant findings were found (21%). Of the 3 bivariate and multivariate findings, 2 indicated that Black youths reported more depressive symptoms and lower self-esteem than Latino or White youths. These and the other significant finding occurred only at the baseline assessment, suggesting that Black youths alleviated their symptomatology and improved their self-esteem by the second assessment. Because the youths were recruited from programs at gay-focused community or college organizations, the programs may have helped the Black youths work through their emotional distress between the baseline and 6-months assessments. If true, these data justify the need for such programs. However, the programs did not affect the Black youths' discomfort with homosexuality during the duration of the study.

The prevalent hypothesis in the literature posits ethnic/racial differences in gay-related stress and health-related outcomes, with Black and Latino individuals experiencing more gay-related stress and poorer health-related outcomes than White peers. We found differences in internal gay-related stress, but with Black youths experiencing more stress than both Latino and White youths. Similarly, differences in emotional distress were found between Black as compared with Latino or White youths. Our data indicate that Black and Latino youths cannot be classified or treated as if they are from the same population (e.g., "ethnic/racial minorities," "non-White"). Although Latino youths may experience ethnic/racial discrimination, these findings suggest that their cultural and historical experiences regarding gay-related stress differ from those of Black youths.

The current study found that Latino and White youths were often nonsignificantly different from each other, but that when differences were identified, both groups differed from Black youths (e.g., discomfort with others knowing). The similarity between Latino and White youths may result from the fact that the majority of both Latino and White youths were raised as Roman Catholic, whereas the Black youths were predominantly raised Protestant (Rosario, Yali, Hunter, & Gwadz, 2006). Thus, the observed differences between Black youths relative to Latino and White youths may be a function of religious upbringing. Future research needs to examine whether religious upbringing may account for ethnic/racial disparities in gay-related stress and health outcomes. If it does find differences, subsequent research would need to identify what it is about the different religious upbringings that may account for Catholic versus Protestant differences (e.g., attitudes, beliefs, or norms), as well as differences with other religious backgrounds. This research is especially needed for LGB individuals because too little current information is available about religion among LGB individuals (Rodriquez & Ouellette, 2000; Rosario, Yali, et al., 2006; Woods, Antoni, Ironson, & Kling, 1999).

Our data on LGB individuals indicate the need for more ethnic/racial comparisons that are sensitive to religious differences. We did not support the prevalent hypothesis in the literature. At best, our findings question whether the hypothesis might be too narrow in scope. In essence, by failing to consider religion, the hypothesis may be missing an important cultural component that is not captured by such crude markers as ethnic and racial classification. Future studies, therefore, should assess potential ethnic/racial disparities as well as comparisons that combine ethnic/racial classification with religious classification. Specifically, the prevalent hypothesis that Blacks and Latinos experience more gay-related stress and poorer health than Whites may have to give way to a hypothesis that crosses ethnic/racial background by religious upbringing and, in the process, considers the overall traditionalism, conservatism, or rigidity of religions on the LGB individual's experience of gay-related stress (especially internal gay-related stress) and poor health-related outcomes.

Limitations

Our study has limitations that should be minimized as much as possible by future studies. First, our sample size was modest. Despite this fact, we had sufficient statistical power to detect a medium effect (Cohen, 1988), given our observed effect sizes. However, we do encourage larger samples, especially to examine the combined effects of ethnic/racial background by religious upbringing. Lastly and as already indicated, our youths were recruited from gay-focused programs at community-based or college organizations, although many LGB youths may not attend such settings. Because so few samples of LGB youths of diverse ethnic/racial background are available in the literature, the generalizability of our data to the population of LGB youths is unknown. Therefore, we strongly recommend replication of the findings with LGB youths recruited from other locations (e.g., suburban areas and urban areas other than New York City) and from non–gay-focused venues (e.g., the general student population at high schools and colleges). Clearly, samples must contain sufficient numbers of LGB individuals of ethnic/racial minority backgrounds (including Asians) to permit empirical examination of hypotheses.

REFERENCES

American Psychiatric Association. (1987). *Diagnostic and statistical manual of mental disorders* (3rd ed., rev.). Washington, DC: Author.

Austin, S. B., Ziyadeh, N., Fisher, L. B., Kahn, J. A., Colditz, G. A., & Frazier, A. L. (2004). Sexual orientation and tobacco use in a cohort study of US adolescent girls and boys. *Archives of Pediatric and Adolescent Medicine, 158,* 317–322.

Blake, S. M., Ledsky, R., Lehman, T., Goodenow, C., Sawyer, R., & Hack, T. (2001). Preventing sexual risk behaviors among gay, lesbian, and bisexual adolescents: The benefits of gay-sensitive HIV instruction in schools. *American Journal of Public Health, 91,* 940–946.

Bontempo, D. E., & D'Augelli, A. R. (2002). Effects of at-school victimization and sexual orientation on lesbian, gay, and bisexual youths' health risk behavior. *Journal of Adolescent Health, 30,* 364–374.

Cohen, J. (1988). *Statistical power analysis for the behavioral sciences* (2nd ed.). Hillsdale, NJ: Erlbaum.

Crouch, J. L., Hanson, R. F., Saunders, B. E., Kilpatrick, D. G., & Resnick, H. S. (2000). Income, race/ethnicity, and exposure to violence in youth: Results from the National Survey of Adolescents. *Journal of Community Psychology, 28,* 625–641.

Derogatis, L. R. (1993). *BSI, Brief Symptom Inventory: Administration, scoring and procedures manual.* Minneapolis, MN: National Computer Systems.

Diaz, R. M. (1998). *Latino gay men and HIV: Culture, sexuality, and risk behavior.* New York: Routledge.

Dubé, E. M., & Savin-Williams, R. C. (1999). Sexual identity development among ethnic sexual-minority male youths. *Developmental Psychology, 35,* 1389–1398.

Faulkner, A. H., & Cranston, K. (1998). Correlates of same-sex sexual behavior in a random sample of Massachusetts high school students. *American Journal of Public Health, 88,* 262–266.

Fergusson, D. M., Horwood, L. J., & Beautrais, A. L. (1999). Is sexual orientation related to mental health problems and suicidality in young people? *Archives of General Psychiatry, 56,* 876–880.

Garofalo, R., Wolf, C., Wissow, L. S., Woods, E. R., & Goodman, E. (1999). Sexual orientation and suicide attempts among a representative sample of youth. *Archives of Pediatric and Adolescent Medicine, 153,* 487–493.

Goodenow, C., Netherland, J., & Szalacha, L. (2002). AIDS-related risk among adolescent males who have sex with males, females, or both: Evidence from a statewide survey. *American Journal of Public Health, 92,* 203–210.

Greene, B. (1998). Family, ethnic identity, and sexual orientation: African American lesbians and gay men. In C. J. Patterson & A. R. D'Augelli (Eds.), *Lesbian, gay, and bisexual identities in families: Psychological perspectives*. New York: Oxford University Press.

Greenwood, G. L., Paul, J. P., Pollack, L. M., Binson, D., Catania, J. A., Chang, J., et al. (2005). Tobacco use and cessation among a household-based sample of US urban men who have sex with men. *American Journal of Public Health, 95*, 145–151.

Harawa, N. T., Greenland, S., Bingham, T. A., Johnson, D. F., Cochran, S. D., Cunningham, W. E., et al. (2004). Associations of race/ethnicity with HIV prevalence and HIV-related behaviors among young men who have sex with men in 7 urban centers in the United States. *Journal of Acquired Immune Deficiency Syndromes, 35*, 526–536.

Herek, G. M., Cogan, J. C., Gillis, J. R., & Glunt, E. K. (1997). Correlates of internalized homophobia in a community sample of lesbians and gay men. *Journal of the Gay and Lesbian Medical Association, 2*, 17–25.

Hershberger, S. L., & D'Augelli, A. R. (1995). The impact of victimization on the mental health and suicidality of lesbian, gay, and bisexual youths. *Developmental Psychology, 31*, 65–74.

Huebner, D. M., Rebchook, G. M., & Kegeles, S. M. (2004). Experiences of harassment, discrimination, and physical violence among gay and bisexual men. *American Journal of Public Health, 94*, 1200–1203.

Icard, L. (1986). Black gay men and conflicting social identities: Sexual orientation versus racial identity. *Journal of Social Work and Human Sexuality, 4*, 83–93.

Irwin, T. W., & Morgenstern, J. (2005). Drug-use patterns among men who have sex with men presenting for alcohol treatment: Differences in ethnic and sexual identity. *Journal of Urban Health, 82* (Suppl 1), i127–i133.

Johnson, J. H., & McCutcheon, S. M. (1980). Assessing life stress in older children and adolescents: Preliminary findings with the Life Events Checklist. In I. G. Sarason & C. D. Spielberger (Eds.), *Stress and anxiety* (Vol. 6). New York: Wiley.

Kilpatrick, D. G., Ruggiero, K. J., Acierno, R., Saunders, B. E., Resnick, H. S., & Best, C. L. (2003). Violence and risk of PTSD, major depression, substance abuse/dependence, and comorbidity: Results from the National Survey of Adolescents. *Journal of Consulting and Clinical Psychology, 71*, 692–700.

Loiacano, D. K. (1989). Gay identity issues among Black Americans: Racism, homophobia, and the need for validation. *Journal of Counseling & Development, 68*, 21–25.

Martinez, D. G., & Sullivan, S. C. (1998). African American gay men and lesbians: Examining the complexity of gay identity development. *Journal of Human Behavior in the Social Environment, 1*, 243–264.

Meyer, I. H. (1995). Minority stress and mental health in gay men. *Journal of Health and Social Behavior, 36*, 38–56.

Meyer, I. H. (2003). Prejudice, social stress, and mental health in lesbian, gay, and bisexual populations: Conceptual issues and research evidence. *Psychological Bulletin, 129*, 674–697.

Meyer, I. H., & Dean, L. (1995). Patterns of sexual risk behavior and risk taking among young New York City gay men. *AIDS Education and Prevention, 7* (Suppl), 13–23.

Meyer-Bahlburg, H. F. L., Ehrhardt, A. A., Exner, T. M., & Gruen, R. S. (1994). *Sexual Risk Behavior Assessment Schedule—Youth*. Unpublished Measure. (Available from H. F. L. Meyer-Bahlburg, HIV Center for Clinical and Behavioral Studies, New York State Psychiatric Institute, 1051 Riverside Drive, Unit 15, New York, NY 10032, meyerb@childpsych.columbia.edu.)

Mills, T. C., Paul, J., Stall, R., Pollack, L., Canchola, J., Chang, Y. J., et al. (2004). Distress and depression in men who have sex with men: The Urban Men's Health Study. *American Journal of Psychiatry, 161*, 278–285.

National Institute of Mental Health. (1992). *Diagnostic interview schedule for children: Child informant (interview about self)*. Rockville, MD: Author.

Nungesser, L. (1983). *Homosexual acts, actors, and identities*. New York: Praeger.

Paul, J. P., Catania, J., Pollack, L., Moskowitz, J., Canchola, J., Mills, T., et al. (2002). Suicide attempts among gay and bisexual men: Lifetime prevalence and antecedents. *American Journal of Public Health, 92*, 1338–1345.

Pilkington, N. W., & D'Augelli, A. R. (1995). Victimization of lesbian, gay, and bisexual youth in community settings. *Journal of Community Psychology, 23*, 34–56.

Remafedi, G., French, S., Story, M., Resnick, M. D., & Blum, R. (1998). The relationship between suicide risk and sexual orientation: Results of a population-based study. *American Journal of Public Health, 88*, 57–60.

Robin, L., Brener, N. D., Donahue, S. F., Hack, T., Hale, K., & Goodenow, C. (2002). Associations between health risk behaviors and opposite-, same-, and both-sex sexual partners in representative samples of Vermont and Massachusetts high school students. *Archives of Pediatric and Adolescent Medicine, 156*, 349–355.

Rodriguez, E. M., & Ouellette, S. C. (2000). Gay and lesbian Christians: Homosexual and religious identity integration in the members and participants of a gay-positive church. *Journal for the Scientific Study of Religion, 39*, 333–347.

Rosario, M., Hunter, J., & Gwadz, M. (1997). Exploration of substance use among lesbian, gay, and bisexual youth: Prevalence and correlates. *Journal of Adolescent Research, 12*, 454–476.

Rosario, M., Hunter, J., Maguen, S., Gwadz, M., & Smith, R. (2001). The coming-out process and its adaptational and health-related associations among gay, lesbian, and bisexual youths: Stipulation and exploration of a model. *American Journal of Community Psychology, 29*, 133–160.

Rosario, M., Rotheram-Borus, M. J., & Reid, H. (1996). Gay-related stress and its correlates among gay and bisexual male adolescents of predominantly Black and Hispanic background. *Journal of Community Psychology, 24*, 136–159.

Rosario, M., & Schrimshaw, E. W. (2006). Sexual behavior among adolescents: The role of the family, schools, and media in promoting sexual health. In K. Freeark & W. S. Davidson, II (Eds.), *The crisis in youth mental health: Critical issues and effective programs. Volume 3: Issues for families, schools, and communities*. New York: Praeger.

Rosario, M., Schrimshaw, E. W., & Hunter, J. (2004a). Ethnic/racial differences in the coming-out process of lesbian, gay, and bisexual youths: A comparison of sexual identity development over time. *Cultural Diversity and Ethnic Minority Psychology, 10*, 215–228.

Rosario, M., Schrimshaw, E. W., & Hunter, J. (2004b). Predictors of substance use over time among gay, lesbian, and bisexual youths: An examination of three hypotheses. *Addictive Behaviors, 29*, 1623–1631.

Rosario, M., Schrimshaw, E. W., & Hunter, J. (2006). A model of sexual risk behaviors among young gay and bisexual men: Longitudinal associations of mental health, substance abuse, sexual abuse, and the coming-out process. *AIDS Education and Prevention, 18*, 444–460.

Rosario, M., Schrimshaw, E. W., Hunter, J., & Gwadz, M. (2002). Gay-related stress and emotional distress among gay, lesbian, and bisexual youths: A longitudinal examination. *Journal of Consulting and Clinical Psychology, 70*, 967–975.

Rosario, M., Yali, M. A., Hunter, J., & Gwadz, M. (2006). Religion and health among lesbian, gay, and bisexual youth: An empirical investigation and theoretical explanation. In A. M. Omoto & H. S. Kurtzman (Eds.), *Sexual orientation and mental health: Examining identity and development in lesbian, gay, and bisexual people*. Washington, DC: American Psychological Association.

Rosenberg, M. (1965). *Society and adolescent self-image*. Princeton, NJ: Princeton University Press.

Rotheram-Borus, M. J., Rosario, M., Van Rossem, R., Reid, H., & Gillis, R. (1995). Prevalence, course, and predictors of multiple problem behaviors among gay and bisexual male adolescents. *Developmental Psychology, 31*, 75–85.

Russell, S. T., Driscoll, A. K., & Truong, N. (2002). Adolescent same-sex romantic attractions and relationships: Implications for substance use and abuse. *American Journal of Public Health, 92*, 198–202.

Russell, S. T., Franz, B. T., & Driscoll, A. K. (2001). Same-sex romantic attraction and experiences of violence in adolescence. *American Journal of Public Health, 91*, 903–906.

Russell, S. T., & Joyner, K. (2001). Adolescent sexual orientation and suicide risk: Evidence from a national study. *American Journal of Public Health, 91*, 1276–1281.

Safren, S. A., & Heimberg, R. G. (1999). Depression, hopelessness, suicidality, and related factors in sexual minority and heterosexual adolescents. *Journal of Consulting and Clinical Psychology, 67*, 859–866.

Savin-Williams, R. C. (1994). Verbal and physical abuse as stressors in the lives of lesbian, gay male, and bisexual youths: Associations with school problems, running away, substance abuse, prostitution, and suicide. *Journal of Consulting and Clinical Psychology, 62*, 261–269.

Savin-Williams, R. C. (1996). Ethnic- and sexual-minority youth. In R. C. Savin-Williams & C. M. Cohen (Eds.), *The lives of lesbians, gays, and bisexuals: Children to adults*. Forth Worth, TX: Harcourt Brace.

Schrimshaw, E. W., Rosario, M., Meyer-Bahlburg, H. F. L., & Scharf-Matlick, A. A. (2006). Test-retest reliability of self-reported sexual behavior, sexual orientation, and psychosexual milestones among gay, lesbian, and bisexual youths. *Archives of Sexual Behavior, 35*, 220–229.

Shaffer, D., & Gould, M. (1986). *Study of completed suicides in adolescents: Progress report*. Washington, DC: National Institute of Mental Health.

Siegel, K., & Epstein, J. A. (1996). Ethnic-racial differences in psychological stress related to gay lifestyle among HIV-positive men. *Psychological Reports, 79*, 303–312.

Singh, G. K., & Yu, S. M. (1996). Trends and differentials in adolescent and young adult mortality in the United States, 1950 through 1993. *American Journal of Public Health, 86*, 560–564.

Stall, R., Paul, J. P., Greenwood, G., Pollack, L. M., Bein, E., Crosby, G. M., et al. (2001). Alcohol use, drug use and alcohol-related problems among men who have sex with men: The Urban Men's Health Study. *Addiction, 96*, 1589–1601.

Stokes, J. P., & Peterson, J. L. (1998). Homophobia, self-esteem, and risk for HIV among African American men who have sex with men. *AIDS Education and Prevention, 10*, 279–292.

Stokes, J. P., Vanable, P. A., & McKirnan, D. J. (1996). Ethnic differences in sexual behavior, condom use, and psychosocial variables among Black and White men who have sex with men. *The Journal of Sex Research, 33*, 373–381.

Thiede, H., Valleroy, L. A., MacKellar, D. A., Celentano, D. D., Ford, W. L., Hagan, H., et al. (2003). Regional patterns and correlates of substance use among young men who have sex with men in 7 US urban areas. *American Journal of Public Health, 93*, 1915–1921.

Udry, J. R., & Chantala, K. (2002). Risk assessment of adolescents with same-sex relationships. *Journal of Adolescent Health, 31*, 84–92.

Valleroy, L. A., MacKellar, D. A., Karon, J. M., Rosen, D. H., McFarland, W., Shehan, D. A., et al. (2000). HIV prevalence and associated risks in young men who have sex with men. *Journal of the American Medical Association, 284*, 198–204.

Waldo, C. R., McFarland, W., Katz, M. H., MacKellar, D., & Valleroy, L. A. (2000). Very young gay and bisexual men are at risk for HIV infection: The San Francisco Bay Area Young Men's Survey II. *Journal of Acquired Immune Deficiency Syndromes, 24*, 168–174.

Williams, T., Connolly, J., Pepler, D., & Craig, W. (2005). Peer victimization, social support, and psychosocial adjustment of sexual minority adolescents. *Journal of Youth and Adolescence, 34*, 471–482.

Williamson, I. R. (2000). Internalized homophobia and health issues affecting lesbians and gay men. *Health Education Research, 15*, 97–107.

Woods, T. E., Antoni, M. H., Ironson, G. H., & Kling, D. W. (1999). Religiosity is associated with affective and immune status in symptomatic HIV-infected gay men. *Journal of Psychosomatic Research, 46*, 165–176.

Xia, Q., Osmond, D. H., Tholandi, M., Pollack, L. M., Zhou, W., Ruiz, J. D., et al. (2006). HIV prevalence and sexual risk behaviors among men who have sex with men: Results from a statewide population-based survey in California. *Journal of Acquired Immune Deficiency Syndromes, 41*, 238–245.

Health Disparities and People With Disabilities

Introduction

People with disabilities face a number of inequities in health. A new approach to global health must ensure that an inclusive approach prevails, allowing this population to experience equity in access to the resources and opportunities deemed essential to the achievement of equity in health. As Linton (1998) explains, the population of people with disabilities is large and diverse, including those using various devices and aids to negotiate the physical environment—whether because of conditions at birth, those resulting from accidents/mishaps, or the aging process, as well as those with mental and emotional conditions, and people living with HIV/AIDS. A full discussion of the characteristics, needs, and disparities in health experienced by this large and diverse group of people with disability will not be presented in this context. Instead, the objectives of this chapter are to (1) define the complexity of understanding health disparities for people with disabilities; (2) describe the relationship between disability and health; (3) explore the access to health care inequities that exist for people with disabilities; (4) describe the relationship between unemployment and the benefits that are and are not available to people with disabilities; and (5) discuss the future research and policy changes that are necessary for improving access to health care for people with disabilities.

Complexity of Disability

If we strive to understand disability from a social constructionist perspective or from a minority model point of view, we begin to see that the disabled community may be one of the most complex populations to define or describe for a number of reasons. First, there is no one specific icon, leader,

Richard M. Keller and Joe P. King

or voice unanimously accepted by people with disabilities. Compare this fact with other groups seeking equality. Think about Dr. Martin Luther King, Jr., and his speeches and protest marches. Think about the images of Matthew Shepard and the rallying effects that his brutal death had on the Lesbian, Gay, Bisexual, and Transgender community. Now try to recall a similar person, image, set of words, or an event that capture the civil rights struggle for the disabled community. If you failed to recall such an event, person, or moment of communication, you are not alone. The failure to agree on a defining icon may be one of the most pervasive failures of the disabled rights movement.

Secondly, it is difficult to arrive at an inclusive definition of disability that is acceptable to all members and groups within the disabled community. We have legal definitions such as the one established by the Americans with Disabilities Act (ADA) of 1990. Although the ADA's definition is seemingly widely accepted, the host of court cases focusing on whether or not an individual meets the conditions of the definition and the myriad of contradictory court decisions speak to the fact that the definition remains unclear.

We could revert to the medical model and define conditions that describe disability or we could ask people to self-identify as being disabled. Reverting to the medical model would not be tolerated by those people with disabilities who are actively involved in the civil rights movement; and, an individual's self-identification as being disabled lacks unity as well. Since an individual can experience disability in a highly idiomatic fashion and there are so many different physical or mental circumstances that can lead one to be defined as an individual with a disability, there is a relative lack of unity in identifying people who might be considered, by themselves or by others, disabled.

Past research has attempted to explore this identity paradox. For example, Toms-Barker, and Maralani (1997) inquired about disability-related conditions and the ways in which the presence of such conditions affect various household and parenting tasks. Despite their self-report of diagnosed medical conditions and functional limitations, several respondents indicated that they do not consider themselves to be a person with a disability. Similarly, in a 1986 Harris Poll, persons with disabilities were asked a series of questions related to their self-views. Almost half of the respondents did not think of themselves as disabled or handicapped and did not think that other people would think so either.

Relationship Between Health and Disability

Dr. Olkin (1999) describes this relationship elegantly. We quote her extensively for this reason with permission:

> ... one of the problems being the blurry distinction between disability and illness. To illustrate this, think of two continua, one representing health and the other disability. The two continua are not parallel but get closer as severity increases on each one; that is, the two concepts of health and disability are related but they are neither completely coincidental nor orthogonal. The left end of the disability continuum might include nearsightedness or some degree of color blindness. People with such relatively minor loss of functioning would rarely be considered 'disabled' by either their own or other people's definition. Moving to the middle of the disability continuum we might find mild

cerebral palsy (CP) or minimal aftereffects of polio. At the right end of this continuum we could place those more serious disabilities that involve significant degrees of impairment in several major life functions; an example might be amyotrophic lateral sclerosis (ALS or "Lou Gehrig's Disease"). The other continuum, the health continuum, focuses on the overall health status of an individual. Its left end is quite separate from that of the disability continuum. Placed there are minor, routine, and temporary ailments such as colds. Slightly to the right on the health continuum are ailments such as the flu or ear infections—ailments that, under certain conditions, can lead to more serious complications. The middle of this continuum might include ailments such as Kartagener syndrome (where the heart is located on the right side of a person's body causing the crowding of other organs) or lower-level spinal cord injury. Examples of ailments that could be found at the right end of the health continuum might include Duchenne muscular dystrophy (MD) and some conditions leading to dwarfism (there are more than 150 such conditions, but a few of them are fatal). It is possible to have a disability—for example, CP—and also be considered in excellent health. However, more serious disabilities often compromise an individual's health. For example, as mobility and movement decrease, certain health problems such as decubitus ulcers, urinary track infections, and pneumonia increase. These secondary health conditions—that is, the ailments—are usually the cause of any eventual death, not the disability per se. Conversely, the ailments that are found at the extreme right end of the health continuum often begin to impair an individual's ability to perform some of life's major functions; in short, compromised health begets disability. So the overlap between disability and illness becomes increasingly important as the conditions on either or both of the continua increase in severity. It is probably not possible to come up with a definition of disability that includes only disability and not illness, and vice versa. (Olkin, 1999)

Beyond the question of the relationship between an individual's health and their disability, there are additional complexities. The experience of functional limitation and the reactions to and strategies to manage disability related concerns may be different for each individual and should be examined on a case-by-case basis. For example, if we were to examine the experience of an individual with a functional limitation such as blindness, we would be better served by first considering the manifestation of the individual's disability. One individual might be congenitally blind. A second individual might be adventitiously blind due to sudden trauma or injury. And still yet, a third individual might have acquired his/her blindness later in life as a result of a slow, degenerative eye disease such as retinopathy or glaucoma. It is clear to see that the experiences and adjustment to the same functional limitation are likely to be quite different for these three individuals.

The complexity and nuance expressed on a case-by-case basis by persons who might or might not be considered disabled may be a partial explanation for the minimal traction of the related civil rights movement. Without real civil rights that are enforced, real change is not likely to take root. In an environment where discrimination is still socially accepted, the resultant unequal lives with respect to employment, social opportunities, and other important areas such as access to health care is understandable yet intolerable. And yet, this describes the enduring and socially accepted discrimination against people with disabilities in our country and in our world. People with disabilities continue to be thought of only through their impairments and not through the discrimination-laden lives they live. In addition, some view disability as medical, and believe medical matters should be kept private. The end result is the reality of less than equal opportunities to access and benefit from health care.

Physical Access to Health Care

A major concern of those with physical disability is physical access and integration to health care facilities and providers. A great concern for persons with disabilities is actually being able to get to the facilities that provide health care and related services—whether the dentist, pharmacist, health clinic, and other related health care services.

Persons with disabilities, while generally content with the quality of care they receive, periodically confront barriers in the pursuit of these services. Anecdotal evidence points to barriers which include lack of physical access to buildings where health care is provided; lack of internal access to offices, rooms, and medical equipment; lack of meaningful communication around medical concerns or medications; and lack of alternative format materials about medical procedures or medication information—to name a few.

Disability Rights Advocates conducted a study of 400 participants with disabilities (Markwalder, 2005), and their results confirm and quantify the above mentioned anecdotal reports seen on TV news magazines, newspaper articles, and community discussions. Some of the findings are as follows: 17% of people who have mobility impairments have difficulty with the main entrance to their doctors' office; 29% of persons with mobility impairments report having difficulty in waiting rooms; 33% of persons with mobility impairments have difficulty with accessible exam rooms; 43% of persons who use wheelchairs have difficulty using exam chairs; 69% of persons who use wheelchairs have difficulty using exam tables; 60% of persons who use wheelchairs have difficulty being weighed because the scales are not accessible; 45% of persons who use wheelchairs report difficulty using X-ray equipment; 26% of persons who are deaf report difficulty getting interpreters for medical appointments; 98% of persons who have visual impairments report not receiving provider lists in accessible formats; 90% of individuals with visual impairments report not receiving educational materials in accessible formats; 95% of individuals with visual impairments report not receiving medical history forms in accessible formats; 59% of persons with learning disabilities and 64% of those with cognitive disabilities report that their providers communicate with someone else in the room and not directly with them; and, 79% of those with cognitive disabilities report receiving not enough time to discuss their symptoms to their health care provider and ask questions that are necessary (Markwalder).

Faced with these inequities, it is sometimes difficult for individuals with disabilities to consider how best to respond to these dilemmas. There are probably many reasons that make it difficult to consider how to develop a variety of optional responses to the conflict situations. First, the power differential in the relationship is likely to make the individual with the disability hesitant to speak out and potentially be perceived as troublesome or critical by the health care provider. Secondly, people with disabilities have in many cases learned the patient role and are likely to remain docile and passive while pursuing medical care. Finally, it is possible that the importance of getting the medical situation attended to in a timely and effective manner supercedes their inclination to advocate for their rights. They might simply consider this battle not worth fighting and take a pass on the conflict at hand.

Notwithstanding the pressures not to advocate for one's self when faced with barriers to equal access to health care, several lawsuits have been filed against health care providers on the basis of discrimination. It is beyond the scope of this chapter to review all the related legal actions and findings, but a glance at an example or two seems in order. For example, *DeVinney v. Maine Medical Center* was a case where Maine Medical Center refused to provide a qualified sign language interpreter or other accommodations such as hearing aids for a deaf patient. This patient was in a suicidal state in a psychiatric ward. The U.S. Attorney's office and the Department of Justice sought changes in hospital policy, damages on behalf of the plaintiff, and civil penalties (Enforcing the ADA: A Status Report, October–December 1997). Although this case was settled out of court, subsequently, several states enacted higher standards related to the provision of sign language interpretation and other related accommodations for medical appointments and procedures. The concept of equity in access to health care certainly does not seem to have been in the forefront of the health care providers' treatment of this individual.

Another discrimination action sought to secure the rights of an individual to be treated by a health care provider in a manner equal to other patients and not in a different and more costly setting solely on the basis of the disability. In the case of *Bragdon v. Abbott*, a dentist refused to fill a cavity of an asymptomatic AIDS patient. The dentist agreed to attend to the patient, but only in a hospital setting with more controls and with increased cost. The question before the Supreme Court was whether AIDS limited a major life activity, specifically reproduction. The plaintiff, a woman, argued not being able to reproduce inhibited a major life activity and therefore deserved protections under the Americans with Disabilities Act. The Supreme Court decided in her favor, finding that reproduction was a major life activity under the Americans with Disabilities Act. Therefore, health care providers are not permitted to refuse service to an individual with a disability based on an assumption of direct threat. Direct threat must be based upon objective evidence of such a threat.

If we can comfortably consider reproduction as a major life activity, we may then contemplate the right of people with disabilities to reproduce or pressing this further to be born. A long-standing dispute is whether or not an individual with a disability has the right to reproduce and potentially bear children with disabilities. Forced sterilization has been conducted throughout the years and in many countries. We need not limit our examination of this social policy to infamous persons such as Hitler, although his first murders were over one-quarter of a million people with disabilities in addition to sterilizing nearly half a million (Paradis & Wolinsky, 1999). This dispute has been a source of discrimination for centuries and has come to the U.S. Supreme Court both before and after the passage of the Americans with Disabilities Act. The ability of the eugenics movement to influence such basic rights such as the right to reproduce remains alive and well even today. Embryos continue to be screened out on the basis of the potential to express a disability in the infant. In Australia, for example, doctors screen out embryos that carry the gene for deafness (Weiss, 2003). On the other hand, and quite on the contrary, another recent trend is that there are also couples that request embryos that have a genetic predisposition to produce a child with a disability. This allows parents with disabilities to have children with disabilities (Geller, 2006). The extreme polarity on this topic captures the diametrically opposed views on the struggle between those that consider people with disabilities an essential part of a diverse tapestry of humanity and those that continue to consider disability a depraved expression of life and one which should be sequestered away or eliminated. If people with disabilities should not be born or should be eliminated after being born, why should the dominant society express concern for health care of people with disabilities?

Transportation for the disabled is a significant issue for persons with disabilities. Adequate access to public transportation is essential for transportation to access employment, health care, and the general community. Transportation barriers are one reason why some persons with disabilities cannot become employed (Wehman, Wilson, Parent, Sherron-Targett, & McKinley, 2000). Contrasting urban and rural areas, in 1996, 35% of rural fixed-route vehicles for public transportation were accessible, as opposed to 60% in urban public transportation systems. Although, rural areas have limited public transportation services, urban areas have more transportation services available. However, there are concerns about the limitations of the schedules, as they fail to adequately meet the needs of persons with disabilities who may wish to travel at odd hours or for night shifts, etc ... (Wehman, Wilson, Targett, West, Bricout, & McKinley, 1999).

Another study found that persons who were younger and had more mobility issues demonstrated greater dissatisfaction with paratransit (personalized public transportation) than others. While this study was focused primarily on satisfaction with one transit system, and used a small sample (Denson, 2000), its conclusions should serve as notice to public transportation systems around the nation. Any inequity in the paratransit system, or the mere fact that no paratransit system need provide transportation outside of the same areas where regular public transportation systems travel, creates difficulties for people with disabilities especially when they live in or desire to travel in more rural areas. The travel related concerns certainly have a negative impact on people with disabilities in a variety of important life activities, including the pursuit of health care.

Health Insurance, Benefits, and Employment

There is also a relationship between unemployment and the benefits that are and are not available to people with disabilities in places such as the United States. The situation people with disabilities face in the United States may serve to illustrate key issues with regard to ensuring the health and access to health care for people with disabilities.

The cost of health care has risen substantially in the last few decades. In 1970, $75.1 billion dollars were spent on health care; in 2004, $1.877 trillion dollars were spent on health care (Smith, Cowan, Heffler, Catlin, & National Health Accounts Team, 2006). Unfortunately, persons and families with disabilities are more likely to live with lower incomes than persons and families without disabilities, which may make access to health care more difficult. A family with a person with a disability has $36,197 in average income, while a family without a person with a disability has an average income of $54,515. Families with at least one member with a disability are three times more likely to receive lifeline assistance (42.8%) than families with no members with disabilities (14.2%). The poverty rate for a family with a person with a disability is higher (12.8%) than a family without a person with a disability (7.7%). In a family who has two or more persons with a disability, the poverty rate rises to 16.5% (U.S. Census Bureau, 2005a).

A study by Hanson, Neuman, Dutwin, and Kasper (2003) examined specific health care and insurance related issues impacting persons with disabilities. Study results were of great concern. Of the 1,505 participants, almost three fourths used family and friends to assist in the performance of activities of daily living (ADL; e.g., eating, bathing, dressing); and fewer than 10% had professional sources of care such as a home health aid. This raises questions about the quality and consistency of care. A person with a disability may not be able to rely on family members or friends to provide care throughout the years. The quality of care might also be inferior, as it is unlikely that these family members or friends are appropriately trained. If this care is substandard, persons with disabilities risk hospitalization, institutionalization, or increased risk for developing other health related issues.

Research has shown there is considerable risk in having professionals deliver services as well. Oktay and Tompkins (2004) showed 30% of disabled participants in one study suffered some abuse by their primary personal assistant (PA; 30%), while a majority suffered abuse from other PA providers (61%). The most reported method of abuse was verbal from their primary PA (18%). Twenty-nine percent reported verbal abuse and theft from other PAs. Other forms of abuse were less prominent for primary PA providers: 6% reported neglect, 5% poor care, 10% physical abuse, 3% sexual abuse, and 8% extortion. Abuse from other PA providers increased for most other forms of abuse. Twenty-six percent reported neglect, 21% poor care, 9% physical abuse, 8% sexual abuse, and 15% extortion. While the study had a low sample size ($N = 84$), results were consistent with other research, and still provide good data as a means to gauge abuse for this at-risk population. Considering the personal nature of care provided and the extensive need (e.g., help with activites of daily living was needed by 94% of participants, including help with dressing by 94%, continence by 85%, mobility by 77%, and feeding by 57%: Oktay & Tompkins, 2004), any abuse could be extremely damaging to the physical and emotional well-being of the client, not to mention disrupting the quality and continuity of health care.

Persons with disabilities tend to use the health care system more frequently than persons without disabilities. Ninety percent of the participants in the Hanson et al. (2003) study had visited a physician in the last 6 months. One third of participants visited an emergency room in the same amount of time. Nearly nine in ten participants used a prescription drug regularly, and in higher rates than the general populace. People in fair and poor health reported more use of medical services than those in better health. Of those who reported fair and poor health, almost 66% visited a physician four or more times in the last 6 months, while for those who reported being in good or very good health, only 40% reported seeing a physician in the last 6 months. People with disabilities use the health care system more frequently than the general population, but less frequently than recommended by health care providers. This might have a negative impact on health status and might be linked to their medical coverage and its limitations. While many people have some form of health insurance, it may not provide adequate coverage for all of their medical needs. In Hanson et al. (2003), 95% of the sample had some access to health insurance. This is due to enrollment in programs such as Supplemental Security Income (SSI) and Social Security Disabilty Income (SSDI), which give them access to Medicaid and Medicare, respectively. Of the participants that were insured, Medicaid insured 44% and Medicare insured 43%, including the 14% who had both Medicaid and Medicare, and 14% with supplemental private insurance. Thirty three percent of those with insurance had some sort of private insurance. When the groups are broken down further, 30% rely exclusively on Medicaid, 15% exclusively on Medicare, and 19% on private insurance alone.

Although persons with disabilities have good access to health insurance, they may not have access to all the services necessary. People with disabilities are four times more likely to have special needs not covered by their health insurance. In addition, persons with severe disabilities are more likely to have needs not covered by insurance than those with less severe disabilities (Harris & Associates, 2000).

Employment

One of the areas related to the issue of access to medical coverage is the issue of employment. Many people look to their employer for assistance with the costs of medical coverage, but persons with disabilities have been consistently unemployed and underemployed as compared with their nondisabled counterparts. U.S. Census Bureau (2005b) results indicated that only 37.5% of all persons with disabilities between the ages of 16 and 64 were employed. The employed people with disabilities who responded were distributed across varying disabilities as follows: 47.2% with sensory disabilities, 31.8% with physical disabilities, and 28.7% of with mental disabilities. This unemployment rate contrasts poorly with the population without disabilities, which has a 74.4% employment rate.

The reasons for this have been thought to be a result of poor economic conditions and negative attitudes towards those with disabilities (Couch, 1994). People with disabilities are interviewed fewer times for jobs (Johnson & Heal, 1976), and employers continue to not hire persons with disabilities (Hernandez, Keys, Balcazar, & Drum, 1998). Todd (1993) noted individuals with disabilities stress there are too few employment opportunities. Not only is there lack of employment, but persistent discrimination, lack of access to accessible transportation, and lack of reasonable accommodations at workplaces that further hinder employment (LaPlante, 1997). Stereotyping and discrimination are still prevalent after more than 15 years after the passage of the Americans with Disabilities Act. Unemployment, underemployment, and inequality in job compensation are a reality for persons with disability in the workforce. This forces those with disabilities to turn to government for financial support, and contributes to their lower socioeconomic status (Gouvier, Sytsma-Jordan, & Mayville, 2003).

Social Security, Supplemental Security, and Medicare

Social Security provides money for the elderly and certain persons with disabilities to sustain themselves. The program for the disabled is called Social Security Disability Income (SSDI). The requirements for this are in three categories: A person who becomes disabled before turning 24 is required to have worked one and a half of the the last 3 years. A person between the ages of 24 and 31 is required to have worked at least half of the time, between the ages of 21 and acquisition of disability. A person over 31 years old is required to have worked 5 out of the last 10 years. Specific requirements for SSDI need to be assessed by the Social Security Offices. There are requirements for people around specific ages to have worked and contributed to the Social Security System (Social Security Administration, 2005a).

Supplemental Security Income (SSI) is different. There are no work requirements for SSI. It is for people who are disabled, blind, or age 65 and older. It allows people to get money to help sustain them, they must be disabled under federal rules, and have an income including resources below $2,000, or $3,000 if a person is married, although there are several exceptions. The income of a spouse may be included, and if a person is a minor (under 18) some of their parents' income and resources may be included in the calculation of benefits (Social Security Administration, 2005b).

The Medicare Program

Understanding Medicare can assist professionals and beneficiaries, allowing them to advise people with disabilities as to the best resources available to them. There are distinct differences between the health care programs Medicaid and Medicare, including how they serve persons with disabilities. Medicare is a federally funded and administered program that provides services to persons over the age of 65 and those who have permanent disabilities under the age of 65. To be eligible, one must be 65 years old and have the client or the client's spouse to have paid into the Social Security system. Some people who become disabled before the age of 65 and cannot work may be eligible for Medicare, but they must wait 29 months to receive benefits. This requirement can be waived for those with life threatening conditions such as end-stage renal disease (kidney failure) or amyotrophic lateral sclerosis (ALS or Lou Gehrig's disease). In addition, a person whose parents received Social Security benefits and acquires a severe permanent disability before the age of 22 is eligible for Medicare, although a waiting period applies to that person as well. Spouses and dependents can continue to receive benefits after the death of the primary beneficiary (Williams, Claypool, & Crowley, 2005).

Work Incentives

Beginning in 1999, people with disabilities could begin to work and not lose certain benefits. This allows a person with a disability to maintain a way of life and the health insurance benefits that accompany being employed. A person with a disability may also explore through employement the extent to which they can manage and adapt to work.

Social Security and Medicare. In most cases people on Medicare can keep their benefits, at least temporarily while attempting to return to work. The first 9 months of working is called a trial work period. In this time, a person keeps their full Social Security benefits, including Medicare. During a trial work period an individual must make more than $640 a month, or a person who owns his or her own business must earn $640 in profits or spend more than 80 hours running the business.

The trial work period continues until one has worked 9 months within a 60-month period. Also, the trial work period ends after 9 months (Social Security Administration, 2007).

After that period, an extended period of eligibility begins. An individual can continue to work and maintain their benefits as long as their work is not deemed substantially gainful employment. Substantially gainful employment is defined as earning more than $900 a month, or $1,500 for a blind individual. An individual who has previously been determined as an individual with a disability, for benefits purposes, can attempt to work and then return to benefits status without a new determination of disability. This extended period of eligibility lasts for 36 months (Social Security Administration, 2007).

If an individual's income exceeds the substantial threshold, he or she has 5 years to ask for benefits to be reinstated. As long as one is within this time frame, he or she will not have to fill out an application and will not have to wait for their disability status to be reviewed until receiving benefits. A person can also remain on Medicare while not receiving SSDI, for 93 months after the trial work period. During these 93 months, Medicare Part A is still free along with the other benefits. After those 93 months, a person can pay a monthly premium for Medicare Part A. In addition, an individual who is working may deduct his or her disability related expenses from their income when determining eligibility for services (Social Security Administration, 2007).

Supplemental Security Income and Medicaid

Supplemental Security Income (SSI) is for those people who have little or no resources. A person who works may continue to receive payments until his or her earnings exceed the SSI income limit. This limit is set by each state; an individual needs to contact his or her local Social Security office to determine the limit that is applicable for their state. If payments stop based on earnings exceeding the amount set, and the individual subsequently stops working because of their disability, the payments can be reinstated again without completing a new application. Like SSDI, a person can deduct disability related expenses from his or her earnings. In addition, if a person has a plan to achieve self-sufficiency, the money he or she uses for this can be deducted from their earnings. Students can earn up to $1,500 a month, and up to $6,100 a year—without affecting SSI payments, although a person must be under 22 and in a school or training program on a regular basis (Social Security Administration, 2007).

Generally, an individual's Medicaid coverage continues until his or her income reaches a certain threshold. This is also determined by the states. Although, if their health care costs are higher than the income threshold, they can continue to receive Medicaid benefits. In most states, Medicaid coverage continues if the individual needs it to continue employment, is unable to afford similar insurance, continues to have a disabling condition, and continues to meet the other SSI requirements. A person's case will be reviewed periodically to ensure these requirements are being met (Social Security Administration, 2007).

A Final Comment on Issues of Benefits and Health Care

A question arises as to whether or not the models described herein, available in the United States, are viable for ensuring income and economic stability for persons with disabilities, as well as equity in health care. However, if the care that people access reflects discrimination, and the context for their overall lives and care is one that reflects discrimination, then what more needs to be done in the United States to move us toward equity in health for persons with disabilities? Also, is the model of benefits and health care described one that might provide a guide and map for other countries? What improvements are needed? Might other countries and models serve to inform and improve what is done in the United States? In addition, might it be possible that the ideal model ensuring equity in health care has yet to emerge? These are just some of the questions that arise from what has been presented; providing answers to such questions is beyond the scope of this chapter.

Future Directions

The material presented in this chapter suggests the need for several improvements to ensure access and use of health care by persons with disabilities. The suggested future efforts are not intended to be exhaustive, rather we hope that they encourage others to think through the dilemmas and systematic barriers for people with disabilities with respect to equity in health care. Although some of the suggestions are provided as measures that people with disabilities can directly take up, this is in no way meant to indicate that the inequity that people with disabilities face is their fault or that they need to bear the burden of repairing systems that are not working properly. These suggestions are meant to provide people with disabilities an active role in the improvement of their own lives.

Psychologists can continue to investigate ways in which stigma and negative attitudes toward people with disabilities can be reduced in our society—specifically, by professional and nonprofessional persons working in the delivery of health care components. Initial research could focus on identifying major sources of these negative aspects of behavior that could lead to the development of psycho-educational interventions in service of this positive change.

It is also important to investigate through research those mechanisms contributing to disparities in medical advising and counseling, resulting in inequities for people with disabilities in the health care system. Such research should focus on how best to assist health care providers in managing stressful and high volumes of inquiry, while at the same time providing strategies for individualized approaches with enough flexibility to respond more individually to the various needs of different clients with disabilities.

Professional organizations and sponsoring boards should be encouraged to explicitly codify their commitment to the goal of equitable health care for persons with disabilities. This could include a commitment to no longer tolerating the provision or establishment of health care facilities that fail to provide physical access, as well as a commitment to equity in the provision of all health care related communications, including oral and written forms, ensuring equitable access for persons with disabilities. Additionally, training programs should explicitly commit to the inclusion of specific courses that foster greater understanding of the needs and barriers faced by people with disabilities with respect to the receipt of all aspects of health care. For persons already working in the field of health care, continued education should include similar mandatory educational offerings.

Research needs to address the difficulties that people with disabilities experience in advocating for their own equal access with respect to health care. Among the goals of such research could be the goal of developing psycho-educational interventions designed to provide people with disabilities options to respond when faced with conflicts as a result of facing barriers in health care delivery. There could be additional outcome research to explore the efficacy of the educational efforts and their potential positive impact in ensuring the equity of health care for people with disabilities.

Additional research could be developed to contribute to the understanding of the complex interactions of employment and health care for people with disabilities. This could include examining not only psychological factors, but also financial factors. Some of the participants could include people with disabilities, employers, and governmental agencies such as the Social Security Administration.

Conclusion

Given this chapter's discussion of the complexity of health disparities for people with disabilities, the relationship between disability and health, inequities in access to health care, description of the unemployment and other benefits that are and are not available to people with disabilities, and future research and policy changes that are necessary for improving access to health care for people with disabilities, final comments are in order.

A disabled rights movement is needed that focuses upon all that is essential to ensure equitable access to health care and moves the diverse communities of people with disabilities toward equity in health. Ideally, this occurs within a larger movement toward the achievement of equity in health for all, being led by a diverse body of professionals, nonprofessionals, and consumers who collaboratively work toward fulfillment of this vision, making it a tangible reality. Calls for equity in access to health care, will ideally come from a collective of diverse voices who recognize and appreciate the needs of people with disabilities and work alongside them to ensure that their needs are included in any agenda to bring about equity.

By highlighting the complexity of health disparities for people with disabilities, illustrating the links between disability and health, inequities in access to health care, unemployment and benefits issues, and spelling out needed research and policy changes, this chapter may serve as a template for what the collaborative teams working within a larger movement for attaining equity need to know. This chapter spells out the a basic body of knowledge needed, while, in the ideal situation, people with disabilities will also be on the team and sitting at the table, working alongside those committed to the vision of equity. If we as a nation and a global community ultimately share the burden of ill health, then perhaps we should share the responsibility for collaboratively working together to bring about equity. The pervasive discrimination, lack of access, inequitable health care, and even abuse that many people with disability currently experience suggests the urgency of such collaborative work within a larger movement for the achievement of equity in health for all.

REFERENCES

Americans with Disabilities Act of 1990, Public Law No. 101-336, § 2, 104 Stat. 328 (1991).
Bragdon v. Abbott, 524 U.S. 624 (1998).

Couch, R. H. (1994). Living with disability in Central America. Special issue: Vocational evaluation and work adjustment in international rehabilitation. *Vocational Evaluation & Work Adjustment Bulletin, 27*, 82–87.

Denson, C. R. (2000). Public sector transportation for people with disabilities: A satisfaction survey. *Journal of Rehabilitation, 66*, 29–37.

Devinny v Maine Medical Center,1998 WL 271495 (D. Me. 1998).

Enforcing the ADA: A status report, October–December 1997. (1997). Retrieved February 09, 2007, from http://www.usdoj.gov/crt/ada/octdec97.htm

Geller, A. (2006, December 22). Docs' designer defect baby. *New York Post Online Edition.* Retrieved February 09, 2007, from http://www.nypost.com/seven/12222006/news/regionalnews/docs_designer_defect_baby_regionalnews_andy_geller.htm

Gouvier, W. D., Sytsma-Jordan, S., & Mayville, S. (2003). Patterns of discrimination in hiring job applicants with disabilities: The role of disability type, job complexity, and public contact. *Rehabilitation Psychology, 48*, 175–181.

Hanson, K. W., Neuman, P., Dutwin, D., & Kasper, J. D. (2003). Uncovering the health challenges facing people with disabilities: The role of health insurance. *Health Affairs.* Retrieved January 21, 2007, from http://content.healthaffairs.org/cgi/content/full/hlthaff.w3.552v1/DC1

Harris, L., & Associates. (1986). *Disabled Americans' self perceptions: Bringing disabled Americans back into the mainstream.* A survey conducted for the International Center for the Disabled, New York.

Harris, L., & Associates. (2000). *2000 Survey of Americans with disabilities.* A survey conducted for the National Organization on Disability, New York.

Hernandez, B., Keys, C., Balcazar, F., & Drum, C. (1998). Construction and validation of the Disability Rights Attitude Scale: Assessing attitudes toward the Americans with Disabilities Act (ADA). *Rehabilitation Psychology, 43*, 203–218.

Johnson, R., & Heal, L. (1976). Private employment agency responses to the physically handicapped applicant in a wheelchair. *Journal of Applied Rehabilitation Counseling, 7*, 12–21.

LaPlante, M. P. (1997). *The context of employment statistics and disability. Data needs, employment statistics, and disability policy.* Presentation. Retrieved December 12, 2003, from http://dsc.ucsf.edu/reps/forum2/present.html

Linton, S. K. (1998). *Claiming disability: Knowledge and identity.* New York: New York University Press.

Markwalder, A. (2005) *A call to action: A guide for managed care plans serving Californians with disabilities.* Berkeley, CA: Disability Rights Advocates.

Oktay, J. S., & Tompkins, C. T. (2004). Personal assistance providers' mistreatment of disabled adults. *Health & Social Work, 29*, 177–188.

Olkin, R. (1999). *What psychotherapists should know about disability.* New York: Guilford Press.

Paradis, L. W., & Wolinsky, S. (1999). *Forgotten crimes: The Holocaust and people with disabilities.* Berkelely, CA: Disability Rights Advocates.

Smith, C., Cowan, C., Heffler, S., Catlin, A., & National Health Accounts Team. (2006). National health spending in 2004: Recent slowdown led by prescription drug spending. *Health Affairs, 25*, 186–196.

Social Security Administration. (2005a). *Disability benefits.* Washington, DC: U.S. Government Printing Office. (Publication No. 05-10701-EN).

Social Security Administration. (2005b). *Supplemental security income.* Washington, DC: U.S. Government Printing Office. (Publication No. 05-11000).

Social Security Administration. (2007). *Working while disabled.* Washington, DC: U.S. Government Printing Office. (Publication No. 05-10095).

Todd, S. (1993). Reflecting on change: Consumers' views of the impact of the All-Wales strategy. *Mental Handicap, 21*, 128–136.

Toms-Barker, L., & Maralani, V. (1997). *Challenges and strategies of disabled parents: Findings from a national survey of parents with disabilities.* Berkeley, CA: Through the Looking Glass.

U.S. Census Bureau. (2005a). *Disability and American families: 2000.* Retrieved from the U.S. Census Bureau Web site: http://www.census.gov

U.S. Census Bureau. (2005b). *American community survey* [Data file; S1801]. Retrieved from the U.S. Census Bureau Web site: http://www.census.gov

Wehman, P. P., Wilson, K. P., Parent, W. P., Sherron-Targett, P. M., & McKinley, W. (2000). Employment satisfaction of individuals with spinal cord injury. *American Journal of Physical Medicine & Rehabilitation, 79*, 161–169.

Wehman, P. P., Wilson, K. P., Targett, P. M., West, M., Bricout, J., & McKinley, W. (1999). Removing transportation barriers for persons with spinal cord injuries: An ongoing challenge to community reintegration. *Journal of Vocational Rehabilitation, 13*, 21–30.

Weiss, R. (2003, July 14). Screening embryos for deafness. *The Washington Post*, A06.

Williams, B., Claypool, H., & Crowley, J. S. (February, 2005). *Navigating Medicare and Medicaid, 2005. A resource guide for people with disabilities, their families, and their advocates.* Menlo Park, CA: Henry J. Kaiser Family Foundation.

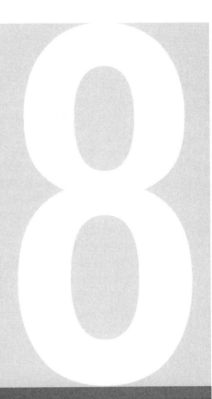

Closing the Education and Health Gaps—Addressing Dual Inter-Related Disparities Through Effective Engagement

Classroom-Based Interventions to Reduce Academic Disparities Between Low-Income and High-Income Students

Introduction

Denise E. Ross
and Yemonja Smalls

According to the National Center for Children in Poverty (NCCP; 2006), there are approximately 42.5 million poor and low-income[1] children in the United States. For the 40% who are school age (NCCP), academic disparities between low-income and high-income students are all too common. The National Center for Educational Statistics (NCES; 2005) reports that fourth-graders from low-income families are at least two times more likely to fail at reading and math than their peers who are not from low-income families (see Figure 26.1). Such academic disparities can persist through secondary school, resulting in dropping out of school and sustaining a low-income lifestyle as an adult. These data suggest that schooling plays a critical role in preventing early academic failure and future economic challenges for low-income students. As such, identifying effective academic interventions is important when addressing disparities between low-income and high-income children.

Among the many district, school, and classroom solutions that exist to address the academic needs of low-income students, increasing the number of academic interactions between teachers and students is a potentially viable intervention. Research suggests positive correlations between the

---

[1]According to the NCCP (2006), families and children are "poor" if their household income is below the federal poverty threshold. They are "low-income" if their household income is less than twice the federal poverty threshold. In this chapter, we use the term "low-income" to describe all children whose families are defined as either poor or low-income.

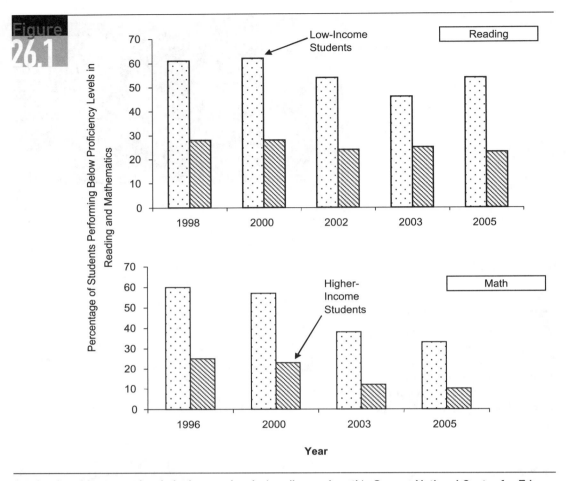

Figure 26.1

Academic achievement levels by income levels (reading and math). *Source:* National Center for Educational Statistics (2006).

rate of teacher–student academic interactions and rates of students' academic success (Greenwood, Hart, Walker, & Risley, 1994; Greer, 2002; Sutherland & Wehby, 2001). These interactions, called *learn units,* are basic measures of instruction that, when accumulated, impact student learning. That is, when teachers present high numbers of accurate and rapid learn units, students respond correctly to instruction more frequently and achieve more instructional objectives (Albers & Greer, 1991; Greer, McCorkle, & Williams, 1989; Ingham & Greer, 1992; Keohane & Greer, 2005; Lamm & Greer, 1991; Selinske, Greer, & Lodhi, 1991). The purpose of the current chapter is to discuss the research on learn units and its implications for improving academic outcomes for low-income students.

A *learn unit* is a construct describing an *interlocking* sequence of teacher and student behaviors that comprise an instance of instruction and learning. For instance, a teacher may say "What is 2 + 2?" wait a few seconds while students say "Four," and then say "Good. 2 + 2 is four." The teacher then records if the response was correct or incorrect,

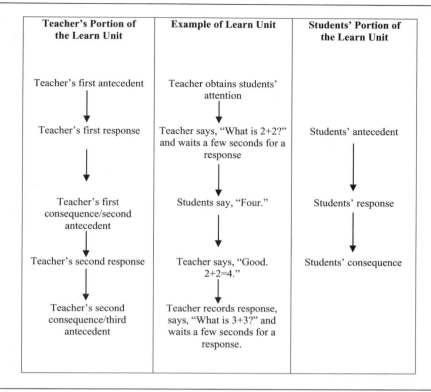

Illustration of a learn unit.

and presents the sequence of behaviors again. In Figure 26.2, which illustrates the learn unit applied to the above example, the students' portion of the learn unit consists of the following behaviors: (1) the teacher presents an instruction to the students (this is the students' antecedent), (2) the students respond to the instruction during a brief pause (the students' response to the antecedent), and (3) the teacher contingently praises or corrects the students' responses—praise for a correct response or a correction for an incorrect response (the students' consequence for their response).

In the same example, the teacher's portion of the learn unit consists of the following behaviors: (1) the teacher obtains the student's attention (the teacher's antecedent), (2) the teacher presents an instruction to the students (the teacher's response to obtaining the students' attention), and (3) the student responds correctly or incorrectly (the teacher's consequence for their presentation of the antecedent). This example constitutes a single learn unit for a teacher with his or her students. The entire sequence is called a "learn" unit because both the teacher and the student stand to learn from the interaction: the students potentially learn an academic response and the teacher learns to change her own behavior based on her interaction with the student. Learn units can occur across lengthy or brief responses (i.e., essays or algebraic equations), and can be presented vocally, on worksheets (Singer-Dudek & Greer, 2005), or via computers (Emurian, 2004).

Research indicates that the number of learn units or academic interactions a teacher has with students each day has a cumulative effect on student learning (Greenwood,

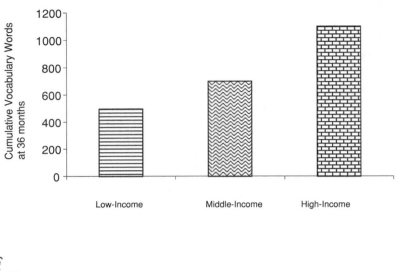

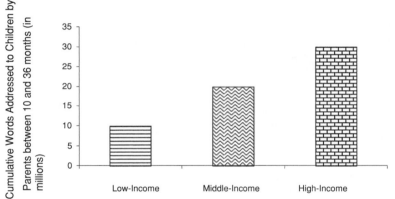

Cumulative vocabulary words at 36 months of age; cumulative words addressed to children by their parents between 10 and 36 months of age. *Source:* Adapted from Hart and Risley (1995).

Hart, et al., 1994; Greer, 2002; Heward, 1994; Johnson & Layng, 1994). That is, when students receive a frequent number of learn units, they learn more, and when they receive infrequent learn units, they learn less (Heward). Thus, one learn unit or academic teacher–student interaction may not seem significant. However, the absence or presence of a number of learn units on a daily basis has a cumulative effect on learning, much like saving small amounts of money results in a steady increase in one's savings balance.

The accumulation of interactions that produces learning actually begins in infancy with low-income children having fewer language interactions with their parents than higher-income children. Hart and Risley (1995) report a 2.5-year long study during which they followed the language experiences of 7-month old infants from low-income, middle-class, and high-income families until the infants were 36 months old. At 36 months of age, they found differences in vocabulary growth for each group, with low-income children using approximately 500 words, middle-class children using approximately 700 words, and high-income children using approximately 1100 words.

Based on their data, they projected that during the first 36 months of life, children of low-income families heard 10 million words from their parents, children of middle-income families heard 20 million words, and children of high-income families heard 30 million words. Differences in vocabulary growth were also predictors of the children's performance on standardized tests of reading, math, and language in first grade, with low-income children continuing to perform significantly lower than the other participants. Figure 26.3 illustrates the disparities in vocabulary growth for all three groups.

In a follow-up study with elementary and middle school students, Greenwood, Hart, et al. (1994) found that in elementary school, low-income students were academically engaged in basic reading and math 24 minutes less each day than high-income students (*academic engagement* is the amount of time students participate in tasks known to produce learning). In middle school, low-income students were academically engaged in basic subjects 12 minutes less each day than high-income students. Based on their data, they projected that the cumulative effect was a difference of 365 fewer hours of engagement for low-income students at the completion of elementary school, and 475 fewer hours of engagement for low-income students at the completion of middle school. Figure 26.4 illustrates hours of academic and non-academic learning time in elementary and middle school by income level.

There were also positive correlations between the amount of academic engagement and reading skills. Low-income students, who were the least academically engaged, began first grade .3 grade levels behind their high-income peers in reading. By sixth grade, they were reading at a grade level of 3.8 and their high-income peers were reading at a grade level of 7.3—a difference of 3.5 grade levels. By eighth grade, they were reading at a grade level of 5.5 and their higher-income peers were reading at a grade level of 11.3—a difference of 5.8 grade levels. Greenwood, Hart, et al. (1994) concluded that if academic growth continued at these rates, low-income students would need an additional 1.6 years of schooling to achieve the same academic levels as their higher-income peers. Figure 26.5 illustrates the cumulative hours of academic engagement upon completion of elementary and middle school and the corresponding reading achievement by income level.

These data suggest several key points about the cyclical nature of academic disparities for low-income students. First, beginning at infancy, children from low-income families have fewer educational experiences to prepare them for schooling than high-income students do. Second, the lack of early educational experiences has a cumulative effect on learning, which is maintained by schools educating low-income students. Additionally, the amount of time that low-income children spend on academic tasks quantifies the cumulative delays they experience. In other words, children from low-income families fail academically because they enter school behind their peers and, as such, must learn more than their peers do, but in less time (Engelmann, 1999). Finally, the cycles begin again as low-income students become adults and raise their own children; that is, their children begin school with the same disadvantages that their parents had. Figure 26.6 illustrates the cyclical process leading to poor academic performance for some children from low-income communities.

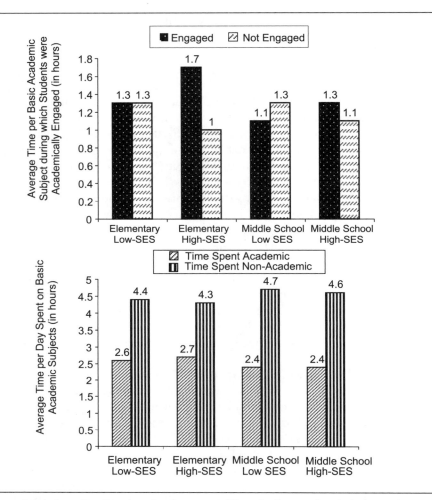

Academic and non-academic learning time/academic engaged time by income level at elementary and middle school. *Source:* Adapted from Greenwood et al. (1994).

An Intervention: Increased Learn Units

The research described above on academic interactions between teachers and students demonstrated that low-income students received one-third of the number of academic interactions that their high-income peers received (Greenwood, Hart, et al., 1994; Hart & Risley, 1995). It also indicated positive correlations between rates of academic interactions and academic achievement (Greenwood et al.). However, this research suggests another key point about academic intervention: Academic interactions between students and teachers may be alterable and can possibly increase academic achievement (Greenwood, 1999). In other words, successful teaching of low-income students may require that teachers present large quantities of instruction within a limited period in order to make

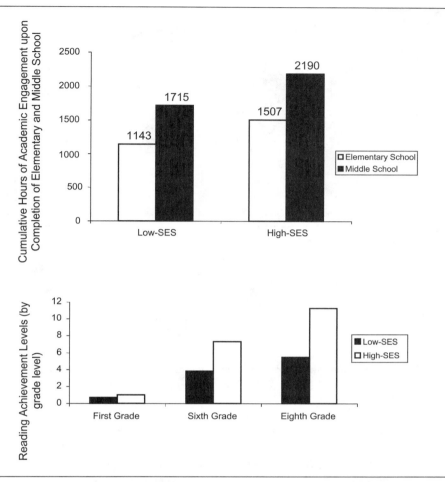

Cumulative hours of academic engagement upon completion of elementary and middle school by income level; reading achievement by income level. *Source:* Adapted from Greenwood et al. (1994).

up for decreased academic interactions. In the current chapter, we suggest that increasing *learn units* is a possible intervention for addressing academic disparities.

Research on the learn unit began with academic engagement or academic engaged time (AET), which is the amount of time that students actively participate in tasks known to result in academic gains. Research on AET showed positive correlations between the amount of AET students received and the size of their academic gains (see Sammons, Hill, & Mortimore, 1995, for a review of this research). Research on AET also showed that specific conditions increased it (Greenwood, Horton, & Utley, 2002). However, AET was a time-based measure and, as such, could not account for the quality and number of interactions between teachers and students (Heward, 1994).

Additional research suggested that AET was comprised of several interactions between teachers and students called *opportunities-to-respond* (OTR). An OTR occurred when a teacher presented a question or instruction and then waited a few seconds for students to respond. Research suggested that students learned more information when

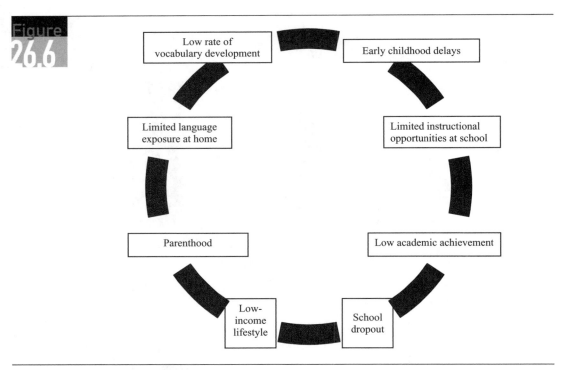

Cycle of academic disparities for low-income students. *Source:* **Adapted from Greenwood et al. (1994).**

teachers presented sufficient numbers of OTR. For instance, Sutherland and Wehby (2001) reported positive correlations between the numbers of OTR received by students with behavior disorders and subsequent reductions in their behavior problems along with increases in learning. Similarly, Greenwood, Hart, et al. (1994) reported that increasing opportunities to respond for low-income students resulted in greater amounts of academic engagement and, consequently, academic achievement. However, research showed that the learn unit, which included the teacher's consequence to the students' responses, produced more learning than OTR alone (Albers & Greer, 1991; Heward, 1994).

Subsequent research built on the concept of measuring academic engaged time by counting the presence or absence of learn units (Albers & Greer, 1991; Emurian, 2004; Emurian, Hu, Wang, & Durham, 2000; Greer, 1994, 2002; Greer et al., 1989; Greer, Keohane, & Healy 2002; Ingham & Greer, 1992; McDonough & Greer, 1999; Selinske et al., 1991). Learn units (see Figure 26.2 for an example) consist of three-term contingencies (a teacher's direction, students' response, and a teacher's contingent consequence) for students and interlocking three-term contingencies for teachers. Greer (2002) termed the measure "learn unit" since both teachers and students "learn" from the interaction in a symbiotic manner. That is, as students respond to teachers' instruction and teachers, in turn, respond to their students' behaviors, the effectiveness of teachers' instruction and students' behaviors from moment-to-moment is isolated. The research background of the learn unit identified those components of the learn unit that were functionally related to increases in student learning. Table 26.1 outlines this research.

Table 26.1	Research Base for Learn Unit	
	Seminal Studies	**Findings**
	Madsen, Becker, Thomas (1968)	Contingent teacher approvals and disapprovals correspond with decreases and increases in student behavior.
	Greenwood et al. (1994)	Students who receive high numbers of opportunities to respond also have increased correct responses to instruction.
	Greer, McCorkle, & Williams (1989); Lamm & Greer (1991); Selinke, Greer, & Lodhi (1991)	Three separate school-wide replications that showed correlations between high numbers of formal observations of learn units by supervisors, and increased productivity for teachers, increased contingent consequences given by teachers during instruction, and increased learning for students with disabilities.
	Ingham & Greer (1992)	More accurate teaching occurs when teachers are given feedback about the rate and accuracy of their learn units instead of nonspecific feedback such as "Nice work."
	Albers & Greer (1991); Ingham & Greer (1992)	Antecedent presentations are more effective when they were unambiguous.
	Albers & Greer (1991); Ingham & Greer (1992)	Student learning increases when teachers follow a student's response with contingent praise or a correction.
	McDonough & Greer (1999)	When correcting incorrect responses, teachers should present the initial direction/question again, and then provide another response opportunity. However, responses during corrections should not be contingently praised and corrected.
	Greer et al. (1989); Linhart-Kelly & Greer (1997); Ingham & Greer (1992); Selinske et al. (1991)	Faster and higher rates of learn unit presentations result in increased correct responses and objectives achieved.
	Bahadourian et al. (2005); Emurian (2004)	Instruction that includes learn units is effective in college classrooms and when used with computerized instruction.

Implications for Instructing Individuals From Low-Income Backgrounds

Teach Teachers to Identify and Present Learn Units Based on Current or Scripted Curricula: Presenting learn units should be easy—the academic question or direction is presented by the teacher, computer, or worksheet; the students have a brief opportunity to respond; and the teacher or computer contingently praises or corrects the students' response. However, there are at least two reasons why this can be challenging. First, teachers come to classrooms with their own set of responses to students that they may have used for years. If these responses are not unambiguous antecedents, praise for correct responses, and corrections for incorrect responses, then changing them can require practice. Second, many instructional materials do not include learn units, and they must be modified to include them. Yet, being able to identify and present learn units is the crux of this intervention. Therefore, using an outside observer who models the presentation of learn units and then ensures that the teacher's presentation is reliable is essential. In the Comprehensive Application of Behavior Analysis to Schooling (CABAS®) schools, teacher trainers use the *Teacher Performance Rate and Accuracy (TPRA)* instrument to ensure that each component of the learn unit is presented accurately and fluently (see Ross, Dudek–Singer, & Greer, 2005, for a description).

Conduct Baseline Measures and Then Increase Rate, Accuracy, and Number of Learn Units Presented. Research on the learn unit and on academic engagement showed that during baseline measures, teachers presented very few learn units (Albers & Greer, 1991; Bahadourian, Tam, Greer, & Rosseau, 2005; Greenwood et al., 2002). Collecting baseline data is important, therefore, to ensure that the number of learn units increases. However, it is also important because the total number of learn units that each group of students receives should be individualized based on the students' needs. Additionally, the rate at which they are presented depends on the size and type of response students are required to give. For example, students who speak their responses will be able to respond faster and more frequently within a class period than students who must write their responses. As a result, the target number of learn units and the increments by which it must increase depend on the students and should be initially determined from the baseline number of learn units that a teacher already presents.

Ensure Accuracy With Ongoing Checks. Ingham and Greer (1992) found functional relationships between the rate and accuracy of learn unit presentations, and the number of objectives achieved by students, and the number of correct responses students had when compared to nonspecific feedback. They also found that the rate and accuracy of learn unit presentations during observations predicted the rate and accuracy of learn unit presentations when formal observations were not conducted. Therefore, to ensure the accuracy of learn unit presentations, regular checks must be conducted, preferably with a formal observational instrument such as the TPRA.

Use Materials and Tactics That Automatically Increase Learn Units. As previously mentioned, many instructional materials are not designed to automatically produce learn units. However, Direct Instruction Programs such as Corrective Reading or Reading Mastery (Engelmann, 1999; Engelmann & Bruner, 2003) or computerized programs such as Headsprout (Layng, Twyman, & Stikeleather, 2004) are programmed to present learn units. In other cases, response cards (cards on which students write their answers), choral responding (a group of students responds simultaneously), and peer tutoring, among other tactics, can be used with a teachers' existing curriculum to increase the learn units students receive.

Use Instructional Arrangements That Increase Them. Greenwood et al. (2002) found that the following instructional arrangements facilitate academic engagement: One-to-one and small instructional groupings; worksheets, paper/pencil, computers and other media, workbooks, and readers; and teachers standing in front or to the side of individual students. The following instructional arrangements did not facilitate academic engagement: cleaning up and putting away, transitions between activities, discussion, and lecture. Therefore, teachers can facilitate learning by arranging instruction to include those situations that promote academic engagement.

Post Visual Displays of Data (Monitoring). Research on self-monitoring suggests that when individuals collect data on their behavior, then they also change their behavior based on the data (Petscher & Bailey, 2006). Having teachers record the total number of learn units they present and the total number of correct responses from students on a weekly basis can help them increase their learn units. Further, for some students, recording the number of correct responses they have can change their behaviors.

Use Components of the Learn Unit to Analyze Student Failure (Greer, 2002; Keohane & Greer, 2005; Ross et al., 2005). When students fail to answer correctly during a few learn units within a single lesson, teachers should use the learn unit components to change their responses. While there are many questions that can be answered based on the learn unit (see Greer, 2002 for a complete description), they generally include the following:

1. Analyzing the teacher's direction/question: Are the materials and the vocal or written instructions clear, unambiguous?
2. Analyzing the student's responses: Does the student have the prerequisite skills to perform the behavior?
3. Analyzing the consequence: Does the consequence (i.e., praise) sufficiently motivate the student to perform the behaviors?

If these questions are sufficiently answered and if the learn unit is being presented correctly, the source of learning problems may be elsewhere (see Greer, 2002 for a description).

Models of Schooling

This section highlights models of schooling that measure learn units and/or academic engagement, including the CABAS® model of schooling (Greer, 2002), Juniper Gardens Children's Project (JGCP; Greenwood, 1999), and the Morningside Academy (Johnson & Layng, 1994). This section is primarily included to illustrate the practice of measuring instruction with learn units. However, it is also included to underscore the importance of a school culture that supports the use of learn units as a measure school effectiveness.

The Comprehensive Application of Behavior Analysis to Schooling (CABAS®). Is a systems approach to teaching that measures its effectiveness primarily by students' responses to learn units. To date, the CABAS® model has been implemented with infants, children, and adolescents with and without developmental disabilities (Greer, 2002). Curricula are selected or modified to increase learn units. Additionally, teachers receive ongoing training and support to identify and present sufficient numbers of accurate learn units based on students' individual needs. During instruction, teachers change their teaching behaviors to increase students' correct responses to learn units. Following instruction, daily and weekly trends in learn units are measured for each classroom, curricular area, and student in the following areas: (1) The total number of learn units presented by teachers, (2) the total number of correct and incorrect responses to learn units by students,

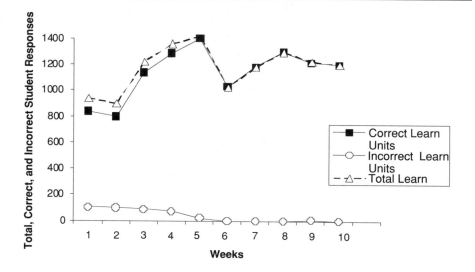

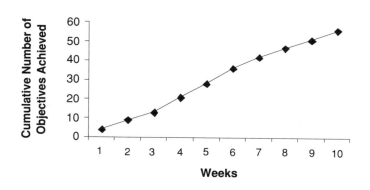

Visual displays of total, correct, and incorrect learn units; visual display of cumulative objectives achieved.

(3) the total number of objectives achieved, and (4) the average number of learn units required to master a single objective (called "learn units to criterion").

Teachers and schools analyze visual displays or graphs of these data for trends in specific directions. Figure 26.7 displays hypothetical learn unit data for one school. The *total number of learn units* and the total number of correct respones presented by teachers should increase over time as teachers acquire expertise and students acquire foundational skills. The *total number of objectives achieved* is displayed on a cumulative graph; steeper slopes demonstrate more objectives achieved, and flat slopes demonstrate fewer objectives achieved. Finally, the *average number of learn units to criterion* indicates how quickly students are achieving curricular objectives. That is, it is more desirable for a student or group of students to achieve more objectives with fewer learn units because learn units represent instructional time; teachers whose students achieve more objectives with fewer learn units are teaching more information in less time—a need for low-income students (Engelmann, 1999). See Greer (2002) for a description of CABAS® and its research base.

Juniper Gardens Children's Project

Juniper Gardens Children's Project (JGCP) began in the 1960s at the University of Kansas to provide education solutions for low-income, inner-city children. Research in the JGCP has contributed instructional tactics to improve the educational outcomes of students with and without disabilities, including classwide peer tutoring (Greenwood, Delquadri, & Hall, 1989), ecological observation (Greenwood et al., 2002), and incidental teaching (Hart & Risley, 1978). However, Greenwood (1999) noted that while improvement was observed across a number of JGCP research programs, academic engagement was the constant feature associated with improvement. Consequently, the JGCP focused on engagement to design and measure interventions that produced change because it was readily alterable by teachers, parents, and peers.

For example, classwide peer tutoring (CWPT) was one intervention developed to increase engagement. During CWPT, students present learn units to each other, thus doubling the total number of learn units that students receive when compared to those presented by a teacher (Greenwood, 1999). Greenwood et al. (1989) found that CWPT resulted in reduced placement in special education and dropping out of high school when long-term effects for an experimental group were compared to long-term effects for at-risk and typically-developing control groups. They attributed their outcomes to increased OTR. Other researchers reported similarly successful outcomes (Arreaga-Mayer, 1998).

Morningside Model

The Morningside Academy is an elementary and middle school program that serves students with and without learning disabilities who are failing to make adequate academic gains. The model of schooling on which it is based is the Morningside Model (Johnson & Layng, 1994), which teaches components of complex skills until students can perform them accurately, quickly, and until the complex skills emerge without direct instruction. To date, Morningside Academy learners gain at least two grade levels per school year, increase their time on-task endurance from 1 to 3 minutes to 20 minutes or more, and perform in the 65th percentile of their peer group on national norms for standardized tests. Johnson and Layng attribute their outcomes to increased opportunities for learner performance via teacher-student interactions.

Conclusion

This chapter discussed the role of effective teaching in decreasing academic disparities between low- and high-income students. Specifically, research on academic engagement (a construct used to describe the amount of time students spend on tasks known to promote learning) showed that low-income students were academically engaged one third of the time that high-income students were engaged (Greenwood, Hart, et al., 1994). Subsequent research suggested that academic engagement was comprised of multiple academic interactions between teachers and students called *learn units* (Greer, 2002). A learn unit is a basic measure of teaching and learning. It is comprised of (1) A teacher's direction or question followed by a brief pause, (2) a student's response to the teacher's question, and (3) an immediate consequence given by the teacher and contingent upon the way the student responded (praise for a correct response, and a correction for an incorrect response). Research shows that when teachers present high numbers of accurate learn units, students have more correct responses to instruction, achieve more objectives, and have higher test scores (Albers & Greer, 1991; Bahadourian et al., 2005; Emurian, 2004; Emurian et al., 2000; Greer, 1994, 2002; Greer et al., 1989; Greer et al., 2002; Ingham & Greer, 1992; McDonough & Greer, 1999; Selinske et al., 1991). Based on this information, in this chapter we recommended that teachers present learn units more frequently by modifying their current instructional behaviors, and by using curricula and tactics such as Direct Instruction, Precision Teaching, and response cards, which all increase learn units. This chapter also reviewed components of programs that effectively use learn units to instruct students.

The learn unit also has many other potential benefits for instruction. First, it provides continuous feedback about students to teachers. Each response by a student lets a teacher know how well they instructed the student during the prior academic interaction. For instance, if a student responds incorrectly to a question during a particular lesson, teachers can measure the effectiveness of their instruction by measuring students' responses to subsequent learn units during the same lesson. In fact, Greer (2002) says that a "true" learn unit is comprised of two sequential teacher–student interactions, which allows the teacher and the student to "learn" from the first interaction and to change their behaviors during the second one. Johnson and Layng (1994) suggested that the effective component of the teacher–student interaction is that teachers can change their instruction immediately.

Second, the learn unit is useful for evaluating cost effectiveness. That is, cost measures can be obtained by dividing the total cost of an instructional program by the total number of learn units, total number of objectives achieved, and gains on standardized tests. These calculations can then be used to assess the cost effectiveness of the learn unit when compared to baseline measures, or the cost effectiveness of the learn unit across schools or classrooms. For instance, Ross, Wilson, and Goodman (2004) found that Direct Instruction was more cost-effective than a comparison program for a middle school when cost per learn unit and cost per achieved objective were calculated. Other potential benefits include decreased behavior problems (Sutherland & Wehby, 2001) and reduced referrals for special education, since regular education teachers are addressing the needs of failing students (Losen & Orfield, 2002).

In closing, while this chapter presented research on the learn unit, the discussion was probably more cursory than in depth. Specifically, we did not discuss the extensive supports needed for the ongoing presentation of learn units in schools. For instance, in CABAS® schools, teachers use research-based instruction and curricula that follow a logical sequence; a positive classroom environment is used to manage students' behaviors; and teachers function as strategic scientists of instruction by using existing research findings to make instructional decisions. Similarly, in the Morningside Academy, all students learn component skills of complex behaviors until they are fluent; later, teachers present real-life, complex applications of mastered instructional material. In other words, there is a culture of support for using learn units during instruction (i.e., a critical mass of teachers and ongoing supervision). This is important because individual teachers will probably not present learn units without support (nor can they impact student achievement given the magnitude of academic problems experienced by low-income students).

While school reform literature frequently recommends school- and district-wide reforms such as increased funding for low-income schools and financial incentives to attract good teachers, the role of effective classroom instruction cannot be overemphasized when addressing academic disparities between low- and high-income students. In some ways, the role of a teacher in helping to ameliorate the current educational crisis for low-income students is analogous to the role of a doctor in a health crisis. In health crises, the public demands greater expertise from doctors and other medical professionals who work closely with those in need. In the same way, the crisis of low academic achievement for millions of poor and low-income students requires instructional expertise from those who work most closely with them—teachers. In fact, we think that teaching is vital to reducing the academic disparities that plague millions of low-income children who are experiencing academic failure.

REFERENCES

Albers, A. E., & Greer, R. D. (1991). Is the three term contingency trial a predictor of effective instruction? *Journal of Behavioral Education, 1*, 337–354.

Arreaga-Mayer, C. (1998). Increasing active student responding and improving academic performance through classwide peer tutoring. *Intervention in School and Clinic, 3*, 89–94, 117.

Bahadourian, A. J., Tam, K. Y., Greer, R. D., & Rousseau, M. K. (2005). The effects of learn units on student performance in two college courses. *International Journal of Behavioral Consulting and Therapy, 2*(2), 245–265.

Emurian, H. H. (2004). A programmed instruction tutoring system for Java: Consideration of learning performance and software self-efficacy. *Computers in Human Behavior, 20*, 423–459.

Emurian, H. H., Hu, X., Wang, J., & Durham, D. (2000). Learning Java: A programmed instruction approach using Applets. *Computers in Human Behavior, 16*, 395–422.

Engelmann, S. (1999). The benefits of direct instruction: Affirmative action for at-risk students. *Educational Leadership, 57*, 77–78.

Engelmann, S., & Bruner, E. C. (2003). *Reading mastery classic: Level 1*. Columbus, OH: SRA/McGraw Hill.

Greenwood, C. R. (1999, Fall). Reflections on a research career: Perspective on 35 years of research at the Juniper Gardens Children's Project. *Exceptional Children, 66*(1), 7–21.

Greenwood, C. R., Carta, J. J., Kamps, D., Terry, B., & Delquadri, J. (1994). Development and validation of standard classroom observation systems for school practitioners: Ecobehavioral assessment systems software (EBASS). *Exceptional Children, 61*, 197–210.

Greenwood, C. R., Delquadri, J., & Hall, R. V. (1989). Longitudinal effects of classwide peer tutoring. *Journal of Educational Psychology, 81*, 371–383.

Greenwood, C. R., Hart, B., Walker, D. I., & Risley, T. (1994). The opportunity to respond and academic performance revisited: A behavioral theory of developmental retardation and its prevention. In R. Gardner, D. M. Sainato, J. O. Cooper, T. E. Heron, W. L. Heward, J. Eshelman, et al. (Eds.), *Behavior analysis in education: Focus on measurably superior education*. Pacific Grove, CA: Brooks/Cole.

Greenwood, C. R., Horton, B. T., & Utley, C. A. (2002). Academic engagement: Current perspective on research and practice. *The School Psychology Review, 31*, 328–349.

Greer, R. D. (1994). The measure of a teacher. In R. Gardner, D. M. Sainato, J. O. Cooper, T. E. Heron, W. L. Heward, J. Eshelman, et al. (Eds.), *Behavior analysis in education: Focus on measurably superior education*. Pacific Grove, CA: Brooks/Cole.

Greer, R. D. (2002). *Designing teaching strategies: An applied behavior analysis systems approach*. New York: Academic Press.

Greer, R. D., Keohane, D., & Healy, O. (2002). Quality and comprehensive applications of behavior analysis to schooling. *The Behavior Analyst Today, 3*, 120–132. Retrieved December 22, 2003, from http://www.behavior-analyst-online.org/BAT/BAT-32.pdf

Greer, R. D., McCorkle, N. P., & Williams, G. (1989). A sustained analysis of the behaviors of schooling. *Behavioral Residential Treatment, 4*, 113–141.

Hart, B., & Risley, T. R. (1978). Promoting productive language through incidental teaching. *Education and Urban Society, 10*, 407–429.

Hart, B., & Risley, T. R. (1995). *Meaningful differences in the everyday experiences of young American children*. Baltimore: Brookes/Cole.

Heward, W. L. (1994). Three "low-tech" strategies for increasing the frequency of active student response during group instruction. In R. Gardner, D. M. Sainato, J. O. Cooper, T. E. Heron, W. L. Heward, J. Eshelman, et al. (Eds.), *Behavior analysis in education: Focus on measurably superior education*. Pacific Grove, CA: Brooks/Cole.

Ingham, P., & Greer, R. D. (1992). Changes in student and teacher response in observed and generalized settings as a function of supervisor observations. *Journal of Applied Behavior Analysis, 25*, 153–164.

Johnson, K. R., & Layng, T. V. J. (1994). The Morningside model of generative instruction. In R. Gardner, D. M. Sainato, J. O. Cooper, T. E. Heron, W. L. Heward, J. Eshelman, et al. (Eds.), *Behavior analysis in education: Focus on measurably superior education*. Pacific Grove, CA: Brooks/Cole.

Keohane, D. D., & Greer, R. D. (2005). Teachers' use of a verbally-governed algorithm and student learning. *International Journal of Behavioral Consultation and Therapy, 1*(3), 252–271.

Lamm, N., & Greer, R. D. (1991). A systematic replication of CABAS in Italy. *Journal of Behavioral Education, 1*, 427–444.

Layng, T. V. J., Twyman, J. S., & Stikeleather, G. (2004). Selected for success: How *Headsprout Reading Basics*™ teaches beginning reading. In D. J. Moran & R. W. Malott (Eds.), *Evidence-based educational methods*. San Diego, CA: Elsevier.

Linhart-Kelly, I., & Greer, R. D. (1997, May). *Rate mastery and the long-term maintenance of sight words*. Paper presented at the 23rd Annual International Conference of the Association for Behavior Analysis, Chicago, IL.

Losen, D. J., & Orfield, G. (2002). *Racial inequity in special education*. Boston: Harvard Education Press.

Madsen, C. H., Jr., Becker, W. C., & Thomas, D. K. (1968). Rules, praise, and ignoring—Elements of elementary classroom control. *Journal of Applied Behavior Analysis, 1*, 139–150.

McDonough, S. H., & Greer, K. D. (1999). Is the learn unit a fundamental measure of pedagogy? *The Behavior Analyst, 22*, 5–16.

National Center for Children in Poverty. (2006). *Low-income children in the United States: National and state trend data (1994–2004)*. New York: Columbia University, Mailman School of Public Health. Retrieved March 8, 2006, from National Center for Children in Poverty On-line: http://www.nccp.org/pub_nst06.html

National Center for Educational Statistics. (2005). *National assessment of educational progress*. Washington, DC: U.S. Department of Education. Retrieved March 7, 2006, from National Center for Educational Statistics Reports Online: http://nces.ed.gov/nationsreportcard/nde/viewresults.asp

Petscher, E. S., & Bailey, J. S. (2006). Effects of training, prompting, and self-monitoring on staff behavior in a classroom for students with disabilities. *Journal of Applied Behavior Analysis, 39*, 215–226.

Ross, D. E., Dudek-Singer, J., & Greer, R. D. (2005). The Teacher Performance Rate and Accuracy Scale (TPRA): Training as evaluation. *Education and Training in Developmental Disabilities, 40*, 411–423.

Ross, D., Wilson, C. L., & Goodman, J. (May, 2004). *Learn unit analysis of a model to improve reading skills of diverse learners using behavioral reading curricula*. Paper presented at the 30th Annual International Conference of the Association for Behavior Analysis, Boston, MA.

Sammons, P., Hill, J., & Mortimore, P. (1995). *Key characteristics of effective schools: A review of effective schools research*. Retrieved July 9, 2006, from http://eric.ed.gov/ERICDocs/data/

ericdocs2/content_storage_01/0000000b/80/24/0a/5e.pdf Washington, DC: U.S. Department of Education.

Selinske, J., Greer, R. D., & Lodhi, S. (1991). A functional analysis of the comprehensive application of behavior analysis to schooling. *Journal of Applied Behavior Analysis, 24*, 107–117.

Singer-Dudek, J., & Greer, R. D. (2005). A long-term analysis of the relationship between fluency and the training and maintenance of complex math skills. *The Psychological Record, 55*(3), 361–376.

Sutherland, K. S., & Wehby, J. H. (2001). Exploring the relationship between increased opportunities to respond to academic requests and the academic and behavioral outcomes of students with EBD: A review. *Remedial and Special Education, 22*(2), 113–121.

Cultivating Academic Ability Through Exposure to Supplementary Education

27

**Beatrice L. Bridglall
and Edmund W. Gordon**

The reciprocal relationship between education and health is well known. Numerous studies have shown the correlation between higher levels of education and improved levels of health in all parts of the world. It may not be surprising that in third-world and developing countries, life expectancy rates are highest among those who have the highest levels of education (Evans, Whitehead, Diderichsen, Bhuiya, & Wirth, 2001). Even in nations with very high levels of educational attainment, such as modern Japan for example, "the differentials between prefectures in education among women continue to maintain a strong association with prefecture-level life expectancy at age 40 years" (Evans et al., 2001, p. 8). It seems that it is education and not simply economic status that plays a role in health promotion. (It could also be argued that people and societies with higher levels of education and health may also have higher economic power.)

Further, it appears that higher levels of education seem to influence morbidity and mortality by lowering the risks of obesity, substance abuse, infectious diseases, popular acceptance of poor health practices, and pro-sedentary tendencies (Smedley, Stith, & Nelson, 2003; Smedley & Syme, 2000). Clearly, those who are serious about their education are on the "road to health," a path that leads to a lifetime of opportunities (Nantulya, Semakafu, Muli-Musiime, Massawe, & Munyetti, 2001). Numerous studies have also shown that there is a strong relationship in the opposite direction: people's health has a strong impact on their levels of academic achievement (Birch & Gussow, 1970; Bourdieu, 1986; Miller, 1995).

Educators who wish to develop academic ability and health professionals who wish to foster the adoption and maintenance of healthy behaviors encounter similar problems in modifying attitudes and behaviors. In their respective domains, educators and health professionals both recognize that (1) current levels of knowledge dissemination are insufficient to achieve their goals; (2) self-affirming attitudes and behaviors need to be shaped and reinforced (Glanz, Lewis, & Rimer, 1996); (3) self-regulation and a sense of self-efficacy (Bandura, 1986) must be developed; and (4) there is insufficient awareness of the amount and quality of time that must be invested in attaining high levels of health and academic achievement (Resnick, 1999). Clearly, these problems go beyond the simple dissemination of information to finding ways (including those that are culturally sensitive) of influencing people's capacity and disposition to utilize information and services to change their behavior (Freire, 1973).

These parallels between aspects of public health and education frame our notion of supplementary education, some times referred to as complementary education (Weiss, Kreider, Lopez, & Chatman, 2005) as an approach to the reduction of discrepancies in educational achievement between underrepresented students and their Asian American and European American counterparts. This focus on informal pedagogical intervention as a supplement to formal schooling is informed by current practices in health maintenance where we have known for sometime that changes in attitudes, behaviors, and life conditions do complement medical treatment in the prevention of disease and the maintenance of good health.

Informed parents, scholars, and educators have known for some time now that schools alone cannot enable or ensure high academic achievement (Bridglall & Gordon, 2001; Coleman et al., 1966; Wilkerson, 1985). James Comer asserts this position more forcefully in *Waiting for a Miracle: Why Our Schools Cannot Solve Our Problems—And How We Can* (1997). Colloquial knowledge among many parents "in the know" reflects awareness that there are a number of things that occur outside of school that appear to enable schooling to work. Examples can be found in the many education related opportunities that affluent and academically sophisticated parents make available to their children, such as travel, dance lessons, scouting, tutoring, and summer camp. In 1966, James Coleman concluded that differences in the family backgrounds of students, as opposed to school characteristics, accounted for the greatest amount of variance in their academic achievement. In related works, Mercer (1973) and Wolf (1966, 1995) posited that it is the presence of family environmental supports for academic development that may explain this association between family status and student achievement. They made the now obvious point that books, positive academic role models, help with homework, and a place to study in the home are associated with school achievement.

It appears that the most academically successful populations (primarily European Americans and Asian Americans with mid to high socioeconomic status [SES] backgrounds) tend to have combinations of strong home and school resources to support their academic development (Massey, Charles, Lundy, & Fischer, 2003). The least successful groups (African American, Latina/o American, Native American, and the poor) have on average a much weaker combination of home and school resources (Birch & Gussow, 1970; College Board, 1999; Miller, 1995; Reardon, 2003; West, Denton, & Germino-Hausken, 2000). There is converging empirical evidence that gaps in knowledge and skills between European American and Asian American students and their African American, Hispanic, and Native American peers surface before kindergarten and continue throughout the elementary, secondary, and postsecondary years (Reardon, 2003; West, Denton, & Germino-Hausken, 2000). For example, substantial gaps between the scores of black and white students on the National Assessment of Educational Progress tests in math, science, and reading have been documented since the early 1970s when data was first collected. These gaps are prevalent not only within school, but also out of school and between schools (Everson & Millsap, 2005; Reardon, 2003). Some of the consequences of these gaps are further reflected in the pronounced minority underrepresentation among high achievers in selective colleges, universities, and professional schools and the over-representation of African American students, particularly males, in special education and Latinos in English language learning programs (Miller, 1995).

Several theoretical perspectives have emerged to explain achievement gaps at all levels of education. Bowen and Bok (1998) suggest that the achievement gap can be partially explained by inadequacies in high school preparation. Yet others conclude that the underrepresentation of high-achieving students of color is solely due to the behavior and characteristics of these students. The seemingly intractable gap however, cannot be completely explained by student characteristics or lack of academic preparation. There is emerging evidence of the influence of other variables. Maton, Hrabowski, and Schmitt (2000) suggest that this persistent underperformance may be attributable to students' academic and social isolation, lack of exposure to support, motivation, monitoring, and advisement, and for those who perform below the norm, weaknesses in their knowledge and skill development (Treisman, 1990, 1992). Other factors identified as influencing the discrepancies in academic achievement include broad family characteristics such as parental warmth, discipline, language use, marital status, mental health, home environment, parent–child interaction, and socioeconomic status (SES) (usually a composite of parental income, education, and occupational prestige (Barber, 2000; Brooks-Gunn & Markman, 2005).

In the second issue of *Pedagogical Inquiry and Praxis* (Gordon, 2001), we referenced Bourdieu's (1986) notion that varieties of human development capital[1] are among the resources necessary for effective schooling. We argued that access to these varieties of capital is unequally distributed, yet it is this access that enables a wide variety of supplementary education experiences. It is the inferred association between access to human development capital and supplementary education, and between supplementary education and the effectiveness of education, that led to the inclusion of supplementary education as a component of our advocacy for the affirmative development of academic ability.

The idea of supplementary education (Bridglall & Gordon, 2001) is based on the premise that beyond exposure to the school's formal academic curriculum, high academic achievement is closely associated with exposure to family and community-based activities and learning experiences that occur outside of school. For low-SES and non-Asian students of color, these opportunities are generally underutilized. In the home environment, for example, high achieving students benefit from literate adults, home computers, books, magazines, journals, and the academic assistance and encouragement of older siblings and parents. In terms of community resources, the combination of local library privileges, mentoring and tutoring programs, peer-based study groups, Saturday and/or after-school academies, and participation in various folk and cultural events and faith-based activities, influence the development of proactive and engaged dispositions toward academic learning.

---

[1]Bourdieu asserts that health, social networks, educated humans, money, membership, and culture are forms of capital which are invested in the development of successfully educated persons.

In general, high degrees of congruency between the values promulgated at school, at home, and in a student's immediate community are associated with high academic achievement. What may be equally critical are students' perceptions that what happens at school matters and is consistent with what parents and other family members consider important (Wilkerson, 1985). This is conveyed through expectations, physical provisions for academic pursuits, attitudes toward intellectual activity, and the models that are available for children to emulate. Participation in supplementary education activities may contribute to the development of a sense of membership in high-performance learning communities and shared values for the importance of academic achievement for personal fulfillment, community development, and social and political upward mobility.

Supplementary Education Defined

We define supplementary education as the formal and informal learning and developmental enrichment opportunities provided for students outside of school and beyond the regular school day or year. Some of these activities may occur inside the school building but are beyond those included in the formal curriculum of the school. After-school care, perhaps the most widespread form of supplementary education, includes the special efforts that parents exert in support of the intellective and personal development of their children (Bridglall & Gordon, 2001). These efforts may range from provisions for good health and nutrition to extensive travel and deliberate exposure to socialization to life in the academy, as well as to mediated exposure to selected aspects of both indigenous and hegemonic cultures. Many activities, considered routine in the settings in which they occur, are nonetheless thought to be implicitly and deliberately engaged in to ensure adequate intellective and academic development of young people. These routines include reading to and with one's children; dinner table talk and inclusion in other family discussions of important issues; exposure to adult models of behaviors supportive of academic learning; active use of the library, museums, community and religious centers as sources of information; help seeking from appropriate sources; and investments in reference and other education materials (Gordon, 1999).

In a related but different domain are efforts directed at influencing children's choice of friends and peers; guiding and controlling use of their spare time; guiding and limiting their time spent watching television; and encouraging their participation in high-performance learning communities. Thus, we find a wide range of deliberate and incidental activities that serve to supplement the more formal and systematically structured learning experiences provided through schooling. These more intentional child development practices are no doubt dually responsive to the folk knowledge of academically sophisticated families and the empirically derived knowledge of experts in child development and education.

Rationale for Supplementary Education

We have found no evidence that specific individuals or groups have formally agreed on the name or need for the components of what we call supplementary education. It seems that over time parents have come to realize that schools are limited in their ability to address all of the needs of individual children. Those of us who are parents can recall situations in which our own children have experienced difficulty with school subjects and we have felt the need to hire tutors or seek the help of counselors. Many of us have had experience with children who were in trouble or were disturbed in some way (beyond our capacity to help or endure) and we have sought guidance for them and/or ourselves. Most of us who are able and well informed will, almost automatically, seek out the additional help that our children need. In less critical situations, many of the things we do quite naturally for recreation or cultural pleasure, or out of anxious concern for the optimal development of our children, are implicitly supplemental to schooling. The problem is that not all children have parents who know how or are well positioned to do these things. In advocating increased access to supplementary education, we are arguing for making available and accessible, to all children, those supplements that many of us automatically provide to ensure the effectiveness of education for our own children.

The Need for Supplementary Education

Studies of high-achieving students, many of whom have been exposed to a wide range of supplementary education efforts, show that they seem to actively engage in school events and extracurricular activities; identify with high achievement values; have good study skills and other learner behaviors; demonstrate personal skills such as independence, interpersonal facility, and flexibility; and maintain positive ties with adults (parents and mentors) and peers who continually advocate high expectations for achievement. These students tend to come from adequately resourced families and experience less housing mobility and greater social stability than their lower achieving counterparts. Support for their intellectual and personal development appears to flow from parents, peers, and school environments that encourage and expect high academic achievement.

Obviously, some of these circumstances and conditions are school dependent. Mastery of the academic content of schooling may be disproportionately a function of exposure to and participation in effective schooling. With the exception of a relatively small number of students who are effectively educated at home, we see strong and adequate schooling as an essential feature of modern societies. However, much of what it means to be an educated and intellectively competent person involves attitudes, appreciations, dispositions, tacit knowledge, and metacognitive abilities that depend on good schooling and good out-of-school activities and experiences that support academic learning. Thus we argue that those cultural and social factors associated with academic learning are as important as the substance of what is to be learned and the processes by which it is to be learned. Consequently, those of us concerned with replicating the circumstances and conditions associated with high academic achievement need to focus on creating positive social and psychological conditions for academic learning inside and outside of schools. This includes developing and implementing cooperative and supportive learning experiences, explicating and mediating the critical demands of academic learning situations, organizing tutorial and study groups, using mentoring and athletic coaching models, and creating ubiquitously high expectations. We must also be aware of the need to reduce the dissonance between hegemonic and ethnic minority cultural identities as is reflected in the phenomenon described as fear of "acting white" (Fordham & Ogbu, 1986) and fear of stereotype confirmation (Steele, 1997).

In addition, given that students are greatly influenced by the social contexts in which they develop, their academic achievement and competencies may be dependent upon the extent to which their social contexts, both natural and contrived, support desired ends. Some of these essential contextual supports have been described as various forms of human and social capital that enable and facilitate academic learning and personal development. The necessary human capital includes adults and peers who themselves are sources of know-how and are models of the behaviors and achievements that students can emulate. The social capital is represented in the networks of support, the connections to sources of information and resources, and the expectations of the group to which a person belongs. For students who are not naturally exposed to academically demanding environments, parents as well as educators will need to create high-performance learning communities (whether they are in the form of families, peer groups, classrooms, social groups, or institutions) where serious academic work is respected, standards are explicit, and high achievement is rewarded. Some parents may need help in developing the capacity to advocate for and access varieties of human development resource capital and to place these at the disposal of their children's academic and personal development. We advocate the following targeted strategies:

1 The facilitation of cooperative learning cadres among students and social environments that nurture academic achievement as instrumental to personal and political agency.
2 The implementation of specific interventions designed to enhance students' skills and understanding, including
   ■ socialization to the demands of serious academic engagement;
   ■ metacognitive competence and metacomponential strategies—an understanding of how one thinks and learns, and strategies to use this understanding in the self-regulation of one's learning behavior; and
   ■ diagnostically-targeted instruction and remediation.
3 The development of facility in the use of electronic and digital technology for accessing various types of information, resources, and extended learning experiences.
4 The academic and political socialization to the requirements and rewards of high levels of achievement as instruments of personal agency and social responsibility.

The last strategy suggests that for low SES students and/or students of color, negative school experiences such as low-level tracking, persistent failure, and manifestations of racism can result in failure to develop positive self-concepts and the outright rejection of aspirations for academic achievement. These reactions may be ameliorated through school-, community-, peer-, and family-mediated supplementary education interventions that allow students to grasp the relevance of education not only for potential individual gains in future careers, but also as a means for developing an informed understanding of issues of social justice and for recognizing academic abilities as vehicles for political advocacy and action (Gordon & Meroe, 2005). Moreover, familiarity with how knowledge and skills can be used in the struggle for emancipation and justice can add an element of politicalization as an instrument of pedagogy. In the process, students can be socialized to their responsibility for personal agency and the empowerment of others, as well as for an understanding of the potential relationships between academic mastery and their own political agendas (agency). Raised political consciousness can be seen as a particular form of supplementary education (Gordon, 2005) and as an organizing principle for the creation of high-performance learning communities among subaltern populations.

Taxonomy of Supplementary Education

Related types of supplementary education include those that are implicit (parenting, nutrition, family talk, parental employment, decision making, reading along with the children, socialization and acculturation, social networks, travel, and environmental supports (Mercer, 1973; Wolf, 1966), and those that are explicit (academic development, tutorials, advocacy, remediation, one-on-one tutoring SAT preparation, Saturday academies, specialized services, socio-cultural and child-centered social groups). These interventions are further impacted by the ethos of students' homes and communities, cultural and socioeconomic demographics, the economic and cultural infrastructure students and families may or may not have access to, incidental and informal experiences, formal and explicit exposure to high-performance learning communities, aspirations, expectations, and access to available resources. As indicated throughout this discussion, these interventions can be directed at students who are performing academically at different levels and achievement ranges: to those who are at risk of underachievement and to those who are high achievers.

Conclusion

Efforts to improve schools on a wide-scale basis for students from the least successful groups have produced many positive results, but there continue to be formidable obstacles to eliminating the differentials in academic achievement between students from high status and low status families. Several in-school initiatives have been identified that may contribute to the closing of achievement gaps but we are not sanguine that schooling alone will solve the problem (Gordon, 2001). We need to consider concentrated efforts at introducing a wide variety of supplementary education opportunities for low-income minority families and communities. It may be simplest to start with an initiative that has already taken root. After-school programs are among the most widespread forms of supplementary education, and are being reconceptualized as opportunities to influence the narrowing of the pervasive academic achievement gap between majority and some ethnic minority student groups. The After School Corporation (TASC), for example, cited some of the educational impacts of this form of supplementary education (TASC, 1999). They include improved academic performance and school behavior, improved attendance and graduation rates, improved family relationships, and decreased pregnancy and drug use rates. Although the after-school movement addresses a range of student needs, it is giving increased attention to the academic development of students. This direction should be encouraged.

School districts and communities that serve low-income populations and families of color might well take a page from Koreatown in Los Angeles, where some 300 agencies provide supplementary education services, most requiring payment by parents (Bhattacharya, 2005). Not only do many more communities need to have such services readily available, but consideration must also be given to ways of involving families within their ability to pay. While we are sensitive to the problem of placing additional financial burdens on already hard-pressed families, Gordon (1999) has raised the possibility that a parent's decision to invest in supplementary education may be an important part of the treatment. When parents extend themselves or even make sacrifices to make an extra education service available, the message to their children is that parents consider this to be important. In a proposal currently being considered for funding, the possibility is raised for organizations like ASPIRA, NAACP, The Urban League, Jack and Jill, The Links, faith-based institutions, and so on, to become local community sponsors of supplementary activities, with the cost subsidized by philanthropic or public sources. The core idea here is that if supplements to schooling are important (if not essential), we must find ways to ensure the availability of such services independent of family status.

REFERENCES

Bandura, A. (1986). *Social foundations of thought and action: A social cognitive theory*. Englewood Cliffs, NJ: Prentice-Hall.

Barber, N. (2000). *Why parents matter: Parental investment and child outcomes*. Westport, CT: Bergin & Garvey.

Bhattacharya, M. (2005). Community support for supplementary education. In E. W. Gordon, B. L. Bridglall, & A. S. Meroe (Eds.), *Supplementary education*. New York: Rowman & Littlefield.

Birch, H., & Gussow, J. D. (1970). *The disadvantaged child: Health, nutrition and school failure*. New York: Harcourt Brace.

Bourdieu, P. (1986). The forms of capital. In J. Richardson (Ed.), *Handbook of theory and research for the sociology of education*. Westport, CT: Greenwood.

Bowen, W. G., & Bok, D. (1998). *The shape of the river: Long-term consequences of considering race in college and university admissions*. Princeton, NJ: Princeton University Press.

Bridglall, B. L., & Gordon, E. W. (2001). *The idea of supplementary education (Pedagogical Inquiry and Praxis, No. 3)*. New York: Institute for Urban and Minority Education, Teachers College, Columbia University.

Brooks-Gunn, J., & Markman, L. B. (2005). The contribution of parenting to ethnic and racial gaps in school readiness. *The Future of Children, 15*(1), 139–168.

Coleman, J. S., Campbell, E. Q., Hobson, C. J., McPartland, J., Mood, A. M., Weinfeld, F. D., et al. (1966). *Equality of educational opportunity*. Washington, DC: U.S. Government Printing Office.

College Board. (1999). *Reaching the top: A report of the National Task Force on Minority High Achievement*. New York: The College Entrance Examination Board.

Comer, J. (1997). *Waiting for a miracle: Why our schools can't solve our problems—And how we can*. New York: Dutton.

Evans, T., Whitehead, M., Diderichsen, F., Bhuiya, A., & Wirth, M. (Eds.). (2001). *Challenging inequities in health: From ethics to action*. New York: Oxford University Press.

Everson, H. E., & Millsap, R. E. (2005). The impact of extracurricular activities on standardized test scores. In E. Gordon, B. Bridglall, & A. S. Meroe (Eds.), *Supplementary education*. New York: Rowman & Littlefield.

Fordham, S., & Ogbu, J. U. (1986). Black students' school success: Coping with the burden of "acting white." *The Urban Review, 18*(3), 176–206.

Freire, P. (1973). *Education for critical consciousness*. New York: Seabury Press.

Glanz, K., Lewis, F. M., & Rimer, B. K. (Eds.). (1996). *Health behavior and health education: Theory, research, and practice* (2nd ed.). San Francisco: Jossey-Bass.

Gordon, E. T. (2005). Academic politicalization: Supplementary education from black resistance. In E. W. Gordon, B. L. Bridglall, & A. S. Meroe, (Eds.), *Supplementary education*. New York: Rowman & Littlefield.

Gordon, E. W. (1999). *Education and justice: A view from the back of the bus*. New York: Teachers College Press.

Gordon, E. W. (2001). *The affirmative development of academic ability (Pedagogical Inquiry and Praxis, No. 2)*. New York: Institute for Urban and Minority Education, Teachers College, Columbia University.

Gordon, E. W., & Meroe, A. S. (2005). Supplementation and supplantation as alternative education strategies. In E. W. Gordon, B. L. Bridglall, & A. S. Meroe (Eds.), *Supplementary education*. New York: Rowman & Littlefield.

Massey, D., Charles, C., Lundy, G., & Fischer, M. (2003). *The source of the river: The social origins of freshmen at America's selective colleges and universities*. Princeton, NJ: Princeton University Press.

Maton, K., Hrabowski, F. A., III, & Schmitt, C. (2000). African American college students excelling in the sciences: College and postcollege outcomes in the Meyerhoff Scholars Program. *Journal of Research in Science Teaching, 37*(7), 629–654.

Mercer, J. (1973). *Labeling the mentally retarded: Clinical and social system perspectives on mental retardation*. Berkeley: University of California Press.

Miller, L. S. (1995). *An American imperative: Accelerating minority educational advancement*. New Haven, CT: Yale University Press.

Nantulya, V. M., Semakafu, A. M., Muli-Musiime, F. Massawe, A., & Munyetti, L. (2001). Tanzania: Gaining insights into adolescent lives and livelihoods. In T. Evans, M. Whitehead, F. Diderichsen, A. Bhuiya, & M. Wirth (Eds.), *Challenging inequities in health: From ethics to action*. New York: Oxford University Press.

Reardon, S. (2003). *Sources of educational inequality: The growth of racial/ethnic and socioeconomic test score gaps in kindergarten and first grade*. Population Research Institute Paper No. 03-05R, University Park: Pennsylvania State University.

Resnick, L. B. (1999). From aptitude to effort: A new foundation for our schools. *American Educator, 23*(1), 14–17.

Smedley, B. D., Stith, A. Y., & Nelson, A. R. (Eds.). (2003). *Unequal treatment: Confronting racial and ethnic disparities in health care*. Washington, DC: National Academies Press.

Smedley, B. D., & Syme, S. L. (Eds.). (2000). *Promoting health: Intervention strategies from social and behavioral research*. Washington, DC: National Academies Press.

Steele, C. (1997). A threat in the air: How stereotypes shape intellectual identity and performance. In J. L. Eberhardt & S. T. Fiske (Eds.), *Confronting racism: The problem and the response*. Thousand Oaks, CA: Sage.

The After School Corporation (TASC). (1999). *After school programs: An analysis of need, current research and public opinion*. Paper prepared for TASC by the National Center for Schools and Communities. Fordham University, New York.

Treisman, P. U. (1990). A study of the mathematics performance of Black students at the University of California, Berkeley. In H. B. Keynes, N. D. Fisher, & P. D. Wagreich (Eds.), *Mathematicians and education reform*. Proceedings of the July 6–8, 1988 workshop, Issues in Mathematics Education, Conference Board of Mathematical Sciences. Providence, RI: American Mathematical Society, Mathematical Association of America.

Treisman, P. U. (1992). Studying students studying calculus: A look at the lives of minority mathematics students in college. *College Mathematics Journal, 23*(5), 362–372.

Weiss, H. B., Kreider, H., Lopez, M. E., & Chatman, C. M. (2005). *Preparing educators to involve families: From theory to practice*. Thousand Oaks, CA: Sage.

West, J., Denton, K., & Germino-Hausken, E. (2000). *America's kindergartners*. Government report. National Center for Educational Statistics, Washington, DC.

Wilkerson, D. A. (1985). *Educating all our children*. Westport, CT: Mediax.

Wolf, R. M. (1966). The measurement of environments. In A. Anastasi (Ed.), *Testing problems in perspective*. Washington, DC: American Council on Education.

Wolf, R. M. (1995). The measurement of environments: A follow-up study. *Journal of Negro Education, 64*(3), 354–59.

A Supplementary Education Model Rooted in an Academic, Community, and Faith-Based Coalition: Closing the Education and Health Gaps

28

Angela Campbell
and Barbara C. Wallace

Introduction

As the current Teachers College home page on the World Wide Web announces to all national and international visitors, the achievement of educational equity is a moral imperative for the 21st century. Within this vision, there is a role for the idea of supplementary education, as Bridglall and Gordon explained in chapter 27. Indeed, Gordon, Bridglall, and Meroe (2005) and others (Bhattacharyya, 2005; Bridglall, 2005; Meroe, 2005) have more than justified the rationale for how models of supplementary education are needed in order to achieve educational equity and close the achievement gap between Blacks/Hispanics and Whites.

This chapter will describe the context for and subsequent development, implementation, evaluation, and refinement of a supplementary education program. This program came into being through the systematic building of an academic, community, and faith-based coalition, as described in this chapter. This process, and the results of an evaluation of the supplementary education model for its 5 year anniversary, are described in this chapter.

Background to the Challenge of Closing the Academic Achievement and Health Gaps

There is a body of work that highlights how the health and academic achievement gaps are inextricably inter-related, given the links between academic achievement, employment, socioeconomic status (SES), access to multiple resources, and health outcomes. For example, level of education can determine future employment, while employment can determine socioeconomic status and access to health care as well as mortality and morbidity across the life span (Diderichsen, Evans, & Whitehead, 2001). Thus, the extent to which both the academic achievement gap and health gap influence broader developmental outcomes across the life span emerges as quite significant, as numerous researchers assert (Evans, Whitehead, Diderichsen, Bhuiya, & Wirth, 2001).

The 1954 *Brown v. Board of Education* decision was both a unanimous decision, as well as a reconfirmation of America's promise "that all men are created equal' and that in the field of education, the doctrine of "separate but equal is inherently unequal." On May 17, 1954, the Supreme Court proclaimed, "separate educational facilities are inherently unequal." This ruling overturned *Plessy v. Ferguson*'s doctrine of "separate but equal" which stood as the law since 1896. Evidence that *Brown*'s promises remain unfulfilled for most minority students is acutely apparent, as detailed by the National Association for the Advancement of Colored People (NAACP; 2005). First, schools remain largely segregated by race, especially in urban areas, and school funding is unequal—with far fewer dollars spent on low-income, minority students. The teachers in high-poverty, high-minority schools are often poorly trained in curriculum and instruction, classroom management, and cultural sensitivity; yet, these teachers have larger classrooms with fewer resources. Minority students are more often assigned to low track, remedial courses, and to special education. Minority students have fewer opportunities to take advanced honor and AP courses, which are often required for postsecondary education. Minority students drop out of school at higher rates than their white counterparts. They are also more frequently suspended or expelled from school, and, as a result, are more likely to enter the juvenile justice system (NAACP, 2005). Thus, the challenge of eliminating inequities and closing gaps remains a challenge and reality over five decades since the historic 1954 *Brown v. Board of Education* ruling.

Beyond historic legal rulings, more recent legislation also draws attention to the realities of persisting inequities and gaps in academic achievement by race/ethnicity. On January 8, 2002 President Bush signed No Child Left Behind into law. This law was to provide every boy and girl in America with a high-quality education regardless of his or her income, ability, or background (Paige, 2002). Hence, contemporary legislation also compels us to engage in systematic efforts to improve academic achievement and to close the gap.

Furthermore, Black students continue to lag behind White students on every standardized test, including the National Assessment of Educational Progress (NAEP) and the SAT (The Education Trust, 2001). To eliminate the achievement gap that separates low-income and minority students from other students, we must understand how the effects of poverty and family background are overwhelming; but with a new winning combination of tools and strategies employed by educators the achievement gap can be lessened (The Education Trust, 2002). Parents and community leaders have come to realize that schools are limited in their ability to address all of the needs of individual children (Gordon, Bridglall, & Meroe, 2005). As Bridglall and Gordon (2005, p. 275) argue, "supplementary education is a well-established and an implicitly effective instrumentality of high levels of academic achievement" (p. 275).

One Response to the Challenge: Development of Goldquest

Given this background, Goldquest was developed in New Rochelle, New York as a community-based supplementary educational program, starting as an after-school and summer program in 2001. Goldquest represents the efforts of an academician—the program founder and first author—to forge a coalition with community and faith organizations. With the support of the local NAACP, the program was eventually located in a Baptist church that serves a largely African American congregation, while the program has attracted not only African American youth, but also Hispanics, Whites and Asians— while also disseminating program components out into other educational settings in the larger New Rochelle, New York community.

Key Theories Guiding Goldquest Program Development

In addition to a burgeoning literature on supplementary education (see Bridglall, 2005; Bridglall & Gordon, chapter 27, this volume; Gordon et al., 2005; Gordon & Meroe, 2005; Meroe, 2005), a number of theories guided the development of the Goldquest program, as summarized in Table 28.1. These may each be discussed in relation to the development of the Goldquest program.

First, Prochaska and DiClemente's (1983, 1992; Prochaska, DiClemente, & Norcross, 1992; Prochaska, Redding, & Evers, 1997) Transtheoretical model (TTM) and stages of change (SOC) integrate processes and principles of change, drawing upon major theories of intervention. Also, within the TTM there are processes of change that are the overt and covert activities that individuals use to progress through the stages of change (Prochaska et al., 1997). Knowledge of these processes was important in responding to "where students were" with regard to changing their academic- and health-related behaviors. A consideration of these processes contributed to the creation of many of the Goldquest program's activities, interventions, and strategies used with students.

Second, "self-efficacy," with its application to educational theory, is beginning to replace self-esteem as a key focus for educators, having long been valued by those focused on behavior change. Bandura (1977a) characterizes self-efficacy as a construct in social cognitive theory that is also one of the most widely used. Self-efficacy is more than knowing what to do. It is one's perceptions of one's own ability to organize cognitive, social, and behavioral traits into actions.

Both confidence and cognitive skills are necessary to carry out the action successfully. It is argued that self-efficacy can be increased when beneficial interventions are implemented (Bandura, 1986). Bandura (1986) proposed that the self-efficacy models might appeal to health behavior practitioners because one's level of self-efficacy can be improved over time. Four principal sources of information can be used to modify self-efficacy: (1) performance attainments (previous experiences with the particular task); (2) vicarious experiences (watching other people perform a task); (3) verbal persuasion; and (4) physiological state, such as being nervous, tense, or relaxed. As Bandura (1977a) argues, of the four sources of information, performance attainments have the greatest impact on a person's level of self-efficacy. Students' firm belief in their efficacy to manage

Table 28.1   The Framework for the Process of Developing and Implementing the Goldquest Supplementary Education Program

FOLLOWING THE WORK OF PROCHASKA AND DICLEMENTE (1983, 1992)*

The Stages of Change for Students in Goldquest

- Precontemplation, or not thinking about change
- Contemplation, or thinking about change
- Preparation, or having determined to change
- Action, taking action to change <6 month
- Maintenance, or maintaining taking action for change >6 months

The Processes of Change

- Consciousness raising, or learning new facts, ideas, and tips that support the healthy behavioral change
- Dramatic relief, or experiencing the negative emotions (fear, anxiety, worry) that go along with unhealthy behavioral risks
- Self-reevaluation, or realizing that the behavioral change is an important part of one's identity as a person
- Environmental reevaluation, or realizing the negative impact of the unhealthy behavior or the positive impact of the healthy behavior on one's proximal social and physical environment
- Self-liberation, or making a firm commitment to change
- Helping relationships, or seeking and using social support for the healthy behavioral change
- Counterconditioning, or substituting healthier alternative behaviors and cognitions for the unhealthy behaviors
- Contingency management, or increasing the rewards for the positive behavioral change and decreasing the rewards of the unhealthy behaviors
- Stimulus control, or removing reminders or cues to engage in the unhealthy behavior and adding cues or reminders to engage in the healthy behavior
- Social Liberation, or realizing that the social norms are changing in the direction of supporting the healthy behavioral change

FOLLOWING THE WORK OF BANDURA (1977a, 1986, 1997)

Social Cognitive Theories: Four Primary Sources of Information to Modify Students' Self-Efficacy

- Performance attainments, or previous experiences with the particular task
- Vicarious experiences, or watching other people perform a task
- Verbal persuasion
- Physiological state, such as being nervous, tense, or relaxed

FOLLOWING THE WORK OF FAWCETT ET AL. (1997)

An Evaluation Framework and Four Phases of Coalition Development Used in Developing and Implementing Goldquest

- Planning, in which a vision, mission statement, objectives, strategies, and action plans are developed
- Intervention, in which coalition staff and membership take action with targets and agents of change in relevant sectors of the community such as schools or other organizations
- Changes in the community that reduce risk and enhance protective factors
- Changes in intermediate and ultimate outcomes, such as reported use of substances and other community-level indicators.

*(Prochaska, Redding, & Evers, 1997)

their own motivation and learning activities provides the staying power for achievement, and enhances performance accomplishments (Bandura, 1994).

Hence, self-efficacy theory justifies Goldquest, as a supplementary education program seeking to close both the health and academic achievement gap, focusing on performance attainments, vicarious experiences, the use of verbal persuasion, and paying attention to students' physiological state (such as learning to be relaxed). Bandura's self-efficacy theory emerges as playing an invaluable role in the design and implementation of the Goldquest program—whether influencing the focus on performance attainments on practice and actual achievement tests, the emphasis placed on role modeling, or the teaching of deep breathing for relaxation.

Third, Fawcett et al.'s (1997) evaluation framework and identification of the four phases of coalition development can serve to organize the presentation of the process of developing and implementing the Goldquest program. These four phases involved the following: (1) *Planning,* in which a vision, mission statement, objectives, strategies, and action plans are developed; (2) *Intervention,* in which coalition staff and membership take action with targets and agents of change in relevant sectors of the community such as schools or other organizations; (3) *Changes in the Community* that reduce risk and enhance protective factors; and (4) *Changes in Intermediate and Ultimate Outcomes,* such as reported use of substances and other community-level indicators.

The first phase of coalition development included planning with strategic partners in New Rochelle, New York—the planned site of the Goldquest supplementary education program—in light of the communities' characteristics and realities. New Rochelle has been called "The Queen City of the Sound," being located in New York State. It has a population of 72,182. This town has a Mayor, a City Manager, and six part-time City Council Members. The City of New Rochelle Public School System has seven elementary schools, two middle schools, and one high school. The SAT scores by school district, 1996–1997 in Westchester County, NY showed that the highest verbal and math mean scores were in the cities of Scarsdale, (1,223 mean), Chappaqua (1,201 mean) and Edgemont (1,194 mean). The lowest verbal and math means are in Mount Vernon (870 mean), Elmsford (940 mean), and New Rochelle (1,001 mean) (Westchester County Department of Planning, 2001). Low income and minority students are primarily located in the cities of Mount Vernon, Elmsford, and New Rochelle.

Given the need for a program in the New Rochelle community to address the achievement gap, the NAACP was identified as a key partner in the *planning phase.* The New Rochelle Chapter of the National Association for the Advancement of Colored People (NAACP) is a nonprofit civil rights organization that was established in 1921 with the objective of ensuring that African Americans residing in New Rochelle, New York experience political, social, economic, and educational equality. The National NAACP is the oldest civil rights organization in the United States with a history of working at the national, regional, and local level to secure civil rights through advocacy. The NAACP has worked successfully with allies of all races who believe in and stand for the principles on which the organization was formed. The NAACP was attractive (to the academically-rooted Goldquest founder, Angela Campbell) as a coalition partner, given their historical role in the nation.

The phase of *intervention* required another key partner—Shiloh Baptist Church. There were already links between the local NAACP leadership and the leadership of the Shiloh Baptist Church. Shiloh Baptist Church had served the New Rochelle community for over a century. The Sunday school, which is essential to this church, encourages young children to engage in structured religious instruction, and has existed over 100 years. This church has various youth programs that are run by active parents and grandparents of the congregation and has over 400 active members, including many children who are not only involved in the various youth groups but also participate in the weekly worship activities that occur each Sunday. For the stage of deploying the *intervention*, they seemed to be an ideal coalition member.

The program founder attended a service at Shiloh Baptist Church during April 2001, first meeting with the Pastor and the NAACP Executive Board member before the service. At that time, the program founder was invited to tell the congregation about the intent to help to close the achievement gap in New Rochelle. During the announcement phase of the service, the program founder told the congregation about the intention to start a college preparation program that would allow middle school students an opportunity to improve their health and educational achievement (we later added high school students), emphasizing how the goal was to motivate these youth, while also having parents involved. What was implied was the manner in which the program would be seeking to move students across the *stages of change* (see Table 28.1) so that they might began to take action to improve their health and educational achievement. The founder, standing ever so briefly in the church, presented information concerning the achievement gap, sharing the SAT and other health statistics, as an act that was consistent with *consciousness raising* and evoking their concerns—so they might move into a *preparation* and/or *action stage* (see Table 28.1) for specifically helping the founder start a new supplementary education program. After the brief presentation of facts to evoke their concerns, and possibly allow those present to emerge all sharing common concerns, the founder received a standing ovation. Support and the common ground of sharing a common concern seemed more than apparent. Next, Pastor Jimmie Brown asked that the pilot after-school program occur at the church.

A discussion of and evaluation of the eventual Goldquest program that took shape and what it accomplished may best serve to illustrate Fawcett et al.'s (1997) last two phases of coalition development: (3) *Changes in the Community* that reduce risk and enhance protective factors; and (4) *Changes in Intermediate and Ultimate Outcomes*, such as reported use of substances (e.g., alcohol, illicit drugs) and other community-level indicators. In this case, the question at hand involves what changes were brought about by the Goldquest program, including changes in intermediate and ultimate outcomes. The available, but limited data on the program piloted in 2000 will be presented here, in order to answer this central question.

The Emergent Program

Goldquest emerged in 2000 as an educational organization, featuring a community-based supplementary after-school program developed through the systematic building of an academic, community, and faith-based coalition. Goldquest's focus is on developing the physical and intellectual growth of students 8–17 years old (3rd–12th grades) living in Southern Westchester County, while improving the academic achievement and health of minority students in Southern Westchester. More specifically, the organization's main mission is to reduce the academic achievement gap minority students experience relative to their White and higher SES peers by teaching effective study and test-taking techniques, providing preparation for standardized testing, and supporting students through the college application process (i.e., research, completing applications and essays, and identifying sources of financial assistance). Goldquest is located within and works in collaboration with Shiloh Baptist Church, while enjoying a coalition with other community-based organizations in New Rochelle, New York, including working in collaboration with the New Rochelle Public School District and the local NAACP.

The Goldquest guiding philosophy involves building bridges that foster strong relationships between youth, families, and communities, in order to foster positive education and health outcomes for youth, while moving local communities toward closing the achievement gap—as measured by tests such as the SAT. The focus of Goldquest is to effectively engage (see Ross & Smalls, chapter 26, this volume) students in the learning and academic achievement process by teaching, training, and coaching students with regard to how to improve their study skills, become more focused on academic achievement, and make healthier life choices for an overall goal of decreasing the academic achievement gap, as well as the health gap. Goldquest relies on a personalized program that accepts where a student is, academically and personally, given his or her stage of change, and then goes on to individually design for each student a recommended program of intervention to address his or her academic performance needs; this is pursued by working on an individual basis with students, while also using small groups (teams), as well as individual tutoring, as warranted.

A main area of focus for Goldquest is to help students improve their test taking skills, specifically for the SATs and PSAT tests. Goldquest works with students as early as the third grade in order to foster and improve their study skills and test-taking skills; and to spur them on to research and focus on college and professional careers, including all steps of the college application and financial aid/scholarship process.

To accomplish goals, Goldquest relies upon a staff that is mostly part time and includes certified teachers. Key staff include the Executive Director (the first author, Dr. Angela Campbell), a Director, maintenance member, and an on-call nutritionist. Other volunteer staff includes college interns and upper high school students who come in 2–3 days each week, serving as role models for younger students and providing tutoring and other supportive services.

What is being accomplished is also something rather distinct in focus. Goldquest is the only after-school program for middle and high school students in Southern Westchester County that has a focus on closing the racial/ethnic achievement gap, fostering high academic success, maximizing PSAT and SAT test performance through early, repeated practice in advance of the test used for college applications, and extensive preparation for the college application and financial aid/scholarship process. Indeed, no other program exists to our knowledge in the larger New York metropolitan region that involves middle school children in PSAT/SAT/ACT test preparation, making us unique.

We seek to meet the needs of students of all ages and grade levels in the program by allowing them access to and working with them in a computer lab, thereby also seeking to close the digital divide within this country by providing access to technology as a potential powerful catalyst to promote learning. We also partner with parents. We encourage parents to learn from and inspire one another. We have also designed our program to specifically meet the needs of Black male students, and at times, have had a majority of participants with these demographics—allowing us to refine methods tailored to meet their needs. In this manner, we feel we showcase and promote some of the best practices in the education community.

Key Program Features

Goldquest has important program features to accomplish its mission. First, there are rules. We refer to these as the 5 "C" words that tell students what they are not to do during their time together: NO CRITICIZING, NO COMPLAINING, NO COMPARING, NO COMPETING, AND NO CONTENDING. We review the definitions of each of the words and practice implementing these into the class work. Each student is handed a sheet with the words on them and is asked to give examples of how to not perform this behavior. Secondly, we use teams. All students are expected to meet as a team once per week for 2 hours. The use of teams allows many processes of change to be invoked, as summarized in Table 28.1, and reiterated here: Consciousness raising, or learning new facts, ideas, and tips that support the healthy behavioral change—potentially from one's buddy or peer in a study group. It also develops helping relationships, or seeking and using social support for the healthy behavioral change, given the friendship with one's buddy that typically develops. Third, we use communication logs. Communication logs are used to promote fellowship for classmates. Every week students are given a student to call and discuss a specific topic that we will talk about on the radio. When students have communicated with the person on the list they both receive extra marbles, as a form of contingency management (see more in the following paragraphs), and they are asked to sit next to that person during the following class.

Twelve Program Components

There are also 12 key program components: Marbles, Practice SAT, Math of the Day, Word of the Day, Math Game, Word Game, Deep Breathing, The Radio Show, Activity Sheets, Peer Tutoring, NAACP Peer Teaching, and NAACP Membership. All of these are explained in further detail:

1. **Marbles** involves the application of contingency management in the classroom, as students receive either systematic rewards or punishments that are contingent on their performance of a behavior that is under their control. We use marbles to reward or punish behavior. Students can anticipate that as a consequence of their behavior he/she will gain or lose marbles. The first author will actually walk around the classroom with a large cup full of marbles. Each student has a cup. Marbles are placed in their cup to reward behavior, and some behaviors result in the loss of marbles. The student who accumulates the most marbles by the end of the class receives a reward. This emerged as highly effective in shaping behavior consistent with academic achievement. This is also consistent with the kind of effective teaching and academic engagement of which Ross and Smalls speak (in chapter 26 of this volume), as a key feature of Goldquest, and one they assert is associated with student improvement, given the evidence they cite.

2. **Practice SAT** is a core program component and involves students experiencing the real Standardized Assessment Test (SAT) at the local high school, and continuing to take

practice tests until 11th grade. This is consistent with the work of Bandura (1977b, 1986, 1997) and his Social Cognitive Theory, seeking to impact the self-efficacy of students, raising self-efficacy via the key source of *performance attainments*, or the accumulation of experiences with a particular task. We also fostered *consciousness raising*, providing facts about the importance of doing well on achievement tests for gaining college admission. Eventually, the ACT was also added as a vital practice test. The first author has found that when students are exposed to both the SAT in January and the ACT in April or June they are likely to feel more relaxed during the first real test date during October of the 10th grade.

3. Math of the Day involves each student being given a one-page math sheet with problems on various topics. All sheets are collected and reviewed by the instructor, using the results to determine that upon which to focus for that day. A student can get up to 6 marbles if he or she has persevered in the activity. This component is consistent with the use of contingency management, as well as consciousness raising, or learning new facts, ideas, and tips that support the healthy behavioral change.

4. The Word of the Day responds to the challenge of getting students to read. Word of the Day involved students being given at the beginning of the class a word from the SAT or ACT on a sheet. The word is defined and they are asked to use it in a sentence and to write an essay using that word. The sheet is turned in and the student receives 6 marbles for turning in this sheet. This fourth Goldquest component combines many elements such as contingency management, as well as enhancing performance to support increases in self-efficacy.

5. The Math Game strives to increase student self-efficacy with regard to performance attainments (see Table 28.1) in math. At the end of class the students sat in a circle; a leader would begin a rhythm that the students kept up by tapping on their thighs; the instructor would give a math problem, and going around the group clockwise, the student would be expected to give a correct answer and initiate a new math problem for the next student. The rhythm served the purpose to give each person a time frame for answering the question. If they exceeded the time frame they were eliminated from the competition. After playing the game at the end of each class, typically, for 15 minutes, there would be one winner who would receive an additional 10 marbles.

6. The Word Game similarly strives to assist students in increasing their self-efficacy and operates in pretty much the same fashion as the math game. However, in this case, the instructor would give a word to the student who began first. The rhythmic tapping would proceed. The student starting would be expected to give a new word with the last letter in the word the instructor gave. The last letter would be the first letter in the new word. This game was also done for 15 minutes at the end of each class. Those who did not perform the task correctly would be eliminated, while a winner would emerge by the end and receive 10 marbles.

All of the components described thus far are consistent with Ross and Smalls' discussion (chapter 26 of this volume) of how academic engagement translates into the amount of time students spend on tasks known to promote learning. As a result of these activities occurring each day of program attendance, students experience a kind of academic engagement comprised of multiple academic interactions (or learn units to use the term described by Ross and Smalls).

7. Deep Breathing, as another program component, enhances student self-efficacy with regard to noting their physiological arousal (see Table 28.1). During the initial student assessments we found that students became distracted and bored. They seemed to yawn a lot and were unable to stay still. I introduced a breathing exercise to accompany classical music. Children take deep rhythmic breaths to slow down their activities and open their minds for learning.

8. The Radio Show evolved because of Napoleon K. Holmes—an early community activist in the New Rochelle community. He was one of six people to be arrested in the 1970s during the labor disputes of the union, getting black workers employed. He became interested in this program and would take young members on his weekly radio show "The Holmes Way." When he was diagnosed with lung cancer in 2002 and had a short period to live, he asked the first author to take over his radio segment. When he died July 2002, she visited the radio station in New Rochelle and asked Mr. Don Stevens if she could start a radio segment that would feature the students of the program as cohosts. Since she would need time to get the students ready she asked to run the show bi-weekly for 1 hour beginning at 6:00 p.m. on Mondays. We started the show "Diamonds in the Rough" September 2002. The radio shows have health related, community activity, and educational issues that we discuss in the Goldquest program. When the middle school students are featured in the program they are given literature regarding the topic and they write essays prior to the show. The show gives our students an ability to be a part of a live broadcast and respond to callers during the hour show. Parents of the middle school students pick their children up from the show and often are smiling and kissing their children for the radio show participation. The radio broadcasts allowed Goldquest to gain in popularity.

9. The Daily Activity Sheets provide students with key organizational skills. As suggested in Table 28.1 with regard to improving performance attainments, we see these daily activity sheets as key to improving self-efficacy for academic achievement. Students must engage in active planning with regard to how they will spend and organize their time at Goldquest for that day. Perhaps they plan to finish their homework and begin studying for the various assessments. We view the activity sheets as also involving the process of consciousness raising, or learning new facts, ideas, and tips that support the healthy behavioral change, as cited in Table 28.1. Activity sheets also support Self-reevaluation, or realizing that the behavioral change is an important part of one's identity as a person and must be nurtured and maintained through self-organization—facilitated by the activity sheets.

10. Peer Tutoring is key, since tutoring allows vicarious learning to be introduced as a potential source for increasing self-efficacy. Students that have been involved in the program are told that one day they will be peer tutors for younger students. They understand that this program is a "gifting" program. Students accept the gift of service from tutors during the middle school years in the program and they will then give that gift of service to students in the future. The peer tutoring program has been quite successful since we have been able to utilize students that have been in the program from the middle school years. All tutors are high school sophomores, juniors or seniors. The tutors dedicate a minimum of 4 hours per week during the school week. Peer tutors have created positive bonds between the high school and middle school students. I find that the older students feel responsible for keeping the students focused and motivated to be successful.

11. NAACP Peer Teaching is carried out by older peers who first joined Goldquest from the outside in January 2005 as part of an Adopt-An-After School Program. The state conference of the NAACP Youth and College Division had approved this program as a way to have the Board Members of Youth Councils visit after-school programs and teach children about the goals and mission of the NAACP. Thus, the NAACP Youth Council of New Rochelle included youth of the ages of 14 to 17 who were developing leadership skills and ended up attending the Goldquest supplementary after-school program. They came into the program once a week for 1 hour. Four of these youth leaders take turns teaching classes on various topics relating to youth getting involved in civic and political affairs. They effectively engage in what we call *NAACP Peer Teaching*, as youth leaders. Civic and volunteer activities have spun off from the NAACP Peer Teaching activities, including letter-writing campaigns, soup kitchen events, and our radio show.

Many joined us for a Youth Health Symposium on April 2, 2005. Our Youth Health Symposium provided members with the knowledge to take action in our community to address health disparities. After a subsequent letter-writing campaign, the youth began to bond even more and respond to requests for action. We reviewed the *Healthy People 2010* set of objectives to discern logical steps for taking actions to reduce the health gap in New Rochelle and in this country.

12. NAACP Membership is also stressed, with the students having been exposed to the NAACP Peer Teachers, as youth leaders. Pertinent activities include getting involved in the NAACP Youth Council's hosting of the twice-per-month "Diamonds In The Rough" radio show on the WVOX–1460 AM station, which has also brought Goldquest attention and praise. We have conducted shows that empower young people to become involved in political and social actions. (Recordings of all shows are available upon request from the first author). We also record public service announcements to inform our community about our monthly meetings, and special events. After every event we have an informational session that informs the community about our goals and objectives of that event. For example, we hosted our First Annual Health Symposium on Saturday, April 2, 2005, and on Monday, April 4, 2005 we hosted a review of that event from 6 to 7 p.m. on WVOX–1460 AM. *The Sound Report, Journal News* and *County Press* are our local newspapers in New Rochelle. We always write press releases and ask for reporters to attend our events. When reporters are unavailable to attend we critique our own event and send pictures and an article to the newspapers to run.

Following and applying what is suggested in Table 28.1, *NAACP Membership*, as a program component, combines several processes of change that positively impact our youth: Consciousness raising, or learning new facts, ideas, and tips that support healthy behavioral change; Environmental reevaluation, or realizing the negative impact of the unhealthy behavior or the positive impact of the healthy behavior on one's proximal social and physical environment—as discussed by youth on the radio; Helping relationships, or seeking and using social support for the healthy behavioral change, even as they reach out to the listening radio audience and seek social support for healthy behavior change; youth also have access to the experience of Social Liberation, or realizing that the social norms are changing in the direction of supporting the healthy behavioral change; finally, with regard to increasing student self-efficacy, the radio show allows vicarious experiences of witnessing others committed to community service, community activism, and community leadership. Moreover, they get to practice the use of verbal persuasion.

Awards Reflecting Positively Upon Goldquest

The New Rochelle Branch of the NAACP was the winner for Outstanding Branch at the 2004 New York State Conference and the 2005 Best Youth Council of the Northeast Region—being indicative of the recognition we have received, suggesting our success in coalition building and implementing a supplementary education program of value.

These awards may best serve to illustrate Fawcett et al.'s (1997) last two phases of coalition development (see Table 28.1): (3) *Changes in the Community* that reduce risk and enhance protective factors; and (4) *Changes in Intermediate and Ultimate Outcomes*, such as the community-level indicator of having an outstanding branch engaged in valuable activities worthy of reward and recognition. However, to further determine changes and outcomes, we next present data from a Spring 2006 program evaluation, using quantitative and qualitative methods.

Goldquest Evaluation at the Five Year Anniversary

The program components of the radio show, math of the day, peer tutoring, marbles, practice SAT, word of the day, word game, NAACP membership, NAACP peer teaching, math game, deep breathing, and activity sheets were all evaluated via a survey in early 2006.

A survey was created based on the Goldquest program components, including a scale that assessed whether there was participation in a particular program component, and allowing a rating of each program component, and a rating of the impact of that program component upon the student; both a parent and student version was created. The resulting surveys were mailed (1 for the parent and 1 for the child) to 324 parent–child pairs who had attended some portion of the Goldquest program from 2000 to 2005. We obtained (13 incomplete) only 83 matched parent-child pairs for data analysis.

Students completing the survey ranged in age from 11 to 22 years of age. The average age of the students in the sample was 16 years (mean $= 16.06$, $SD = 2.33$). The sample was 42.17% male ($N = 35$) and 58% female ($N = 48$). Regarding racial demographics for the sample, 56% of the sample was African American ($N = 56$, 67.5), 12% Hispanic ($N = 10$), and 18.1% White ($N = 15$), as well as including some other ($N = 2$, 2.0 %).

Survey results ($n = 83$) showed that the majority of students participated in the Practice SAT test (84.3%, $n = 70$), followed by the contingency management activity of receiving Marbles (74.70%, $n = 62$), then the Radio Show activity at 67.50% ($n = 56$), Math of the Day at 63.90% ($n = 53$), and the Word of the Day at 62.70% (52). The students' mean rating (4.61, $SD = .58$) of the program quality, overall, suggested it was valued as close to "very good"—on a Likert scale of 1 (very poor) to 6 (excellent).

Students' ratings of program components (1 = very poor to 6 = excellent) showed that Radio Show participation ($n = 56$, 67.50%) improved oratory skills at a good to very good level (mean = 4.84, $SD = .92$), and also promoted a more positive outlook for the students (mean 4.71, .98). Also, a majority of students reported Math of the Day ($n = 53$, 63.90%) improved their test grades in math (mean = 4.81, $SD = .83$) and math grades (mean = 4.78, $SD = .96$), while the Word Game ($n = 53$, 63.90%) and Word of the Day ($n = 52$, 62.70%) improved their English grades (mean = 4.85, $SD = .86$), and English test scores (mean = 4.67, $SD = .85$). For the Activity Sheets ($n = 50$, 60.2%), the majority of students reported that their study skills improved (mean = 4.49, $SD = .83$), their attitude doing homework improved (mean = 4.60, $SD = .91$), and test-taking attitude improved (mean = 4.78, $SD = .91$). Deep Breathing ($n = 50$, 60.2%) reduced stress during test taking fairly well (mean = 3, $SD = 1.35$).

Students were also asked to rate the program impact upon them. Overall, for students' program impact ratings, the mean was 4.17 ($SD = .92$), or closest to "helped some." The program components having the greatest impact upon them were performing better on tests (mean = 4.84, $SD = 1,03$), and encouragement to take the ACT/SAT before 10th grade (4.61, $SD = 1.5$). Despite the intended program focus on health, students rated the impact of the program for helping take better care of health only at 3.83 ($SD = 1.41$), or at "barely had an impact" to "helped me some." Similarly, parents also felt the program had the greatest impact on their child with regard to "encouraging to take the ACT/SAT before 10th grade" at 5.04 ($SD = 1.07$) or "helped a lot." And, parents also rated the program impact on their child as close to "helped a lot" (4.69, $SD = .96$) in the area of performing better on tests.

Parent and Student Recommendations for Program Improvement: Thoughts and Feelings

Parents and student were asked an opened-ended question regarding what recommendations they could offer the program to improve. Students stated they feel they can achieve their goals, get into the college they want, and felt the program will provide them with the tools they need to succeed. Some students wanted access to the Internet on program computers. Parents as well as students wanted the Goldquest classes to have more teachers and professional instructors. Parents also wanted outside resources that could be used to allow their children to remain as participants in the Goldquest program. Most parents have the ability to start their child in the program, but are unable to pay for the entire school year. Parents will often ask the Director about funding streams to allow their children to continue in the program.

From Goldquest to Academic Pathways

Since a year ago, when the 2006 survey was conducted and analyzed, the supplementary education program became a nonprofit 501(c)(3) organization. As a result of pursuing this path, we had to change our name, becoming the supplementary education program now known as Academic Pathways. As Academic Pathways, we have been able to secure several small grants from various funding sources. Any funding that a student receives from Academic Pathways is divided by the number of remaining months in the school year. This should allow the program to avoid discontinuity in student participation, due to parental problems paying for the program. Recipients of the resulting scholarships must have completed a minimum of one month of good attendance, and attended at least 80% of all classes.

Instead of directly increasing the number of teachers and professional instructors, more older high school students have been added, who now tutor twice per week—on 1 day receiving community service hours and for the other day receiving pay. Tutors need money to get to the program and return home. The tutors enjoy a situation that allows community service and some monetary benefit.

Another recommendation was that the computers at the program add Internet access. The first author met with the Pastor of Shiloh Baptist Church and several Board Members about this. The decision was made to facilitate access to the Internet through the service provider they were using. Now that we have full functional Internet privileges, students are able to work on potential college scholarships, college essays, and personal statements after school at a more relaxed pace—going beyond the focus we had in our special summer boot camp focused on the college application process.

We also now hold our program 5 days per week, whereas for the first 5 years we met Monday through Thursday. At the start of the school year in Fall 2006, we made this change, informing all potential students via e-mail that we would be open 5 days per week. This extra day allows parents to enjoy a program that is deemed a stable after school activity.

Academic Pathways also provides customized services in the larger New Rochelle community. In October 2006 the first author was asked by another church to start a program for their youth. The response was the development of a Saturday Program, offering SAT and ACT standardized test preparation program for the middle and high school students that attend this church. At present, an attempt is being made to engage these students in the process of attending monthly NAACP meetings so they, too, can become a part of the leadership and community service components deemed essential to their development. Such participation also creates additional opportunities to interact with these students, fostering stronger links with the students. Recently, the Saturday Program students have been encouraged to attend at least 1 day per week the primary 5-day-per-week program housed at the Shiloh Baptist church, experiencing a tutoring session in a subject of their choice. The students that have started to obtain the additional weekday tutoring sessions have also started to attend community service events such as the Radio Show and NAACP meetings.

Conclusion

Goldquest has evolved into Academic Pathways, becoming a stable feature of the New Rochelle, New York community, and providing an important service designed to help close the achievement and health gaps; however, we appear to be having a significant impact on academic achievement only from students' self-reports. The 5-year anniversary evaluation of the original Goldquest program was able to capture the voices of only 83 parent–child pairs of participants from among the 324 we have served in some measure since our founding in 2000. Nonetheless, the results of the five-year anniversary evaluation were informative and useful, allowing us to further refine and improve the program—leading to the establishment of a nonprofit 501(c)(3) organization—Academic Pathways.

In considering what has been presented in this chapter, a number of limitations of the 5-year anniversary evaluation must be kept in mind. First, as a participant–observer, the first author and founder who created Goldquest was also evaluating it, suggesting the potential for bias. Also, the 5-year anniversary survey was given to a small sample of convenience in a survey with a low response rate. It is possible that those who did not respond may have provided a more negative evaluation of the Goldquest program; or, that volunteers had certain characteristics, including wanting to please or gain the admiration of the researcher. Also, the survey utilized self-report data, which may have been subject to recall bias. The use of a parent to report and rate what they believe their child received in the program helps to give validity to students' self-report data; but these data, too, may be subject to recall bias—or reflect the peripheral involvement of parents in not knowing every detail of their child's involvement in Goldquest.

At the core of the initial vision was the intent to impact SAT achievement test scores, hence, to some extent, the founder emerges feeling validated. The program component involving SAT practice tests was rated as having the highest impact. The program origins emerged as the program's strengths. A clearer vision for addressing health now seems warranted. Also, the recommendations of students and parents provided a guide for how to further improve and evolve—shaping the current program and helping to plot the trajectory for future growth. This trajectory involves facing the challenge of better integrating projects that allow students to experience a significant impact in the domain of health.

Through the dissemination of models such as Academic Pathways, the goal is to realize the promise of equity for all embodied in the *Brown v. The Board of Education* decision, and in the much newer No Child Left Behind legislation. The goal is to move communities of learners toward the achievement of educational equity, as well equity in health—as the moral imperative of this century. This imperative necessitates building coalitions among academics, community groups such as the NAACP, and faith-based organizations such as Shiloh Baptist Church, as illustrated in this chapter. Hopefully, the model described in this chapter, though supported by evidence that is only suggestive, within a study with many limitations, will inspire others to develop coalitions in their communities to launch supplementary education programs tailored for their community setting.

REFERENCES

Bandura, A. (1977a). Self-efficacy: Toward a unifying theory of behavioral change. *Psychological Review*, *84*(2), 191–215.

Bandura, A. (1977b). *Social learning theory*. Englewood Cliffs, NJ: Prentice-Hall.

Bandura, A. (1986). *Social foundations of thought & action: A social cognitive theory*. Englewood Cliffs, NJ: Prentice-Hall.

Bandura, A. (1994). Self-efficacy. In V. S. Ramachaudran (Ed.), *Encyclopedia of human behavior* (Vol. 4). New York: Academic Press.

Bandura, A. (1997). *Self-efficacy: The exercise of control*. New York: W. H. Freeman and Company.

Bhattacharyya, M. (2005). Community support for supplementary education. In E. Gordon, B. Bridglall, & A. Meroe (Eds.), *Supplementary education: The hidden curriculum of high academic achievement.* Lanham, MD: Rowman & Littlefield.

Bridglall, B. (2005). Varieties of supplementary education intervention. In E. Gordon, B. Bridglall, & A. Meroe (Eds.), *Supplementary education: The hidden curriculum of high academic achievement.* Lanham, MD: Rowman & Littlefield.

Bridglall, B., & Gordon, E. (2005). The institutionalization of supplementary education. In E. Gordon, B. Bridglall, & A. Meroe (Eds.), *Supplementary education: The hidden curriculum of high academic achievement.* Lanham, MD: Rowman & Littlefield.

Diderichsen, F., Evans, T., & Whitehead, M. (2001). The social basis of disparities in health. In T. Evans, M. Whitehead, F. Diderichsen, A. Bhuiya, & M. Wirth (Eds.), *Challenging inequities in health: From ethics to action.* New York: Oxford University Press.

Education Trust, The. (2001, May 23). States can close the achievement gap by decade's end. *Ed Watch Online.* Retrieved August 3, 2002, from http://www.edtrust.org

Education Trust, The. (2002, August 4). The funding gap: Low-income and minority students receive fewer dollars. *Ed Watch Online.* Retrieved March 8, 2003, from http://www.edtrust.org

Evans, T., Whitehead, M., Diderichsen, F., Bhuiya, A., & Wirth, M. (Eds.). (2001). *Challenging inequities in health: From ethics to action.* New York: Oxford University Press.

Fawcett, S., Lewis, R., Andrews, A., Francisco, V., Richter, K., Williams, E., et al. (1997). Evaluating community coalitions for prevention of substance abuse: The case of Project Freedom. *Health Education & Behavior, 24*(6), 812–828.

Gordon, E., Bridglall, B., & Meroe, A. (Eds.). (2005). *Supplementary education: The hidden curriculum of high academic achievement,* Lanham, MD: Rowman & Littlefield.

Gordon, E., & Meroe, A. (2005). Supplementation and supplantation as alternative education strategies. In E. Gordon, B. Bridglall, & A. Meroe (Eds.), *Supplementary education: The hidden curriculum of high academic achievement.* Lanham, MD: Rowman & Littlefield.

Meroe, A. (2005). Supplementary education, the negotiation of sociocultural marginality and the uses of reflexivity. In E. Gordon, B. Bridglall, & A. Meroe (Eds.), *Supplementary education: The hidden curriculum of high academic achievement.* Lanham, MD: Rowman & Littlefield.

National Association for Advancement of Colored People (NAACP). (2005). *Brown fifty years and beyond: Promise and progress.* An NAACP Advocacy Report.

Paige, R. (2002, April). *No Child Left Behind: What to know & where to go: Parents' guide to No Child Left Behind: A new era in education.* Washington, DC: U.S. Department of Education.

Prochaska, J., & DiClemente, C. (1983). Stages and processes of self-change of cigarette smoking: Toward an integrative model of change. *Journal of Consulting and Clinical Psychology, 51*(3), 390–395.

Prochaska, J., & DiClemente, C. (1992). Stages of change in the modification of problem behaviors. *Progress in Behavior Modification, 28,* 183–218.

Prochaska, J., DiClemente, C., & Norcross, J. (1992). In search of how people change: Applications to addictive behaviors. *American Psychologist, 47*(9), 1102–1114.

Prochaska, J., Redding, C., & Evers, K. (1997). The transtheoretical model and stages of change: Social cognitive theory. In K. Glanz, F. Lewis, & B. Rimer (Eds.), *Health behavior and health education: Theory, research & practice.* San Francisco: Wiley.

Westchester County Department of Planning. (2001). Databook 2001: Westchester County, New York. Retrieved April 7, 2004, from http://www.westchestergov.com/planning/research/main.htm

So No Child Is Left Behind: A Peer Mentoring/Tutoring Program for At-Risk Urban Youth Attending a College Preparatory High School

29

Adrienne Chew
and Barbara C. Wallace

Introduction

The goal of achieving equity in health for all remains inextricably tied to the achievement of educational equity. Education may be the most important form of early prevention and intervention to ensure the very best health outcomes across the life span, while impacting adult employment, socioeconomic status, as well as morbidity and mortality. Thus, in conceptualizing how to attain educational equity for all, and close the achievement gap between those excelling and those currently being left behind, the kind of paradigm shift being called for throughout this book may need also occur within the field of education. Within the desired paradigm, collaborations among administrators, teachers, mentors, peers, and parents—as members of a common school culture and community—will be essential, along with a common vision and commitment to educational equity for all. Also, within the desired paradigm, a vision that both appreciates diversity and values fair play and equity in ensuring access to educational opportunities so all achieve their highest potential is vitally needed, while totally abandoning any blame-the-victim or deficit-oriented approaches. In this manner, common themes run throughout the discourse on how to achieve both equity in health for all, and educational equity.

Some view the goal of achieving educational equity as embodied in the federal legislation known as The No Child Left Behind Act of 2001 (NCLB). NCLB underscores the need to develop the full potential of all students. The goal is to have all students reach the *proficient* or *advanced* level. As a consequence, every school professional in America is being challenged to work for the success of struggling at-risk students. At-risk students are in danger of being left behind, whether by virtue of lagging in their academic achievement test scores, grades, rates of retention, or graduation rates. Instead of at-risk, ideally, we see students as being in need of appropriate social and other supports in order to develop their full potential as students toward the goal of achieving equity for all. High schools in America, especially in large urban cities, are being challenged to accomplish this goal, necessitating that they attend to the needs of those most at-risk. The vision of NCLB is for all students to know and demonstrate mastery of academic content standards in reading and math, taught by highly qualified teachers, using research-based instruction and teaching methods (Office of Vocational and Adult Education, 2003). Thus, urban high schools are being challenged to take up the mission step by step that follows from this vision.

In ensuring that no child is left behind, special attention must be paid to those currently lagging the furthest behind—at-risk urban African American students. In urban cities, the greatest challenge in closing the academic achievement gap emerges as involving the task of meeting the needs of at-risk African American male students, in particular. In this regard, Roderick (2003) found that African American male students began to lag behind their female peers across the transition from eighth to ninth grade, suggesting yet another academic achievement gap within the group of African Americans—one based on gender. Roderick also found that African American male students tended to be viewed more negatively by teachers. In addition, the consequences of this gap were far-reaching, given how twice as many males as females ended up dropping out of high school (Roderick). The challenge that Roderick describes requires a meaningful and effective response. Montecel, Cortez, and Cortez (2004) discuss the same dropout crisis for Hispanic students, as well as the need for a new paradigm and approach to preventing dropouts, echoing the call for effective responses.

Among the responses being described in the literature, there are those deemed desirable, such as urban school leaders also being multicultural leaders—bringing sensitivity to the needs of the diverse members of their student bodies (Gardiner & Enomoto, 2006). Other responses are deemed less desirable, such as urban school districts' over-reliance on punitive measures involving the police and criminal justice system to prevent school dropout, as the most common response, despite no evidence of effectiveness in reducing dropout rates (Hoyle & Collier, 2006).

Agents internal to the school environment may be seen as capable of playing a powerful role in preventing not only school dropout, but also in intervening much earlier on in the high school experience to prevent the experience of students failing ninth-grade classes. In this manner, teachers, counselors, administrators, coaches, parents, and peers each may have a role to play in ensuring no child is left behind.

The teaching strategies of some high school teachers may also be at issue. However, apparently, school leadership in urban settings is currently failing to adequately appreciate the importance of instructional initiatives for early grade intervention and dropout prevention (Hoyle & Collier, 2006). Again, not surprisingly, where lack of attention is being paid to instructional initiatives, dropout rates remain unchanged (Hoyle & Collier, 2006).

In the search for points for early prevention and intervention, it is important to acknowledge the magnitude of the transition facing ninth-grade boys and girls, entering the novel setting of a high school, especially in large urban high school settings. Ninth grade is the most critical point to intervene and prevent students from losing motivation, and failing.

The experience of caring and supportive relationships in the new high school setting may help young people succeed. Such supportive relationships may foster strong commitments on the part of students to remain in the high school setting, the development of positive values with regard to the role of schooling in their lives, and foster the evolution of social competencies that are important for the successful negotiation of the high school environment. Patterns of success in high-performing high schools include such relationships and connections. Also key to success are collaborative instruction and collaborative leadership (Cooper, Ponder, Merritt, & Matthews, 2005).

Given the contemporary imperative that no child is left behind, this chapter describes the implementation and evaluation of a peer mentoring program for at-risk ninth-grade students. The program was established to ensure the academic achievement of at-risk students attending a college preparatory high school in an urban setting by connecting high-achieving high school students with at-risk ninth-grade students in mentoring relationships that included the provision of tutoring in major subject areas. Within the model implemented, school leadership also sought to collaborate with teachers in improving instruction. The rationale for developing a peer mentoring program, the multitude of factors operating in influencing student academic achievement, the process of developing a model peer mentoring program, and the results of a quantitative and qualitative evaluation of the program will be presented in this chapter.

Why a Peer Mentoring Program?

Numerous authors provide powerful support for the value and role of peer mentoring in improving academic achievement for at-risk students (Barton-Arwood, Jolivette, & Massey, 2002; Bisland, 2001; Burgsthaler & Cronheim, 2001; Du Bois, Holloway, Valentine, & Harris, 2002; Harris & Jones, 1999; Perez & Dorman, 2001; Reiser, Petry, & Amitag, 1989; Stader & Gagnepain, 2000; Swap, Leonard, Shields, & Abrams, 2001). At the same time, many other factors impact achievement (Roderick & Camburn, 1999), including skill level, motivation, peer influences, level of expectations, monitoring at school and home, and teaching effectiveness (p. 335). The work of Thompson, Warren, and Carter (2004) uncovered the need to address teacher attitude, expectations, and instructional practices that are detrimental to student achievement. There is a need for administrators to identify all high school teachers in need of professional development to strengthen instructional practices and to change any deficit-oriented mind-sets brought to their perception of at-risk students—as endorsed by numerous authors (Avery, 1999; Darling-Hammond, 1999; Kaplan & Owings, 2001; Windschitl, 2002; Ybarra & Hollingsworth, 2001). Meanwhile, a peer mentoring program constitutes a valuable approach, while others are surely also needed to improve academic outcomes.

Thus, with the first author serving as an administrator at a college preparatory high school located in an urban center—Central High School in Philadelphia (CHS) Pennsylvania, the decision was made to introduce mentoring for incoming probationary and at-risk ninth-grade students. The goal was to offer the social support deemed necessary for a successful transition from eighth to ninth grade, as students entered high school. Peer mentoring was seen as holding the potential to break the cycle of early failure for ninth-grade students, particularly the most at-risk male African American students. It was felt that peer mentoring could create the foundation for early social and academic success among at-risk students, since mentoring is an effective intervention to provide students with opportunities to create academic and social success.

The approach implemented also applied selected, programmatic components from NCLB. The components were highly qualified teachers, a focus on academic standards, an analysis of assessment data, and an assessment of teaching methods in classrooms to improve instruction. The primary author, an administrator at the high school, believed that reducing failure would not occur with one sole solution focusing only on students, only on teachers, or only on parents. Instead, the challenge of reducing failure was seen as multifaceted.

Important Background on the Setting

CHS was established in 1836. It is the second oldest continuous high school in the nation. The first author was one of three assistant principals whose role is to support the principal and his administration of CHS. Alumni of CHS are many, including artist Thomas Eakins and comedian Bill Cosby. The alumni remain active and financially supportive of the school, providing many resources. The operating budget for the school in 2003–2004 was $12 million, in addition to the funds separately designated for special education, desegregation, and Title I. The 2002 Merit Award–winning Home and School Association schedules monthly meetings and fosters active parental involvement. Hence, in many respects, CHS is unique as a well-endowed public school providing college preparation, while enjoying illustrious alumni support. Within the city of Philadelphia, to gain entrance to CHS is a privilege and honor, while also suggesting the pressure to succeed that admitted students may feel.

Demographics and School Culture

During the 2003–2004 school year, total school enrollment in grades 9–12 was 2,400 with a diverse student population of 41% White, 33% African American, 21% Asian, and 5% Hispanic. The gender breakdown was 49% male and 51% female students. Enjoying a culture and climate perceived by the faculty as positive, CHS students were generally inspired and motivated through their middle-school education, although 137 of them failed major subjects. The faculty and staff members totaled 161 including cafeteria and custodial staff.

Annually at Open House during the preceding May, the president's address includes a message that indicates that CHS students are capable of the academic challenge, but they must do the work, ask for help when needed, get involved in activities, and be respectful to all. The atmosphere of individuality and respect from the educational leader is immediately obvious within the school culture. Student activities before and after school include publications, varsity and junior varsity sports, award-winning art and music programs, and over 80 clubs (e.g., poetry, skateboarding, chess, and a forum for diversity). Every ethnic group has an organization for expression of its culture and a voice in the school community. Community service is a school requirement for all students.

Traditions at CHS also foster various continuous student activities and functions, such as proms, homecoming dances, and football games. In addition, CHS has a tradition of designating classes by class number. During the 2004–2005 school year when the peer mentoring model was introduced and evaluated, the 266th class was scheduled to graduate in 2007—coincidentally, the year of this chapter being published. Being identified with their class number, class spirit, tradition, socialization, and academic promise are characteristics the administrators promote for the students of each incoming class.

It is within this context that the peer mentoring model was introduced so as to make a difference in the academic and social dilemmas of at-risk students with exceptional academic capabilities in the 266th class. Permission to conduct this study at CHS was granted by the Northwest Regional Superintendent and the School District of Philadelphia Office of Research and Evaluation. The chapter first author believed students who were at risk for academic failure disconnected early from school and the social spirit CHS tries to impart. The process of failing courses seemed to result in isolation. Unfortunately, such failures prevented students from being eligible to participate in sports and other social activities, further compounding isolation. CHS became a stressful place for such failing students and, therefore, harmful to the cognitive, social, and overall growth of students at risk, as others have suggested (Manning & Baruth, 1996).

The first author began an intervention after determining that the practices of the institution, or lack thereof, resulted in a problem for at-risk students. Social support was deemed an intervention that could positively influence high school students who were at risk of school failure (Richman, Rosenfeld, & Bowen, 1998).

High Expectations for Students and the First Author's Role as Assistant Principal

Prior to acceptance to CHS, records showed the high academic potential of the students admitted. Acceptance to CHS generated an expectation and belief that all students would do well. This was a misconception, however, because many students did struggle.

Prior to the implementation of the peer mentoring intervention, the chapter first author reviewed archival data of 50 randomly selected ninth-grade students, searching for potential primary characteristics of ninth-grade students critical to the study at CHS. She found elementary and middle school information showing consistent attendance, above-average standardized test scores in third, fifth, and seventh grades, as well as intellectual giftedness. The general range of teacher comments on elementary report cards included the following: "hard-worker," "demonstrated good citizenship and behavior," and "has leadership potential." Students previously enjoyed good grades not only in academic areas but also in music, art, and physical education. In essence, they could be called "Renaissance children." Grades were consistently A's and B's from elementary through middle school. Most students were from two-parent families. Comments on reports from faculty at elementary and middle schools indicated parents had been "supportive and involved with their students at home and in their elementary and middle schools."

A CHS Middle States evaluation survey of students conducted in 2000 determined that exactly 50% of the school population lived in the Philadelphia area for their entire lives. Every conceivable family configuration existed among families who responded to this survey. In the same survey, it was found that 60% of CHS students lived with both parents and 34% lived with only one parent. The average student household income was $40,000. Thus, CHS's at-risk students may be somewhat unique, being drawn from a school containing students with such characteristics and backgrounds.

The meaning of "at-risk" varies among educators and situations. Historically, "at-risk" has meant that the student was not likely to graduate from high school (Slavin, 1989). Those considered at-risk were students admitted to CHS who exhibited failure at the first marking period of high school, potentially being at risk for not graduating from CHS, losing a well-earned opportunity.

CHS has a continuous history of student perseverance, endurance, excellence, and fame. The high standards of academic excellence have remained unchanged through the years. The diversity and range of courses continue to grow at CHS. The CHS 2003 *Central Yearbook* reports, "It remains the place where prominent leaders of tomorrow are trained and memories of yesterday are taught" (p. 262).

The school received approximately 4,000 applications during the 2003–2004 school year. The principal reviewed each application and made the final decision on all CHS freshmen. All students and potential at-risk students were admitted based on the principal's optimistic judgment that the students could succeed. At-risk students identified in this study were admitted to CHS based on the criteria of seventh-grade Terra Nova standardized test scores at or above the 88th percentile in both reading and math. Applicants met the seventh-grade criteria of A's and B's in major subjects with a possible C in one subject, as well as excellent attendance and behavior. The eighth-grade student applicant also submitted a current proficient, handwritten one-page essay on a topic of the applicant's choice.

Students were admitted to CHS, and all Philadelphia public schools, based solely on the report card grades and standardized test scores they earned during seventh grade. Incoming at-risk students received one or more grades of C, D, or F in major subjects during eighth grade. This indicated low major subject performance in eighth grade, however, and potential academic problems at CHS. Administrators at CHS were concerned about any sudden reversal in middle school academic performance during the eighth grade. Students were expected to maintain high academic performance levels throughout middle school before coming to CHS.

Based on students' performance in eighth grade, administrators of the school identified potential at-risk students with C's, D's, or F's in major subjects and placed them on probation status before they began their first academic school year at CHS. During the summer months of 2003, the chapter first author spent time meeting with 20 students and their parents, discussing those students' significantly low performance in eighth grade. Table 29.1 disaggregates incoming probationary at-risk students for 2 years, 2002 and 2003. Both Table 29.1 and 29.2 reveal data that indicate African Americans were among the highest number of probationary students.

During the meetings with probationary students and their parent(s), the first author inquired, "What happened to your academic performance in eighth grade?" Naturally, there were varied responses such as the following: "I played around"; "I knew I was in high school"; "I was not serious about my work"; and "I did not study." The students who were interviewed did not state that middle school academic work was difficult. With the exception of their eighth-grade marks, these students had A's, B's, and possibly a C in elementary and middle school grades as well as the required CHS standardized test scores.

Table 29.1	Incoming Students on Probation by Race, September 2002 ($N = 20$) and 2003 ($N = 7$)							
	African American		White		Hispanic		Asian	
Year	M	F	M	F	M	F	M	F
2002	8	4	3	0	0	2	3	0
2003	3	3	1	0	0	0	0	0

The first author informed both the student and parent that the ninth grader was entering CHS on probation based his or her performance in eighth grade. The primary purpose of the individual interviews was giving the student and parents a "pep talk." Most importantly, the tone was kept positive and encouraged the student to envision a personal reversal from lower performance in eighth grade to higher academic performance at CHS.

Introducing Peer Mentoring at CHS as Prevention and Intervention

The first author did not "blame the victim" or assume a deficit-oriented mind-set. Instead, a personal and professional commitment was made to help at-risk learners achieve their potential (Manning & Baruth, 1995). This reflected a deep personal commitment to the position that "No Child in the Class of 2007 was to be Left Behind." Moreover, the decision was made to implement a peer mentoring program at CHS as vital prevention and intervention, enjoying the support of the school administration.

Peer Mentoring Program Participants: At-Risk Ninth Graders

Ninth-grade students demonstrating failing performance during the first report period of the 2003–2004 school year were targeted for involvement in the peer mentoring project. The sample consisted of 137 ninth-grade students or 21.7% of the 632 students in the freshman class, including the 20 students who entered CHS on probation, 14 of whom demonstrated failing performance in the first marking period. Table 29.2 identifies by gender and ethnicity the 2003–2004 ninth-grade at-risk students who failed major subjects at the end of the first marking report period. African Americans were identified as having the highest percentages of failure at the end of the first report period.

During a second 45-minute orientation assembly meeting, the first author allowed mentees to ask questions about their prospective mentors and what their mentoring objectives were. The goals for the program were clearly laid out, focusing on students' receipt of the support and knowledge they needed to pass all their major subject areas.

Key Procedures: Implementing and Monitoring Interventions

To facilitate appropriate student engagement and more student learning the first author implemented interventions supported by research. Interventions included (a) the formal

Table 29.2	Ninth-Grade Students Failing During First Report 2003–2004 by Gender and Ethnicity									
	White		Afr. Am.		Asian		Hispanic		Am. Ind.	
Gender	No.	%	No.	%	No.	%	No.	%	No.	%
Male	22	16	31	23	8	6	10	7	1	1
Female	10	7	38	28	8	6	9	6	0	0

Note. Afr. Am. = African American; Am. Ind. = American Indian. $N = 137$ ninth-grade students.

assignment of peer mentors for incoming probationary ninth-grade students and ninth-grade students failing at the end of the first report card period; (b) ongoing formal and informal supervisory observations and recommended changes in instruction for teachers of ninth-grade teachers of major subjects; and (c) monitoring of student participation in the School District of Philadelphia (SDP) school-based after-hours support program entitled "credit recovery." Students attending the credit recovery school-based program can recover credits towards reversing their failing grade. However, a full discussion of all of these interventions is beyond the scope of this chapter, and only component (a), the peer mentoring program, will be focused upon in this context. Quantitative data on student failure in major subject areas and qualitative interview data (mentees, teachers, parents of mentees) will be presented and discussed in order to assess the impact of the peer mentoring program at CHS.

Data Collection Procedures: School Records

The chapter first author collected grade reports from the first through the fourth marking periods during the 2003–2004 school year. The principal was actively involved in the project, making records of grade reports for all marking periods available from the 2002–2003 school year, as well as across the 2003–2004 school year. This data was deemed vital for assessing the impact of instituting the peer mentoring program across the academic year 2003–2004.

Other Data Collection Procedures: Pre- and Post-Intervention Surveys/Guides

Together, the chapter authors created brief pre-intervention and post-intervention surveys for mentors and mentees, collecting self-report data. Beyond basic demographics, the survey asked student to respond to the following items: My strongest Major Subject areas are listed below along with my last grade . . . ; What type of student would you be most interested in mentoring? Please describe some of the characteristics you would most enjoy below (i.e., an athlete, orchestra member, etc. . . .); How do you rate the importance of initiating a new student peer-mentoring program for incoming freshmen?; How important is it to you that you receive some portion of your community service credit for serving as a peer mentor during the 2003–2004 academic year?; What extracurricular activities or athletics do you currently enjoy or anticipating joining?; From your perspective, what can a student mentor do to help an incoming freshman student?).

The pre-intervention surveys were distributed in early March 2004, after students returned parental informed consent and their own minor consent forms. The pre-intervention surveys guided the process of creating mentor–mentee pairs. Post-intervention surveys for mentors and mentees posed questions about what the students experienced during the mentoring period. This information was used to determine the quality of the mentoring relationships.

Interview Data Collection: Guiding Questions

Interview guides were also created, adding structure to face-to-face interviews conducted with selected ninth-grade students, their teachers, and parents, facilitating further assessment of the perception of at-risk students' needs and the impact of the peer mentoring intervention. The first author conducted interviews during the school advisory period, lunches, teacher prep periods, and after-school credit recovery program, while also interviewing parents by telephone.

Procedures for Selecting and Training Mentors

Of the 410 mentoring pre-intervention surveys distributed to upperclassmen, only 240 were returned for a 58% response rate. This may have reflected student's self-perceptions regarding their ability to serve as mentors. After selections were made by the first author as to who was qualified to serve as a peer mentor, based on the information students' submitted, a total of 142 upperclassmen (mentors) from grades 10, 11, and 12 eventually formally entered the CHS peer mentoring program—including 45 seniors, 60 juniors, and 37 sophomores.

The first author conducted a pre-intervention training in the auditorium for peer mentors. This training was held in the morning. One 45-minute orientation-training session was conducted with the potential peer mentors. Training included discussion of the goals and objectives of the program, time management, communication skills and methods, the role of the mentor, and support services intended (Redmond, 1990). A daily intervention of student-to-student peer mentoring centered on the provision of a successful student to help an at-risk student. Mentors were to help mentees consider school expectations for managing the high school workload, learning study skills, tutoring, test taking, and approaching assignments for a particular teacher or subject matter. Additionally mentors were to refer at-risk students to a counselor, the health office, an administrator, or a teacher to answer any more serious concerns.

Quite simply a peer mentor was expected to be a friend or student consultant who could provide a "safety net" so an at-risk student did not "fall through the cracks" or experience academic failure, while providing vital social support and collaboration during the learning process. Upperclassmen would receive 30 hours of community service by mentoring a ninth-grade student.

In addition to face-to-face interactions, the peer mentor was expected to seek to meet the needs of probationary and at-risk students through electronic mentoring, via the Internet through e-mail and/or text messaging—as daily communication between student and student mentor was deemed essential and anticipated to increase over time.

Other Key Procedures Involving Other School Resources

The other resources deemed necessary to implement the planned intervention of a peer mentoring program for at-risk ninth-grade students were the time and cooperation of students, faculty, and parent(s)/guardian(s). The peer mentoring intervention model was reviewed and approved by the principal of CHS. Prepared to change, the faculty at CHS recognized and accepted the need to improve instructional practices as addressed in NCLB recommendations. With this support, the actual implementation and evaluation for the peer mentoring program occurred across the 2003–2004 academic year.

Instituting the Structure of the Peer Mentoring Program: Time Line

From the third week in March 2004 through June 2004, the student mentors met their mentees approximately three times a week during a 35- or 45-minute morning advisory period. Mentors and their mentees met in one of three locations—the lunchroom, tutoring room, or library. During this time period, there were four student mentors who had been assigned to ninth-grade students who withdrew from the study. The mentors elected to remain in the program and participated as assistants to other peer mentors and mentees.

During the study period of March 2004 to June 2004, students committed approximately 105–135 minutes per week. Multiplied by 11 weeks, a total of approximately 19 to 25 hours were devoted by each mentor to the mentee from March to June. At the conclusion of the mentoring program, the first author provided all participants with a celebration at the school for their efforts and commitment to mentoring.

Evaluation of the Peer Mentoring Model

Study Hypothesis

It was hypothesized that the introduction of peer mentoring to identified at-risk students in ninth grade at CHS would result in a decrease in the rate at which students failed major subjects (i.e., below the passing grades of 65, or D)—when comparing ninth-grade students' grades in school year 2002–2003 and 2003–2004. In addition, it was hypothesized that the post-intervention survey data would indicate and further substantiate a positive impact from participation in the peer mentoring program.

Results of the Quantitative Evaluation Using School Records

Examining *second report period grades* served to provide a pre-intervention picture of the nature of ninth-grade failures—both the year before the peer mentoring intervention was put in place across the 2003–2004 academic year, and before any effect of the peer intervention might be expected to manifest; this was because, at the second report period, no peer mentoring activities had begun for the 2003–2004 academic school year. For ninth-grade students at second report in the school year 2002–2003, the mean number of subjects failed by students was 1.79 with a standard deviation of 1.02. And, for ninth-grade students at second report in the school year 2003–2004 the mean number of

| Table 29.3 | CHS Ninth-Grade Students Failing One to Five Major Subjects at Second Report in 2002–2003 and 2003–2004 |

	Number of Major Subjects Failed									
	1		2		3		4		5	
Year	No.	%	No.	%	No.	%	No.	%	No.	%
2002–2003 ($N = 628$)	98	15.6	49	7.8	25	4.0	13	2.1	3	<1
2003–2004 ($N = 632$)	74	11.7	63	10.0	20	3.2	7	1.1	3	<1

Note: In 2002–2003, there were 338 instances of major subject failure for 188 students; in 2003–2004, there were 303 instances of major subject failure for 167 students.

subjects failed by students was 1.81 with a standard deviation of 0.93. Most importantly, the total number of ninth-grade students who failed a major subject was 188 within a class of 628 in 2002–2003, and 167 within a class of 632 in 2003–2004. To put this pre-intervention data in further perspective, a two-proportion z-test of the number of students who failed major subjects at the *second report card period* in academic years 2002–2003 and 2003–2004 was performed. Results showed no significant difference ($z =$ 1.39, p-value $= .08$) in the proportion of students who failed at the *second report period* in academic years 2002–2003 and 2003–2004, suggesting a useful pre-intervention indicator. See Table 29.3.

However, to test the study hypothesis, the key comparison is between the 2002–2003 and 2003–2004 academic school year student failures for major subjects at the *fourth report card period*; this was deemed the best post-intervention indicator of any effects for the 2003–2004 academic year peer mentoring intervention. For ninth-grade students' failing at *fourth report card period* in 2002–2003, the mean number of subjects failed was 1.84 with a standard deviation of 1.24, while in 2003–2004, the mean was 2 with a standard deviation of 1.28. More specifically, the total number of students failing the *fourth report card period* was 147 students in a class of 619 (23.7%) in 2002–2003 versus 113 students in a class of 623 (18.1%) in 2003–2004. A two-proportion z-test of the number of students who failed major subjects at the *fourth report card period* in academic years 2002–2003 and 2003–2004 was performed to test the study hypothesis. Analysis produced a z-test statistic of $z = 2.37$ and a p-value of .008, achieving significance ($p < .01$), indicating a significantly smaller proportion of students failed major subjects in the 2003–2004 school year—the year of the peer mentoring intervention. As hypothesized, peer mentoring emerged as having an impact when comparing major subject failures across the two academic years for the *fourth report card period*. See Table 29.4.

Moreover, the greatest impact of peer mentoring was upon those most at risk. Most noteworthy were the failures in the major subject areas of science and math for African American male students, as shown in bold in Table 29.5 at the *fourth report card period* for academic years 2002–2003 and 2003–2004. At the 2002–2003 school *fourth report card period*, 24 (13%) African American males failed math, whereas in 2003–2004 15 (9%) African American males failed math. Similarly, at the 2002–2003 *fourth report card period*, 17 (9%) African American males failed science, while in the 2003–2004 school year 9 (5%) African American males failed science. See Table 29.5.

Table 29.4	CHS Ninth-Grade Students Who Failed One to Five Major Subjects at Fourth Report in 2002–2003 and 2003–2004									

	Number of Major Subjects Failed									
	1		2		3		4		5	
Year	No.	%	No.	%	No.	%	No.	%	No.	%
2002–2003 ($N = 619$)	87	14.1	28	4.5	10	1.6	13	2.1	9	1.5
2003–2004 ($N = 623$)	59	9.5	20	3.2	17	2.7	9	1.5	8	1.3

Note: In 2002–2003, there were 270 instances of major subject failure for 147 students; in 2003–2004, there were 226 instances of major subject failure for 113 students.

Results Using Post-Intervention Survey Data

The mentors' post-intervention survey data were also analyzed, ascertaining their perceptions of the mentoring experience. Limitations of these data include lack of detailed information on students' demographics, limiting data analysis. Furthermore, from among the 142 peer mentors, only 74 surveys were returned. Findings showed that mentors had provided the most academic support in the subject areas of math (67%) and science (45%). Also, 77% of the student mentor-mentee pairs met approximately two to three times a week during the advisory period. The majority of mentors (78%) rated their experiences of mentoring as valuable to very valuable, and 76% felt it was beneficial or very beneficial to the mentee—suggesting the mentoring experience as a positive, useful experience. Also noteworthy, only 35% felt it was extremely important or very

Table 29.5	Major Subject Failures of Ninth-Grade Students by Gender and Race/Ethnicity for the Fourth Report in 2002–2003 and 2003–2004															

	FW		FAA		FH		FA		MW		MAA		MH		MA	
Subject	N	%	N	%	N	%	N	%	N	%	N	%	N	%	N	%
English																
2002–2003	2	1.0	4	2.0	2	1.0	0	0.0	6	3.0	13	6.7	3	1.5	2	1.0
2003–2004	5	2.9	2	1.1	1	0.5	0	0.0	7	4.0	11	6.5	2	1.1	1	0.5
Social Studies																
2002–2003	2	1.0	9	4.6	2	1.0	0	0.0	4	2.0	8	4.0	1	0.5	3	1.5
2003–2004	7	4.0	10	5.9	2	1.1	1	0.5	5	2.9	9	5.3	1	0.5	0	0.0
Math																
2002–2003	10	5.2	15	7.8	5	2.6	3	1.5	9	4.7	24	12.5	5	2.6	4	2.0
2003–2004	10	6.5	18	10.7	2	1.1	1	0.5	12	7.1	15	8.9	3	1.7	3	1.7
Science																
2002–2003	5	2.6	13	6.7	3	1.5	3	1.5	8	4.1	17	8.8	4	2.0	4	2.0
2003–2004	6	3.5	9	5.3	3	1.7	2	1.1	5	2.9	9	5.3	3	1.7	2	1.1

Note: Data in 2002–2003 are for 147 students who failed 192 major subject courses. Data for 28 failing students on the specific major courses they failed were missing from office files. Data in 2003–2004 are for 113 students who failed 168 major subject courses. F = female; M = male; W = White; AA = African American; H = Hispanic; A = Asian.

important to receive credit for community service by mentoring. Finally, a majority of mentors (62%) gave the program an overall rating of excellent or very good.

Suggestions were obtained regarding how to improve the program via an open-ended question. Recurrent themes regarding weaknesses involved problems with attendance, time allotted, scheduling, and the need for more information from the teacher about the mentees' major subject performance—as mentors wanted to know if the mentee was actually learning the material the mentor was covering. Knowing such information would have influenced how the mentors addressed their mentees' achievement problems.

For mentees, out of the original 137 ninth graders, with 4 leaving the program, and a remaining possible 133 post-intervention surveys, only 76 surveys were returned. Mentees concurred with mentors, for the most part, that the subject areas of major focus were math (48%) and science (30%). Also, mentees (79%) met with their mentors two to three times a week during the advisory period, and 79% reporting having complied with attendance requirements. The majority of mentees (79%) indicated that the mentoring experience was valuable to very valuable for them. A majority rated (70%) the mentoring experience as helpful to very helpful, and felt that (75%) the mentoring program was very important to extremely important in helping them.

Furthermore, they believed the most important things their mentors did to help them were to (a) review their subject material; (b) enhance the mentees' skills in various ways; and (c) increase their knowledge. Also, an analysis of the open-ended question (Was there anything you feel you did not get from your mentor?), elicited the following sample comments: "She does not come much"; "Late at times"; "She didn't do anything"; "I needed more explanations from my mentor"; "More time and visits"; "More tutoring"; "I wanted to be pushed harder"; "More space and rooms available"; "A mentor that spoke the same language as I."

The post-intervention survey data served to reinforced findings from the analysis of the data for the fourth-period report card, indicating that math and science were the areas of greatest focus among the peer mentor–mentee pairs; and, consistent with this, as was shown in Table 29.5 African American males experienced the greatest impact from peer mentoring in the subject areas of math and science.

Results Using Qualitative Interview Data

Qualitative data were also available for data analysis, given interviews conducted with students, teachers, and parents. This data further compliments the body of quantitative findings discussed thus far.

Data From Student Interviews. The demographics of the at-risk students ($N = 34$) interviewed during the intervention were 12 White, 14 African American, 4 Asian, and 4 Hispanic students. The gender breakdown was 15 male and 19 female students. Pertinent and recurrent themes are presented here.

During interviews, students revealed low self-esteem, wanting to try harder, and a lack of engagement with their teachers in the classroom. The students made statements that "middle school was easier." Their top five common concerns had to do with the transition to CHS: they were coping with the change in the school environment (larger); doing more homework; having difficulty meeting standards at the new high school; felt they needed to study more; and, experienced the loss of personal authority and leadership roles.

Twenty-two students said their failure at CHS was their first. Two students responded that they ruined their parents' upcoming summer because they might have to go to summer school. Ten believed parents were disappointed with them. Three other students said that failing is "an embarrassment," "a shock," and that they "can't handle it." Ten students felt overwhelmed and intimidated by the workload, and two mentioned feelings of obligation to parents and family.

The majority ($n = 30$) of students said their performance could improve with studying more, staying focused in class, and learning how to take notes. Two students stated they "already studied hard" and that better time management was key to their improvement. One student expressed that his behavior "got in the way of performing well," as "I should have paid attention instead of focusing on other stuff." Another stated, "I'm trying my best, I can do no more."

Twenty-five mentees mentioned their mentors in a positive light. Specific comments included that the mentor was "very helpful," "always friendly," and "caring." "We e-mailed each other daily," was another comment included. Instant messaging on the Internet was also a popular form of communication, or "tele-mentoring" by cell or telephone. Explicitly mentioned was that "mentors were persons whom they could ask for help." Five students stated that their mentors gave advice on where else they could go for help (e.g., counselor, parent, teacher, or tutoring after school).

Seven students stated that asking for help did not bother them. Five students indicated that mothers were asked for help more than fathers. Fathers seemed not to be home frequently enough to ask for help. Four students mentioned "feeling good in class," when asking for help. One student commented, "Some students just sit there and don't ask. I ask." In contrast, another student commented, "I don't feel smart asking. I feel kind of stupid." "Awkward," "weird," and "shy" were other words used by students to describe their feelings about asking for help. Asking can be difficult, and as one student explained, "It depends on your level of comfort with the teacher and mentor."

Twelve students said that positive responses from the teacher helped them the most (i.e., the kind of contingencies Ross & Smalls discuss in chapter 26 as a function of teachers' engagement with students). When asked if teachers could do anything differently to promote more student achievement, most students initially took the blame themselves for not doing well. They explained failure as their own fault. Yet, when asked what teachers could do differently during instruction, one student responded that his teacher did not "break it down" and "he talks to the blackboard and paces too much." Ten students noted that their teachers just "keep on talking too fast. How can we keep up?" Another student responded with, "Teachers in middle school are more aware of their students and know what each person is capable of and try to meet their needs." Several students wanted the teacher to help the student pay more attention. Comments such as, "He loses me," "breezes through," and "maybe they could call on me sometimes" were frequent. Finally, two said, "Sometimes classes are too large. How can teachers help everyone?" In this manner, students seemed to be crying out for the experience of being engaged by teachers, even as they offered explanations for why this was lacking, yet still needed it.

Twenty-nine students were concerned that their middle school did not prepare them well. Never having to do homework in eighth grade was a predominate concern of students. Twelve students responded that they "did not study much" or "in middle school if you knew a little, you were smart." They said that they did not have to study much in their former schools. "Middle school was smaller, but the diversity of cultures here is nice," said another student. Ten students referred to the size of the school as a factor during their freshman year. One student intimated that sexuality becomes an issue in high school: "You may want a different type of personal relationship, and friends judge you based on your choice."

Twenty students mentioned new surroundings, adjusting to the size of their high school environment, and the schedule of the school as factors that they needed to overcome. Four mentioned the subjects of math and English, as well as reading many different types of literature, as obstacles. Three said "time management," "trying to please," and "troubles with friends and parents" were problematic. Five believed that not paying attention and apathetic behaviors (laziness, boredom, indifference) were their personal issues.

All students believed CHS was a friendly place, a friendly environment in which to socialize and make friends. One student stated, "There is every type of person here. You'll find someone to fit in with." Three students stated that, even though they were able to make friends, "a failing grade will keep you from joining CHS clubs." Five students indicated how their mentors made them feel welcomed.

All students were hopeful during the interview. Fifteen believed that, if they worked harder and, if necessary, they went to summer school, they could succeed at CHS. Seven believed that next year would be easier because they will know what to expect with the amount of required work. Four believed that taking summer courses and tutoring would help their performance next year. One student said, "I can't do what I did. . . . I did not work hard. However, you have to be motivated to motivate yourself." Another stated, "My Mom wanted me to go here. I wanted to go to another school." Finally a student openly shared, "I just want to come back and get a second chance."

These responses indicated that high school issues are complex, and the middle schools may not have adequately prepared students for the transition. Meanwhile, some students did indicate that their current teachers could help improve students' achievement.

Data From Teacher Interviews. Due to teacher time constraints, only 13 (52%) of 25 teachers who were also observed teaching by the first author (results of which are beyond the scope of this chapter) were interviewed during the study period. Four teachers of English, four teachers of Biology, three teachers of Algebra I, and two teachers of World History signed consent forms and agreed to an interview with the first author. Themes emerged as they expressed their feelings about students who failed major subjects.

Teachers' themes included noting how failing ninth-grade students often lacked study skills, had bad organizational skills, poor time management, and poor writing skills. Some teachers held the belief that some at-risk students simply did not belong there, while some did belong at CHS. Teachers stated that failing students did not do enough work, did not do homework, and were under-prepared for the high school curriculum.

With 27 years of experience teaching science and math, one teacher said that most at-risk students did not understand that this school is a college preparatory program and there was much studying needed to reach goals. He also said that at-risk students could learn content material, but had not mastered necessary analytical skills. He noted how students must learn to organize their materials, simplify, and state the required information.

Also, ninth graders often found the transition to CHS from their middle school to be overwhelming. He also noted that the biggest challenge to help low-performing students was to let them know they could do the work and to guide them towards what was needed for achievement. When asked about the effects teaching methodology had on at-risk students, the same teacher responded with, "The mode of instruction does affect teaching, yet teachers have to teach to the average population, and it is hard to reach those individuals failing, due to the large number of students." Thus, class size seemed to negatively impact the process of engaging students and providing positive reinforcement to students.

He continued by stating that sometimes using supplemental materials is helpful for failing students. Additionally, cooperative learning groups and differentiated materials can be beneficial instructional methods for at-risk students. This response indicated receptivity to help in improving student performance, perhaps through cooperative learning groups.

With 20 years of experience teaching English, another teacher said, "At-risk students have the capability to do well, but do not have the knowledge to manipulate the curriculum and compete with high achieving students." She continued by stating that the challenge lay in developing their willingness to put forth the commitment. At times, a student felt badly when he or she was unsuccessful, intimating a role for the low self-esteem of at-risk students. This teacher also believed that the mode of instruction affected at-risk students who had difficulty with a variety of teachers and lecture styles not commonly used in most middle schools: "Most ninth graders had been used to hands-on instruction," she explained.

Another English teacher said that most at-risk students have the basic skills to be in an academic school; "They just need more self-discipline, fine-tuning of skills, and personal attention." The teacher also said that at-risk students tend to have questionable social skills, both aggressive and attention getting, and the opposite, quiet and lonely. And, "At-risk students understand the importance of their education, but view what they are learning as 'stupid,' with topics of no innate sense of importance." This English teacher also said, "The mode of instruction affects at-risk students. The authoritarian style of teaching is not good for them. These students need cognitive reinforcement and more of the teachers asking, 'What can I do for you?'" Finally, this teacher said it is important for teachers to give at-risk students respect so they will respond to the teacher as an individual. The last perspective recognizes that instruction must be student-centered and related to meaningful activities that best engage students.

One history teacher believed the mode of instruction should be differentiated so all are engaged and that "they have the talent to do the work." This history teacher expressed, "Differentiated instruction would give all a chance to learn, using student centered activities, group work, and teacher-guided discussions." Another history teacher expressed that instruction does not have to be differentiated. "We do not group kids," and "I wanted to go to a higher level," and "Kids in the middle need challenging, too."

Three teachers mentioned peer mentoring as a source of support. However, one stated, "Failing African American males would benefit more from same-sex African American mentors." Other comments were as follows: "Some students lack confidence and are unsure of how to find help"; "There is a gap in writing and grammar for failing students"; "Most are African American males who don't perform well in class"; and "Maybe students were not asked to perform in middle school. Now they have to."

In sum, many of the interviewed teachers found that students needed to be more organized and study more, needed to put forth commitment, and that they lacked analytical skills. Further, the teachers found it hard to teach failing students due to large classes of 33 students that do not allow for the personalized attention these students required. They all seemed interested, however, in helping students achieve more. Parents were seen as a resource for helping the student when contacted early by the teacher.

Data From Parent Interviews. Twenty-seven parents returned informed consent forms and agreed to participate in a 10- to 15-minute telephone interview. However, due to parental time constraints, the first author was able to contact and interview only seven (26%) parents after many telephone calls, leaving messages, and having only some parents respond. Recurrent themes emerged and are reported here.

Sample recurrent themes emerging from these parent interviews involved parents commenting on how their children had "inconsistent study habits and skills," were coping with the "challenges of high school," and "the heavier school workload." While describing their ninth graders, parents' specific opinions were quite revealing. One parent observed, "She came from a small school and immediately found more freedom." Another parent stated, "It was like she was a deer in the headlights." A third parent asked, "What do we do when you have a child who does not have the skills?" One parent admitted, "I felt helpless." Another parent witnessed how "trying to keep up with projects, due dates, and the amount of homework was challenging for him." Two parents admitted that not much time was spent on homework, or it was a rushed effort. One parent thought her child was being responsible in the way he studied and did all homework. All seven parents believed the average amount of time their children spent doing homework was 2 hours per school night. One parent explained, "More time for homework was needed, but he had after-school responsibilities, too." Four parents said their children's mentors were very helpful with homework.

All seven parents believed their children had academic strengths in middle school. However, their prominent strengths were replaced by more prominent weaknesses during the CHS ninth-grade year. One parent shared this about her child: "I think he could have done a lot better. He sings, draws, and plays the flute. He wants to apply himself better, and he understands education is the key." All seven parents intimated the first ninth-grade year in high school constituted a lesson learned. One said, "There is nowhere to go but up. Now is the time to become responsible to do the things to move forward."

In this manner, students, teachers, and parents emerge as having given honest responses as part of this study.

Discussion

The findings in this study are consistent with those of prior researchers. For example, research by Steinberg, Dornbusch, and Brown (1992) showed that academic support and social guidance, especially among African American males, are essential for at-risk students to reverse failure and become successful. They believed students who receive both parental and peer academic support are more likely to have academic success. Bronfenbrenner (1979) believed moving to a new school was an "ecological transition" that encompassed changes in setting and roles. He saw the high school student face multiple challenges of a new physical environment, new teachers, and different expectations with new peers. Supporting students in transition to high school was essential for success. This study adds to the body of literature making these essential points.

If Central High School is "the place where prominent leaders of tomorrow are trained and memories of yesterday are taught" (CHS 2003 *Central Yearbook*, 2003, p. 262), then for at-risk African American ninth graders there is also the risk of accumulating painful memories of personal failure—perhaps for the first time in their life. In this manner, this study's findings support those of Roderick (2003) who found that African American male students begin to lag behind their female peers across the transition from eighth to ninth grade. The findings add to a body of research underscoring how African American males may face the greatest risk of failing in our nation's schools. However, in the evaluation presented in this chapter, those at greatest risk also emerged as the greatest beneficiaries of peer mentoring, especially in the subject areas of math and science.

Toward the goal of further reducing the risk faced by all, this chapter presented in detail an evidence-based approach to reducing disparities in academic achievement, even as the study presented was only a suggestive pilot with many limitations. Limitations involved the mentoring program possibly being compromised by students leaving the study period early or not attending scheduled sessions. Other limitations involved the decision to compare students across two different school years (2002–2003 and 2003–2004) to ascertain the impact of the mentoring program across the 2003–2004 academic school year—a common methodology but not necessarily the ideal one to discern effects of the mentoring intervention. Another limitation involves the relatively small number of participants in the actual mentoring program. Also, there was no random assignment of students to the mentoring intervention. This limits the extent to which the study findings can be generalized to students other than those similar to or actually attending CHS. Moreover, CHS is a unique public school and college preparatory high school, enjoying a long legacy, alumni support, and an endowment, further limiting the extent to which findings may generalize.

Also, the mentoring intervention did not begin early in the school year. Mentoring was not begun in response to the very first signs that a student was at-risk for failing a major subject, such as a failing or poor grade on their first assignments, homework, or tests in the very first weeks of the school year. Instead, only after ninth graders had already failed major subjects in earlier report card periods did peer mentoring begin for them during the third and fourth report card periods.

Given these limitations, the post-intervention survey data were seen as important in further ascertaining the impact of the peer mentoring program. However, these surveys lacked detailed demographic data, also limiting data analysis.

The strength of the study is that it occurred in the real world context of a school, suggesting how others might adapt the model to their real world school environments and how research in such complex settings can produce meaningful findings that are likely to be relevant to others working in the real world. Another strength of the study involved the selected interviews with students, parents, and teachers; these were viewed as important sources of qualitative data, helping to determine the impact of the peer mentoring program, and perceptions of the characteristics and needs of failing ninth-grade students. This qualitative data was seen as rich, and further augmenting the quantitative data—even though there were limitations here, too, given obstacles to greater participation in the interviews experienced by mentees, their teachers, and parents.

What emerges from this body of data is the manner in which peer mentoring programs may potentially play a valuable role in helping to close the academic achievement gap, especially as it is experienced by African American males, and with regard to their math and science achievement, in particular.

Of note, a full discussion of the observational data collected when the first author observed the classroom instruction of 25 teachers of at-risk ninth graders, and how interventions were done with teachers, was deemed beyond the scope of this chapter. However, it is vital for school leadership to address teacher attitudes, expectations, and instructional practices. For these may be found to be detrimental to student achievement—including teacher failure to engage at-risk students. Ross and Smalls (chapter 26, this volume) underscored the importance of teachers engaging students, while the comments of students interviewed in this chapter also points toward critical failures to engage students. It is vital that the professional development of teachers include a focus on their becoming competent at academic engagement, consistent with Ross and Smalls highlighting the experience of multiple academic interactions between teachers and students, including how: (1) a teacher's direction or question is followed by a brief pause; (2) there is a student response to the teacher's question; and (3) an immediate consequence given by the teacher that is contingent upon the way the student responded (praise for a correct response, and a correction for an incorrect response)—that is, the delivery of a "learn unit" to use the term deployed by Ross and Smalls. If teachers engage students using this evidence-based approach, then they will be delivering the kind of engagement the students in this study asked for in their interviews. Thus, we concur with the conclusion of Ross and Smalls that "the crisis of low academic achievement for millions of poor and low-income students requires instructional expertise from those who work most closely with them—teachers."

We would also add a role for diversity training. For, also pertinent is how teachers may possibly view at-risk students or members of a diverse student body. As Ross and Smalls noted in chapter 26, "teachers come to classrooms with their own set of responses to students that they may have used for years. If these responses are not unambiguous antecedents, praise for correct responses, and corrections for incorrect responses, then changing them can require practice." Undesirable responses may include the kind of negative views of students held by teachers, as Roderick (2003) noted, specifically in regard to African American male students. It is the responsibility of school administrators to identify all high school teachers in need of interventions, including those needing diversity training coupled with training in how to academically engage all students in an equitable manner. Differential reinforcement of student behavior in the classroom by race and gender is not acceptable. School administers may need to provide and/or direct teachers to attend professional development to strengthen not only instructional practices, but also to change deficit-oriented mind-sets among teachers and staff. Instead of perceiving and focusing upon student deficits, or holding negative views of certain students based on race or gender, an approach that values diversity and seeks to see and positively reinforce student strengths is vitally needed on the part of teachers. It is the responsibility of school leaders, administrators, and principals to ensure that their teaching staff receives the training needed so all shift to a new paradigm—one that holds the potential to bring about educational equity for all.

Conclusion

It is at the level of the individual school administrator, or principal, that we can invest the greatest hope for the establishment and success of prevention and intervention strategies for at-risk youth. The school leader can set the tone and provide positive, passionate, dynamic, caring, multiculturally sensitive leadership that seeks to ensure that no child is left behind, while creating and sustaining the school culture consistent with this stance, and insisting that teachers are trained to effectively engage with students.

Toward the fulfillment of the vision of principals providing such leadership, this chapter has provided principals (and other school leaders) with an evidence-based model for ensuring no child is left behind. While the evidence is based on a pilot and is only suggestive, given the limitations of the study, the chapter serves to point school leaders toward a viable means of prevention and intervention. Ideally, principals will respond by drawing upon those agents internal to the school setting, enlisting high-achieving peers and allowing them to receive credit for community service in exchange for mentoring their at-risk peers. High-achieving peers emerge through this study as invaluable resources that can be brought to bear to ensure that no child is left behind at the critical junction of ninth grade in a new high school setting—as they, too, can meaningfully engage with their peers and both role model and reinforce behaviors consistent with academic achievement. Meanwhile, the instructional and professional development needs of teachers are not to be ignored, nor are the responsibilities of parents.

Finally, this chapter serves as an invitation to others to embrace the challenge which the chapter first author now faces: to replicate and establish a successful peer mentoring program in a setting that lacks the legacy, alumni, and funding of a CHS. The first author is now the first Principal of the Academy at Palumbo, in Philadelphia in the first year of this school's existence, having only a ninth-grade class and small group of teachers; each year a new class will be added so we become a fully functioning high school with all grades. Perhaps by virtue of implementing much of what is stressed in this chapter, the first class enjoyed a 100% promotion (to 10th grade) rate. No child was left behind in this academic preparatory high school.

However, this chapter's message is also directed toward those who may be in urban schools plagued by violence and other social ills. Today, all too often, school violence spills over into surrounding communities, and community violence spills over into schools. This is commonplace, with both students and teachers being assaulted on a regular basis by violent students. However, despite this disturbing contemporary reality, the first step toward a solution may start with a vision. This chapter offers a vision for all schools—one where diversity is accepted, respected, and expressed, while all agree to focus on a common goal: achieving educational equity for all so no child is left behind. This also means the equitable engagement of all students by all teachers. From such a vision, a mission follows that must unfold step by step through collaborative partnerships among all parties involved in the school setting. One highly recommended step is the establishment of peer mentoring programs. Through this chapter, peer mentoring emerges as an invaluable tool, allowing us to benefit from readily available resources internal to our varied, diverse school settings and cultures, while allowing mentors/students to engage in community service.

REFERENCES

Avery, P. (1999). Authentic assessment and instruction. *Social Education, 63*(6), 368–373.

Barton-Arwood, S., Jolivette, K., & Massey, N. G. (2002). Mentoring with elementary age students. *Intervention in School and Clinic, 36*(1), 36–39.

Bisland, A. (2001). Mentoring: An educational alternative for gifted students. *Gifted Child Today, 24*(4), 22–25.

Bronfenbrenner, U. (1979). *The ecology of human development: Experiments by nature and design.* Cambridge, MA: Harvard University Press.

Burgsthaler, S., & Cronheim, D. (2001). Supporting peer-peer and mentor-protégé relationships on the Internet. *Journal of Research on Technology in Education, 34*, 56–72.

Central High School. (2003). *Central yearbook.* Philadelphia: Author.

Cooper, J. E., Ponder, G., Merrit, S., & Matthews, C. (2005). High-performing high schools: Patterns of success. *NASSP Bulletin, 89*(645), 2–23.

Darling-Hammond, L. (1999). Educating teachers for the next century: Rethinking practice and policy. In G. Griffin (Ed.), *The education of teachers: Ninety-eighth yearbook of the National Society for the Study of Education* (Part I). Chicago: University of Chicago Press.

DuBois, D. L., Halloway, B. E., Valentine, J. C., & Harris, C. (2002). Effectiveness of mentoring programs for youth: A meta-analytic review. *American Journal of Community Psychology, 30*(2), 157–198.

Gardiner, M. E., & Enomoto, E. G. (2006). Urban school principals and their role as multicultural leaders. *Urban Education, 41*(6), 560–584.

Harris, J., & Jones, G. (1999). A descriptive study of telementoring among students, subject matter experts, and teachers: Message flow and function patterns. *Journal of Research on Computing in Education, 32*, 36–53.

Hoyle, J. R., & Collier, V. (2006). Urban CEO superintendents' alternative strategies in reducing school dropouts. *Education and Urban Society, 39*(1), 69–90.

Kaplan, L. S., & Owings, W. A. (2001). Personalizing learning to prevent failure. *Principal Leadership, 1*(8), 42–47.

Manning, M., & Baruth, L. G. (1995). *Students at risk.* Boston: Allyn and Bacon.

Manning, M. L., & Baruth, L. G. (1996). Learners at risk: Three issues for educators. *The Clearing House, 69*, 239–241.

Montecel, M. R., Cortez, J. D., & Cortez, A. (2004). Dropout-prevention programs: Right intent, wrong focus, and some suggestions on where to go from here. *Education and Urban Society, 36*(2), 169–188.

Office of Vocational and Adult Education. (2003). *No Child Left Behind and high schools.* Retrieved July 18, 2003, from http://www.ed.gov/nclb/overview/introduction/guide

Perez, S., & Dorman, S. M. (2001). Enhancing youth achievement through telementoring. *Journal of School Health, 71*(3), 122–123.

Redmond, S. P. (1990). Mentoring and cultural diversity in academic settings. *American, Behavioral Scientist, 34*(2), 188–200.

Reiser, E., Petry, C., & Amitag, M. (1989). *A review of programs involving college students as tutors or mentors in grades K-12.* Washington, DC: Policy Studies Associates.

Richman, J. M., Rosenfeld, L. B., & Bowen, G. L. (1998). G.I. social support for adolescents at risk of school failure. *Social Work, 43*, 309–321.

Roderick, M. (2003). What's happening to the boys? Early high school experiences and school outcomes among African American male adolescents in Chicago. *Urban Education, 38*(5), 538–607.

Roderick, M., & Camburn, E. (1999). Risk and recovery from course failure in early years of high school. *American Educational Journal, 36*, 303–343.

Slavin, R. E. (1989). Students at risk of school failure: The problem and its dimensions. In R. E. Slavin, N. L. Karweit, & N. A. Madden (Eds.), *Effective programs for students at risk.* Needham Heights, MA: Allyn and Bacon.

Stader, D., & Gagnepain, F. G. (2000). Mentoring: The power of peers. *American Secondary Education*, *28*(3), 28–32.

Steinberg, L., Dornbusch, S. M., & Brown, B. B. (1992). Ethnic differences in adolescent achievement: An ecological perspective. *American Psychologist*, *47*(6), 723–729.

Swap, W., Leonard, D., Shields, M., & Abrams, L. (2001). Using mentoring and storytelling to transfer knowledge in the workplace. *Journal of Management Information*, *18*(1), 93–114.

Thompson, G., Warren, S., & Carter, L. (2004). It's not my fault: Predicting high school teachers who blame parents and students for low achievement. *The High School Journal*, *87*(3), 5–15.

Windschitl, M. (2002). Framing constructivism in practice as negotiation of dilemmas: An analysis of the conceptual, pedagogical, cultural and political challenges facing teachers. *Review of Educational Research*, *72*, 131–175.

Ybarra, S., & Hollingsworth, J. (2001). Increasing classroom productivity. *Leadership*, *31*(1), 34–35.

A Model for Comprehensive Community-Wide Asthma Education Using Partnerships and the Public School Curriculum

Betty Perez-Rivera
and Natalie Langston-Davis

Introduction

Approximately 20 million people in the United States have asthma; including 9 million children (American Academy of Allergy, Asthma and Immunology, 2006). This disease is associated with a significant degree of morbidity and mortality. Asthma is the cause of 5,000 deaths annually in this country (American Lung Association, 2005). It is the most common chronic disease among children and in 2003 resulted in 12.8 million missed school days (American Lung Association). During the same year there were 24.5 million workdays lost for adults secondary to asthma (American Lung Association).

Although the prevalence of asthma has stabilized in recent years it continues to have an essential impact on American health care expenditures. According to estimates from the American Lung Association there are 16.1 billion dollars of health care costs attributed to asthma each year (American Lung Association, 2005). Asthma was the primary diagnosis for 12.7 million physician office visits in 2002 and 1.9 million emergency room visits (American Lung Association).

The statistics are even more striking when racial differences are examined. The 2003 prevalence of asthma was 39% higher in the African American population than the Caucasian population (American Lung Association, 2005). Mortality from asthma among African Americans (3.4 per 100,000) was three times the rate in the Caucasian population (1.2 per 100,000); African American females had the highest mortality rate (3.4 per 100,000) (American Lung Association). The mortality rate of Latino-Americans was similar to the mortality rate of Caucasian Americans (1.3 per 100,000) (American Lung Association). During the period between 1997 and 1998 African American children had asthma mortality rates 4.6 times higher than both Caucasian and Latino children (Akinbami & Schoendorf, 2002).

Multiple factors have been suggested to explain the disparity in asthma prevalence and morbidity between the African American and Caucasian populations. However, the single factor that may confound the effect of all the others is economic disadvantage. Nationwide, 33% of African American children, 28% of Latino children, 10% of Asian children and 10.5% of Caucasian children live in poverty (National Center for Children in Poverty, 2005). In 2003 the Children's Defense Fund reported that almost 1 million African American children in the United States lived in extreme poverty with an after-tax income of less than one-half the federal poverty line. Thus, many African American children with asthma and their families are coping with the reality of a chronic disease within a foundation of true financial adversity.

The most basic health consequence of poverty is the absolute negative impact on access to medical care. In fact, the typical cofactors of child poverty, such as parental unemployment and low parental education, produce a compound destructive effect on a child's overall health status (Bauman, Silver, & Stein, 2006). Without consistent access to a primary care provider, asthmatic patients will rely on the acute care they are able to receive in the emergency department. A dependence on emergency management of asthma completely counteracts the continuous and quality care that is required to ensure successful treatment of the asthmatic patient's condition.

During primary care visits, health care providers are able to review the components of successful asthma management with the patient, such as peak flow monitoring and review of the asthma action plan (Lieu et al., 1997). Lack of access to quality health care is a distinct barrier to successful asthma management for millions of impoverished children.

While it is true that poverty may act as an obstacle to adequate asthma care and management, it is not likely the sole barrier. There are sub-factors present that are equally as damaging to the goal of effective asthma care. These additional factors are typically a consequence of the impoverished life but are more rapidly amenable to change and instruction once they are recognized.

The National Institutes of Health's National Heart, Lung, and Blood Institute (NHLBI) has long emphasized the need for patient education, realizing the importance of education to the improvement of clinical outcomes. Studies have shown that asthma education can have a significant impact on hospitalization rates, productivity, school days and workdays lost, and improvement in the patient's overall quality of life (Peterson, Strommer-Pace, & Dayton, 2001).

Growing concern for the high prevalence of asthma led NHLBI to increase their emphasis on asthma education, resulting in the creation of the National Asthma Education and Prevention Program (NAEPP). This program was created to help patients gain a better understanding of the impact of asthma and to enhance their ability to control the disease through active self-management (American Lung Association, 2005). "The NAEPP is a multidisciplinary coalition of private sector and governmental groups, co-ordinated by the National Heart, Lung, and Blood Institute (NHLBI) of the National Institutes of Health. It seeks to reduce asthma-related illness and death and to enhance the quality of life of asthma patients" (National Institutes of Health, 1997). Asthma education programs have been designed to help improve clinical outcomes for the asthma patients, many of them taking place within the clinical setting (Liu & Feekery, 2001).

An ideal setting for the identification of barriers for adequate asthma care lies at the interface of the provider and the patient. Providers sometimes struggle to get the message of asthma management across to the patients and their families. While communication between provider and patient is paramount for the proper management of asthma, time constraints during a clinical visit can limit the provider's ability to answer questions and clarify misconceptions about asthma.

Studies evaluating a number of clinical sites and their ability to provide comprehensive asthma education for the patients show that while a large number of providers advocate for increased patient education, many are unable to provide the necessary information. For example, a lack of financial compensation for patient education has been reported as a contributing factor in the decreased levels of patient and family education (Peterson et al., 2001). There are limitations to the therapeutic alliance as it relates to asthma care and the things that can be done to make asthma education more effective and constructive for both provider and patient.

Community education may be the next logical course of action. Community education about asthma may take place in medical clinic settings, schools, and other community settings via outreach. The resulting comprehensive approach to providing community-wide asthma education may also need to utilize educational programs that are interactive.

A study by Liu and Feekery (2001) indicates that while most methods of asthma education can have positive outcomes, the interactive educational programs have had the best results. Interactive programs are more conducive to learning and provide patients and their families with more opportunities to ask questions and gain a better understanding about asthma (Liu & Feekery, 2001). The authors further state that face-to-face interactive programs are most effective for short-term as well as for long-term retention of information, helping patients by changing attitudes and behaviors in conjunction with decreasing asthma severity, asthma morbidity scores, and patient and caregiver anxiety.

Given this background and introduction, The Children's Health Fund's Childhood Asthma Initiative (CAI) targets two subgroups within New York City's medically-indigent population—homeless families served by the New York Children's Health Project (NYCHP) and residents of low-income housing utilizing the South Bronx Health Center for Children and Families (SBHCCF), a Community Pediatrics Program of the Children's Hospital at Montefiore Medical Center. Within the context of the work being done by the CAI, this chapter will (1) present pertinent historical background on the CHF and details on the partnerships allowing the work of the CAI to go forth, both at the SBHCCF and the NYCHP; (2) offer three case studies of asthmatic patients and their parents that highlight the contemporary asthma education challenge; (3) describe the work of the CAI and our models of interactive community asthma education; (4) introduce the CAI model for integrating asthma education into the public school literacy and science curriculums; and (5) offer emergent principles and recommendations for others to follow for creating a comprehensive community-wide health education initiative. Overall, what is introduced through this chapter is an innovative model of interactive comprehensive community-wide health education focused on increasing asthma awareness via partnerships, community collaborations, and the public school curriculum.

Pertinent Historical Background: The Role of Partnerships and Collaborations

The Children's Health Fund (CHF) was cofounded in 1987 through a partnership between singer/songwriter Paul Simon and pediatrician/child advocate Irwin Redlener, MD—largely in response to a crisis in New York City where 9,400 children were living in homeless shelters and welfare hotels around the city. The core of what CHF does is to "partner" with major academic medical centers to address the kinds of crises to which Paul Simon and Dr. Redlener originally responded in founding the organization. Advocating for the creation of policies and public programs that will benefit the health care of children in need is another core function of CHF. Evolving into a national network, the CHF is committed to providing health care to the nation's most medically underserved children through the development of innovative pediatric programs and guaranteed access to high quality health care. There are currently 19 programs in the CHF's National Network—extending from inner-city areas such as Los Angeles and Chicago, to small towns in West Virginia and the Mississippi Delta, to what is considered their flagship sites in New York City. Starting in 1987, the focus in New York City was to ensure that very vulnerable children received comprehensive, consistent, quality health care. The result has been the establishment of models deemed suitable for both urban and rural areas across the country. Often the provision of this quality care includes making it available to at-risk children and adolescents via mobile medical units, fixed-site clinics, and school-based sites. To date, more than one million health care visits to at-risk children and families in rural and urban areas have been completed.

Consistent with the value placed upon partnerships and collaborations in addressing disparities in health (see Hayes, chapter 13, and Kwong, Ho-Asjoe, Chung, & Wong, chapter 14, this volume), the CHF partners with New York's Montefiore Medical Center in order to deliver both ongoing and new programs, serving approximately 10,000 disadvantaged or at-risk children and their families annually. Through CHF's flagship programs at the South Bronx Health Center for Children and Families (SBHCCF), considered the "medical home" for the South Bronx community and the New York Children's Health Project (NYCHP), the Childhood Asthma Initiative is able to reach the most medically under-served populations in low-income housing or one of New York City's family homeless shelters, providing services regardless of their ability to pay or immigration status. These services fill the needs of an at-risk community, one where, historically, there were inadequate community health resources. CHF is now celebrating its 20th year of providing services to the most at-risk medically underserved populations.

Among the New York-based programs and services that the CHF has evolved and currently provides, the Childhood Asthma Initiative (CAI) is considered its largest special initiative born out of partnerships and consistent with new guidelines issued in 1997 on asthma management (National Institutes of Health, 1997). The CHF launched the CAI in December 1997 to empower families to successfully manage childhood asthma. The CHF's CAI responds to patient needs and the challenges identified by providers and educators within the South Bronx community. However, as we shall see later in this chapter, partnerships and collaborations with community leaders, public schools, and the teachers delivering standard curriculum—and willing to adapt and enhance the curriculum to include asthma education—are also key.

Understanding the comprehensive needs of asthma patients and their families is crucial to developing educational programs for families. The CHF is committed to providing such services for families. With this in mind, the CAI was specifically created. This initiative is a comprehensive, multidisciplinary model that consists of four integrated components: (1) quality clinical care for asthma patients; (2) community and provider education regarding asthma diagnosis, treatment, and prevention; (3) the delivery of psychosocial services; and (4) evaluation for enhancement of programs and quality assurance. The aim of these components is to reduce the medical, educational, and psychological risk factors for this chronic disease.

In compliance with NHLBI guidelines (National Institutes of Health, 1997), a main focus of CAI's educational component is to provide hands-on, interactive workshops for children, parents, teachers and health care and childcare providers—fostering an asthma-friendly community through community education in the South Bronx. Innovative educational programs have been created to address issues of health literacy, the patient's and the family's lack of confidence in communicating problems to the provider, and the ability of the patients and their families to take control of asthma through effective management of their environmental triggers. Our interactive educational workshops engage patients in dialogue and pertinent hands-on interactive educational activities, while providing a supportive and informational session that emphasizes the importance of active self-management. The workshops enhance understanding about the characteristics, symptoms, environmental triggers, and medications for asthma. The CAI has made substantial progress towards creating an asthma-friendly community by reaching nearly 4,000 people through asthma education and outreach to schools, community organizations, and public housing facilities (2003–2005). Schools, community organizations, and public housing facilities emerge as essential partners in implementing a community-wide health education model for increasing asthma awareness.

The CAI team is rooted in collaborative workshop relationships among members of a transdisciplinary team—which includes a pediatrician, a doctor of education specializing in health and behavior, a research specialist, and various other health professionals. The team has developed a number of curricula that are highly replicable and suitable for a variety of audiences, venues, and time restrictions. An important component of these community activities involves educating families about the importance of having a primary care provider, how and when to access health care, and the availability of fixed-site primary care and asthma care at the SBHCCF and at the New York Children's Health Project via mobile medical units.

Through the work of the CAI, outreach and interventions with families include active encouragement to speak with medical providers about asthma and to follow instructions related to asthma medications. The educational programs serve to increase awareness about the impact of asthma in medically-underserved communities of the South Bronx, as well as empower families to take control of asthma through active management of their environmental triggers. Families and parents may be the most important partners who are essential to ensuring the implementation of appropriate asthma management for the benefit of their children.

The CAI also conducts outreach to elected officials and community leaders as well as collaborates with several organizations to further disseminate information about asthma, thus encouraging community leaders to play an active role in enhancing community understanding through an increase in educational programs. Thus, partnerships that are vital to a community-wide health education program, such as one focusing on increasing asthma awareness, includes those with elected officials and community leaders.

Illustrative Case Examples

Three cases are provided in order to illustrate the contemporary asthma education challenge that exists in the South Bronx. The cases reveal some of the misconceptions about asthma, highlighting the importance of providing asthma education. Within the cases (italicized), all of the names and other key identifying data have been changed to protect the privacy of the patients and their families. Each case is followed by commentary (non-italicized), highlighting key emergent issues.

Case Study #1

Angelica Morales and her mother Gail are waiting for Angelica's pediatrician in the clinic's waiting area. Ms. Morales is in the middle of chastising her daughter as Dr. Johnson walks in. Dr. Johnson overhears Ms. Morales saying, "I should never have allowed you to go to that camp." Ms. Morales appears extremely upset, while Angelica sits quietly and withdrawn on the examination table. Angelica, a chubby and pleasant 10-year-old, is breathing very deeply and has audible nasal congestion. Dr. Johnson proceeds to examine Angelica and finds that she has diffuse wheezing in all of her lung fields. Angelica is started on a nebulizer treatment while Dr. Johnson talks to Ms. Morales about what happened to bring Angelica to the clinic that afternoon. Ms. Morales states that Angelica was playing with the other children at her day camp earlier that day when she "started to have an asthma attack." Ms. Morales begins to explain that she never wanted Angelica to go to the camp but her daughter begged her to be able to play with the other children. Ms. Morales goes on to say that, "Angelica doesn't understand that she is not like other children because she has asthma" and she has to be "extra careful." Ms. Morales asks Dr. Johnson if she will be able to stop Angelica's asthma attack and she vows that she will keep Angelica at home for the rest of the summer "so her asthma won't act up."

Not many diseases are able to produce the level of anxiety and uncertainty that asthma can. Even the manner in which an acute exacerbation of asthma is spoken about reveals much about the general trepidation surrounding this disease. Asthma is said to "attack," immediately invoking an image of the asthma patient being overcome by a formidable and unconquerable opponent. There is a certain element of validity to the apprehension attributed to asthma. A severe asthma exacerbation may literally take the breath away. However, it is possible to control asthma; but parents tend to focus on the relatively short-term period of asthma exacerbation rather than the possibility of asthma control—taking a passive and reactive role in their child's health.

Ms. Morales exhibits a prominent health belief held by many of the patients and parents seen by the CAI. Parents often express an unwillingness to let their children participate in sports and other activities for fear that this will bring on an asthma attack. In many instances this is done despite the presence of other conditions, such as obesity, that would benefit from physical activity. Consequently, the children are bereft of the opportunity to interact with their peers and may suffer consequences such as social stigmatization and impairment in quality of life (Merikallio, Mustalahti, Remes, Valovirta, & Kaila, 2005). For fear of causing the patient harm, parents fall victim to their own beliefs, often exhibiting a sort of learned helplessness when it comes to their child's health. Patients and caregivers must consistently be given the positive message that asthma control is possible, in order to combat the widespread, negative belief that there is nothing that can be done to ward off an asthma attack.

There are medications that help to control the symptoms of persistent asthma so that these children are able to participate in activities in the same manner as other children without asthma. The asthma pump is very well known as a rescue medication during acute episodes; however, the other available asthma control medications are not given an equal-value position in the asthmatic patient's daily management. It is clear that the message must be changed in order for patients and their families to fully understand that it is possible for asthma to be controlled and the asthma patient does not have to be subject to the whim and capriciousness of the dreaded "asthma attack."

Case Study #2

Dennis Roberts is a 16-year-old boy coming for an initial visit to the clinic. He and his parents, along with his 4-year-old brother have been living in a shelter in the Bronx for the past 15 months. Dennis came to the shelter clinic today for an employment clearance letter for a summer job he will start next month. Dennis has not had a clinic visit with his own primary care doctor since entering the shelter.

Dennis is accompanied by his father for the visit. Both father and son are smiling and talking playfully as Dr. Rosado enters the room. Dennis says that he needs to get his employment letter back today so he can be sure to start his job on time. Dr. Rosado states that he will have to ask some questions and perform a physical examination before he can fill out the form. He begins by asking Dennis and his father if Dennis has any current or past medical problems. Mr. Roberts' initial reply is, "No," but he quickly adds, "Well, he does have asthma, but it's not the chronic type."

Dr. Rosado explains that asthma is a chronic disease and needs regular monitoring by a health care provider. Dr. Rosado asks about current medications. Dennis says that he is on an asthma pump and some other medicine called "Pulmicort"; he says that this medication is also a pump but he "hardly ever takes it." Mr. Roberts add that he does not want his son taking "all of that medicine with too many side effects."

When asked how often he has daytime and nighttime symptoms, Dennis says he is not bothered by his asthma in the night and he only gets his asthma during the day when he walks up the stairs at school and when he plays baseball with his team after school 4 days out of the week. He also has symptoms on "really hot days." In those cases he will use his pump if he remembered to bring it. Mr. Roberts nods in agreement at his child's responses.

In order for the provider–patient relationship to be effective it is essential for the provider to identify and discuss the patient's own understanding of his condition. Many asthmatic patients and their families do not perceive asthma as an ongoing condition. It is believed that asthma is something that "comes and goes" and needs to be treated only when there is a problem. Medications that are meant to control asthma symptoms, like Pulmicort, are not used because they are viewed as unnecessary.

Some patients refuse to take inhaled corticosteroid medications (i.e., Pulmicort, Aerobid, Flovent, Flovent Rotadisk, Asmanex Twisthaler, Asmacort) because they perceive the potential side effects as more risky than their actual asthma symptoms (Boulet, 1998). Often the patient's concept of their condition is influenced by their culture's perception of illness and disease (Flores, 2002).

Case Study #3

Joyce Vega is returning today for a follow-up checkup for her 2½-year-old son, Manuel. Manuel was diagnosed with mild persistent asthma a couple of months ago. In the short period since his diagnosis, Manuel has had four visits to the emergency room. During the last emergency room visit Manuel was hospitalized for 2 days. The ER physicians and residents that took care of Manuel all noted the same observation—Ms. Vega did not have any of the medications prescribed for Manuel. In fact she did not seem to know the names of the medications. The doctor had prescribed a bronchodilator (serving to relax the muscles around the airways during an asthma attack, such as Albuterol, Alupent, Atrovent, Brethine, Ipatroprium, Metaproteronol, Metaprel, Proventil, Salbutamol, Terbutaline, Theophylline, Theodur, Ventolin), and a controller medication (such as the inhaled corticosteroids, whether AeroBid, Azmacort, Beclovent, Flovent, Pulmicort, Vanceril) for Manuel during his last visit; however, it was no surprise to Dr. Martin, the pediatrician, that Manuel's mother was so forgetful. During most of their clinic visits, Ms. Vega could readily be described as very distracted—as she seems today.

Ms. Vega is struggling to control Manuel and his 4-year-old brother while trying to hold onto their 2-month-old sister, as Dr. Martin enters the room. Ms. Vega has been living in a domestic violence shelter for the past 7 months. Dr. Martin asks how she has been since the last time she was in the clinic and Ms. Vega begins to explain how "crazy busy" she has been "trying to keep up with all the appointments" she has. "I need to look for housing and keep up with my welfare appointments or they're gonna cut me off!" she exclaims. Dr. Martin nods her head in understanding and gives Ms. Vega a moment to air out her frustrations. After a moment of venting, Ms. Vega turns to Dr. Martin and announces that she needs refills for the medications prescribed for Manuel during the last visit. She was "so busy with all of the appointments" that she could not get them filled.

Caring for a child with asthma requires a heightened recognition of the disease's symptoms and knowledge of how to handle an acute exacerbation, particularly if the child is classified with persistent symptoms. These are difficult tasks for anyone to master; but, if parents are also dealing with many outside stressors, then this may diminish their capability to react in an effective capacity if their child has any acute asthma symptoms (Rand, 2002). The fact that many children with asthma come from impoverished backgrounds increases the likelihood that their parents are struggling with daily issues of unemployment, lack of housing options, domestic and other interpersonal violence, and inadequate food supply.

The presence of such stressors and the additional stress of a child's chronic illness may cause some parents to become depressed. A 2004 study by researchers from Johns Hopkins School of Medicine examined the affect of maternal depression on the adherence to prescribed asthma therapy for inner-city children residing in Baltimore, Maryland and Washington, DC (Bartlett, Krishnan, Riekert, Butz, & Rand, 2004). Study results indicated that mothers with a high number of symptoms of depression reported having more difficulty with their children's prescribed medications and more trouble performing daily activities because of the stress associated with having an asthmatic child. These mothers also reported having less understanding about the purpose or use of the asthma medication.

The Work of CAI and our Models of Interactive Community Asthma Education

As the cases illustrate, parents and families need viable health education materials that are ethnically and culturally appropriate and can reach those with low literacy as well as those who speak English or Spanish—being linguistically appropriate. The cases also illustrate how medical providers could benefit from having education tools to use in their offices to use in face-to-face interactions to educate parents and families on how to understand and manage asthma (i.e., track symptoms, medications, and other management strategies). Ideally, this might be an educational tool that is engaging, having illustrations, and providing a means of impacting parental knowledge, attitudes, and behaviors consistent with bringing about effective asthma management for their child.

Creation of Ethnically and Culturally Appropriate Health Education Materials

In response to such needs, the Children's Health Fund (CHF) has a long history of creating many health education materials, while the Childhood Asthma Initiative (CAI) has specifically created materials focused on asthma education. For example, as an innovative tool for family and community health education, the Family Asthma Guide was created in 2000, serving as a model for what constitutes an ethnically and culturally sensitive source of information, containing illustrations, being accessible for those with low literacy, while written in English and Spanish; most important, the guide introduces readers to the National Heart, Lung, and Blood Institute (NHLBI) asthma guidelines. Annually, 15,000 copies of the Family Asthma Guide are printed and distributed nationally within the CHF's National Network and internationally, reaching programs as far away as Canada and Puerto Rico. It is a powerful tool that meets the needs of physicians in medical settings, and the needs of health educators, outreach workers, and educators in group and classroom settings.

Multiple CAI Program Components and Ethnically and Culturally Appropriate Curricula

There are multiple key elements of the Childhood Asthma Initiative (CAI) community education program. Our models for providing interactive community asthma education respond to the reality of serious asthma knowledge deficits and beliefs that hinder asthma medication compliance. At the same time, we seek to be in compliance with NHLBI guidelines (National Institutes of Health, 1997), providing hands-on, interactive workshops and curricula for children, parents, teachers, and health care/child care providers, toward the goal of creating an asthma-friendly community in the South Bronx. These multiple CAI program components and models may be summarized, serving to illustrate the dimensions of a multicomponent community-wide asthma education initiative, including the importance of ethnically and culturally appropriate curricula.

Asthma Create, Read, Educate, Write (C.R.E.W.)

The Asthma Create, Read, Educate, Write (C.R.E.W.) is a two-session curriculum developed by CAI to teach school-age children about asthma and asthma management in a fun, interactive, hands-on learning environment. Younger aged children construct airway models made of clay or drawings to learn about the anatomy of the lung and to fully understand the physiology of asthma. They are given the opportunity to share experiences and talk about the areas in their environment (i.e., home, school, after-school programs) where they may find some of the triggers (i.e., dust mites, animals, cockroaches, mould, pollen, smoke, cold air, exercise, etc.) for asthma. The characteristics, symptoms, triggers, and types of medications for asthma are discussed in detail. Students finish their participation in the workshops by seeing a video and joining in on a question and answer segment.

One-Hour Asthma Sessions

These 1-hour asthma sessions are provided to teach school-aged children in the South Bronx about asthma when time constraints do not allow for a full Asthma C.R.E.W. workshop. These sessions are also provided to undergraduate college and graduate students who are studying health education, so that they can disseminate information about asthma within their communities.

Asthma Forums

Asthma forums are group education workshops designed to educate homeless and housed parents about asthma. The curriculum developed by the CAI team includes asthma symptoms, triggers, medications, and the importance of having a medical home. Parents are encouraged to discuss challenges of taking care of children with asthma as well as share anecdotes of things that have been helpful for them in managing indoor allergens (i.e., dust mites, pets).

The Integration of Asthma and Music Education

Music is just one more of the innovative methods of teaching asthma that we use to teach children about the impact of asthma in their lives. The music and educational programs allow students to learn about asthma while participating in music and recreational activities. There are two types of music programs available for the students (discussed in the next two paragraphs), allowing students to learn how to strengthen their lungs by incorporating breathing exercises into the workshop, while also increasing their asthma management knowledge.

Harmonica Workshops team-up CAI staff with musicians to teach children about asthma and how harmonica playing can help strengthen their lungs. The two-session curriculum includes an asthma lesson and an interactive session when students "jam" with the musicians.

Asthma and Music Workshops involve a four-session workshop with the CAI team and professional musicians. Students learn to control their breathing while playing the recorder, a wind instrument. They also learn about asthma and how to put together effective presentations for community learning. This workshop is more detailed, allowing the students an opportunity to explore the different aspects of asthma in depth. Students prepare materials that allow them to present what they have learned. In addition, they learn a few simple songs that they share with other classes, primarily students with asthma. Again parents, school administration, and other classes are invited to participate and ask questions at the end of the presentations.

Other Education and Outreach Components Utilized to Foster Information Dissemination

Professional Training is available to shelter staff and other service professionals who are interested in teaching the community about asthma. The professional training has been offered at the New South Bronx Police Athletic League (P.A.L.) and in various health education classes at various colleges in New York City.

Train the Trainer Workshops for Professionals are provided to increase the number of qualified health and childcare givers who are able to provide asthma education to the community. Additional trainings are provided to community leaders/community members who are interested in peer education.

Clinical Outreach Activities for Public Housing in the South Bronx are outreach activities designed to educate families about asthma, making them aware of the resources available to them and linking them to health centers (e.g., South Bronx Health Center for Children and Families) where they can receive treatment for their child's asthma.

Other Recommendations to Physicians. Culture may influence multiple aspects of the patient's medical care including compliance with prescribed medications and maintenance of follow-up appointments. Patients may seek the care of nonmedical providers and utilize the alternative treatments that are recommended such as herbal home remedies. It is important for physicians to seek an understanding about their patient's culture and use that understanding to direct the interaction and communication with the patient and family during the clinic visit.

The Integration of Asthma Education Into the Public School Literacy and Science Curriculums

CAI has forged a close relationship with New York City public schools, community after-school programs, and community-based organizations. Discussions with teachers, parent coordinators, and school administrators revealed the schools' hesitation to include asthma education as part of their scheduled activities for fear that it would interfere with the daily academic requirements of the students. With increased pressure for teachers to prepare students for standardized testing, teachers are most reluctant to give up valuable classroom instruction time. This reality threatened to limit CAI's access to the children. It was important to find a viable solution that would best suit the needs of all involved.

The Role of Asthma Education Within the Curriculum Expansion Project

The solution came with the creation of the literacy expansion curriculum for elementary school students and the science expansion curriculum for high school students. This program is innovative and groundbreaking in that it does not take away from classroom instruction. On the contrary, it enhances students' experiences by engaging them in special projects that allows them to learn about asthma while doing some of their regular academic activities.

Unlike other programs on asthma, this one does not focus its attention only on the asthmatic child. Because learning about asthma is a community endeavor, the curriculum expansion is made available to all students. With the prevalence levels so high in the South Bronx, it is likely that students who do not have asthma themselves either have a family member with asthma or know someone who has the disease. It is, therefore, important to provide asthma education just as one would provide instruction on all academic subjects. As health education is not a continual part of the New York City academic curriculum, the literacy and science curriculum expansions become a prime vehicle for providing health education specific to asthma and asthma management. Such curriculum expansions may help to promote changes in attitudes and behaviors at an early age. The components of the asthma curriculum expansion program may be described, in brief.

Asthma Curriculum for Public Schools: Expansion to the Literacy Curriculum for Elementary School Children. This is a 2-week expansion to the literacy curriculum of elementary school children that has been used at several schools in the South Bronx. The curriculum allows students to conduct group research on the characteristics, symptoms, triggers, medication, and management of asthma. Prior to the start of the project period, teachers participate in an adult Asthma Forum (described earlier in this chapter) so that they can also become familiar with the multiplicity of and confounding factors surrounding asthma. This is important because teachers who do not fully understand what they need to do when a child starts to experience asthma symptoms may often ask the parents to keep the child at home. This may potentially further negatively impact the school engagement of the child and financial productivity of the child's family via lost school days for the child and lost work days for the parents, respectively. This also adds to the increased anxiety and helplessness felt by the families. As so many of these are families that already experience severe economic hardships, lost work days could further devastate the stability of the family unit.

Students use self-expression, research, and collaborative learning to present their findings at a culminating "publishing party." The children are encouraged to use their creativity to put together presentations based on what they learn about asthma. Students collect information and present it in various forms such as posters, poetry, stories, informational papers, role-plays, interviews, or experiential accounts. Parents are encouraged to participate in the gathering of information and invited to attend the school presentations given by the students.

The most important aspect of this curriculum is that it does NOT disrupt the academic process. Asthma education is incorporated into the daily academic activities. Ongoing pre- and post-intervention testing allows CAI to determine how many participants have increased their knowledge of asthma as a result of the curriculum expansion.

Asthma Curriculum for Public Schools: Expansion to the Science Curriculum for High School Students. This is a similar 2-week expansion incorporated into the science curriculum for high school students with emphasis on learning the anatomy and physiology of the lung as well as the impact that asthma has on the body. Great care was taken to make sure that the curriculum addressed many of the literacy and science standards requirements for students. The following are specific areas of the English and Language Arts as well as Science educational standards that are addressed through the use of this curriculum. Each standard is approached with a focus on incorporating asthma education. For Reading, the pertinent standards are **Standard E1a**, to read twenty-five books of the quality and complexity illustrated in a sample reading list; and **Standard E1c**, to read and comprehend informational materials. For Writing, the applicable standards are **Standard E2a**, to produce a report of information; **Standard E2b**, to produce a response to literature; and **Standard E2d**, to produce a narrative procedure. For the Speaking, Listening, and Viewing domain, the relevant standards are **Standard E3b**, to participate in group meetings; and **Standard E3c**, to prepare and deliver an individual presentation. Within the Conventions, Grammar, and Usage of the English Language area, the following standard applies: **Standard E4b**, to analyze and subsequently revise work to improve its clarity and effectiveness.

There are also pertinent performance standards for science and math. The area of Scientific Connections and Applications include **Standard S4c**, to demonstrate understanding of personal health; and **Standard S4d**, to demonstrate understanding of science as a human endeavor. Within the area of Statistics and Probability Concepts the pertinent standards include **Standard M4a**, to collect and organize data to answer a question; **Standard M4b**, to display data; and **Standard M4c**, to make statements and draw simple conclusions based on data.

Implementation and Results. Across the academic years 2004–2005 and 2005–2006, for 2 consecutive years the asthma pertinent curriculum has been incorporated into the literacy curriculum for 110 third-grade and 466 fourth-grade students; and the science curriculum of 84 ninth- and tenth-grade students, combined. Students successfully presented accurate asthma facts. Pre- and post-tests showed that student knowledge had increased by 59% after participation in the literacy or science curriculum. This begins to suggest how this component of our model is evidence-based, even as we plan to continue to collect and publish data.

Going Beyond the School Curriculum. After completion of the curriculum expansion program, health educators returned to the schools to provide an additional 27 workshops that reached 226 parents and school staff members. In this manner, the goal is to impact the entire school culture and to effectively respond to asthma as a school- and community-wide health issue, requiring all to be educated and involved in asthma education and management.

Emergent Principles and Recommendations

Principles for how to go about responding to disparities in health emerge from the experiences of both the Children's Health Fund (CHF) and the work of the Childhood Asthma Initiative (CAI), in particular. These also constitute recommendations we offer to others in communities seeking to take action in response to contemporary health crises impacting at-risk populations.

The Creative Partnering of Cofounders and Coleaders

Explore, initiate, and value the potential of partnerships between entertainers (e.g., singer/song-writer Paul Simon) and professionals (e.g., pediatrician/child advocate, Irwin Redlener, MD) or other community representatives in the process of cofounding and providing ongoing coleadership for new organizational entities (e.g., the Children's Health Fund). The new organizational entities created may also enjoy a new freedom in taking fresh approaches, or engaging in social action to bring about social justice (i.e., ensuring the vulnerable find access to equitable quality health care). The presence of an entertainer may help to attract the attention of other generous individuals, especially at event fundraisers, as well as donations from corporations and foundations, while the government should also assume their responsibility to contribute—even if in lesser amounts relative to that of the private donors attracted to the new cause.

A Central Role for Organizational and Academic Medical Center Partnerships/Collaborations

Given the focus on health, forge a partnership with a major academic medical center (such as the New York Montefiore Medical Center) and maximize the potential benefits of the medical center's presence and sense of responsibility to its surrounding vulnerable communities (such as the Montefiore Medical Center's South Bronx Health Center for Children and Families, SBHCCF), while also meeting its potential to provide services, including embracing those who cannot pay and may be immigrants.

Respond to Specific Health Disparities/Issues as New Needs Arise via New Initiatives

In response to new national priorities or guidelines the National Heart, Lung, and Blood Institute guidelines put out by the National Institutes of Health in 1997 create new initiatives to address a pressing new health disparity or to meet new emergent health needs (such as rising asthma rates and the Childhood Asthma Initiative). It is important for organizations (such as the Children's Health Fund) to demonstrate their capacity to grow and flexibly respond to new and emergent health crises, concerns, or needs.

Deploy Transdisciplinary Teams to Design, Implement and Evaluate Ethnically, Culturally, and Linguistically Appropriate and Engaging Health Education Materials and Interactive Face-to-Face Educational Programming

Draw upon the work of transdisciplinary teams (e.g., a pediatrician, a doctor of education specializing in health and behavior, a medical anthropologist, a research specialist, and various other health education professionals) to develop health education materials and curricula that are ethnically, culturally, and linguistically appropriate (such as the *Family Asthma Guide*); perspectives reflective of and/or representing the community must also be brought to the table to review and approve all materials. Health education materials must also be engaging and use illustrations, so as to meaningfully engage learners and maximize learning. Ethnically, culturally and linguistically appropriate materials as well as interactive face-to-face educational programming are also seen as absolutely vital in addressing health issues such as asthma management. Finally, the evaluation of all educational materials and programming is crucial, allowing for quality assurance, and information that can lead to further improvement, or support wider dissemination.

Collaborate With Diverse Community Organizations, Representatives and Leaders to Ensure Broad Community Buy-In and to Maximize Community-Wide Dissemination

Work with diverse community organizations (e.g., medical clinics, public housing, public schools, community organizations), community representatives (e.g., elected officials, medical providers, parents and families with children with asthma), and community leaders (e.g., school principals, teachers) to ensure broad-base participation in the health education projects being created, adequate community buy-in, and to maximize community-wide dissemination of the projects. These community collaborations are key to ensuring that what has been created for purposes of community health education actually evolves into what constitutes comprehensive community-wide health education.

Conclusion

This chapter introduced a model of hands-on face-to-face interactive comprehensive community-wide health education focused on increasing asthma awareness via partnerships and the public school curriculum. Specifically, this chapter provided historical background on the Children's Health Fund, key partnerships, the work of the Childhood Asthma Initiative (CAI), case studies of asthmatic patients highlighting the contemporary asthma education challenge, and the work of the CAI in response to this challenge—specifically, our materials and models for hands on, face-to-face, interactive community asthma education. Of special note is the work of CAI integrating asthma education into the public school literacy and science/math curriculums. Finally, five emergent principles and recommendations were offered for others to follow for creating an innovative model of comprehensive community-wide health education, such as our initiative seeking to increase asthma awareness and improve asthma management.

The component of the model involving integrating asthma education into the public school literacy and science/math curriculums has supportive evidence, showing substantial increases in asthma knowledge. Consistent with the other chapters in this section (i.e., Ross & Smalls; Campbell & Wallace; and Chew & Wallace, chapters 26, 28, and 29, this volume), *engagement* emerges as vital in producing significant increases in asthma knowledge; in this case, engagement means participation in hands-on, face-to-face, interactive asthma education, while doing things such as having students make presentations, or create products/publications based on what they learned, or integrating music into the learning process.

While other chapters in this volume (see Woo, chapter 18, and other chapters in Part V) highlight a role for online interactive multimedia technology, an important role remains for interactive face-to-face educational programming. The value of interactive face-to-face educational programming emerges as having great value, especially when the goal is to ensure acquisition of the knowledge, attitudes, and skills necessary for achieving compliance to asthma medication and management regimens. Such compliance can be lifesaving, as well as decrease emergency room visits, missed school days by children, and missed workdays by parents. Face-to-face interactions that achieve adequate engagement may result in the desired acquisition of knowledge, attitudes, and behavior consistent with asthma management.

As another measure suggestive of our success in having a community-wide impact, CAI reached approximately 4,000 people through asthma education and outreach to schools, community organizations, and public housing facilities from 2003 through 2005. Our success is also reflected in our expanding reach. CAI plans to market this innovative approach pioneered in the South Bronx for public schools across New York City. This school-based program component was also implemented in Washington, DC in Spring 2006, where the prevalence of asthma is also a major concern—showing how our being a part of the Children's Health Fund's National Network allows for dissemination to other urban and potentially rural areas. Students and families in the Washington, DC area have demographics similar to those in the New York City area, suggesting the logic in this first extension project in this urban area. The infusion of asthma education into the school curricula effectively serves to increase the number of people with formal asthma education. Teachers can use this valuable new interactive approach to learning about a practical community health issue impacting a multitude of community and family members in order to help students excel overall academically.

Meanwhile, there is great value in the overall model of community-wide health education focusing on increasing asthma awareness implemented by the CAI. The educational programs created by CAI have had a positive impact, based on our active involvement in implementation and dissemination, allowing us to observe how the services motivate patients to become involved in their care.

There is also a role for a variety of diverse professionals in promoting community-wide health education focusing on increasing asthma awareness. A health educator, for example, associated with a primary care facility (such as the South Bronx Center for Children and Families, SBCCF, of the New York Montefiore Medical Center) can help the community by providing the connection to clinical care. Overall, our work evolving, implementing, and disseminating the model of comprehensive community-wide health education focused on increasing asthma awareness serves to corroborate the value placed on face-to-face interactive educational programming, as indicated by others (Liu & Feekery, 2001).

We look forward to the expansion of our work in this regard, while recommending that others consider the value of this model of face-to-face interactive comprehensive community-wide health education in addressing serious disparities in health, targeting communities in need, as this chapter serves to illustrate. The five principles and corresponding recommendations we have put forth may serve as a guide to others in this process.

REFERENCES

Akinbami, L. J., & Schoendorf, K. C. (2002). Trends in childhood asthma: Prevalence, health care utilization and mortality. *Pediatrics, 110*, 315–322.

American Academy of Allergy, Asthma and Immunology. (2006). *Asthma statistics.* Retrieved June 9, 2006, from www.aaaai.org/media/resources/media_kit/asthma_statistics.stm

American Lung Association. (2005). *Trends in asthma morbidity and mortality.* New York: Author, Epidemiology and Statistics Unit, Research and Program Services.

Bartlett, S. J., Krishnan, J. A., Riekert, K. A., Butz, A., & Rand, C. (2004). Maternal depression and adherence to therapy in inner-city children with asthma. *Pediatrics, 113*, 229–236.

Bauman, L. J., Silver, E. J., & Stein, R. (2006). Cumulative social disadvantage and child health. *Pediatrics, 117*, 1321–1328.

Boulet, L. P. (1998). Perception of the role and potential side effects of inhaled corticosteroids among asthmatic patients. *Chest, 113*, 587–592.

Children's Defense Fund. (2003). *Number of Black children in extreme poverty hits record high.* Author. Family Income and Jobs-Reports.

Flores, G. (2002). Culture and the patient–physician relationship: Achieving cultural competency in health care. *Journal of Pediatrics, 136*, 14–23.

Lieu, T. A., Quesenberry, C. P., Capra, A. M., Sorel, M. E., Martin, K. E., & Mendoza, G. R. (1997). Outpatient management practices associated with reduced risk of pediatric asthma hospitalization and emergency department visits. *Pediatrics, 100*, 334–341.

Liu, C., & Feekery, C. (2001). Can asthma education improve clinical outcomes? An evaluation of a pediatric asthma education program. *Journal of Asthma, 38*(3), 269–278.

Merikallio, V. J., Mustalahti, K., Remes, S. T., Valovirta, E. J., & Kaila, M. (2005). Comparison of quality of life between asthmatic and healthy school children. *Pediatric Allergy and Immunology, 16*, 332–340.

National Center for Children in Poverty. (2005). Who are America's children in poverty? Retrieved December 2006, from www.nccp.org/publications/pub_684.html

National Institutes of Health (NIH). (1997). Updated asthma guidelines released. Retrieved July 24, 2007, from http://www.nih.gov/news/pr/feb97/nhlbi-24.htm

Peterson, M. W., Strommer-Pace, L., & Dayton, C. (2001). Asthma patient education: Current utilization in pulmonary training programs. *Journal of Asthma, 28*, 261–267.

Rand, C. S. (2002). Adherence to asthma therapy in the preschool child. *Allergy, 57*(S74), 48–57.

Conclusion: The Future of the Field of Equity in Health

31

Barbara C. Wallace

This edited volume set out to launch a new field of equity in health, as a new global approach to inequities in health. The chapters in this volume served to delineate the parameters of the emergent field—one rooted in the need to move *From InEquity in Health to Equity In Health* and spur a global civil rights movement across the 21st century in response to injustice in health. The edited volume serves as a tool for training global leaders for this movement who may work collaboratively on transdisciplinary teams. Diverse members of transdisciplinary teams may include policy makers, funders, government officials, researchers, interventionists, epidemiologists, health care administrators, leaders in health care insurance systems, physicians, psychologists, health educators, social workers, nurses, anthropologists, sociologists, economists, demographers, lawyers, teachers, computer/information technology specialists, community health workers, or peer educators who work alongside community members.

At the very beginning of this book, it is noted how this is the time of milestones and the weeding out of destructive forces (Ayeboafo, 2005). It is the intention of the work to be a milestone by launching a new field of equity in health, and to weed out any destructive forces that have grown within the prevailing approaches to health. Herein, we have declared a clearing in which something new may manifest, as some new growth. This volume also reflects an ongoing shifting in the discourse from a primary discussion about health disparities to one that will increasingly focus on issues of social justice, the right to health, and especially how to achieve and sustain equity in health for all—in particular as this means new policies, procedures, and the redistribution of wealth and access to resources and opportunities.

The Making of a Movement: Guiding Metaphors

Fields of knowledge, theory, and practice may recall the natural fields known to the indigenous people around the world as places where they grow their crops. Indigenous people farming their lands have practiced careful selection of the crop to grow—given the nature of the growing environment, crop rotation to keep the earth as healthy as possible, and systematic careful weeding. They weed out that which starts to grow, but is seen as undesirable in facilitating crops growing to their full potential.

Accepting this metaphor offers an opportunity to raise questions within the context of health disparity, inequity, and equity. First, to what extent do we exercise the same level of care when it comes to those fields of knowledge, theory, and practice that are near and dear to us? Do we practice careful selection of what to grow, or the research to conduct, or the intervention to deliver—given the nature of the environment, or full consideration of the nature of the bio–psycho–social–environmental–cultural context?

Second, do we practice anything akin to crop rotation so that which we seek to grow, nurture, and produce emerges as healthy as possible, capable of reaching its highest or full potential—all by virtue of knowing when the signs in the bio–psycho–social–cultural–environmental context are telling us to "rotate" or change what we do, or which crops we grow? Do we conduct the kind of assessments and discern the signs that might tell us to "rotate" to a particular theory or approach, or to rotate back to yet another? Do we discern when it may be appropriate to deploy just parts or elements of theories or approaches to ensure maximum growth, including deploying creative combinations that address just some dimension or serve to address all dimensions of the bio–psycho–social–cultural–environmental context? The result might be the deployment of integrated theories, approaches, models, and interventions; a menu of integrated theories and evidence-based approaches. Such menus of options or viable alternatives could be drawn upon as we practice a kind of "crop rotation." The foundation or rationale for what we decide to do might vary, as we rotate from one rationale to another—as embodied in one or more theories or evidence-based approaches. Rotation might also result as a function of the diverse ways of thinking represented on transdisciplinary teams where collaboration in decision making prevails, and the rationale for what we do might come from a particular perspective or multiple perspectives at any given time (e.g., legal, economic, sociological, medical, psychiatric).

Third, do we know when it is time to engage in systematic weeding out of that which has grown in a field? Moreover, are we able to acknowledge when it is time to use fire to burn entire sections of our fields that are so overgrown with weeds that such a measure is needed to create a clearing for new growth?

Finally, to what extent do the fields of which we speak also reflect our own inner psychic space? Are our identities intertwined with old paradigmatic theories that are like weeds choking our ability to think from the multiple perspectives that are brought to the table when a transdisciplinary team meets alongside community members?

Are the fields about which we speak reflections of our organizations, academic disciplines, universities, health care systems, countries, and global community? What has overgrown and become a destructive force in need of being weeded out? Is the destructive force in need of being weeded out a remnant of the old paradigm of hierarchical domination and oppression—whether an individual or cultural or institutionalized form of white supremacy, privilege, racism, homophobia, heterosexism, classism, sexism, ageism, or oppression of people with disabilities?

Such a metaphor may guide us with regard to what we must do in making a movement. With regard to the making of a 21st century civil rights movement—one seeking to ensure the human right to health, social justice, and forging of equity in health for all—it has been suggested that the means and methods of a contemporary movement may be quite different from the past (Billings, 2007). Instead of the huge marches of the prior 20th century, a contemporary civil rights movement may involve our use of new technologies now available and in wide use—cellular telephones and text messaging, for example, as well as the Internet. Consider the following: If millions of Americans seeking to support their preferred candidate on the show American Idol can vote via text messaging 10 times a day, even every day, across a specified period of time (Billings), then what is possible within a civil rights movement for health? Through the additional combined use of television, the media, the Internet, blogs, chat rooms, and e-mail, mass mobilization in a new civil rights movement across the 21st century is attainable.

As emphasized repeatedly in the introduction to this book, citing numerous authors, it is a new era, a turning point, or a time where a tipping point has been reached in our history. "It is that time, in this place" (Ayeboafo, 2005)! What if it is such a time? It may very well be that it is time for us to ask for what we want, as vital action, holding in mind the vision of what is desired. For example, you ask for an entire nourishing meal, but are only offered an appetizer. You accept the appetizer, eat it, and then ask for the entire meal. At least you have made it to the table and been offered something to eat, yet not all that you want, nor an equitable share. Taking the action of asking for what one wants, in this case, resulted in receiving just some portion of it; this represents progress. However, the task is to then ask for what one wants again and again, while acknowledging the progress being made step by step by step. The vision maintained is of sitting at the table as a recipient of a full course meal, finally having achieved equal access to opportunity (Sayegh, 2007).

Airhihenbuwa (2005) has offered a metaphor of people at an outside gathering eating freely from a huge buffet, sitting comfortably at tables, while those who are hungry and perhaps even homeless walk by, observing. Integrating the metaphor above (Sayegh, 2007) with Airhihenbuwa's imagery, we arrive at a fuller picture of the social-environmental-cultural context. The context includes those who have enjoyed privilege having so much access to opportunity that they could literally gorge on it, stuffing themselves until they are obese or sick. Meanwhile, there are those who are starving and excluded from access to opportunity, as resources are not shared or equitably distributed.

To build a movement for equity in health for all, multiple steps must be taken. One possible step is for those who are hungry and long denied access to ask for what they want: a place at the table; to sit and eat a full course meal; and, to be able to witness the manifestation of the vision of what they want—such as equal access to all desired opportunities and the equitable distribution and sharing of abundant resources within the global community. Another possible step, indeed, the ideal first step, involves people with privilege taking social action for social justice and freely feeding the hungry and ensuring housing for the homeless, ensuring they have access to a whole meal; and, access to all it takes to ensure the right to health.

Ensuring the right to health follows from a new paradigm—one based on non-hierarchical equality. This non-hierarchical equality may become the foundation for bringing about equity in health for all across the 21st century. Indeed, as suggested in the introduction of this volume, thirteen principles should drive what we do within the field of equity in health, as well as drive and direct the steps and actions we take within an overall global civil rights movement for equity in health for all. More specifically, the field of equity in health is driven by thirteen guiding principles reflective of contemporary forces serving to bring about change:

1) The Drive for a Major Paradigm Shift;
2) The Drive for New Models of Health Care and Training;
3) The Drive for New Theories, Perspectives, and Identities;
4) The Drive for Evidence-Based Approaches;
5) The Drive for Transdisciplinary Teams and Community-Based Participatory Research;
6) The Drive for Globalization and Global Collaboration;
7) The Drive for Cultural Competence and Cultural Appropriateness;
8) The Drive for Health Literacy and Linguistic Appropriateness;
9) The Drive to Ensure the Right to Health;
10) The Drive for Social Justice and Acknowledgment of Forces in the Social Context;
11) The Drive to Protect and Support the Most Vulnerable;
12) The Drive to Repair Damage, Restore Trust, and Take Responsibility; and
13) The Drive to Redistribute Wealth and Access to Opportunity.

By way of elaboration, beyond the drive for a major paradigm shift to bring about non-hierarchical equality, for example, there must also be a drive for the creation of new models of health care (medical and public) and training, going beyond a focus on disease to a focus on prevention and all that it takes to ensure mental, emotional, physical, and spiritual health—taking a holistic approach. There must also be a drive for the creation of new theories, as well as the forging of new perspectives and new identities—ultimately leading to new integrated theories and multiple perspective being brought to bear on health issues by those with identities sensitive to how there are multiple realities and diverse cultures around the globe.

There is also a need for new evidence-based approaches, ultimately leading to menus of evidence-based approaches to various health challenges. Additionally, the creation of transdisciplinary teams that include and work alongside community members, while valuing and engaging in community-based participatory research, is critical to our success. And, there must also be a drive for globalization—one newly defined as the actualization of our potential to have a sense of interdependence, an awareness of how "what affects one affects all," while working collaboratively within our global community.

There is also the imperative that we all possess cultural competence and ensure cultural appropriateness in all that we do—policy, procedures, research, interventions; we must seek out such training ourselves and then train others. In the same vein, there must be a drive ensuring we meet people where they are and effectively engage them in light of their health literacy, while all materials and interventions are linguistically appropriate; meanwhile, all are trained to be able to do this. There is also the contemporary push to ensure the right to health, as an absolute core value that gets actualized in all that we do. There is also a call for social justice and full acknowledgement of those forces operating in the social context. Another key value is reflected in the need to protect and support the most vulnerable, allowing special attention to be paid to special populations—those historically dominated, oppressed, and denied access to opportunity.

There is also a drive to repair the damage done, as most poignantly reflected in the experiences of those historically dominated, oppressed, and denied access to opportunity, as well as for restoration of the trust lost, while we take responsibility for what must be done and do it, in light of pertinent history. Finally, given the prior principles, not surprisingly, there is the compelling force to redistribute wealth and access to opportunity. Collectively, the thirteen principles are effectively driving the global civil rights movement for equity in health for all.

The Future

The future is holding the potential for tremendous transformation and change. The future is holding us all accountable and responsible for what manifests, for the future ultimately depends upon all of us—our individual cumulative actions, those of our professions, organizations, institutions, governments, and global community. We can maximize the moment as a milestone, turning point, tipping point, or new era, and move toward equity in health for all. We can sit together on transdisciplinary teams, while enjoying the presence of community members at the table who sit as our equals; and, we can ensure that those who have been excluded and denied access, heretofore, are adequately represented—especially the most vulnerable and historically the most dominated and oppressed. Perhaps, only together can such a diverse collective envision the kind of future that "will work" for us all, as we go on to collaborate in taking social action for social justice and manifest a 21st century global civil rights movement for equity in health for all.

REFERENCES

Airhihenbuwa, C. O. (2005, November 9). *On being comfortable with being uncomfortable: Centering an Africanist vision in our gateway to global health.* Presidential address delivered at the 53rd Annual Meeting of the Society of Public Health Education, Philadelphia, PA.

Ayeboafo, N. K. (2005). *Tigare speaks: Lessons for living in harmony.* Philadelphia: StarSpirit Press.

Billings, D. (2007, April 11). *The challenge.* A presentation at the Drop the Rock-Update 2007: Will the new governor change the Rockefeller drug laws? Hunter College of the City University of New York, New York.

Sayegh, G. (2007, April 11). *Who are the criminals and who is being punished?* A presentation at the Drop the Rock-Update 2007: Will the new governor change the Rockefeller drug laws? Hunter College of the City University of New York, New York.

Index

SPRINGER PUBLISHING COMPANY

Health Promotion and Aging

Fourth Edition

Practical Applications for Health Professionals

David Haber, PhD

"...[this book] should be on the bookshelf of every student and every professor in any one of the health disciplines...[it] is a resource that pulls together everything that a health provider would need to know about promoting health and quality of life for older adults."

—From the Foreword by **Barbara Resnick**, PhD, FAAN

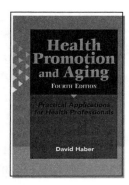

Continuing to advocate for health professionals becoming health educators and a more informed, healthier aging population, David Haber has updated this fourth edition with discussion and analysis of major issues and topics in the field, including:

- A critique of the MyPyramid Food Guide
- How to change medical encounters into health encounters
- Descriptions of model health programs
- A review of the 2006 Surgeon General's Report on secondhand smoke
- Critical analysis of Medicare Part D
- The benefits of pet support
- Life review and cognitive fitness
- Appraisals of complementary and alternative practices

Innovative ideas on public policy and aging, examples of stand-out community health advocacy, and a final chapter on the future of the field complete this integrated look at our health, community, and aging.

2007 · 572pp · hardcover · 978-0-8261-8463-4

11 West 42nd Street, New York, NY 10036-8002 • Fax: 212-941-7842
Order Toll-Free: 877-687-7476 • Order Online: www.springerpub.com

SPRINGER PUBLISHING COMPANY

Health Care Politics, Policy, and Services

A Social Justice Analysis

Gunnar Almgren, MSW, PhD

- **Who Has a Right to Health Care?**

- **What Is the Government's Role in Providing Accessible Health Care?**

- **How Are Corporations, Insurance Companies, and Health Care Providers Impacting the Quality of Health Care?**

- **And, Most Importantly, Can We Reform the U.S. Health Care System?**

Students often debate these issues in health care policy or public health courses, yet they do so without the proper knowledge of the underlying structure of the U.S. health care system—or a framework by which it can be judged. Many health care workers entering the system are ill-equipped to address the issues faced in direct health care practice, in part because they have no ability to evaluate it.

In this innovative text, Gunnar Almgren provides all the tools necessary to understand and critique a health care policy in dire need of change. First, he describes the historical evolution of U.S. health care, explaining how the early roles of hospitals, doctors, and nurses still influence today's system. He explains the complex financial aspects of health care, including the concerns of all its major stakeholders. He looks at the government's role in regulating and funding health care, and how that role has expanded and contracted through various political administrations. An entire chapter describes the facilities and services available for the elderly—an issue that will continue to rise in importance as America ages. Finally, he examines the many causes of disparities in the U.S. health care system.

2006 · 352pp · hardcover · 0-8261-0236-0

11 West 42nd Street, New York, NY 10036-8002 • Fax: 212-941-7842
Order Toll-Free: 877-687-7476 • Order Online: www.springerpub.com

SPRINGER PUBLISHING COMPANY

Health Literacy in Primary Care
A Clinician's Guide
Gloria G. Mayer, RN, EdD, FAAN
Michael Villaire, MSLM

At the intersection of health care delivery and practice there lies a large area of patient care with no manual: how to provide the best care to patients who have a critically low level of comprehension and literacy. Because all patients play a central role in the outcome of their own health care, competent health care becomes almost impossible for caregivers when the boundary of low literacy skills is present.

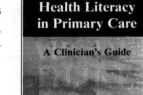

In a concise and well-written format you will learn:

- Common myths about low literacy
- How to recognize patients with low literacy
- Strategies to help patients with low literacy and reduce medical errors
- Cultural issues in health literacy
- Ways to create a patient-friendly office environment
- Guidelines to target and overcome common problems practitioners encounter

This clear, well-written book is packed with examples and tips and will serve as a much needed guide for primary care providers, nurse practitioners, hospital administrators, and others who are looking for ways to improve their communication with patients and provide the most beneficial health care to their low-literacy patients.

Table of Contents

- Understanding Health Literacy
- Creating a Patient-Friendly Environment
- Assessing Patients' Literacy Levels
- Understanding and Avoiding Medical Errors
- Factoring Culture Into the Care Process
- Improving Patient-Provider Communication
- Designing Easy-to-Read Patient Education Materials
- Principles of Writing for Low Literacy

- Using Alternative Forms of Patient Communication
- Interpreters and Their Role in the Health Care Setting
- Designing Easy-to-Read Patient Education Materials
- Principles of Writing for Low Literacy
- Using Alternative Forms of Patient Communication

2007 · 312 pp · Softcover · 978-0-8261-0229-4

11 West 42nd Street, New York, NY 10036-8002 • Fax: 212-941-7842
Order Toll-Free: 877-687-7476 • Order Online: www.springerpub.com

SPRINGER PUBLISHING COMPANY

An Introduction to the US Health Care System

Sixth Edition

Steven Jonas, MD, MPH, FACPM
Raymond L. Goldsteen, DrPH
Karen Goldsteen, PhD, MPH

Completely expanded and updated to account for the latest changes in the U.S. health care system, this bestselling text remains the most concise and balanced introduction to the domestic health care system. Like its predecessors, it provides an accessible overview of the basic components of the system: health care personnel, hospitals and other institutions, the federal government, financing and payment mechanisms, and managed care. Finally, it provides an insightful look at the prospects for health care reform.

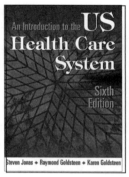

Steven Jonas, a revered expert in public health, has enlisted his colleagues, Drs. Raymond and Karen Goldsteen, to add their expertise in public health and health policy and management to this outstanding volume. All students of health care administration and policy, as well as practicing health professionals who simply want a relatively brief overview of the system, will find it useful.

Partial Table of Contents

Health Care Systems • U.S. Health Care System • Future of the U.S. Health Care System • Health Care Workforce • Physicians • Nursing • Physicians' Assistants • Health Care Workforce Outside the Hospital and Physician Office

Hospitals and Other Health Care Institutions • Hospital Structure • Public General Hospitals • The Hospital in the Present Era • Long-Term Care: The Example of Nursing Homes • Primary and Ambulatory Care • Primary Care • Ambulatory Care

Government and the Health Care System • The Constitutional Basis of Government Authority in Health Care • The Health Care Functions of Government • The Federal Government and the Provision of Health Services • State Governments' Role in Health Services • Local Governments' Role in Health Services • Problems in Public Health

Financing and Payment of Health Care • How Much Is Spent • Where the Money Comes From, Within the System • Where the Money Goes • How the Money Is Paid Out: Providers, Payers, and Payments • Equity of Health Care • Efficiency of Health Care • A National Scorecard

2007 · 292pp · Softcover · 978-0-8261-0214-0

11 West 42nd Street, New York, NY 10036-8002 • **Fax: 212-941-7842**
Order Toll-Free: 877-687-7476 • **Order Online: www.springerpub.com**